SCHAUM'S OUTLINE OF

THEORY AND PROBLEMS

OF

GENETICS

Third Edition

•

WILLIAM D. STANSFIELD, Ph.D.

Emeritus Professor of Biological Sciences
California Polytechnic State University
at San Luis Obispo

•

SCHAUM'S OUTLINE SERIES

McGRAW-HILL, INC.

New York   St. Louis   San Francisco   Auckland   Bogotá   Caracas   Lisbon
London   Madrid   Mexico City   Milan   Montreal   New Delhi
San Juan   Singapore   Sydney   Tokyo   Toronto

WILLIAM D. STANSFIELD has degrees in Agriculture (B.S., 1952), Education (M.A., 1960), and Genetics (M.S., 1962; Ph.D., 1963; University of California at Davis). His published research is in immunogenetics, twinning, and mouse genetics. From 1957 to 1959 he was an instructor in high school vocational in agriculture. He was a faculty member of the Biological Sciences Department of California Polytechnic State University from 1963 to 1992 and is now Emeritus Professor. He has written university-level textbooks in evolution and serology/immunology, and has coauthored a dictionary of genetics.

 This book is printed on recycled paper containing a minimum of 50% total recycled fiber with 10% postconsumer de-inked fiber. Soybean based inks are used on the cover and text.

Schaum's Outline of Theory and Problems of
GENETICS

5 6 7 8 9 10 11 12 13 14 15 16 17 18 19 20 BAW BAW 9 9 8 7 6 5 4

ISBN 0-07-060877-6

Sponsoring Editor, Jeanne Flagg
Production Supervisor, Leroy Young
Editing Supervisors; Meg Tobin, Maureen Walker
Cover design by Amy E. Becker.

Library of Congress Cataloging-in-Publication Data

Stansfield, William D.
    Schaum's outline of theory and problems of genetics / William D.
Stansfield.—3rd ed.
        p. cm.—(Schaum's outline series)
    Includes index.
    ISBN 0–07–060877–6
    1. Genetics—Problems, exercises, etc.   I. Title.   II. Title:
Outline of theory and problems of genetics.
QH440.3.S7   1991
575.1—dc20   90–41479
                                                        CIP

Preface

Genetics, the science of heredity, is a fundamental discipline in the biological sciences. All living things are products of both "nature and nurture." The hereditary units (genes) provide the organism with its "nature"—its biological potentialities/limitations—whereas the environment provides the "nurture," interacting with the genes (or their products) to give the organism its distinctive anatomical, physiological, biochemical, and behavioral characteristics.

Johann (Gregor) Mendel laid the foundations of modern genetics with the publication of his pioneering work on peas in 1866, but his work was not appreciated during his lifetime. The science of genetics began in 1900 with the rediscovery of his original paper. In the next ninety years, genetics grew from virtually zero knowledge to the present day ability to exchange genetic material between a wide range of unrelated organisms. Medicine and agriculture may literally be revolutionized by these recent developments in molecular genetics.

Some exposure to college-level or university-level biology is desirable before embarking on the study of genetics. In this volume, however, basic biological principles (such as cell structures and functions) are reviewed to provide a common base of essential background information. The quantitative (mathematical) aspects of genetics are more easily understood if the student has had some experience with statistical concepts and probabilities. Nevertheless, this outline provides all of the basic rules necessary for solving the genetics problems herein presented, so that the only mathematical background needed is arithmetic and the rudiments of algebra.

The original focus of this book remains unchanged in this third edition. It is still primarily designed to *outline* genetic theory and, by numerous examples, to illustrate a logical approach to problem solving. Admittedly the theory sections in previous editions have been "bare bones," presenting just enough basic concepts and terminology to set the stage for problem solving. Therefore, an attempt has been made in this third edition to bring genetic theory into better balance with problem solving. Indeed, many kinds of genetics problems cannot be solved without a broad conceptual understanding and detailed knowledge of the organism being investigated. The growth in knowledge of genetic phenomena, and the application of this knowledge (especially in the fields of genetic engineering and molecular biology of eucaryotic cells), continues at an accelerated pace. Most textbooks that try to remain current in these new developments are outdated in some respects before they can be published. Hence, this third edition outlines some of the more recent concepts that are fairly well understood and thus unlikely to change except in details. However, this book cannot continue to grow in size with the field; if it did, it would lose its "outline" character. Inclusion of this new material has thus required the elimination of some material from the second edition.

Each chapter begins with a theory section containing definitions of terms, basic principles and theories, and essential background information. As new terms are introduced they appear in boldface type to facilitate development of a genetics vocabulary. The first page reference to a term in the index usually indicates the location of its definition. The theory section is followed by sets of type problems solved in detail and supplementary problems with answers. The solved problems illustrate and amplify the theory, and they bring into sharp focus those fine points without which students might continually feel themselves on unsafe ground. The supplementary problems serve as a complete review of the material of each chapter and provide for the repetition of basic principles so vital to effective learning and retention.

In this third edition, one or more kinds of "objective" questions (vocabulary, matching, multiple choice, true-false) have been added to each chapter. This is the format used for examinations in some genetics courses, especially those at the survey level. In my experience, students often will give different answers to essentially the same question when asked in a different format. These objective-type questions are therefore designed to help students prepare for such exams, but they are also valuable sources of feedback in self-evaluation of how well one understands the material in each chapter. Former chapters dealing with the chemical basis of heredity, the genetics of bacteria and phage, and molecular genetics have been extensively revised. A new chapter outlining the molecular biology of eucaryotic cells and their viruses has been added.

I am especially grateful to Drs. R. Cano and J. Colome for their critical reviews of the last four chapters. Any errors of commission or omission remain solely my responsibility. As always, I would appreciate suggestions for improvement of any subsequent printings or editions.

WILLIAM D. STANSFIELD

Contents

Chapter 1

The Physical Basis of Heredity

GENETICS

Genetics is that branch of biology concerned with heredity and variation. The hereditary units that are transmitted from one generation to the next (inherited) are called **genes.** The genes reside in a long molecule called **deoxyribonucleic acid** (DNA). The DNA, in conjunction with a protein matrix, forms **nucleoprotein** and becomes organized into structures with distinctive staining properties called **chromosomes** found in the nucleus of the cell. The behavior of genes is thus paralleled in many ways by the behavior of the chromosomes of which they are a part. A gene contains coded information for the production of proteins. DNA is normally a stable molecule with the capacity for self-replication. On rare occasions a change may occur spontaneously in some part of DNA. This change, called a **mutation,** alters the coded instructions and may result in a defective protein or in the cessation of protein synthesis. The net result of a mutation is often seen as a change in the physical appearance of the individual or a change in some other measurable attribute of the organism called a **character** or **trait.** Through the process of mutation a gene may be changed into two or more alternative forms called **allelomorphs** or **alleles.**

> **Example 1.1.** Healthy people have a gene that specifies the normal protein structure of the red blood cell pigment called hemoglobin. Some anemic individuals have an altered form of this gene, i.e., an allele, which makes a defective hemoglobin protein unable to carry the normal amount of oxygen to the body cells.

Each gene occupies a specific position on a chromosome, called the gene **locus (loci,** plural). All allelic forms of a gene therefore are found at corresponding positions on genetically similar **(homologous)** chromosomes. The word "locus" is sometimes used interchangeably for "gene." When the science of genetics was in its infancy the gene was thought to behave as a unit particle. These particles were believed to be arranged on the chromosome like beads on a string. This is still a useful concept for beginning students to adopt, but will require considerable modification when we study the biochemical basis of heredity in Chapter 11. All the genes on a chromosome are said to be **linked** to one another and belong to the same **linkage group.** Wherever the chromosome goes it carries all of the genes in its linkage group with it. As we shall see later in this chapter, linked genes are not transmitted independently of one another, but genes in different linkage groups (on different chromosomes) are transmitted independently of one another.

CELLS

The smallest unit of life is the **cell.** Each living thing is composed of one or more cells. The most primitive cells alive today are the bacteria. They, like the presumed first forms of life, do not possess a **nucleus.** The nucleus is a membrane-bound compartment isolating the genetic material from the rest of the cell **(cytoplasm).** Bacteria therefore belong to a group of organisms called **procaryotes** (literally, "before a nucleus" had evolved; also spelled prokaryotes). All other kinds of cells that have a nucleus (including fungi, plants, and animals) are referred to as **eucaryotes** (literally, "truly nucleated"; also spelled eukaryotes). Most of this book deals with the genetics of eucaryotes. Bacteria will be considered in Chapter 12.

The cells of a multicellular organism seldom look alike or carry out identical tasks. The cells are differentiated to perform specific functions (sometimes referred to as a "division of labor"); a neuron is specialized to conduct nerve impulses, a muscle cell contracts, a red blood cell carries oxygen, and so on. Thus there is no such thing as a typical cell type. Fig. 1-1 is a composite diagram of an animal cell showing common subcellular structures that are found in all or most cell types. Any subcellular structure that has a characteristic morphology and function is considered to be an **organelle.** Some of

1

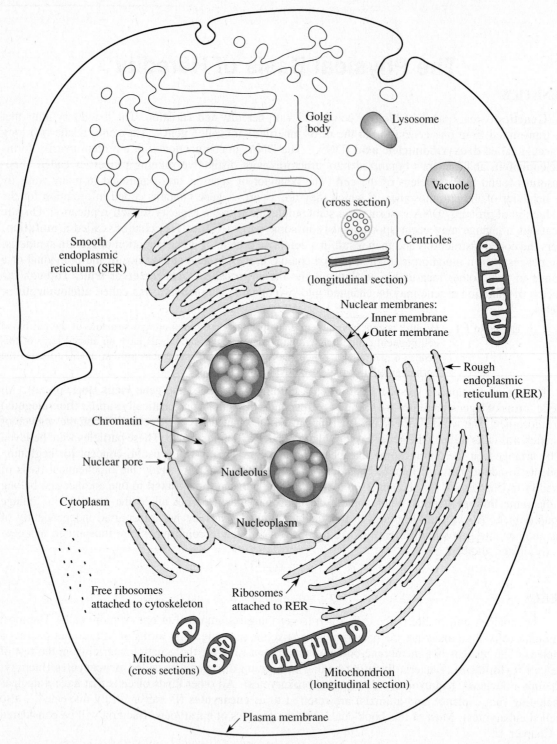

Fig. 1-1. Diagram of an animal cell.

the organelles (such as the nucleus and mitochondria) are membrane-bound; others (such as the ribosomes and centrioles) are not enclosed by a membrane. Most organelles and other cell parts are too small to be seen with the light microscope, but they can be studied with the electron microscope. The characteristics of organelles and other parts of eucaryotic cells are outlined in Table 1.1.

Table 1.1.   Characteristics of Eucaryotic Cellular Structures

Cell Structures	Characteristics
Extracellular structures	A cell wall surrounding the plasma membrane gives strength and rigidity to the cell and is composed primarily of cellulose in plants (peptidoglycans in bacterial "envelopes"); animal cells are not supported by cell walls; slime capsules composed of polysaccharides or glycoproteins coat the cell walls of some bacterial and algal cells
Plasma membrane	Lipid bilayer through which extracellular substances (e.g., nutrients, water) enter the cell and waste substances or secretions exit the cell; passage of substances may require expenditure of energy (active transport) or may be passive (diffusion)
Nucleus	Master control of cellular functions via its genetic material (DNA)
Nuclear membrane	Double membrane controlling the movement of materials between the nucleus and cytoplasm; contains pores that communicate with the ER
Chromatin	Nucleoprotein component of chromosomes (seen clearly only during nuclear division when the chromatin is highly condensed); only the DNA component is hereditary material
Nucleolus	Site(s) on chromatin where ribosomal RNA (rRNA) is synthesized; disappears from light microscope during cellular replication
Nucleoplasm	Nonchromatin components of the nucleus containing materials for building DNA and messenger RNA (mRNA molecules serve as intermediates between nucleus and cytoplasm)
Cytoplasm	Contains multiple structural and enzymatic systems (e.g., glycolysis and protein synthesis) that provide energy to the cell; executes the genetic instructions from the nucleus
Ribosome	Site of protein synthesis; consists of three molecular weight classes of ribosomal RNA molecules and about 50 different proteins
Endoplasmic reticulum	Internal membrane system (designated ER); rough endoplasmic reticulum (RER) is studded with ribosomes and modifies polypeptide chains into mature proteins (e.g., by glycosylation); smooth endoplasmic reticulum (SER) is free of ribosomes and is the site of lipid synthesis
Mitochondria	Production of adenosine triphosphate (ATP) through the Krebs cycle and electron transport chain; beta oxidation of long-chain fatty acids; ATP is the main source of energy to power biochemical reactions
Plastid	Plant structure for storage of starch, pigments, and other cellular products; photosynthesis occurs in chloroplasts
Golgi body (apparatus)	Sometimes called dictyosome in plants; membranes where sugars, phosphate, sulfate, or fatty acids are added to certain proteins; as membranes bud from the Golgi system they are marked for shipment in transport vesicles to arrive at specific sites (e.g., plasma membrane, lysosome)
Lysosome	Sac of digestive enzymes in all eucaryotic cells that aid in intracellular digestion of bacteria and other foreign bodies; may cause cell destruction if ruptured
Vacuole	Membrane-bound storage deposit for water and metabolic products (e.g., amino acids, sugars); plant cells often have a large central vacuole that (when filled with fluid to create turgor pressure) makes the cell turgid
Centrioles	Form poles of the spindle apparatus during cell divisions; capable of being replicated after each cell division; rarely present in plants
Cytoskeleton	Contributes to shape, division, and motility of the cell and the ability to move and arrange its components; consists of microtubules of the protein tubulin (as in the spindle fibers responsible for chromosomal movements during nuclear division or in flagella and cilia), microfilaments of actin and myosin (as occurs in muscle cells), and intermediate filaments (each with a distinct protein such as keratin)
Cytosol	The fluid portion of the cytoplasm exclusive of the formed elements listed above; also called hyaloplasm; contains water, minerals, ions, sugars, amino acids, and other nutrients for building macromolecular biopolymers (nucleic acids, proteins, lipids, and large carbohydrates such as starch and cellulose)

CHROMOSOMES

1. Chromosome Number.

In higher organisms, each **somatic** cell (any body cell exclusive of sex cells) contains one set of chromosomes inherited from the **maternal** (female) parent and a comparable set of chromosomes (homologous chromosomes or **homologues**) from the **paternal** (male) parent. The number of chromosomes in this dual set is called the **diploid** ($2n$) number. The suffix "-ploid" refers to chromosome "sets." The prefix indicates the degree of ploidy. Sex cells, or gametes, which contain half the number of chromosome sets found in somatic cells, are referred to as **haploid** cells (n). A **genome** is a set of chromosomes corresponding to the haploid set of a species. The number of chromosomes in each somatic cell is the same for all members of a given species. For example, human somatic cells contain 46 chromosomes, tobacco has 48, cattle 60, the garden pea 14, the fruit fly 8, etc. The diploid number of a species bears no direct relationship to the species position in the phylogenetic scheme of classification.

2. Chromosome Morphology.

The structure of chromosomes becomes most easily visible during certain phases of nuclear division when they are highly coiled. Each chromosome in the genome can usually be distinguished from all others by several criteria, including the relative lengths of the chromosomes, the position of a structure called the **centromere** that divides the chromosome into two arms of varying length, the presence and position of enlarged areas called "knobs" or **chromomeres,** the presence of tiny terminal extensions of chromatin material called "satellites," etc. A chromosome with a median centromere (**metacentric**) will have arms of approximately equal size. A **submetacentric,** or **acrocentric,** chromosome has arms of distinctly unequal size. The shorter arm is called the **p arm** and the longer arm is called the **q arm.** If a chromosome has its centromere at or very near one end of the chromosome, it is called **telocentric.** Each chromosome of the genome (with the exception of sex chromosomes) is numbered consecutively according to length, beginning with the longest chromosome first.

3. Autosomes vs. Sex Chromosomes.

In the males of some species, including humans, sex is associated with a morphologically dissimilar (**heteromorphic**) pair of chromosomes called **sex chromosomes.** Such a chromosome pair is usually labeled X and Y. Genetic factors on the Y chromosome determine maleness. Females have two morphologically identical X chromosomes. The members of any other homologous pairs of chromosomes (homologues) are morphologically indistinguishable, but usually are visibly different from other pairs (nonhomologous chromosomes). All chromosomes exclusive of the sex chromosomes are called **autosomes.** Fig. 1-2 shows the chromosomal complement of the fruit fly *Drosophila melanogaster* ($2n = 8$) with three pairs of autosomes (2, 3, 4) and one pair of sex chromosomes.

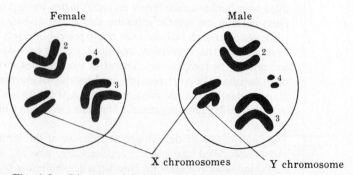

Fig. 1-2.   Diagram of diploid cells in *Drosophila melanogaster*.

CELL DIVISION

1. Mitosis.

All somatic cells in a multicellular organism are descendants of one original cell, the fertilized egg, or **zygote,** through a divisional process called **mitosis** (Fig. 1-3). The function of mitosis is first to construct an exact copy of each chromosome and then to distribute, through division of the original (mother) cell, an identical set of chromosomes to each of the two progeny cells, or daughter cells. **Interphase** is the period between division cycles. When the cell is ready to begin mitosis each DNA molecule (which is an integral part of the chromosome) **replicates,** or makes an exact copy of itself. This copying process produces a chromosome with two identical functional strands called **chromatids,** both attached to a common centromere. Chromatids are sometimes called **sister chromatids** or simply **sisters.** Chromatids become new chromosomes when the centromeric DNA replicates (''divides''); former sisters then become separate chromosomes because they no longer are connected by a common centromere. Each centromere contains a proteinaceous region (the **kinetochore**) to which traction fibers of the **spindle**

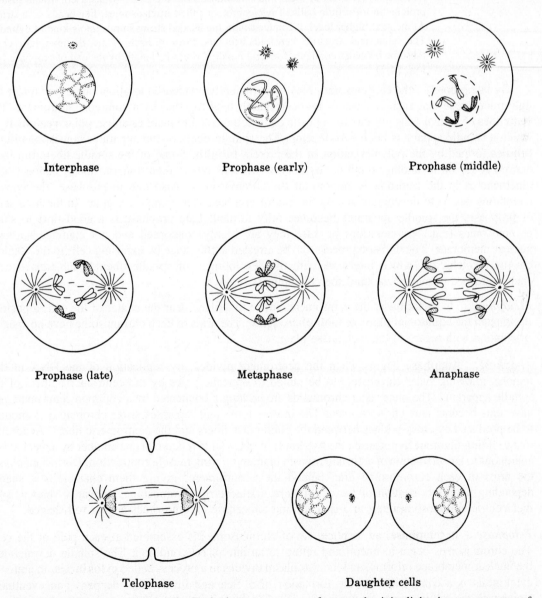

Interphase	Prophase (early)	Prophase (middle)
Prophase (late)	Metaphase	Anaphase

Telophase   Daughter cells

Fig. 1-3.   Mitosis in animal cells. Dark chromosomes are of maternal origin; light chromosomes are of paternal origin. One pair of homologues is metacentric, the other pair is submetacentric.

apparatus become attached. The centromere is a late-replicating segment of a single, double-stranded DNA molecule that is thought to form the backbone of a given chromosome. As long as the centromere remains unreplicated (undivided), copies of the DNA stay connected as sister chromatids. At this stage, the replicated chromosomes are in a very long, attenuated condition and usually cannot be seen in the light microscope as distinct threads. The chromatin material simply appears granular in a stained interphase nucleus.

A mitotic division has four major phases: prophase, metaphase, anaphase, and telophase.

(a) *Prophase.*   In **prophase,** the chromosomes **condense,** becoming visible in the light microscope first as thin threads, and then becoming progressively shorter and thicker.

> **Example 1.2.**   A toy airplane can be used as a model to explain the condensation of the chromosomes. A rubber band, fixed at one end, is attached to the propeller at its other end. As the prop is turned, the rubber band coils and supercoils on itself, becoming shorter and thicker in the process. Something akin to this process occurs during the condensation of the chromosomes. However, as a chromosome condenses, the DNA wraps itself around histone proteins to form little balls of nucleoprotein called **nucleosomes,** like beads on a string. At the next-higher level of condensation, the beaded string spirals into a kind of cylinder. The cylindrical structure then folds back and forth on itself. Thus, the interphase chromosome becomes condensed several hundred times its length by the end of prophase (see Fig. 14-1).

By late prophase, the chromosomes may be sufficiently condensed to allow one to see under the light microscope that each consists of two chromatids held together by a common centromere. The **centrioles** of animal cells migrate to opposite ends of the cell and there establish **polar regions** from which a spindle apparatus begins to develop. The spindle fibers of the apparatus consist of **microtubules** formed by the polymerization of the protein **tubulin.** Some of the spindle fibers run from one polar region to another (continuous fibers), whereas others (centromeric fibers) connect with kinetochores in the centromeric regions of the chromosomes. Also late in prophase, the nuclear membrane begins to degenerate and by the end of prophase it is completely gone. In the final stage of prophase, the spindle apparatus becomes fully formed. Late prophase is a good time to study chromosomes (e.g., enumeration) because they are highly condensed and not confined within a nuclear membrane. The division process can be arrested at this stage by exposing cells to the alkaloid chemical **colchicine,** which interferes with the development of spindle fibers. Such treated cells cannot proceed to metaphase until the colchicine is removed.

(b) *Metaphase.*   In **metaphase,** the centromeres move to a plane near the center of the cell, a position designated the **equatorial plane** or **metaphase plate.** The arms of each chromosome have no specific orientation with regard to the metaphase plate.

(c) *Anaphase.*   **Anaphase** begins when the centromere divides (by replication of the DNA in that region), allowing sister chromatids to be pulled to opposite poles by the centromeric fibers of the spindle apparatus. The once sister chromatids are no longer connected by a common centromere and have thus become new chromosomes. The motive force that separates sister chromatids is thought to be produced by cross-bridges between the continuous fibers and the centromeric fibers. According to the **sliding filament hypothesis,** the two kinds of fibers slide relative to one another by a mechanism analogous to the interaction of actin and myosin filaments during muscle contraction. During anaphase, the arms of each chromosome drag behind their centromere, giving them characteristic shapes depending upon the location of the centromere. Metacentric chromosomes appear V-shaped, submetacentric chromosomes appear J-shaped, and telocentric chromosomes appear rod-shaped.

(d) *Telophase.*   In **telophase,** an identical set of chromosomes is assembled at each pole of the cell. The chromosomes begin to uncoil and return to an interphase condition. The spindle degenerates, the nuclear membrane reforms, and the cytoplasm divides in a process called **cytokinesis.** In animals, cytokinesis is accomplished by the formation of a cleavage furrow that deepens and eventually ''pinches'' the cell in two as shown in Fig. 1-3. Cytokinesis in most plants involves the construction of a **cell plate** of pectin originating in the center of the cell and spreading laterally to the cell wall.

Later, cellulose and other strengthening materials are added to the cell plate, converting it into a new cell wall. The two products of mitosis are called **daughter cells** or **progeny cells** and may or may not be of equal size depending upon where the plane of cytokinesis sections the cell. Thus while there is no assurance of equal distribution of cytoplasmic components to daughter cells, they do contain exactly the same type and number of chromosomes and hence possess exactly the same genetic constitution.

The time during which the cell is undergoing mitosis is designated the **M period.** The times spent in each phase of mitosis are quite different. Prophase usually requires far longer than the other phases; metaphase is the shortest. DNA replication occurs before mitosis in what is termed the **S (synthesis) phase** (Fig. 1-4). In nucleated cells, DNA synthesis starts at several positions on each chromosome, thereby reducing the time required to replicate the sister chromatids. The period between M and S is designated the **G_2 phase** (post-DNA synthesis). A long **G_1 phase** (pre-DNA synthesis) follows mitosis and precedes chromosomal replication. Interphase includes G_1, S, and G_2. The four phases (M, G_1, S, G_2) constitute the life cycle of a somatic cell. The lengths of these phases vary considerably from one cell type to another. Normal mammalian cells growing in tissue culture usually require 18–24 hours at 37°C to complete the cell cycle.

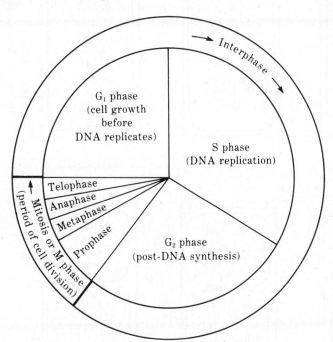

Fig. 1-4.   Diagram of a typical cell reproductive cycle.

2. Meiosis.

Sexual reproduction involves the manufacture of gametes (**gametogenesis**) and the union of a male and a female gamete (**fertilization**) to produce a zygote. Male gametes are **sperms** and female gametes are **eggs,** or **ova** (ovum, singular). Gametogenesis occurs only in the specialized cells (**germ line**) of the reproductive organs (**gonads**). In animals, the testes are male gonads and the ovaries are female gonads. Gametes contain the haploid number (*n*) of chromosomes, but originate from diploid (2*n*) cells of the germ line. The number of chromosomes must be reduced by half during gametogenesis in order to maintain the chromosome number characteristic of the species. This is accomplished by the divisional process called **meiosis** (Fig. 1-5). Meiosis involves a single DNA replication and two divisions of the cytoplasm. The first meiotic division (meiosis I) is a **reductional division** that produces two haploid cells from a single diploid cell. The second meiotic division (meiosis II) is an **equational division**

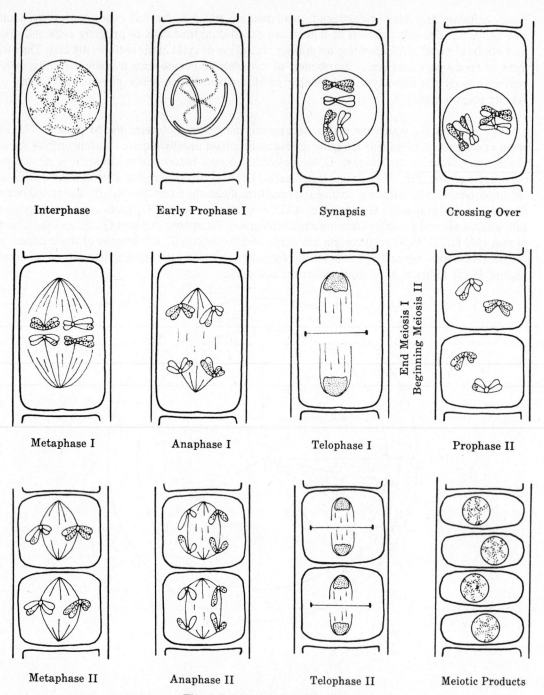

Fig. 1-5.   Meiosis in plant cells.

(mitotislike, in that sister chromatids of the haploid cells are separated). Each of the two meiotic divisions consists of four major phases (prophase, metaphase, anaphase, and telophase).

(a) **Meiosis I.**   The DNA replicates during the interphase preceding meiosis I; it does not replicate between telophase I and prophase II. The prophase of meiosis I differs from the prophase of mitosis in that homologous chromosomes come to lie side by side in a pairing process called **synapsis.** Each pair of synapsed chromosomes is called a **bivalent** (2 chromosomes). Each chromosome consists of two identical sister chromatids at this stage. Thus, a bivalent may also be called a **tetrad** (4 chromatids) if chromatids are counted. The number of chromosomes is always equivalent to the number of centromeres regardless of how many chromatids each chromosome may contain. During synapsis nonsister chromatids (one from each of the paired chromosomes) of a tetrad may break and reunite at one or more corresponding sites in a process called **crossing over.** The point of exchange appears in the microscope as a cross-shaped figure called a **chiasma (chiasmata,** plural). Thus, at a given chiasma, only two of the four chromatids cross over in a somewhat random manner. Generally, the number of crossovers per bivalent increases with the length of the chromosome. By chance, a bivalent may experience 0, 1, or multiple crossovers, but even in the longest chromosomes the incidence of multiple chiasmata of higher numbers is expected to become progressively rare. It is not known whether synapsis occurs by pairing between strands of two different DNA molecules or by proteins that complex with corresponding sites on homologous chromosomes. It is thought that synapsis occurs discontinuously or intermittently along the paired chromosomes at positions where the DNA molecules have unwound sufficiently to allow strands of nonsister DNA molecules to form specific pairs of their building blocks or monomers (nucleotides). Despite the fact that homologous chromosomes appear in the light microscope to be paired along their entire lengths during prophase I, it is estimated that less than 1% of the DNA synapses in this way. A ribbonlike structure called the **synaptonemal complex** can be seen in the electron microscope between paired chromosomes. It consists of **nucleoprotein** (a complex of nucleic acid and proteins). A few cases are known in which synaptonemal complexes are not formed, but then synapsis is not as complete and crossing over is markedly reduced or eliminated. By the breakage and reunion of nonsister chromatids within a chiasma, linked genes become recombined into **crossover-type** chromatids; the two chromatids within that same chiasma that did not exchange segments maintain the original linkage arrangement of genes as **noncrossover-** or **parental-type** chromatids. A chiasma is a cytological structure visible in the light microscope. Crossing over is usually a genetic phenomenon that can be inferred only from the results of breeding experiments.

Prophase of meiosis I may be divided into five stages. During **leptonema** (thin-thread stage), the long, thin, attenuated chromosomes start to condense and, as a consequence, the first signs of threadlike structures begin to appear in the formerly amorphous nuclear chromatin material. During **zygonema** (joined-thread stage), synapsis begins. In **pachynema** (thick-thread stage), synapsis appears so tight that it becomes difficult to distinguish homologues in a bivalent. This tight pairing becomes somewhat relaxed during the next stage called **diplonema** (double-thread stage) so that individual chromatids and chiasmata can be seen. Finally, in **diakinesis** the chromosomes reach their maximal condensation, nucleoli and the nuclear membrane disappear, and the spindle apparatus begins to form.

During **metaphase I,** the bivalents orient at random on the equatorial plane. At **anaphase I,** the centromeres do not divide, but continue to hold sister chromatids together. Because of crossovers, sister chromatids may no longer be genetically identical. Homologous chromosomes separate and move to opposite poles; i.e., whole chromosomes (each consisting of 2 sister chromatids) move apart. This is the movement that will reduce the chromosome number from the diploid ($2n$) condition to the haploid (n) state. Cytokinesis in **telophase I** divides the diploid mother cell into 2 haploid daughter cells. This ends the first meiotic division.

(b) *Interkinesis.* The period between the first and second meiotic divisions is called **interkinesis.** Depending on the species, interkinesis may be brief or continue for an extended period of time. During an extensive interkinesis, the chromosomes may uncoil and return to an interphaselike condition with reformation of a nuclear membrane. At some later time, the chromosomes would again condense and the nuclear membrane would disappear. Nothing of genetic importance happens during interkinesis. The DNA does *not* replicate during interkinesis!

(c) *Meiosis II.* In **prophase II,** the spindle apparatus reforms. By **metaphase II,** the individual chromosomes have lined up on the equatorial plane. During **anaphase II,** the centromeres of each chromosome divide, allowing the sister chromatids to be pulled apart in an equational division (mitotislike) by the spindle fibers. Cytokinesis in **telophase II** divides each cell into 2 progeny cells. Thus, a diploid mother cell becomes 4 haploid progeny cells as a consequence of a meiotic cycle (meiosis I and meiosis II). The characteristics that distinguish mitosis from meiosis are summarized in Table 1.2.

Table 1.2. Characteristics of Mitosis and Meiosis

Mitosis	Meiosis
1. An equational division that separates sister chromatids	1. The first stage is a reductional division which separates homologous chromosomes at first anaphase; sister chromatids separate in an equational division at second anaphase
2. One division per cycle, i.e., one cytoplasmic division (cytokinesis) per equational chromosomal division	2. Two divisions per cycle, i.e., two cytoplasmic divisions, one following reductional chromosomal division and one following equational chromosomal division
3. Chromosomes fail to synapse; no chiasmata form; genetic exchange between homologous chromosomes does not occur	3. Chromosomes synapse and form chiasmata; genetic exchange occurs between homologues
4. Two products (daughter cells) produced per cycle	4. Four cellular products (gametes or spores) produced per cycle
5. Genetic content of mitotic products are identical	5. Genetic content of meiotic products are different; centromeres may be replicas of either maternal or paternal centromeres in varying combinations
6. Chromosome number of daughter cells is the same as that of the mother cell	6. Chromosome number of meiotic products is half that of the mother cell
7. Mitotic products are usually capable of undergoing additional mitotic divisions	7. Meiotic products cannot undergo another meiotic division although they may undergo mitotic division
8. Normally occurs in most all somatic cells	8. Occurs only in specialized cells of the germ line
9. Begins at the zygote state and continues through the life of the organism	9. Occurs only after a higher organism has begun to mature; occurs in the zygote of many algae and fungi

MENDEL'S LAWS

Gregor Mendel published the results of his genetic studies on the garden pea in 1866 and thereby laid the foundation of modern genetics. In this paper Mendel proposed some basic genetic principles. One of these is known as the **principle of segregation.** He found that from any one parent, only one allelic form of a gene is transmitted through a gamete to the offspring. For example, a plant which had a factor (or gene) for round-shaped seed and also an allele for wrinkled-shaped seed would transmit only one of these two alleles through a gamete to its offspring. Mendel knew nothing of chromosomes or meiosis, as they had not yet been discovered. We now know that the physical basis for this principle is in first meiotic anaphase where homologous chromosomes segregate or separate from each other. If the gene for round seed is on one chromosome and its allelic form for wrinkled seed is on the homologous chromosome, then it becomes clear that alleles normally will not be found in the same gamete.

Mendel's **principle of independent assortment** states that the segregation of one factor pair occurs independently of any other factor pair. We know that this is true only for loci on nonhomologous chromosomes. For example, on one homologous pair of chromosomes are the seed shape alleles and on another pair of homologues are the alleles for green and yellow seed color. The segregation of the seed shape alleles occurs independently of the segregation of the seed color alleles because each pair of homologues behaves as an independent unit during meiosis. Furthermore, because the orientation of bivalents on the first meiotic metaphase plate is completely at random, four combinations of factors could be found in the meiotic products: (1) round-yellow, (2) wrinkled-green, (3) round-green, (4) wrinkled-yellow.

GAMETOGENESIS

Usually the immediate end products of meiosis are not fully developed gametes or spores. A period of **maturation** commonly follows meiosis. In plants, one or more mitotic divisions are required to produce reproductive spores, whereas in animals the meiotic products develop directly into gametes through growth and/or differentiation. The entire process of producing mature gametes or spores, of which meiotic division is the most important part, is called **gametogenesis.** In Figs. 1-6, 1-7, and 1-9, the number of chromatids in each chromosome at each stage may not be accurately represented. Refer back to Figs. 1-3 and 1-5 for details of mitotic and meiotic divisions if in doubt. Crossovers have also been deleted from these figures for the sake of simplicity. Thus in Fig. 1-6(a), if two sperm cells appear to contain identical chromosomes, they are probably dissimilar because of crossovers.

1. Animal Gametogenesis (as represented in mammals).

Gametogenesis in the male animal is called **spermatogenesis** [(Fig. 1-6(a)]. Mammalian spermatogenesis originates in the germinal epithelium of the seminiferous tubules of the male gonads (testes) from diploid primordial cells. These cells undergo repeated mitotic divisions to form a population of **spermatogonia.** By growth, a spermatogonium may differentiate into a diploid **primary spermatocyte** with the capacity to undergo meiosis. The first meiotic division occurs in these primary spermatocytes, producing haploid **secondary spermatocytes.** From these cells the second meiotic division produces 4 haploid meiotic products called **spermatids.** Almost the entire amount of cytoplasm then extrudes into a long whiplike tail during maturation and the cell becomes transformed into a mature male gamete called a **sperm cell** or **spermatozoan** (-zoa, plural).

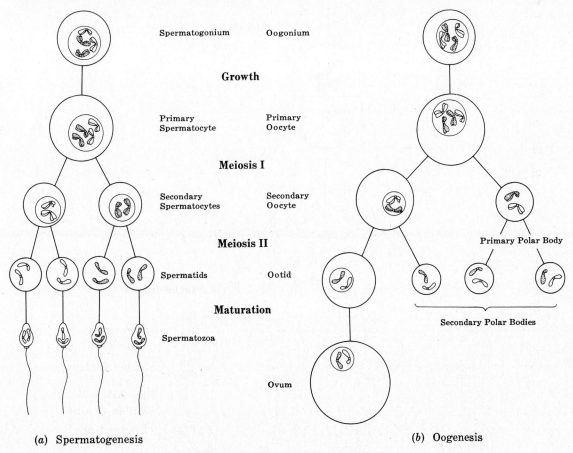

(a) Spermatogenesis (b) Oogenesis

Fig. 1-6. Animal gametogenesis.

Gametogenesis in the female animal is called **oogenesis** [Fig. 1-6(*b*)]. Mammalian oogenesis originates in the germinal epithelium of the female gonads (ovaries) in diploid primordial cells called **oogonia.** By growth and storage of much cytoplasm or yolk (to be used as food by the early embryo), the oogonium is transformed into a diploid **primary oocyte** with the capacity to undergo meiosis. The first meiotic division reduces the chromosome number by half and also distributes vastly different amounts of cytoplasm to the two products by a grossly unequal cytokinesis. The larger cell thus produced is called a **secondary oocyte** and the smaller is a primary **polar body.** In some cases the first polar body may undergo the second meiotic division, producing two secondary polar bodies. All polar bodies degenerate, however, and take no part in fertilization. The second meiotic division of the oocyte again involves an unequal cytokinesis, producing a large yolky **ootid** and a secondary polar body. By additional growth and differentiation the ootid becomes a mature female gamete called an **ovum** or **egg cell.**

The union of male and female gametes (sperm and egg) is called fertilization and reestablishes the diploid number in the resulting cell called a zygote. The head of the sperm enters the egg, but the tail piece (the bulk of the cytoplasm of the male gamete) remains outside and degenerates. Subsequent mitotic divisions produce the numerous cells of the embryo that become organized into the tissues and organs of the new individual.

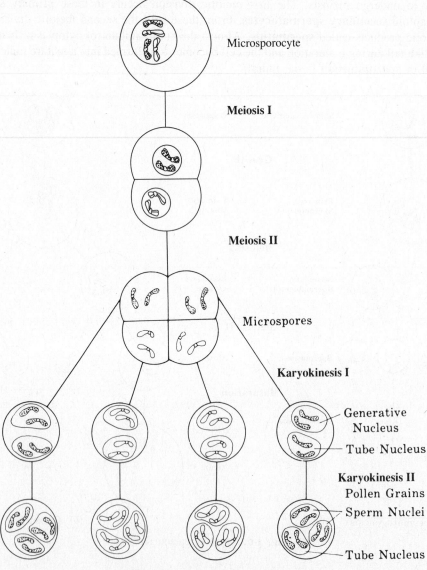

Microsporocyte

Meiosis I

Meiosis II

Microspores

Karyokinesis I

Generative Nucleus

Tube Nucleus

Karyokinesis II
Pollen Grains
Sperm Nuclei

Tube Nucleus

Fig. 1-7. Microsporogenesis.

2. Plant Gametogenesis (*as represented in angiosperms*).

Gametogenesis in the plant kingdom varies considerably between major groups of plants. The process as described below is that typical of many flowering plants (**angiosperms**). **Microsporogenesis** (Fig. 1-7) is the process of gametogenesis in the male part of the flower (**anther,** Fig. 1-8) resulting in reproductive spores called **pollen grains.** A diploid microspore mother cell (**microsporocyte**) in the anther divides by meiosis, forming at the first division a pair of haploid cells. The second meiotic division produces a cluster of 4 haploid **microspores.** Following meiosis, each microspore undergoes a mitotic division of the chromosomes without a cytoplasmic division (**karyokinesis**). This requires chromosomal replication that is not illustrated in the karyokinetic divisions of Fig. 1-7. The product of the first karyokinesis is a cell containing 2 identical haploid nuclei. Pollen grains are usually shed at this stage. Upon germination of the pollen tube, one of these nuclei (or haploid sets of chromosomes) becomes a **generative nucleus** and divides again by mitosis without cytokinesis (karyokinesis II) to form 2 **sperm nuclei.** The other nucleus, which does not divide, becomes the **tube nucleus.** All 3 nuclei should be genetically identical.

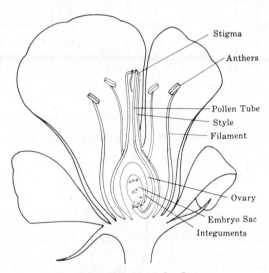

Fig. 1-8.   Diagram of a flower.

Megasporogenesis (Fig. 1-9) is the process of gametogenesis in the female part of the flower (**ovary,** Fig. 1-8) resulting in reproductive cells called **embryo sacs.** A diploid megaspore mother cell (**megasporocyte**) in the ovary divides by meiosis, forming in the first division a pair of haploid cells. The second meiotic division produces a linear group of 4 haploid **megaspores.** Following meiosis, 3 of the megaspores degenerate. The remaining megaspore undergoes three mitotic divisions of the chromosomes without intervening cytokineses (karyokineses), producing a large cell with 8 haploid nuclei (immature embryo sac). Remember that chromosomal replication must precede each karyokinesis, but this is not illustrated in Fig. 1-9. The sac is surrounded by maternal tissues of the ovary called **integuments** and by the megasporangium (**nucellus**). At one end of the sac there is an opening in the integuments (**micropyle**) through which the pollen tube will penetrate. Three nuclei of the sac orient themselves near the micropylar end and 2 of the 3 (**synergids**) degenerate. The third nucleus develops into an **egg nucleus.** Another group of 3 nuclei moves to the opposite end of the sac and degenerates (**antipodals**). The 2 remaining nuclei (**polar nuclei**) unite near the center of the sac, forming a single diploid **fusion nucleus.** The mature embryo sac (**megagametophyte**) is now ready for fertilization.

Pollen grains from the anthers are carried by wind or insects to the **stigma.** The pollen grain germinates into a pollen tube that grows down the **style,** presumably under the direction of the tube nucleus. The pollen tube enters the ovary and makes its way through the micropyle of the ovule into the embryo sac (Fig. 1-10). Both sperm nuclei are released into the embryo sac. The pollen tube and the tube nucleus, having served their function, degenerate. One sperm nucleus fuses with the egg nucleus to form a diploid zygote, which will then develop into the embryo. The other sperm nucleus unites with the fusion nucleus

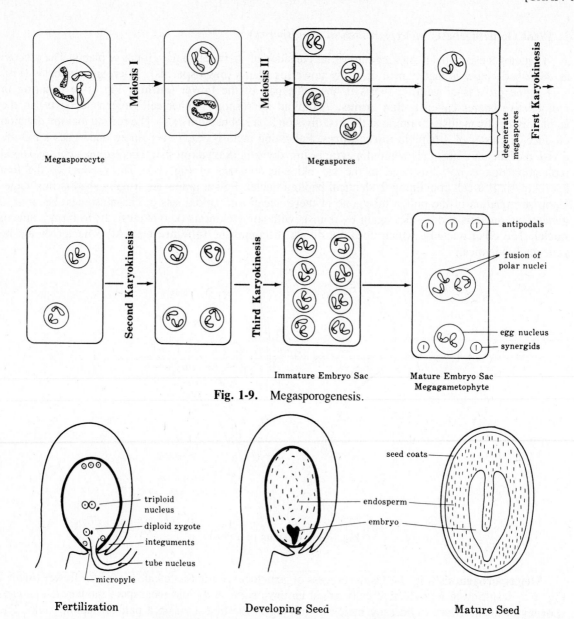

Fig. 1-9. Megasporogenesis.

Fig. 1-10. Fertilization and development of a seed.

to form a triploid (3*n*) nucleus, which, by subsequent mitotic divisions, forms a starchy nutritive tissue called **endosperm.** The outermost layer of endosperm cells is called **aleurone.** The embryo, surrounded by endosperm tissue, and in some cases such as corn and other grasses where it is also surrounded by a thin outer layer of diploid maternal tissue called **pericarp,** becomes the familiar seed. Since 2 sperm nuclei are involved, this process is termed **double fertilization.** Upon germination of the seed, the young seedling (the next sporophytic generation) utilizes the nutrients stored in the endosperm for growth until it emerges from the soil, at which time it becomes capable of manufacturing its own food by photosynthesis.

LIFE CYCLES

Life cycles of most plants have two distinctive generations: a haploid **gametophytic** (gamete-bearing plant) generation and a diploid **sporophytic** (spore-bearing plant) generation. Gametophytes produce gametes which unite to form sporophytes, which in turn give rise to spores that develop into gametophytes, etc. This process is referred to as the **alternation of generations.** In lower plants, such as mosses and liverworts, the gametophyte is a conspicuous and independently living generation, the sporophyte being small and dependent upon the gametophyte. In higher plants (ferns, gymnosperms, and angiosperms), the situation is reversed; the sporophyte is the independent and conspicuous generation and the gametophyte is the less conspicuous and, in the case of gymnosperms (cone-bearing plants) and angiosperms (flowering plants), completely dependent generation. We have just seen in angiosperms that the male gametophytic generation is reduced to a pollen tube and three haploid nuclei (**microgametophyte**); the female gametophyte (**megagametophyte**) is a single multinucleated cell called the embryo sac surrounded and nourished by ovarian tissue.

Many simpler organisms such as one-celled animals (protozoa), algae, yeast, and other fungi are useful in genetic studies and have interesting life cycles that exhibit considerable variation. Some of these life cycles, as well as those of bacteria and viruses, are presented in later chapters.

Solved Problems

1.1. Consider 3 pairs of homologous chromosomes with centromeres labeled A/a, B/b, and C/c where the slash line separates one chromosome from its homologue. How many different kinds of meiotic products can this individual produce?

Solution:

For ease in determining all possible combinations, we can use a dichotomous branching system.

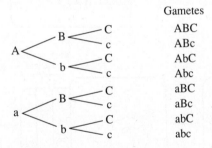

Eight different chromosomal combinations are expected in the gametes.

1.2. Develop a general formula that expresses the number of different types of gametic chromosomal combinations which can be formed in an organism with k pairs of chromosomes.

Solution:

It is obvious from the solution of the preceding problem that 1 pair of chromosomes gives 2 types of gametes, 2 pairs give 4 types of gametes, 3 pairs give 8 types, etc. The progression 2, 4, 8, . . . can be expressed by the formula 2^k, where k is the number of chromosome pairs.

1.3. The horse (*Equus caballus*) has a diploid complement of 64 chromosomes including 36 acrocentric autosomes; the ass (*Equus asinus*) has 62 chromosomes including 22 acrocentric autosomes. (*a*) Predict the number of chromosomes to be found in the hybrid offspring (mule) produced by mating a male ass (jack) to a female horse (mare). (*b*) Why are mules usually sterile (incapable of producing viable gametes)?

Solution:

(a) The sperm of the jack carries the haploid number of chromosomes for its species ($\frac{62}{2} = 31$); the egg of the mare carries the haploid number for its species ($\frac{64}{2} = 32$); the hybrid mule formed by the union of these gametes would have a diploid number of $31 + 32 = 63$.

(b) The haploid set of chromosomes of the horse, which includes 18 acrocentric autosomes, is so dissimilar to that of the ass, which includes only 11 acrocentric autosomes, that meiosis in the mule germ line cannot proceed beyond first prophase where synapsis of homologues occurs.

1.4. When a plant of chromosomal type *aa* pollinates a plant of type *AA*, what chromosomal type of embryo and endosperm is expected in the resulting seeds?

Solution:

The pollen parent produces two sperm nuclei in each pollen grain of type *a*, one combining with the *A* egg nucleus to produce a diploid zygote (embryo) of type *Aa* and the other combining with the maternal fusion nucleus *AA* to produce a triploid endosperm of type *AAa*.

1.5. Given the first meiotic metaphase orientation shown on the right, and keeping all products in sequential order as they would be formed from left to right, diagram the embryo sac that develops from the meiotic product at the left and label the chromosomal constitution of all its nuclei.

Solution:

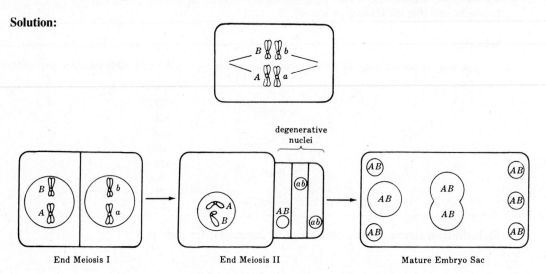

Supplementary Problems

1.6. There are 40 chromosomes in somatic cells of the house mouse. (a) How many chromosomes does a mouse receive from its father? (b) How many autosomes are present in a mouse gamete? (c) How many sex chromosomes are in a mouse ovum? (d) How many autosomes are in somatic cells of a female?

1.7. Name each stage of mitosis described. (a) Chromosomes line up in the equatorial plane. (b) Nuclear membrane reforms and cytokinesis occurs. (c) Chromosomes become visible, spindle apparatus forms. (d) Sister chromatids move to opposite poles of the cell.

1.8. Identify the mitotic stage represented in each of the following diagrams of isolated cells from an individual with a diploid chromosome complement of one metacentric pair and one acrocentric pair of chromosomes.

(a)   (b)   (c)   (d)

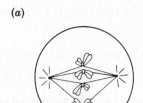
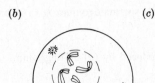
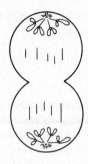
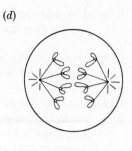

1.9. Identify the meiotic stage represented in each of the following diagrams of isolated cells from the germ line of an individual with one pair of acrocentric and one pair of metacentric chromosomes.

(a)   (b)   (c)

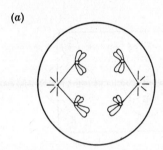
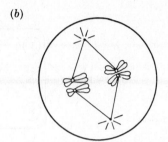
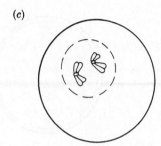

(d)   (e)   (f)

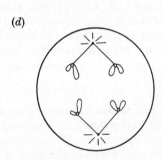
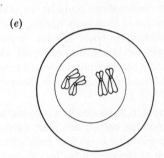
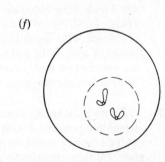

1.10. How many different types of gametic chromosomal combinations can be formed in the garden pea ($2n = 14$)? *Hint:* See Problem 1.2.

1.11. (a) What type of division (equational or reductional) is exemplified by the anaphase chromosomal movements shown below?
(b) Does the movement shown at (i) occur in mitosis or meiosis?
(c) Does the movement shown at (ii) occur in mitosis or meiosis?

(i) 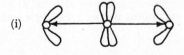   (ii)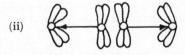

1.12. What animal cells correspond to the 3 megaspores that degenerate following meiosis in plants?

1.13. What plant cell corresponds functionally to the primary spermatocyte?

1.14. What is the probability of a sperm cell of a man ($n = 23$) containing only replicas of the centromeres that were received from his mother?

1.15. How many chromosomes of humans ($2n = 46$) will be found in (a) a secondary spermatocyte, (b) a spermatid, (c) a spermatozoan, (d) a spermatogonium, (e) a primary spermatocyte?

1.16. How many spermatozoa are produced by (*a*) a spermatogonium, (*b*) a secondary spermatocyte, (*c*) a spermatid, (*d*) a primary spermatocyte?

1.17. How many human egg cells (ova) are produced by (*a*) an oogonium, (*b*) a primary oocyte, (*c*) an ootid, (*d*) a polar body?

1.18. Corn (*Zea mays*) has a diploid number of 20. How many chromosomes would be expected in (*a*) a meiotic product (microspore or megaspore), (*b*) the cell resulting from the first nuclear division (karyokinesis) of a megaspore, (*c*) a polar nucleus, (*d*) a sperm nucleus, (*e*) a microspore mother cell, (*f*) a leaf cell, (*g*) a mature embryo sac (after degeneration of nonfunctional nuclei), (*h*) an egg nucleus, (*i*) an endosperm cell, (*j*) a cell of the embryo, (*k*) a cell of the pericarp, (*l*) an aleurone cell?

1.19. A pollen grain of corn with nuclei labeled A, B, and C fertilized an embryo sac with nuclei labeled D, E, F, G, H, I, J, and K as shown below.

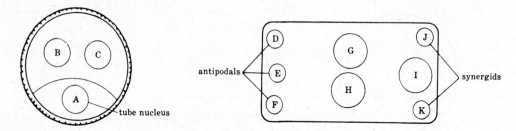

(*a*) Which of the following five combinations could be found in the embryo: (1) ABC, (2) BCI, (3) GHC, (4) AI, (5) CI? (*b*) Which of the above five combinations could be found in the aleurone layer of the seed? (*c*) Which of the above five combinations could be found in the germinating pollen tube? (*d*) Which of the nuclei, if any, in the pollen grain would contain genetically identical sets of chromosomes? (*e*) Which of the nuclei in the embryo sac would be chromosomally and genetically equivalent? (*f*) Which of the nuclei in these two gametophytes will have no descendants in the mature seed?

1.20. A certain plant has 8 chromosomes in its root cells: a long metacentric pair, a short metacentric pair, a long telocentric pair, and a short telocentric pair. If this plant fertilizes itself (self-pollination), what proportion of the offspring would be expected to have (*a*) four pairs of telocentric chromosomes, (*b*) one telocentric pair and three metacentric pairs of chromosomes, (*c*) two metacentric and two telocentric pairs of chromosomes?

1.21. Referring to the preceding problem, what proportion of the meiotic products from such a plant would be expected to contain (*a*) four metacentric pairs of chromosomes, (*b*) two metacentric and two telocentric pairs of chromosomes, (*c*) one metacentric and one telocentric pair of chromosomes, (*d*) 2 metacentric and 2 telocentric chromosomes?

1.22. How many pollen grains are produced by (*a*) 20 microspore mother cells, (*b*) a cluster of 4 microspores?

1.23. How many sperm nuclei are produced by (*a*) a dozen microspore mother cells, (*b*) a generative nucleus, (*c*) 100 tube nuclei?

1.24. (*a*) Diagram the pollen grain responsible for the doubly fertilized embryo sac shown below. (*b*) Diagram the first meiotic metaphase (in an organism with two pairs of homologues labeled *A*, *a* and *B*, *b*) which produced the pollen grain in part (*a*).

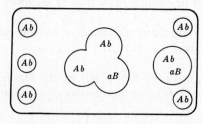

For Problems 1.25–1.28, diagram the designated stages of gametogenesis in a diploid organism that has one pair of metacentric and one pair of acrocentric chromosomes. Label each of the chromatids assuming that the locus of gene *A* is on the metacentric pair (one of which carries the *A* allele and its homologue carries the *a* allele) and that the locus of gene *B* is on the acrocentric chromosome pair (one of which carries the *B* allele and its homologue carries the *b* allele).

1.25. *Oogenesis:* (*a*) first metaphase; (*b*) first telophase resulting from part (*a*); (*c*) second metaphase resulting from part (*b*); (*d*) second telophase resulting from part (*c*).

1.26. *Spermatogenesis:* (*a*) anaphase of a dividing spermatogonium; (*b*) anaphase of a dividing primary spermatocyte; (*c*) anaphase of a secondary spermatocyte derived from part (*b*); (*d*) 4 sperm cells resulting from part (*b*).

1.27. *Microsporogenesis:* (*a*) synapsis in a microsporocyte; (*b*) second meiotic metaphase; (*c*) first meiotic metaphase in the microspore mother cell that produced the cell of part (*b*); (*d*) anaphase of the second nuclear division (karyokinesis) following meiosis in a developing microgametophyte derived from part (*b*).

1.28. *Megasporogenesis:* (*a*) second meiotic telophase; (*b*) first meiotic telophase that produced the cell of part (*a*); (*c*) anaphase of the second nuclear division (karyokinesis) in a cell derived from part (*a*); (*d*) mature embryo sac produced from part (*c*).

Review Questions

Matching Questions   Choose the one best match between each organelle (in the left column) with its function or description (in the right column).

Cell Organelle	**Function or Description**
1. Mitochondria	A. Establishes polar region
2. Centrioles	B. May contain a photosynthetic system
3. Chromosome	C. Site of protein synthesis
4. Hyaloplasm	D. Contains most of cell's DNA
5. Nucleolus	E. Called dictyosome in plants
6. Ribosome	F. Storage of excess water
7. Endoplasmic reticulum	G. Site of Krebs cycle
8. Plastid	H. Site of glycolysis
9. Golgi body	I. Internal membrane network
10. Vacuole	J. RNA-rich region in nucleus

Vocabulary   For each of the following definitions, give the appropriate term and spell it correctly. Terms are single words unless indicated otherwise.

1. Any chromosome other than a sex chromosome.

2. Site on a chromosome to which spindle fibers attach.

3. Adjective applicable to a chromosome with arms of about equal length.

4. Adjective referring to the number of chromosomes in a gamete.

5. Reduction division.

6. Division of the cytoplasm.

7. The first phase of mitosis.

8. The cytological structure on paired chromosomes with which genetic exchange (crossing over) is correlated.

9. Chromosomes that contain enough similar genetic material to pair in meiosis.

10. The period between mitotic division cycles.

True-False Questions   Answer each of the following questions either true (T) or false (F).

1. The phase of the cell cycle in which DNA replicates is designated S.

2. A bivalent or a tetrad is a common feature of mitosis.

3. The immediate product of the first meiotic division in animals is termed a spermatid.

4. A diploid plant cell with the capacity to undergo meiosis is called a microspore.

5. A micropyle is a small intracellular organelle.

6. Double fertilization is a common attribute of angiosperms.

7. Synapsis is a regular occurrence in meiosis.

8. Barring mutation, the genetic content of daughter cells produced by mitosis should be identical.

9. Sister chromatids separate from each other during first meiotic anaphase.

10. None of the products of a meiotic event are expected to be genetically identical.

Multiple-Choice Questions   Choose the one best answer.

1. An organelle present in animal cells but missing from plant cells is   (*a*) a nucleolus   (*b*) a centriole   (*c*) a vacuole   (*d*) a mitochondrion   (*e*) more than one of the above

2. How many spermatids are normally produced by 50 primary spermatocytes?   (*a*) 25   (*b*) 50   (*c*) 100   (*d*) 200   (*e*) 400

3. Humans normally have 46 chromosomes in skin cells. How many autosomes would be expected in a kidney cell?   (*a*) 46   (*b*) 23   (*c*) 47   (*d*) 44   (*e*) none of the above

4. During mitosis, synapsis occurs in the phase called   (*a*) telophase   (*b*) anaphase   (*c*) prophase   (*d*) metaphase   (*e*) none of the above

5. If the genetic endowments of two nuclei that unite to produce the plant zygote are labeled A and B, and the other product of fertilization within that same embryo sac is labeled ABB, then the tube nucleus that was in the pollen tube that delivered the fertilizing male gametes must be labeled   (*a*) A   (*b*) AB   (*c*) B   (*d*) BB   (*e*) none of the above

6. The diploid number of corn is 20. How many chromosomes are expected in the product of the second karyokinesis following meiosis in the formation of an embryo sac?   (*a*) 10   (*b*) 20   (*c*) 30   (*d*) 40   (*e*) none of the above

7. The yolk of a chicken egg serves a nutritive function for the developing embryo. A functionally comparable substance in plants is   (*a*) pectin   (*b*) endosperm   (*c*) cellulose   (*d*) lignin   (*e*) pollen

8. Which of the following cells is normally diploid?   (*a*) primary polar body   (*b*) spermatid   (*c*) primary spermatocyte   (*d*) spermatozoa   (*e*) secondary polar body

9. Upon which two major features of chromosomes does their cytological identification depend?   (*a*) length of chromosome and position of centromere   (*b*) amount of DNA and intensity of staining   (*c*) numbers of nucleoli and centromeres   (*d*) number of chromatids and length of arms   (*e*) chromosome thickness and length

10. In oogenesis, the cell that corresponds to a spermatid is called a(an)   (*a*) ovum   (*b*) egg   (*c*) secondary oocyte   (*d*) oogonium   (*e*) secondary polar body

Answers to Supplementary Problems

1.6.   (*a*) 20,   (*b*) 19,   (*c*) 1,   (*d*) 38

1.7.   (*a*) Metaphase,   (*b*) telophase,   (*c*) prophase,   (*d*) anaphase

1.8.   (*a*) Metaphase,   (*b*) prophase,   (*c*) telophase,   (*d*) anaphase

1.9.   (*a*) 1st anaphase,   (*b*) 1st metaphase,   (*c*) 2nd prophase or end of 1st telophase,   (*d*) 2nd anaphase,   (*e*) 1st prophase,   (*f*) 2nd telophase (meiotic product)

1.10. 128

1.11. (*a*) (i) is an equational division, (ii) is a reductional division;   (*b*) both;   (*c*) meiosis

1.12. Polar bodies

1.13. Microspore mother cell (microsporocyte); both are diploid cells with the capacity to divide meiotically

1.14. $(\frac{1}{2})^{23}$, less than one chance in 8 million

1.15. (*a*) 23,   (*b*) 23,   (*c*) 23,   (*d*) 46,   (*e*) 46

1.16. (*a*) 4,   (*b*) 2,   (*c*) 1,   (*d*) 4

1.17. (*a*) 1,   (*b*) 1,   (*c*) 1,   (*d*) 0

1.18. (*a*) 10,   (*b*) 20,   (*c*) 10,   (*d*) 10,   (*e*) 20,   (*f*) 20,   (*g*) 30,   (*h*) 10,   (*i*) 30,   (*j*) 20,   (*k*) 20,   (*l*) 30

1.19. (*a*) 5;   (*b*) 3;   (*c*) 1;   (*d*) A, B, C;   (*e*) D, E, F, G, H, I, J, K;   (*f*) A, D, E, F, J, K

1.20. (*a*) 0,   (*b*) 0,   (*c*) all

1.21. (*a*) 0,   (*b*) 0,   (*c*) 0,   (*d*) all

1.22. (*a*) 80,   (*b*) 4

1.23. (*a*) 96,   (*b*) 2,   (*c*) 0

1.24. (*a*)   (*b*)

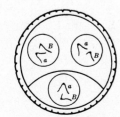
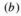
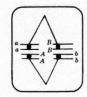

Only one of several possible solutions is shown for each of Problems 1.25–1.28.

1.25. (a) 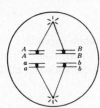 (b) 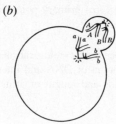 (c) 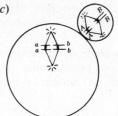 (d)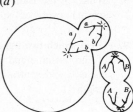

1.26. (a) 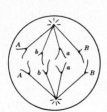 (b) 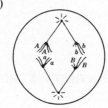 (c) 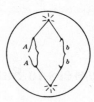 (d)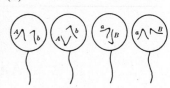

1.27. (a) (b) 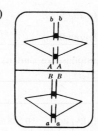 (c) 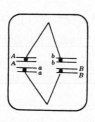 (d)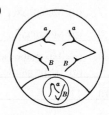

1.28. (a) 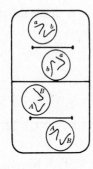 (b) 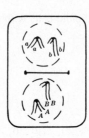 (c) 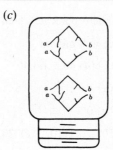 (d)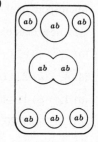

Answers to Review Questions

Matching Questions

1. G   2. A   3. D   4. H   5. J   6. C   7. I   8. B   9. E   10. F

Vocabulary

1. autosome
2. centromere or kinetochore
3. metacentric
4. haploid
5. meiosis
6. cytokinesis
7. prophase
8. chiasma
9. homologues
10. interphase

True-False Questions

1. T   2. F (meiosis) 3. F (secondary spermatocyte)   4. F (microsporocyte or microspore mother cell; megasporocyte or megaspore mother cell)   5. F (opening in integuments for passage of pollen tube into embryo sac) 6. T   7. T   8. T   9. F (second meiotic anaphase)   10. T

Multiple-Choice Questions

1. *b*   2. *d*   3. *d*   4. *e*   5. *a*   6. *d*   7. *b*   8. *c*   9. *a*   10. *e*

Chapter 2

Single-Gene Inheritance

TERMINOLOGY

1. Phenotype.

A **phenotype** may be any measurable characteristic or distinctive trait possessed by an organism. The trait may be visible to the eye, such as the color of a flower or the texture of hair, or it may require special tests for its identification, as in the determination of the respiratory quotient or the serological test for blood type. The phenotype is the result of gene products brought to expression in a given environment.

> **Example 2.1.** Rabbits of the Himalayan breed in the usual range of environments develop black pigment at the tips of the nose, tail, feet, and ears. If raised at very high temperatures, an all-white rabbit is produced. The gene for Himalayan color pattern specifies a temperature sensitive enzyme that is inactivated at high temperature, resulting in a loss of pigmentation.

> **Example 2.2.** The flowers of hydrangea may be blue if grown in acid soil or pinkish if grown in alkaline soil, due to an interaction of gene products with the hydrogen ion concentration of their environment.

The kinds of traits that we shall encounter in the study of simple Mendelian inheritance will be considered to be relatively unaffected by the normal range of environmental conditions in which the organism is found. It is important, however, to remember that genes establish boundaries within which the environment may modify the phenotype.

2. Genotype.

All of the genes possessed by an individual constitute its **genotype.** In this chapter, we shall be concerned only with that portion of the genotype involving alleles at a single locus.

(*a*) *Homozygous.* The union of gametes carrying identical alleles produces a **homozygous** genotype. A homozygote produces only one kind of gamete.

> **Example 2.3.** Uniting gametes:

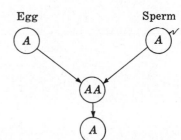

(*b*) *Pure Line.* A group of individuals with similar genetic background (breeding) is often referred to as a line or strain or variety or breed. Self-fertilization or mating closely related individuals for many generations (inbreeding) usually produces a population which is homozygous at nearly all loci. Matings between the homozygous individuals of a **pure line** produce only homozygous offspring like the parents. Thus we say that a pure line "breeds true."

> **Example 2.4.** Pure-line parents: *AA* × *AA*
>
> Gametes: Ⓐ Ⓐ
>
> Offspring: ⒶⒶ

24

(c) *Heterozygous.*   The union of gametes carrying different alleles produces a **heterozygous** genotype. Different kinds of gametes are produced by a heterozygote.

Example 2.5.

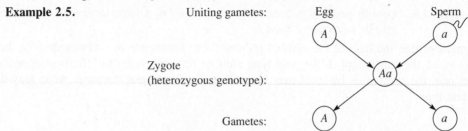

Uniting gametes: Egg   Sperm

(A)   (a)

Zygote
(heterozygous genotype):   (Aa)

Gametes: (A)   (a)

(d) *Hybrid.*   The term **hybrid** as used in the problems of this book is synonymous with the heterozygous condition. Problems in this chapter may involve a single-factor hybrid (monohybrid). Problems in the next chapter will consider heterozygosity at two or more loci (polyhybrids).

ALLELIC RELATIONSHIPS

1. Dominant and Recessive Alleles.

Whenever one of a pair of alleles can come to phenotypic expression only in a homozygous genotype, we call that allele a **recessive** factor. The allele that can phenotypically express itself in the heterozygote as well as in the homozygote is called a **dominant** factor. Upper- and lowercase letters are commonly used to designate dominant and recessive alleles, respectively. Usually the genetic symbol corresponds to the first letter in the name of the abnormal (or mutant) trait.

Example 2.6.   Lack of pigment deposition in the human body is an abnormal recessive trait called "albinism." Using *A* and *a* to represent the dominant (normal) allele and the recessive (albino) allele, respectively, 3 genotypes and 2 phenotypes are possible:

Genotypes	Phenotypes
AA (homozygous dominant)	Normal (pigment)
Aa (heterozygote)	Normal (pigment)
aa (homozygous recessive)	Albino (no pigment)

(a) *Carriers.*   Recessive alleles (such as the one for albinism) are often deleterious to those who possess them in duplicate (homozygous recessive genotype). A heterozygote may appear just as normal as the homozygous dominant genotype. A heterozygous individual who possesses a deleterious recessive allele hidden from phenotypic expression by the dominant normal allele is called a **carrier.** Most of the deleterious alleles harbored by a population are found in carrier individuals.

(b) *Wild-Type Symbolism.*   A different system for symbolizing dominant and recessive alleles is widely used in numerous organisms from higher plants and animals to the bacteria and viruses. Different genetics texts favor either one or the other system. In the author's opinion, every student should become familiar with both kinds of allelic representation and be able to work genetic problems regardless of the symbolic system used. Throughout the remainder of this book the student will find both systems used extensively. Where one phenotype is obviously of much more common occurrence in the population than its alternative phenotype, the former is usually referred to as **wild type.** The phenotype that is rarely observed is called the **mutant type.** In this system, the symbol + is used to indicate the normal allele for wild type. The base letter for the gene usually is taken from the name of the mutant or abnormal trait. If the mutant gene is recessive the symbol would be a lowercase letter(s) corresponding to the initial letter(s) in the name of the trait. Its normal (wild-type) dominant allele would have the same lowercase letter but with a + as a superscript.

Example 2.7.   Black body color in *Drosophila* is governed by a recessive gene *b*, and wild type (gray body) by its dominant allele b^+.

If the mutant trait is dominant, the base symbol would be an uppercase letter without a superscript, and its recessive wild-type allele would have the same uppercase symbol with a + as a superscript.

Example 2.8.   Lobe-shaped eyes in *Drosophila* are governed by a dominant gene *L*, and wild type (oval eye) by its recessive allele L^+.

Remember that the case of the symbol indicates the dominance or recessiveness of the *mutant* allele to which the superscript + for wild type must be referred. After the allelic relationships have been defined, the symbol + by itself may be used for wild type and the letter alone may designate the mutant type.

2. Codominant Alleles.

Alleles that lack dominant and recessive relationships may be called incompletely dominant, partially dominant, semidominant or **codominant.** This means that each allele is capable of some degree of expression when in the heterozygous condition. Hence the heterozygous genotype gives rise to a phenotype distinctly different from either of the homozygous genotypes. Usually the heterozygous phenotype resulting from codominance is intermediate in character between those produced by the homozygous genotypes; hence the erroneous concept of "blending." The phenotype may appear to be a "blend" in heterozygotes, but the alleles maintain their individual identities and will segregate from each other in the formation of gametes.

(*a*) *Symbolism for Codominant Alleles.*   For codominant alleles, all uppercase base symbols with different superscripts should be used. The uppercase letters call attention to the fact that each allele can express itself to some degree even when in the presence of its alternative allele (heterozygous).

Example 2.9.   The alleles governing the M-N blood group system in humans are codominants and may be represented by the symbols L^M and L^N, the base letter (*L*) being assigned in honor of its discoverers (Landsteiner and Levine). Two antisera (anti-M and anti-N) are used to distinguish three genotypes and their corresponding phenotypes (blood groups). Agglutination is represented by + and nonagglutination by −.

Genotype	Reaction with:		Blood Group
	Anti-M	Anti-N	(Phenotype)
$L^M L^M$	+	−	M
$L^M L^N$	+	+	MN
$L^N L^N$	−	+	N

3. Lethal Alleles.

The phenotypic manifestation of some genes is the death of the individual in either the prenatal or postnatal period prior to maturity. Such factors are called **lethal genes.** A fully dominant lethal allele (i.e., one that kills in both the homozygous and heterozygous conditions) occasionally arises by mutation from a normal allele. Individuals with a dominant lethal die before they can leave progeny. Therefore the mutant dominant lethal is removed from the population in the same generation in which it arose. Lethals that kill only when homozygous may be of two kinds: (1) one that has no obvious phenotypic effect in heterozygotes, and (2) one that exhibits a distinctive phenotype when heterozygous.

Example 2.10.   By special techniques, a completely recessive lethal (*l*) can sometimes be identified in certain families.

Genotype	Phenotype
LL, Ll	Normal viability
ll	Lethal

Example 2.11. The amount of chlorophyll in snapdragons (*Antirrhinum*) is controlled by a pair of co-dominant alleles, one of which exhibits a lethal effect when homozygous, and a distinctive color phenotype when heterozygous.

Genotype	Phenotype
C^1C^1	Green (normal)
C^1C^2	Pale green
C^2C^2	White (lethal)

4. Penetrance and Expressivity.

Differences in environmental conditions or in genetic backgrounds may cause individuals that are genetically identical at a particular locus to exhibit different phenotypes. The percentage of individuals with a particular gene combination that exhibits the corresponding character to any degree represents the **penetrance** of the trait.

Example 2.12. In some families, extra fingers and/or toes (polydactyly) in humans is thought to be produced by a dominant gene (P). The normal condition with five digits on each limb is produced by the recessive genotype (pp). Some individuals of genotype Pp are not polydactylous, and therefore the gene has a penetrance of less than 100%.

A trait, although penetrant, may be quite variable in its expression. The degree of effect produced by a penetrant genotype is termed **expressivity**.

Example 2.13. The polydactylous condition may be penetrant in the left hand (6 fingers) and not in the right (5 fingers), or it may be penetrant in the feet and not in the hands.

A recessive lethal gene that lacks complete penetrance and expressivity will kill less than 100% of the homozygotes before sexual maturity. The terms **semilethal** or **subvital** apply to such genes. The effects that various kinds of lethals have on the reproduction of the next generation form a broad spectrum from complete lethality to sterility in completely viable genotypes. Problems in this book, however, will consider only those lethals that become completely penetrant, usually during the embryonic stage. Genes other than lethals will likewise be assumed completely penetrant.

5. Multiple Alleles.

The genetic systems proposed thus far have been limited to a single pair of alleles. The maximum number of alleles at a gene locus that any individual possesses is 2, with 1 on each of the homologous chromosomes. But since a gene can be changed to alternative forms by the process of mutation, a large number of alleles is theoretically possible in a population of individuals. Whenever more than two alleles are identified at a gene locus, we have a **multiple allelic series**.

Symbolism for Multiple Alleles. The dominance hierarchy should be defined at the beginning of each problem involving multiple alleles. A capital letter is commonly used to designate the allele that is dominant to all others in the series. The corresponding lowercase letter designates the allele that is recessive to all others in the series. Other alleles, intermediate in their degree of dominance between these two extremes, are usually assigned the lowercase letter with some suitable superscript.

Example 2.14. The color of *Drosophila* eyes is governed by a series of alleles that cause the hue to vary from red or wild type (w^+ or W) through coral (w^{co}), blood (w^{bl}), eosin (w^e), cherry (w^{ch}), apricot (w^a), honey (w^h), buff (w^{bf}), tinged (w^t), pearl (w^p), and ivory (w^i) to white (w). Each allele in the system except w can be considered to produce pigment, but successively less is produced by alleles as we proceed down the hierarchy: $w^+ > w^{co} > w^{bl} > w^e > w^{ch} > w^a > w^h > w^{bf} > w^t > w^p > w^i > w$. The wild-type allele ($w^+$) is completely dominant and w is completely recessive to all other alleles in the series. *Compounds* are heterozygotes that contain unlike members of an allelic series. The compounds of this series that involve alleles other than w^+ tend to be phenotypically intermediate between the eye colors of the parental homozygotes.

Example 2.15. A classical example of multiple alleles is found in the ABO blood group system of humans, where the allele I^A for the A antigen is codominant with the allele I^B for the B antigen. Both I^A and I^B are completely dominant to the allele i, which fails to specify any detectable antigenic structure. The hierarchy of dominance relationships is symbolized as $(I^A = I^B) > i$. Two antisera (anti-A and anti-B) are required for the detection of four phenotypes.

Genotypes	Reaction with:		Phenotype
	Anti-A	Anti-B	(Blood Groups)
$I^A I^A$, $I^A i$	+	−	A
$I^B I^B$, $I^B i$	−	+	B
$I^A I^B$	+	+	AB
ii	−	−	O

Example 2.16. A slightly different kind of multiple allelic system is encountered in the coat colors of rabbits: C allows full color to be produced (typical gray rabbit); c^{ch}, when homozygous, removes yellow pigment from the fur, making a silver-gray color called chinchilla; c^{ch}, when heterozygous with alleles lower in the dominance hierarchy, produces light gray fur; c^h produces a white rabbit with black extremities called "Himalayan"; c fails to produce pigment, resulting in albino. The dominance hierarchy may be symbolized as follows: $C > c^{ch} > c^h > c$.

Phenotypes	Possible Genotypes
Full color	CC, Cc^{ch}, Cc^h, Cc
Chinchilla	$c^{ch}c^{ch}$
Light gray	$c^{ch}c^h$, $c^{ch}c$
Himalayan	$c^h c^h$, $c^h c$
Albino	cc

SINGLE-GENE (MONOFACTORIAL) CROSSES

1. The Six Basic Types of Matings.

A pair of alleles governs pelage color in the guinea pig; a dominant allele B produces black and its recessive allele b produces white. There are 6 types of matings possible among the 3 genotypes. The parental generation is symbolized P and the first filial generation of offspring is symbolized $\mathbf{F_1}$.

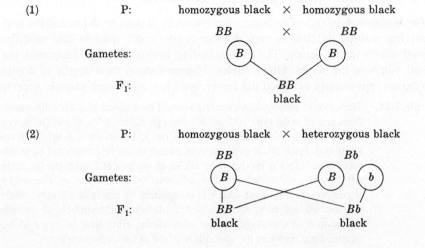

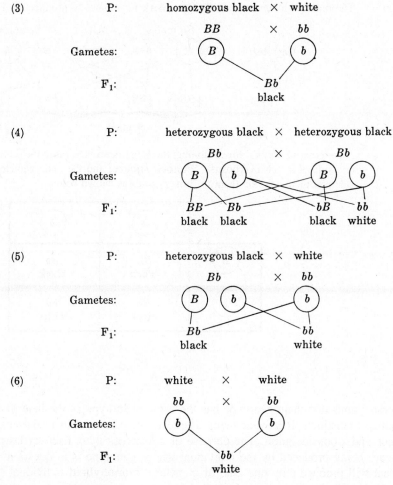

(3)   P: homozygous black × white

                              BB   ×   bb

Gametes: Ⓑ   Ⓑ

F₁: Bb
                               black

(4)   P: heterozygous black × heterozygous black

                         Bb   ×   Bb

Gametes: Ⓑ   Ⓑ   Ⓑ   Ⓑ

F₁: BB   Bb   bB   bb
                   black black   black   white

(5)   P: heterozygous black × white

                         Bb   ×   bb

Gametes: Ⓑ   Ⓑ   Ⓑ

F₁: Bb   bb
                   black   white

(6)   P: white   ×   white

                         bb   ×   bb

Gametes: Ⓑ   Ⓑ

F₁: bb
                               white

Summary of the 6 types of matings:

No.	Matings	Expected F₁ Ratios	
		Genotypes	Phenotypes
(1)	$BB \times BB$	All BB	All black
(2)	$BB \times Bb$	$\frac{1}{2}BB : \frac{1}{2}Bb$	All black
(3)	$BB \times bb$	All Bb	All black
(4)	$Bb \times Bb$	$\frac{1}{4}BB : \frac{1}{2}Bb : \frac{1}{4}bb$	$\frac{3}{4}$ black : $\frac{1}{4}$ white
(5)	$Bb \times bb$	$\frac{1}{2}Bb : \frac{1}{2}bb$	$\frac{1}{2}$ black : $\frac{1}{2}$ white
(6)	$bb \times bb$	All bb	All white

2. Conventional Production of the F₂.

Unless otherwise specified in the problem, the second filial generation (F_2) is produced by crossing the F_1 individuals among themselves randomly. If plants are normally self-fertilized, they can be artificially cross-pollinated in the parental generation and the resulting F_1 progeny may then be allowed to pollinate themselves to produce the F_2.

Example 2.17.   P: BB × bb
                                                     black   white

                                   F₁: Bb
                                                     black

The black F_1 males are mated to the black F_1 females to produce the F_2.

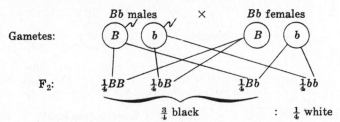

An alternative method for combining the F_1 gametes is to place the female gametes along one side of a "checkerboard" (**Punnett square**) and the male gametes along the other side and then combine them to form zygotes as shown below.

	B	b
B	BB black	Bb black
b	Bb black	bb white

3. Testcross.

Because a homozygous dominant genotype has the same phenotype as the heterozygous genotype, a **testcross** is required to distinguish between them. The testcross parent is always homozygous recessive for all of the genes under consideration. The purpose of a testcross is to discover how many different kinds of gametes are being produced by the individual whose genotype is in question. A homozygous dominant individual will produce only one kind of gamete; a **monohybrid** individual (heterozygous at one locus) produces two kinds of gametes with equal frequency.

Example 2.18.   Consider the case in which testcrossing a black female produced only black offspring.

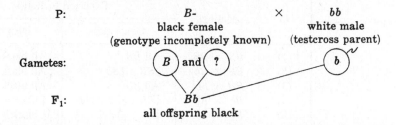

Conclusion: The female parent must be producing only one kind of gamete and therefore she is homozygous dominant BB.

Example 2.19.   Consider the case in which testcrossing a black male produced black and white offspring in approximately equal numbers.

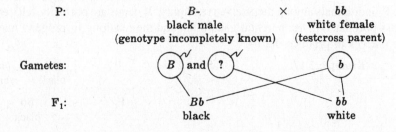

Conclusion: The male parent must be producing 2 kinds of gametes and therefore he is heterozygous *Bb*.

4. Backcross.

If the F_1 progeny are mated back to one of their parents (or to individuals with a genotype identical to that of their parents) the mating is termed **backcross**. Sometimes "backcross" is used synonymously with "testcross" in genetic literature, but it will not be so used in this book.

> **Example 2.20.** A homozygous black female guinea pig is crossed to a white male. An F_1 son is backcrossed to his mother. Using the symbol ♀ for female and ♂ for male (♀♀ = females, ♂♂ = males), we diagram this backcross as follows:
>
> | P: | *BB*♀ | × | *bb*♂ |
> |---|---|---|---|
> | | black female | | white male |
>
> | F_1: | *Bb* ♂♂ and ♀♀ |
> |---|---|
> | | black males and females |
>
> | F_1 backcross: | *Bb* ♂ | × | *BB*♀ |
> |---|---|---|---|
> | | black son | | black mother |
>
> Backcross progeny: $\left.\begin{array}{l}\frac{1}{2}BB \\ \frac{1}{2}Bb\end{array}\right\}$ all-black offspring

PEDIGREE ANALYSIS

A pedigree is a systematic listing (either as words or as symbols) of the ancestors of a given individual, or it may be the "family tree" for a large number of individuals. It is customary to represent females as circles and males as squares. Matings are shown as horizontal lines between two individuals. The offspring of a mating are connected by a vertical line to the mating line. Different shades or colors added to the symbols can represent various phenotypes. Each generation is listed on a separate row labeled with Roman numerals. Individuals within a generation receive Arabic numerals.

> **Example 2.21.** Let solid symbols represent black guinea pigs and open symbols represent white guinea pigs.

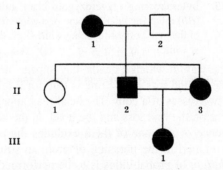

Individuals	Phenotype	Genotype
I1	Black ♀	*Bb*
I2	White ♂	*bb*
III1	White ♀	*bb*
II2	Black ♂	*Bb*
II3	Black ♀	*Bb*
III1	Black ♀	*B-**

* The dash indicates that the genotype could be either homozygous or heterozygous.

PROBABILITY THEORY

1. Observed vs. Expected Results.

Experimental results seldom conform exactly to the expected ratios. Genetic probabilities derive from the operation of chance events in the meiotic production of gametes and the random union of these gametes in fertilization. Samples from a population of individuals often deviate from the expected ratios, rather widely in very small samples, but usually approaching the expectations more closely with increasing sample size.

Example 2.22. Suppose that a testcross of heterozygous black guinea pigs ($Bb \times bb$) produces 5 offspring: 3 black (Bb) and 2 white (bb). Theoretically we expect half of the total number of offspring to be black and half to be white $= \frac{1}{2}(5) = 2\frac{1}{2}$. Obviously we cannot observe half of an individual, and the results conform as closely to the theoretical expectations as is biologically possible.

Example 2.23. Numerous testcrosses of a black guinea pig produced a total of 10 offspring, 8 of which were black and 2 were white. We theoretically expected 5 black and 5 white, but the deviation from the expected numbers which we observed in our small sample of 10 offspring should not be any more surprising than the results of tossing a coin 10 times and observing 8 heads and 2 tails. The fact that at least one white offspring appeared is sufficient to classify the black parent as genetically heterozygous (Bb).

2. Combining Probabilities.

Two or more events are said to be **independent** if the occurrence or nonoccurrence of any one of them does not affect the probabilities of occurrence of any of the others. When 2 independent events occur with the probabilities p and q, respectively, then the probability of their joint occurrence is pq. That is, the combined probability is the product of the probabilities of the independent events. If the word "and" is used or implied in the phrasing of a problem solution, a *multiplication* of independent probabilities is usually required.

Example 2.24. Theoretically there is an equal opportunity for a tossed coin to land on either heads or tails. Let p = probability of heads $= \frac{1}{2}$, and q = probability of tails $= \frac{1}{2}$. In 2 tosses of a coin the probability of 2 heads appearing (i.e., a head on the first toss *and* a head on the second toss) is $p \times p = p^2 = (\frac{1}{2})^2 = \frac{1}{4}$.

Example 2.25. In testcrossing a heterozygous black guinea pig ($Bb \times bb$), let the probability of a black (Bb) offspring be $p = \frac{1}{2}$ and of a white (bb) offspring be $q = \frac{1}{2}$. The combined probability of the first 2 offspring being white (i.e., the first offspring is white *and* the second offspring is white) $= q \times q = q^2 = (\frac{1}{2})^2 = \frac{1}{4}$.

There is only one way in which 2 heads may appear in two tosses of a coin, i.e., heads on the first toss and heads on the second toss. The same is true for 2 tails. There are two ways, however, to obtain 1 head and 1 tail in two tosses of a coin. The head may appear on the first toss and the tail on the second *or* the tail may appear on the first toss and the head on the second. **Mutually exclusive events** are those in which the occurrence of any one of them excludes the occurrence of the others. The word "or" is usually required or implied in the phrasing of problem solutions involving mutually exclusive events, signaling that an *addition* of probabilities is to be performed. That is, whenever alternative possibilities exist for the satisfaction of the conditions of a problem, the individual probabilities are combined by addition.

Example 2.26. In two tosses of a coin, there are two ways to obtain a head and tail.

	First Toss		**Second Toss**		**Probability**
First alternative:	Head (p)	(and)	Tail (q)	=	pq
					(or)
Second alternative:	Tail (q)	(and)	Head (p)	=	qp
			Combined probability	=	$2pq$

$p = q = \frac{1}{2}$; hence the combined probability $= 2(\frac{1}{2})(\frac{1}{2}) = \frac{1}{2}$.

Example 2.27. In testcrossing heterozygous black guinea pigs ($Bb \times bb$), there are two ways to obtain 1 black (Bb) and 1 white (bb) offspring in a litter of 2 animals. Let p = probability of black = $\frac{1}{2}$ and q = probability of white = $\frac{1}{2}$.

	First Offspring		**Second Offspring**		**Probability**
First alternative:	Black (p)	(and)	White (q)	=	pq
					(or)
Second alternative:	White (q)	(and)	Black (p)	=	qp
			Combined probability	=	$2pq$

$p = q = \frac{1}{2}$; hence the combined probability = $2(\frac{1}{2})(\frac{1}{2}) = \frac{1}{2}$.

Many readers will recognize that the application of the above two rules for combining probabilities (independent and mutually exclusive events) is the basis of the binomial distribution, which will be considered in detail in Chapter 7.

Solved Problems

DOMINANT AND RECESSIVE ALLELES

2.1. Black pelage of guinea pigs is a dominant trait; white is the alternative recessive trait. When a pure black guinea pig is crossed to a white one, what fraction of the black F_2 is expected to be heterozygous?

Solution:

As shown in Example 2.17, the F_2 genotypic ratio is $1BB : 2Bb : 1bb$. Considering only the black F_2, we expect $1BB : 2Bb$ or 2 out of every 3 black pigs are expected to be heterozygous; the fraction is $\frac{2}{3}$.

2.2. If a black female guinea pig is testcrossed and produces 2 offspring in each of 3 litters, all of which are black, what is her probable genotype? With what degree of confidence may her genotype be specified?

Solution:

$$\text{P:} \qquad \underset{\text{black female}}{B\text{-}} \qquad \times \qquad \underset{\text{white male}}{bb}$$

$$\text{F}_1\text{:} \qquad \qquad \text{all } Bb = \text{all black}$$

The female parent could be homozygous BB or heterozygous Bb and still be phenotypically black; hence the symbol B-. If she is heterozygous, each offspring from this testcross has a 50% chance of being black. The probability of 6 offspring being produced, all of which are black, is $(\frac{1}{2})^6 = \frac{1}{64} = 0.0156 = 1.56\%$. In other words, we expect such results to occur by chance less than 2% of the time. Since it is chance that operates in the union of gametes, she might actually be heterozygous and thus far only her B gametes have been the "lucky ones" to unite with the b gametes from the white parent. Since no white offspring have appeared in six of these chance unions we may be approximately 98% confident $(1 - 0.0156 = 0.9844$ or 98.44%) on the basis of chance, that she is of homozygous genotype (BB). It is possible, however, for her very next testcross offspring to be white, in which case we would then become certain that her genotype was heterozygous Bb and not BB.

2.3. Heterozygous black guinea pigs (Bb) are crossed among themselves. (a) What is the probability of the first three offspring being alternately black-white-black or white-black-white? (b) What is the probability among 3 offspring of producing 2 black and 1 white in any order?

Solution:

(a)   P: Bb × Bb
                                           black   black

                   F_1: $\frac{3}{4}$ black : $\frac{1}{4}$ white

                   Let p = probability of black = $\frac{3}{4}$, q = probability of white = $\frac{1}{4}$.

                   Probability of black *and* white *and* black = $p \times q \times p = p^2q$,   *or*
                   Probability of white *and* black *and* white = $q \times p \times q = \underline{pq^2}$
                                                   Combined probability = $p^2q + pq^2 = \frac{3}{16}$

(b)   Consider the number of ways that 2 black and 1 white offspring could be produced.

Offspring Order			Probability
1st	2nd	3rd	
Black *and* Black *and* White		= $(\frac{3}{4})(\frac{3}{4})(\frac{1}{4})$	= $\frac{9}{64}$, *or*
Black *and* White *and* Black		= $(\frac{3}{4})(\frac{1}{4})(\frac{3}{4})$	= $\frac{9}{64}$, *or*
White *and* Black *and* Black		= $(\frac{1}{4})(\frac{3}{4})(\frac{3}{4})$	= $\frac{9}{64}$,
		Combined probability	= $\frac{27}{64}$

Once we have ascertained that there are three ways to obtain 2 black and 1 white, the total probability becomes $3(\frac{3}{4})^2(\frac{1}{4}) = \frac{27}{64}$.

2.4.   A dominant gene b^+ is responsible for the wild-type body color of *Drosophila;* its recessive allele b produces black body color. A testcross of a wild-type female gave 52 black and 58 wild type in the F_1. If the wild-type F_1 females are crossed to their black F_1 brothers, what genotypic and phenotypic ratios would be expected in the F_2? Diagram the results using the appropriate genetic symbols.

Solution:

                 P: b^+-♀   × bb♂
                              wild-type female   black male

             F_1: $52bb$ (black) : $58b^+b$ (wild type)

Since the recessive black phenotype appears in the F_1 in approximately a 1 : 1 ratio, we know that the female parent must be heterozygous b^+b. Furthermore, we know that the wild-type F_1 progeny must also be heterozygous. The wild-type F_1 females are then crossed with their black brothers:

        F_1 cross: b^+b♀♀   × bb♂♂
                              wild-type females   black males

        F_2: $\frac{1}{2}b^+b$ wild type : $\frac{1}{2}bb$ black

The expected F_2 ratio is therefore the same as that observed in the F_1, namely, 1 wild type : 1 black.

CODOMINANT ALLELES

2.5.   Coat colors of the Shorthorn breed of cattle represent a classical example of codominant alleles. Red is governed by the genotype C^RC^R, roan (mixture of red and white) by C^RC^W, and white by C^WC^W. (a) When roan Shorthorns are crossed among themselves, what genotypic and phenotypic ratios are expected among their progeny? (b) If red Shorthorns are crossed with roans, and the F_1 progeny are crossed among themselves to produce the F_2, what percentage of the F_2 will probably be roan?

Solution:

(a)

$$P: \quad C^R C^W \times C^R C^W$$
$$\text{roan} \qquad \text{roan}$$

$$F_1: \quad \tfrac{1}{4}C^R C^R \text{ red} : \tfrac{1}{2}C^R C^W \text{ roan} : \tfrac{1}{4}C^W C^W \text{ white}$$

Since each genotype produces a unique phenotype, the phenotypic ratio $1:2:1$ corresponds to the same genotypic ratio.

(b)

$$P: \quad C^R C^R \times C^R C^W$$
$$\text{red} \qquad \text{roan}$$

$$F_1: \quad \tfrac{1}{2}C^R C^R \text{ red} : \tfrac{1}{2}C^R C^W \text{ roan}$$

There are three types of matings possible for the production of the F_2. Their relative frequencies of occurrence may be calculated by preparing a mating table.

	$\tfrac{1}{2}C^R C^R \male$	$\tfrac{1}{2}C^R C^W \male$
$\tfrac{1}{2}C^R C^R \female$	(1) $\tfrac{1}{4}C^R C^R \female \times C^R C^R \male$	(2) $\tfrac{1}{4}C^R C^R \female \times C^R C^W \male$
$\tfrac{1}{2}C^R C^W \female$	(2) $\tfrac{1}{4}C^R C^W \female \times C^R C^R \male$	(3) $\tfrac{1}{4}C^R C^W \female \times C^R C^W \male$

(1) The mating $C^R C^R \female \times C^R C^R \male$ (red $\times$ red) produces only red ($C^R C^R$) progeny. But only one-quarter of all matings are of this type. Therefore $\tfrac{1}{4}$ of all the F_2 should be red from this source.

(2) The matings $C^R C^W \times C^R C^R$ (roan female $\times$ red male or roan male $\times$ red female) are expected to produce $\tfrac{1}{2}C^R C^R$ (red) and $\tfrac{1}{2}C^R C^W$ (roan) progeny. half of all matings are of this kind. Therefore $(\tfrac{1}{2})(\tfrac{1}{2}) = \tfrac{1}{4}$ of all the F_2 progeny should be red and $\tfrac{1}{4}$ should be roan from this source.

(3) The mating $C^R C^W \female \times C^R C^W \male$ (roan $\times$ roan) is expected to produce $\tfrac{1}{4}C^R C^R$ (red), $\tfrac{1}{2}C^R C^W$ (roan), and $\tfrac{1}{4}C^W C^W$ (white) progeny. This mating type constitutes $\tfrac{1}{4}$ of all crosses. Therefore the fraction of all F_2 progeny contributed from this source is $(\tfrac{1}{4})(\tfrac{1}{4}) = \tfrac{1}{16}C^R C^R$, $(\tfrac{1}{4})(\tfrac{1}{2}) = \tfrac{1}{8}C^R C^W$, $(\tfrac{1}{4})(\tfrac{1}{4}) = \tfrac{1}{16}C^W C^W$.

The expected F_2 contributions from all three types of matings are summarized in the following table.

Type of Mating	Frequency of Mating	F₂ Progeny		
		Red	Roan	White
(1) Red × red	$\tfrac{1}{4}$	$\tfrac{1}{4}$	0	0
(2) Red × roan	$\tfrac{1}{2}$	$\tfrac{1}{4}$	$\tfrac{1}{4}$	0
(3) Roan × roan	$\tfrac{1}{4}$	$\tfrac{1}{16}$	$\tfrac{1}{8}$	$\tfrac{1}{16}$
Totals		$\tfrac{9}{16}$	$\tfrac{6}{16}$	$\tfrac{1}{16}$

The fraction of roan progeny in the F_2 is $\tfrac{3}{8}$, or approximately 38%.

LETHAL ALLELES

2.6. The absence of legs in cattle ("amputated") has been attributed to a completely recessive lethal gene. A normal bull is mated with a normal cow and they produce an amputated calf (usually dead at birth). The same parents are mated again.

(a) What is the chance of the next calf being amputated?
(b) What is the chance of these parents having 2 calves, both of which are amputated?

(c) Bulls carrying the amputated allele (heterozygous) are mated to noncarrier cows. The F_1 is allowed to mate at random to produce the F_2. What genotypic ratio is expected in the adult F_2?

(d) Suppose that each F_1 female in part (c) rears one viable calf, i.e., each of the cows that throws an amputated calf is allowed to remate to a carrier sire until she produces a viable offspring. What genotypic ratio is expected in the adult F_2?

Solution:

(a) If phenotypically normal parents produce an amputated calf, they must both be genetically heterozygous.

$$\text{P:} \qquad \underset{\text{normal}}{Aa} \quad \times \quad \underset{\text{normal}}{Aa}$$

F_1:   **Genotypes**   **Phenotypes**

$$\left.\begin{array}{l} \tfrac{1}{4}AA \\ \tfrac{1}{2}Aa \end{array}\right\} \quad \tfrac{3}{4}\ \text{normal}$$

$$\tfrac{1}{4}aa \quad = \tfrac{1}{4}\ \text{amputated (dies)}$$

Thus there is a 25% chance of the next offspring being amputated.

(b) The chance of the first calf being amputated *and* the second calf also being amputated is the product of the separate probabilities: $(\tfrac{1}{4})(\tfrac{1}{4}) = \tfrac{1}{16}$.

(c) The solution to part (c) is analogous to that of Problem 2.5(b). A summary of the expected F_2 follows:

Type of Mating	F_2 Genotypes		
	AA	Aa	aa
$AA \times AA$	$\frac{4}{16}$		
$AA \times Aa$	$\frac{4}{16}$	$\frac{4}{16}$	
$Aa \times Aa$	$\frac{1}{16}$	$\frac{2}{16}$	$\frac{1}{16}$
Totals	$\frac{9}{16}$	$\frac{6}{16}$	$\frac{1}{16}$

All aa genotypes die and fail to appear in the adult progeny. Therefore the adult progeny has the genotypic ratio $9AA : 6Aa$ or $3AA : 2Aa$.

(d) The results of matings $AA \times AA$ and $AA \times Aa$ remain the same as in part (c). The mating of Aa by Aa now is expected to produce $\tfrac{1}{3}AA$ and $\tfrac{2}{3}Aa$ adult progeny. Correcting for the frequency of occurrence of this mating, we have $(\tfrac{1}{4})(\tfrac{1}{3}) = \tfrac{1}{12}AA$ and $(\tfrac{1}{4})(\tfrac{2}{3}) = \tfrac{2}{12}Aa$.

Summary of the F_2:

Type of Mating	F_2 Genotypes	
	AA	Aa
$AA \times AA$	$\frac{3}{12}$	
$AA \times Aa$	$\frac{3}{12}$	$\frac{3}{12}$
$Aa \times Aa$	$\frac{1}{12}$	$\frac{2}{12}$
Totals	$\frac{7}{12}$	$\frac{5}{12}$

The adult F_2 genotypic ratio is expected to be $7AA$ to $5Aa$.

2.7. A bull, heterozygous for a completely recessive lethal gene, sires 3 calves each out of 32 cows. Twelve of the cows have one or more stillborn calves and therefore must be carriers of this lethal gene. How many more carrier cows probably exist in this herd undetected?

Solution:

The probability that a heterozygous cow will not have a stillborn calf in 3 matings to a heterozygous male is calculated as follows: each calf has a $\frac{3}{4}$ chance of being normal; therefore the probability of 3 calves being normal is $(\frac{3}{4})^3 = \frac{27}{64}$. That is, the probability that we will fail to detect a heterozygous (carrier) cow with 3 calves is $\frac{27}{64}$. The probability that we will detect a carrier cow with 3 calves is $\frac{37}{64}$. Let $x = $ number of heterozygous cows in the herd; then $(\frac{37}{64})x = 12$ or $x = 21$ (to the nearest integer). Probably 21 carrier cows exist; since we have detected 12 of them, there are probably 9 carrier cows undetected in this herd.

MULTIPLE ALLELES

2.8. The genetics of rabbit coat colors is given in Example 2.16. Determine the genotypic and phenotypic ratios expected from mating full-colored males of genotype Cc^{ch} to light-gray females of genotype $c^{ch}c$.

Solution:

P: $Cc^{ch} \male\male$ × $c^{ch}c\female\female$
            full color   light gray

F₁:

	C	c^{ch}
c^{ch}	Cc^{ch} full color	$c^{ch}c^{ch}$ chinchilla
c	Cc full color	$c^{ch}c$ light gray

Thus we have a $1:1:1:1$ genotypic ratio, but a phenotypic ratio of 2 full color : 1 chinchilla : 1 light gray.

2.9. The coat colors of mice are known to be governed by a multiple allelic series in which the allele A^y, when homozygous, is lethal early in embryonic development but produces yellow color when in heterozygous condition with other alleles. Agouti (mousy color) is governed by the A allele, and black by the recessive a. The dominance hierarchy is as follows: $A^y > A > a$. What phenotypic and genotypic ratios are expected in the viable F₁ from the cross $A^yA \times A^ya$?

Solution:

P: A^yA × A^ya
            yellow   yellow

F₁:

	A^y	a
A^y	A^yA^y dies	A^ya yellow
A	A^yA yellow	Aa agouti

Since $\frac{1}{4}$ of the progeny dies before birth, we should observe 2 yellow offspring for every 1 agouti (phenotypic ratio of $2:1$). However, the genotypic ratio is a $1:1:1$ relationship. That is, $\frac{1}{3}$ of the viable genotypes should be A^yA, $\frac{1}{3}A^ya$, and $\frac{1}{3}Aa$.

2.10. A man is suing his wife for divorce on the grounds of infidelity. Their first child and second child, whom they both claim, are blood groups O and AB, respectively. The third child, whom the man disclaims, is blood type B. (*a*) Can this information be used to support the man's case? (*b*) Another test was made in the M-N blood group system. The third child was group M, the man was group N. Can this information be used to support the man's case?

Solution:

(*a*) The genetics of the ABO blood group system was presented in Example 2.15. Because the group O baby has the genotype *ii*, each of the parents must have been carrying the recessive allele. The AB baby indicates that one of his parents had the dominant I^A allele and the other had the codominant allele I^B. Any of the four blood groups can appear among the children whose parents are $I^A i \times I^B i$. The information given on ABO blood groups is of no use in supporting the man's claim.

(*b*) The genetics of the M-N blood group system was presented in Example 2.9. The M-N blood groups are governed by a pair of codominant alleles, where groups M and N are produced by homozygous genotypes. A group N father must pass the L^N allele to his offspring; they all would have the N antigen on their red blood cells, and would all be classified serologically as either group MN or N depending upon the genotype of the mother. This man could not be the father of a group M child.

PEDIGREE ANALYSIS

2.11. The black hair of guinea pigs is produced by a dominant gene *B* and white by its recessive allele *b*. Unless there is evidence to the contrary, assume that II1 and II4 do not carry the recessive allele. Calculate the probability that an offspring of III1 × III2 will have white hair.

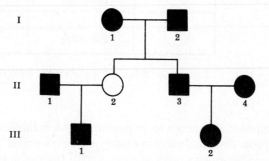

Solution:

Both I1 and I2 must be heterozygous (*Bb*) in order to have the white (*bb*) offspring II2. If III1 or III2 had been white, this would constitute evidence that II1 or II4 were heterozygous. In the absence of this evidence the problem tells us to assume that II1 and II4 are homozygous (*BB*). If the offspring of III1 × III2 is to be white, then both III1 and III2 would have to be heterozygous (*Bb*). In this case, II3 would also have to be heterozygous in order to pass the recessive allele on to III2. Under the conditions of the problem, we are certain that III1 is heterozygous because his parents (II1 × II2) are *BB* × *bb*. We notice that II3 is black. The probability that *black* progeny from I1 × I2 are heterozygous is $\frac{2}{3}$. If II3 is heterozygous, the probability that III2 is heterozygous is $\frac{1}{2}$. If III2 is heterozygous, there is a 25% chance that the offspring of III1 × III2 will be white (*bb*). Thus the combined probability that II3 is heterozygous *and* III2 is heterozygous *and* producing a white offspring is the product of the independent probabilities = $(\frac{2}{3})(\frac{1}{2})(\frac{1}{4}) = \frac{2}{24} = \frac{1}{12}$.

Supplementary Problems

DOMINANT AND RECESSIVE ALLELES

2.12. Several black guinea pigs of the same genotype were mated and produced 29 black and 9 white offspring. What would you predict the genotypes of the parents to be?

2.13. If a black female guinea pig is testcrossed and produces at least one white offspring, determine (*a*) the genotype and phenotype of the sire (male parent) that produced the white offspring, (*b*) the genotype of this female.

2.14. Heterozygous black (*Bb*) guinea pigs are mated to homozygous recessive (*bb*) whites. Predict the genotypic and phenotypic ratios expected from backcrossing the black F_1 progeny to (*a*) the black parent, (*b*) the white parent.

2.15. In *Drosophila*, sepia-colored eyes are due to a recessive allele *s* and wild type (red eye color) to its dominant allele s^+. If sepia-eyed females are crossed to pure wild-type males, what phenotypic and genotypic ratios are expected if the F_2 males are backcrossed to the sepia-eyed parental females?

2.16. The lack of pigmentation, called albinism, in humans is the result of a recessive allele (*a*) and normal pigmentation is the result of its dominant allele (*A*). Two normal parents have an albino child. Determine the probability that (*a*) the next child is albino, (*b*) the next 2 children are albinos. (*c*) What is the chance of these parents producing 2 children, 1 albino and the other normal?

2.17. Short hair is due to a dominant gene *L* in rabbits, and long hair to its recessive allele *l*. A cross between a short-haired female and a long-haired male produced a litter of 1 long-haired and 7 short-haired bunnies. (*a*) What are the genotypes of the parents? (*b*) What phenotypic ratio was expected in the offspring generation? (*c*) How many of the 8 bunnies were expected to be long-haired?

2.18. A dominant gene *W* produces wire-haired texture in dogs; its recessive allele *w* produces smooth hair. A group of heterozygous wire-haired individuals are crossed and their F_1 progeny are then testcrossed. Determine the expected genotypic and phenotypic ratios among the testcross progeny.

2.19. Black wool of sheep is due to a recessive allele *b* and white wool to its dominant allele *B*. A white buck (male) is crossed to a white ewe (female), both animals carrying the allele for black. They produce a white buck lamb that is then backcrossed to the female parent. What is the probability of the backcross offspring being black?

2.20. In foxes, silver-black coat color is governed by a recessive allele *b* and red color by its dominant allele *B*. Determine the genotypic and phenotypic ratios expected from the following matings: (*a*) pure red × carrier red, (*b*) carrier red × silver-black, (*c*) pure red × silver-black.

2.21. In the Holstein-Friesian breed of dairy cattle, a recessive allele *r* is known to produce red and white; the dominant allele *R* is known to produce black and white. If a carrier bull is mated to carrier cows, determine the probability (*a*) of the first offspring being born red and white, (*b*) of the first 4 offspring born being black and white. (*c*) What is the expected phenotypic ratio among offspring resulting from backcrossing black and white F_1 cows to the carrier bull? (*d*) If the carrier bull was mated to homozygous black and white cows, what phenotypic ratio would be expected among the backcross progeny from F_1 cows × carrier bull?

2.22. Consider a cross between two heterozygous black guinea pigs (*Bb*). (*a*) In how many ways can 3 black and 2 white offspring be produced? (*b*) What is the probability from such a cross of 3 black and 2 white offspring appearing in any order?

CODOMINANT ALLELES

2.23. When chickens with splashed white feathers are crossed with black-feathered birds, their offspring are all slate blue (Blue Andalusian). When Blue Andalusians are crossed among themselves, they produce splashed white, blue, and black offspring in the ratio of 1 : 2 : 1, respectively. (*a*) How are these feather traits inherited? (*b*) Using any appropriate symbols, indicate the genotypes for each phenotype.

2.24. Yellow coat color in guinea pigs is produced by the homozygous genotype $C^Y C^Y$, cream color by the heterozygous genotype $C^Y C^W$, and white by the homozygous genotype $C^W C^W$. What genotypic and phenotypic ratios are matings between cream-colored individuals likely to produce?

2.25. The shape of radishes may be long ($S^L S^L$), round ($S^R S^R$), or oval ($S^L S^R$). If long radishes are crossed to oval radishes and the F_1 then allowed to cross at random among themselves, what phenotypic ratio is expected in the F_2?

2.26. The Palomino horse is a hybrid exhibiting a golden color with lighter mane and tail. A pair of codominant alleles (D^1 and D^2) is known to be involved in the inheritance of these coat colors. Genotypes homozygous for the D^1 allele are chestnut-colored (reddish), heterozygous genotypes are Palomino-colored, and genotypes homozygous for the D^2 allele are almost white and called *cremello*. (*a*) From matings between Palominos, determine the expected Palomino : non-Palomino ratio among the offspring. (*b*) What percentage of the non-Palomino offspring in part (*a*) will breed true? (*c*) What kind of mating will produce only Palominos?

LETHAL ALLELES

2.27. Chickens with shortened wings and legs are called "creepers." When creepers are mated to normal birds they produce creepers and normals with equal frequency. When creepers are mated to creepers they produce 2 creepers to 1 normal. Crosses between normal birds produce only normal progeny. How can these results be explained?

2.28. In the Mexican Hairless breed of dogs, the hairless condition is produced by the heterozygous genotype (*Hh*). Normal dogs are homozygous recessive (*hh*). Puppies homozygous for the *H* allele are usually born dead with abnormalities of the mouth and absence of external ears. If the average litter size at weaning is 6 in matings between hairless dogs, what would be the average expected *number* of hairless and normal offspring at weaning from matings between hairless and normal dogs?

2.29. A pair of codominant alleles is known to govern cotyledon leaf color in soybeans. The homozygous genotype $C^G C^G$ produces dark green, the heterozygous genotype $C^G C^Y$ produces light green, and the other homozygous genotype $C^Y C^Y$ produces yellow leaves so deficient in chloroplasts that seedlings do not grow to maturity. If dark-green plants are pollinated only by light-green plants and the F_1 crosses are made at random to produce an F_2, what phenotypic and genotypic ratios would be expected in the mature F_2 plants?

2.30. Thalassemia is a hereditary disease of the blood of humans resulting in anemia. Severe anemia (thalassemia major) is found in homozygotes ($T^M T^M$) and a milder form of anemia (thalassemia minor) is found in heterozygotes ($T^M T^N$). Normal individuals are homozygous $T^N T^N$. If all individuals with thalassemia major die before sexual maturity, (*a*) what proportion of the adult F_1 from marriages of thalassemia minors by normals would be expected to be normal, (*b*) what fraction of the adult F_1 from marriages of minors by minors would be expected to be anemic?

2.31. The Pelger anomaly of rabbits involves abnormal white blood cell nuclear segmentation. Pelgers are heterozygous (*Pp*), normal individuals are homozygous (*PP*). The homozygous recessive genotypes (*pp*) have grossly deformed skeletons and usually die before or soon after birth. If Pelgers are mated together, what phenotypic ratio is expected in the adult F_2?

MULTIPLE ALLELES

2.32. A multiple allelic series is known in the Chinese primrose where A (Alexandria type = white eye) $> a^n$ (normal type = yellow eye) $> a$ (Primrose Queen type = large yellow eye). List all of the genotypes possible for each of the phenotypes in this series.

2.33. Plumage color in mallard ducks is dependent upon a set of 3 alleles: M^R for restricted mallard pattern, M for mallard, and m for dusky mallard. The dominance hierarchy is $M^R > M > m$. Determine the genotypic and phenotypic ratios expected in the F_1 from the following crosses: (*a*) $M^R M^R \times M^R M^R$, (*b*) $M^R M^R \times M^R m$, (*c*) $M^R M \times M^R m$, (*d*) $M^R m \times Mm$, (*e*) $Mm \times mm$.

2.34. A number of self-incompatibility alleles is known in clover such that the growth of a pollen tube down the style of a diploid plant is inhibited when the latter contains the same self-incompatibility allele as that in the pollen tube. Given a series of self-incompatibility alleles S^1, S^2, S^3, S^4, what genotypic ratios would be expected in embryos and in endosperms of seeds from the following crosses?

	Seed Parent	Pollen Parent
(a)	S^1S^4	S^3S^4
(b)	S^1S^2	S^1S^2
(c)	S^1S^3	S^2S^4
(d)	S^2S^3	S^3S^4

2.35. The coat colors of many animals exhibit the "agouti" pattern, which is characterized by a yellow band of pigment near the tip of the hair. In rabbits, a multiple allelic series is known where the genotypes E^DE^D and E^De produce only black (nonagouti), but the heterozygous genotype E^DE produces black with a trace of agouti. The genotypes EE or Ee produce full color, and the recessive genotype ee produces reddish-yellow. What phenotypic and genotypic ratios would be expected in the F_1 and F_2 from the cross (a) $E^DE^D \times Ee$, (b) $E^De \times ee$?

2.36. The inheritance of coat colors of cattle involves a multiple allelic series with a dominance hierarchy as follows: $S > s^h > s^c > s$. The S allele puts a band of white color around the middle of the animal and is referred to as a Dutch belt; the s^h allele produces Hereford-type spotting; solid color is a result of the s^c allele; and Holstein-type spotting is due to the s allele. Homozygous Dutch-belted males are crossed to Holstein-type spotted females. The F_1 females are crossed to a Hereford-type spotted male of genotype s^hs^c. Predict the genotypic and phenotypic frequencies in the progeny.

2.37. The genetics of the ABO human blood groups was presented in Example 2.15. A man of blood group B is being sued by a woman of blood group A for paternity. The woman's child is blood group O. (a) Is this man the father of this child? Explain. (b) If this man actually is the father of this child, specify the genotypes of both parents. (c) If it was impossible for this group B man to be the father of a type O child, regardless of the mother's genotype, specify his genotype. (d) If a man was blood group AB, could he be the father of a group O child?

2.38. A multiple allelic series is known to govern the intensity of pigmentation in the mouse such that D = full color, d = dilute color, and d^l is lethal when homozygous. The dominance order is $D > d > d^l$. A full-colored mouse carrying the lethal is mated to a dilute-colored mouse also carrying the lethal. The F_1 is backcrossed to the dilute parent. (a) What phenotypic ratio is expected in the viable backcross progeny? (b) What percentage of the full-colored backcross progeny carry the lethal? (c) What fraction of the dilute-colored progeny carry the lethal?

PEDIGREE ANALYSIS

2.39. The phenotypic expression of a dominant gene in Ayrshire cattle is a notch in the tips of the ears. In the pedigree below, where solid symbols represent notched individuals, determine the probability of notched progeny being produced from the matings (a) III1 × III3, (b) III2 × III3, (c) III3 × III4, (d) III1 × III5, (e) III2 × III5.

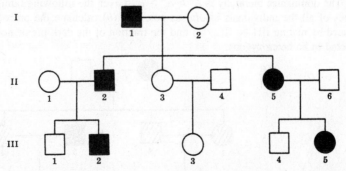

2.40. A single recessive gene r is largely responsible for the development of red hair in humans. Dark hair is largely due to its dominant allele R. In the family pedigree shown below, unless there is evidence to the contrary, assume that individuals who marry into this family do not carry the r allele. Calculate the probability of red hair appearing in children from the marriages (a) III3 × III9, (b) III4 × III10, (c) IV1 × IV2, (d) IV1 × IV3. Solid symbols represent red hair; open symbols represent dark hair.

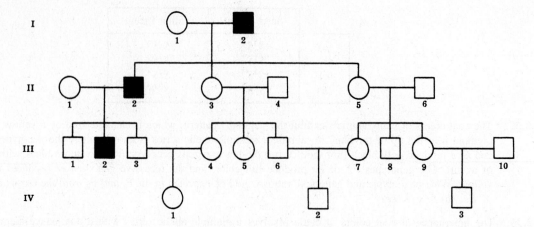

2.41. The gene for spotted coat color in rabbits (S) is dominant to its allele for solid color (s). In the following pedigree assume that those individuals brought into the family from outside do not carry the gene for solid color, unless there is evidence to the contrary. Calculate the probability of solid-colored bunnies being produced from the matings (*a*) III1 × III9, (*b*) III1 × III5, (*c*) III3 × III5, (*d*) IV4 × III6, (*e*) III6 × III9, (*f*) IV1 × IV2, (*g*) III9 × IV2, (*h*) III5 × IV2, (*i*) III6 × IV1. Solid symbols represent solid-colored animals, open symbols represent spotted animals.

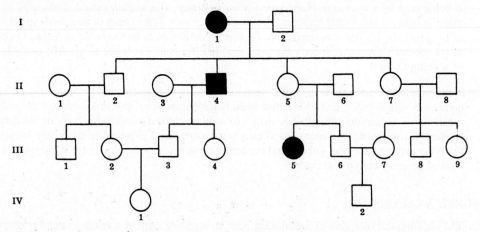

2.42. A multiple allelic series in dogs governs the distribution of coat-color pigments. The allele A^s produces an even distribution of dark pigment over the body; the allele a^y reduces the intensity of pigmentation and produces sable or tan-colored dogs; the allele a^t produces spotted patterns such as tan and black, tan and brown, etc. The dominance hierarchy is $A^s > a^y > a^t$. Given the following family pedigree, (*a*) determine the genotypes of all the individuals insofar as possible, (*b*) calculate the probability of spotted offspring being produced by mating III1 by III2, (*c*) find the fraction of the dark-pigmented offspring from I1 × II3 that is expected to be heterozygous.

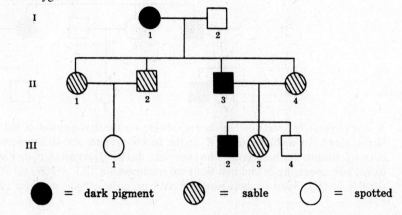

Legend: ● = dark pigment   ▨ = sable   ○ = spotted

Review Questions

Matching Questions   In guinea pigs, black coat color is dominant over white. Match the correct answer in the right column with the question in the left column.

Male		Female		Progeny		
1.	BB	×	BB	= genotypic ratio?	A.	All Bb
2.	BB	×	Bb	= phenotypic ratio?	B.	$\frac{3}{4}$ black : $\frac{1}{4}$ white
3.	BB	×	bb	= genotypic ratio?	C.	All bb
4.	BB	×	Bb	= genotypic ratio?	D.	$\frac{1}{4} BB : \frac{1}{2} Bb : \frac{1}{4} bb$
5.	Bb	×	Bb	= phenotypic ratio?	E.	All white
6.	Bb	×	Bb	= genotypic ratio?	F.	All BB
7.	bB	×	bb	= phenotypic ratio?	G.	$\frac{1}{2}$ white : $\frac{1}{2}$ black
8.	bB	×	bb	= genotypic ratio?	H.	$\frac{1}{2} BB : \frac{1}{2} Bb$
9.	bb	×	bb	= phenotypic ratio?	I.	$\frac{1}{2} Bb : \frac{1}{2} bb$
10.	bb	×	bb	= genotypic ratio?	J.	All black

Vocabulary   For each of the following definitions, give the appropriate term and spell it correctly. Terms are single words unless indicated otherwise.

1. Any measurable or distinctive characteristic or trait possessed by an organism.

2. The genetic endowment of an individual or cell.

3. A cell produced by the union of gametes carrying identical alleles.

4. A cell produced by the union of gametes carrying different alleles.

5. Adjective descriptive of an allele that is not expressed in a heterozygote; also descriptive of the phenotype produced when the allele is homozygous.

6. Any phenotype that is extremely rare in a natural population. (One or two words.)

7. Adjective describing any pair of alleles that interact in the heterozygous condition to produce a phenotype different from those of the respective homozygotes. (One or two words.)

8. Any gene that when homozygous results in death of the individual prior to sexual maturity. (One or two words.)

9. The proportion of individuals of a specified genotype that shows the expected phenotype.

10. The degree of effect produced by a given genotype under a given set of environmental conditions or over a range of environmental conditions.

True-False Questions   Answer each of the following questions either true (T) or false (F).

1. A phenotype is either the product of gene or of environmental influences.

2. Barring mutation, a pure line is expected to breed true to type.

3. An individual with a hybrid genotype or in a carrier state must also be heterozygous.

4. The simplest multiple allelic system consists of 3 alleles.

5. A backcross is equivalent to a testcross.

6.   In pedigrees, circles represent males and squares represent females.

7.   The probabilities of independent events are added to find the probability of their joint occurrence.

8.   Codominant alleles cannot express lethality when homozygous.

9.   Dominant traits are expected to be the most frequent phenotypes in a population.

10. The F_2 generation is conventionally produced by random union of the F_1 gametes.

Multiple-Choice Questions   Choose the one best answer.
Questions 1–5 use the following information. In guinea pigs, black coat color (governed by gene B) is a dominant trait, and white (attributed to allele b) is a recessive trait.

1.   A black female is testcrossed, producing 6 black offspring. The probability that a heterozygous black female would do this by chance alone is approximately   (a) 50%   (b) 25%   (c) 1%   (d) cannot be determined from the information given   (e) none of the above

2.   A mating that is expected to produce 50% homozygotes and 50% heterozygotes is   (a) $BB \times Bb$ (b) $Bb \times Bb$ (c) $bb \times Bb$ (d) two of the above   (e) matings a, b, and c above

3.   When heterozygous black pigs are intercrossed, approximately what fraction of the black progeny are expected to be homozygous?   (a) $\frac{3}{4}$ (b) $\frac{2}{3}$ (c) $\frac{1}{2}$ (d) $\frac{1}{3}$ (e) none of the above

4.   How many genetically different kinds of matings can be made in a population containing these 2 alleles (ignoring reciprocal crosses)?   (a) 4   (b) 6   (c) 8   (d) more than 8   (e) none of the above

5.   When heterozygous black pigs are intercrossed the chance of the first 2 offspring being black is   (a) more than 75%   (b) 56%   (c) 44%   (d) 6%   (e) none of the above

6.   The ABO blood groups of humans are determined by 3 alleles (Example 2.15). How many genotypes are possible for these phenotypes?   (a) 3   (b) 4   (c) 6   (d) 8   (e) none of the above

7.   A mother of blood group O has a group O child. The father could be   (a) A or B or O   (b) O only   (c) A or B   (d) AB only   (e) none of the above

8.   How many different genotypes can exist in a population with the dominance hierarchy $g^a > g^b > g^c > g^d$?   (a) 6   (b) 8   (c) 16   (d) more than 16   (e) none of the above

9.   Snapdragon flowers can be red ($C^r C^r$), pink ($C^r C^w$) or white ($C^w C^w$). When red-flowered plants are crossed to white-flowered plants, the possibility of an F_2 offspring being homozygous is   (a) $\frac{1}{4}$ (b) $\frac{1}{2}$ (c) $\frac{3}{4}$ (d) $\frac{1}{12}$ (e) none of the above

10. When snapdragons with pale-green leaves are intercrossed, their adult progeny consist of approximately 1 dark green: 2 pale green. What portion of all F_2 zygotes are expected to reach sexual maturity?   (a) $\frac{8}{9}$ (b) 0.75   (c) 50%   (d) 66.7%   (e) none of the above

Answers to Supplementary Problems

2.12. $Bb \times Bb$

2.13. (a) bb = white,   (b) Bb

2.14. (a) $\frac{1}{4}BB : \frac{1}{2}Bb : \frac{1}{4}bb$, $\frac{3}{4}$ black : $\frac{1}{4}$ white;   (b) $\frac{1}{2}Bb$ = black : $\frac{1}{2}bb$ = white

2.15. $\frac{1}{2}$ wild-type s^+s : $\frac{1}{2}$ sepia ss

2.16. (a) $\frac{1}{4}$, (b) $\frac{1}{16}$, (c) $2(\frac{3}{4} \times \frac{1}{4}) = \frac{3}{8}$

2.17. (a) Ll female $\times$ ll male, (b) 1 short : 1 long, (c) 4

2.18. $\frac{1}{2}Ww =$ wire-haired : $\frac{1}{2}ww =$ smooth

2.19. $\frac{1}{6}$

2.20. (a) $\frac{1}{2}BB$: $\frac{1}{2}Bb$, all red; (b) $\frac{1}{2}Bb =$ red : $\frac{1}{2}bb =$ silver-black; (c) all $Bb =$ red

2.21. (a) $\frac{1}{4}$, (b) $\frac{81}{256}$, (c) $\frac{5}{6}$ black and white : $\frac{1}{6}$ red and white, (d) 7 black and white : 1 red and white

2.22. (a) 10, (b) $10(\frac{3}{4})^3(\frac{1}{4})^2 = \frac{135}{512}$

2.23. (a) Single pair of codominant alleles
(b) $F^SF^S =$ splashed-white : $F^SF^B =$ Blue Andalusian : $F^BF^B =$ black

2.24. $\frac{1}{4}C^YC^Y =$ yellow : $\frac{1}{2}C^YC^W =$ cream : $\frac{1}{4}C^WC^W =$ white

2.25. $\frac{9}{16}$ long : $\frac{6}{16}$ oval : $\frac{1}{16}$ round

2.26. (a) 1 Palomino : 1 non-Palomino
(b) 100%, $D^1D^1 \times D^1D^1 =$ all D^1D^1 (chestnut); similarly $D^2D^2 \times D^2D^2 =$ all D^2D^2 (cremello)
(c) D^1D^1 (chestnut) $\times D^2D^2$ (cremello)

2.27. Creepers are heterozygous. Normal birds and lethal zygotes are homozygous for alternative alleles. One of the alleles is dominant with respect to the creeper phenotype; the other allele is dominant with respect to viability.

2.28. 4 normal : 4 hairless

2.29. $\frac{9}{15}$ dark-green C^GC^G : $\frac{6}{15}$ light-green C^GC^Y

2.30. (a) $\frac{1}{2}$, (b) $\frac{2}{3}$

2.31. $\frac{1}{2}$ Pelger : $\frac{1}{2}$ normal

2.32. Alexandria type (white eye) $= AA$, Aa^n, Aa; normal type (yellow eye) $= a^na^n$, a^na; Primrose Queen type (large yellow eye) $= aa$

2.33. (a) $\frac{1}{2}M^RM^R$: $\frac{1}{2}M^RM$; all restricted
(b) $\frac{1}{2}M^RM^R$: $\frac{1}{2}M^Rm$; all restricted
(c) $\frac{1}{4}M^RM^R$: $\frac{1}{4}M^Rm$: $\frac{1}{4}M^RM$: $\frac{1}{4}Mm$; $\frac{3}{4}$ restricted : $\frac{1}{4}$ mallard
(d) $\frac{1}{4}M^RM$: $\frac{1}{4}M^Rm$: $\frac{1}{4}Mm$: $\frac{1}{4}mm$; $\frac{1}{2}$ restricted : $\frac{1}{4}$ mallard : $\frac{1}{4}$ dusky
(e) $\frac{1}{2}Mm =$ mallard : $\frac{1}{2}mm =$ dusky

2.34. (a) Embryos $= \frac{1}{2}S^1S^3$: $\frac{1}{2}S^3S^4$
Endosperms $= \frac{1}{2}S^1S^1S^3$: $\frac{1}{2}S^4S^4S^3$
(b) None
(c) Embryos $= \frac{1}{4}S^1S^2$: $\frac{1}{4}S^1S^4$: $\frac{1}{4}S^3S^2$: $\frac{1}{4}S^3S^4$;
Endosperms $= \frac{1}{4}S^1S^1S^2$: $\frac{1}{4}S^1S^1S^4$: $\frac{1}{4}S^3S^3S^2$: $\frac{1}{4}S^3S^3S^4$
(d) Embryos $= \frac{1}{2}S^2S^4$: $\frac{1}{2}S^3S^4$, endosperms $= \frac{1}{2}S^2S^2S^4$: $\frac{1}{2}S^3S^3S^4$

2.35. (a) $F_1 = \frac{1}{2}E^DE$ (black with trace of agouti) : $\frac{1}{2}E^De$ (nonagouti black);
$F_2 = \frac{1}{4}E^DE^D$: $\frac{1}{4}E^De$: $\frac{1}{4}E^DE$: $\frac{1}{16}EE$: $\frac{1}{8}Ee$: $\frac{1}{16}ee$;
$\frac{1}{2}$ nonagouti black : $\frac{1}{4}$ black with trace of agouti : $\frac{3}{16}$ full color : $\frac{1}{16}$ reddish-yellow
(b) $F_1 = \frac{1}{2}E^De$ (nonagouti black) : $\frac{1}{2}ee$ (reddish-yellow);
$F_2 = \frac{1}{16}E^DE^D$: $\frac{3}{8}E^De$: $\frac{9}{16}ee$; $\frac{7}{16}$ nonagouti black : $\frac{9}{16}$ reddish-yellow

2.36. $\frac{1}{4}Ss^h$: $\frac{1}{4}Ss^c$: $\frac{1}{4}s^hs$: $\frac{1}{4}s^cs$; $\frac{1}{2}$ Dutch-belted : $\frac{1}{4}$ Hereford-type spotting : $\frac{1}{4}$ solid color

2.37. (a) The man could be the father, but paternity cannot be *proved* by blood type. In certain cases, a man may be *excluded* as a father of a child [see part (d)]. (b) I^Bi man $\times$ I^Ai woman, (c) I^BI^B, (d) no

2.38. (a) $\frac{2}{5}$ full color : $\frac{3}{5}$ dilute, (b) 50%, (c) $\frac{2}{3}$

2.39. (a) 0, (b) $\frac{1}{2}$, (c) 0, (d) $\frac{1}{2}$, (e) $\frac{3}{4}$

2.40. (a) $\frac{1}{8}$, (b) 0, (c) $\frac{2}{35}$, (d) $\frac{1}{28}$

Note: The solution to 2.40 (c), at top of page 46, serves as an example for solving all parts of 2.40 and 2.41.

Solution to problem 2.40 (c)

	Gametes
III3 is Rr (probability = 1.0)	$\longrightarrow$ $\frac{1}{2}$R : $\frac{1}{2}$r
III4 may be RR (probability = $\frac{1}{2}$)	$\longrightarrow$ all R ($\frac{1}{2}$) = $\frac{1}{2}$R
III4 may be Rr (probability = $\frac{1}{2}$)	$\longrightarrow$ $\frac{1}{2}(\frac{1}{2}$R : $\frac{1}{2}$r) = $\frac{1}{4}$R : $\frac{1}{4}$r
Total R gametes for III4 = $\frac{1}{2} + \frac{1}{4} = \frac{3}{4}$	
Total r gametes for III4 = $\frac{1}{4}$	

Mating table for III3 x III4:

III4 \ III3	$\frac{1}{2}$R	$\frac{1}{2}$r
$\frac{3}{4}$R	$\frac{3}{8}$RR	$\frac{3}{8}$Rr
$\frac{1}{4}$r	$\frac{1}{8}$Rr	$\frac{1}{8}$rr

Summary: $\frac{3}{8}$RR : $\frac{4}{8}$Rr : $\frac{1}{8}$rr

But IV1 is not rr. Therefore, the probability that IV1 is Rr is $\frac{4}{7}$, not $\frac{4}{8}$.

	Gametes
III6 may be Rr (probability = $\frac{1}{2}$)	$\longrightarrow$ $\frac{1}{2}(\frac{1}{2}$R + $\frac{1}{2}$r) = $\frac{1}{4}$R : $\frac{1}{4}$r
III6 may be RR (probability = $\frac{1}{2}$)	$\longrightarrow$ $\frac{1}{2}$(all R) = $\frac{1}{2}$R
Total R gametes for III6 = $\frac{1}{4} + \frac{1}{2} = \frac{3}{4}$	
Total r gametes for III6 = $\frac{1}{4}$	
III7 has the same gametic frequencies as III6	

Mating table for III6 x III7:

III7 \ III6	$\frac{3}{4}$R	$\frac{1}{4}$r
$\frac{3}{4}$R	$\frac{9}{16}$RR	$\frac{3}{16}$Rr
$\frac{1}{4}$r	$\frac{3}{16}$Rr	$\frac{1}{16}$rr

Summary: $\frac{9}{16}$RR : $\frac{6}{16}$Rr : $\frac{1}{16}$rr

But IV2 is not rr. Therefore, the probability that IV2 is Rr is $\frac{6}{15}$, not $\frac{6}{16}$.

The joint probability that IV1 is Rr ($\frac{4}{7}$) and IV2 is Rr ($\frac{6}{15}$) and their mating produces a rr offspring ($\frac{1}{4}$) = $\frac{24}{420} = \frac{2}{35}$.

2.41. (a) $\frac{1}{16}$, (b) $\frac{1}{4}$, (c) $\frac{1}{2}$, (d) $\frac{1}{8}$, (e) $\frac{1}{12}$, (f) $\frac{5}{77}$, (g) $\frac{5}{88}$, (h) $\frac{5}{22}$, (i) $\frac{2}{21}$

2.42. (a) I1 = $A^s a^s$, I2 = $a' a'$, II1 = $a^s a'$, II2 = $a^s a'$, II3 = $A^s a'$, II4 = $a^s a'$, III1 = $a' a'$, III2 = A^s-($A^s a^s$ or $A^s a'$), III3 = $a^s a'$, III4 = $a' a'$, (b) $\frac{1}{4}$, (c) $\frac{2}{3}$

Answers to Review Questions

Matching Questions

1. F   2. J   3. A   4. H   5. B   6. D   7. G   8. I   9. E   10. C

Vocabulary

1. phenotype
2. genotype
3. homozygote (homozygous cell)
4. heterozygote (heterozygous cell)
5. recessive
6. mutant type
7. codominant, incompletely dominant, partially dominant, semidominant
8. lethal gene
9. penetrance
10. expressivity

True-False Questions

1. F (or both)   2. T   3. T   4. T   5. F (only if the backcross involves mating an offspring of dominant phenotype back to a parent with recessive phenotype)   6. F (vice versa)   7. F (multiplied)   8. F (see Example 2.11)   9. F (frequencies of genes are a function of evolutionary forces, such as natural selection)   10. T

Multiple-Choice Questions

1. c   2. e   3. d   4. b   5. b   6. c   7. a   8. e (10 genotypes)   9. b   10. a

Chapter 3

Two or More Genes

INDEPENDENT ASSORTMENT

In this chapter we shall consider simultaneously two or more traits, each specified by a different pair of independently assorting autosomal genes, i.e., genes on different chromosomes other than the sex chromosomes.

Example 3.1. In addition to the coat color locus of guinea pigs introduced in Chapter 2 ($B-$ = black, bb = white), another locus on a different chromosome (independently assorting) is known to govern length of hair, such that $L-$ = short hair and ll = long hair. Any of 4 different genotypes exist for the black, short-haired phenotype: $BBLL$, $BBLl$, $BbLL$, $BbLl$. Two different genotypes produce a black, long-haired pig: $BBll$ or $Bbll$; likewise 2 genotypes for a white, short-haired pig: $bbLL$ or $bbLl$; and only 1 genotype specifies a white, long-haired pig: $bbll$.

A **dihybrid** genotype is heterozygous at 2 loci. Dihybrids form 4 genetically different gametes with approximately equal frequencies because of the random orientation of nonhomologous chromosome pairs on the first meiotic metaphase plate (Chapter 1).

Example 3.2. A dihybrid black, short-haired guinea pig ($BbLl$) produces 4 types of gametes in equal frequencies.

			Gametes	Frequency
	L	=	BL	$\frac{1}{4}$
B				
	l	=	Bl	$\frac{1}{4}$
	L	=	bL	$\frac{1}{4}$
b				
	l	=	bl	$\frac{1}{4}$

A summary of the gametic output for all 9 genotypes involving two pairs of independently assorting factors is shown below.

Genotypes	Gametes in Relative Frequencies
$BBLL$	All BL
$BBLl$	$\frac{1}{2}BL : \frac{1}{2}Bl$
$BBll$	All Bl
$BbLL$	$\frac{1}{2}BL : \frac{1}{2}bL$
$BbLl$	$\frac{1}{4}BL : \frac{1}{4}Bl : \frac{1}{4}bL : \frac{1}{4}bl$
$Bbll$	$\frac{1}{2}Bl : \frac{1}{2}bl$
$bbLL$	All bL
$bbLl$	$\frac{1}{2}bL : \frac{1}{2}bl$
$bbll$	All bl

A testcross is the mating of an incompletely known genotype to a genotype that is homozygous recessive at all of the loci under consideration. The phenotypes of the offspring produced by a testcross reveal the number of different gametes formed by the parental genotype under test. When all of the gametes of an individual are known, the genotype of that individual also becomes known. A monohybrid testcross gives a $1:1$ phenotypic ratio, indicating that one pair of factors is segregating. A dihybrid testcross gives a $1:1:1:1$ ratio, indicating that two pairs of factors are segregating and assorting independently.

Example 3.3. Testcrossing a dihybrid yields a $1:1:1:1$ genotypic and phenotypic ratio among the progeny.

Parents:	$BbLl$	$\times$	$bbll$
	black, short-haired		white, long-haired

F₁:
$\frac{1}{4}BbLl$ black, short-haired
$\frac{1}{4}Bbll$ black, long-haired
$\frac{1}{4}bbLl$ white, short-haired
$\frac{1}{4}bbll$ white, long-haired

SYSTEMS FOR SOLVING DIHYBRID CROSSES

1. Gametic Checkerboard Method.

When 2 dihybrids are crossed, four kinds of gametes are produced in equal frequencies in both the male and the female. A 4×4 gametic checkerboard can be used to show all 16 possible combinations of these gametes. This method is laborious and time-consuming, and offers more opportunities for error than the other methods that follow.

Example 3.4.

P: $BBLL \times bbll$
black, short   white, long

F₁: $BbLl$ = black, short

F₂:

		Male Gametes			
		BL	*Bl*	*bL*	*bl*
Female Gametes	*BL*	*BBLL* black short	*BBLl* black short	*BbLL* black short	*BbLl* black short
	Bl	*BBLl* black short	*BBll* black long	*BbLl* black short	*Bbll* black long
	bL	*BbLL* black short	*BbLl* black short	*bbLL* white short	*bbLl* white short
	bl	*BbLl* black short	*Bbll* black long	*bbLl* white short	*bbll* white long

F₂ Summary:

Proportions	Genotypes	Proportions	Phenotypes
$\frac{1}{16}$	*BB LL*	$\frac{9}{16}$	Black, short
$\frac{1}{8}$	*BB Ll*	$\frac{3}{16}$	Black, long
$\frac{1}{16}$	*BB ll*	$\frac{3}{16}$	White, short
$\frac{1}{8}$	*Bb LL*	$\frac{1}{16}$	White, long
$\frac{1}{4}$	*Bb Ll*		
$\frac{1}{8}$	*Bb ll*		
$\frac{1}{16}$	*bb LL*		
$\frac{1}{8}$	*bb Ll*		
$\frac{1}{16}$	*bb ll*		

2. Genotypic and Phenotypic Checkerboard Methods.

A knowledge of the monohybrid probabilities presented in Chapter 2 may be applied in a simplified genotypic or phenotypic checkerboard.

Example 3.5. Genotypic checkerboard.

$$F_1: \qquad BbLl \qquad \times \qquad BbLl$$
$$\text{black, short} \qquad\qquad \text{black, short}$$

Considering only the B locus, $Bb \times Bb$ produces $\frac{1}{4}BB$, $\frac{1}{2}Bb$, and $\frac{1}{4}bb$. Likewise for the L locus, $Ll \times Ll$ produces $\frac{1}{4}LL$, $\frac{1}{2}Ll$, and $\frac{1}{4}ll$. Let us place these genotypic probabilities in a checkerboard and combine independent probabilities by multiplication.

F_2:

	$\frac{1}{4}LL$	$\frac{1}{2}Ll$	$\frac{1}{4}ll$
$\frac{1}{4}BB$	$\frac{1}{16}BBLL$	$\frac{1}{8}BBLL$	$\frac{1}{16}BBll$
$\frac{1}{2}Bb$	$\frac{1}{8}BbLL$	$\frac{1}{4}BbLl$	$\frac{1}{8}Bbll$
$\frac{1}{4}bb$	$\frac{1}{16}bbLL$	$\frac{1}{8}bbLl$	$\frac{1}{16}bbll$

Example 3.6. Phenotypic checkerboard.

$$F_1: \qquad BbLl \qquad \times \qquad BbLl$$
$$\text{black, short} \qquad\qquad \text{black, short}$$

Considering the B locus, $Bb \times Bb$ produces $\frac{3}{4}$ black and $\frac{1}{4}$ white. Likewise at the L locus, $Ll \times Ll$ produces $\frac{3}{4}$ short and $\frac{1}{4}$ long. Let us place these independent phenotypic probabilities in a checkerboard and combine them by multiplication.

F_2:

	$\frac{3}{4}$ Black	$\frac{1}{4}$ White
$\frac{3}{4}$ Short	$\frac{9}{16}$ Black, short	$\frac{3}{16}$ White, short
$\frac{1}{4}$ Long	$\frac{3}{16}$ Black, long	$\frac{1}{16}$ White, long

3. Branching Systems.

This procedure was introduced in Chapter 1 as a means for determining all possible ways in which any number of chromosome pairs could orient themselves on the first meiotic metaphase plate. It can also be used to find all possible genotypic or phenotypic combinations. It will be the method of choice for solving most examples in this and subsequent chapters.

Example 3.7. Genotypic trichotomy.

		Ratio	Genotypes
	$\frac{1}{4}LL$ =	$\frac{1}{16}$	BB LL
$\frac{1}{4}BB$	$\frac{1}{2}Ll$ =	$\frac{1}{8}$	BB Ll
	$\frac{1}{4}ll$ =	$\frac{1}{16}$	BB ll
	$\frac{1}{4}LL$ =	$\frac{1}{8}$	Bb LL
$\frac{1}{2}Bb$	$\frac{1}{2}Ll$ =	$\frac{1}{4}$	Bb Ll
	$\frac{1}{4}ll$ =	$\frac{1}{8}$	Bb ll
	$\frac{1}{4}LL$ =	$\frac{1}{16}$	bb LL
$\frac{1}{4}bb$	$\frac{1}{2}Ll$ =	$\frac{1}{8}$	bb Ll
	$\frac{1}{4}ll$ =	$\frac{1}{16}$	bb ll

Example 3.8. Phenotypic dichotomy.

		Ratio	Phenotypes
	$\frac{3}{4}$ short =	$\frac{9}{16}$	Black, short
$\frac{3}{4}$ black	$\frac{1}{4}$ long =	$\frac{3}{16}$	Black, long
	$\frac{3}{4}$ short =	$\frac{3}{16}$	White, short
$\frac{1}{4}$ white	$\frac{1}{4}$ long =	$\frac{1}{16}$	White, long

If only one of the genotypic frequencies or phenotypic frequencies is required, there is no need to be concerned with any other genotypes or phenotypes. A mathematical solution can be readily obtained by combining independent probabilities.

Example 3.9.   To find the frequency of genotype *BBLl* in the offspring of dihydrid parents, first consider each locus separately: $Bb \times Bb = \frac{1}{4}BB$; $Ll \times Ll = \frac{1}{2}Ll$. Combining these independent probabilities, $\frac{1}{4} \times \frac{1}{2} = \frac{1}{8}BBLl$.

Example 3.10.   To find the frequency of white, short pigs in the offspring of dihybrid parents, first consider each trait separately: $Bb \times Bb = \frac{1}{4}$ white (*bb*); $Ll \times Ll = \frac{3}{4}$ short (*L*-). Combining these independent probabilities, $\frac{1}{4} \times \frac{3}{4} = \frac{3}{16}$ white, short.

MODIFIED DIHYBRID RATIOS

The classical phenotypic ratio resulting from the mating of dihybrid genotypes is $9:3:3:1$. This ratio appears whenever the alleles at both loci display dominant and recessive relationships. The classical dihybrid ratio may be modified if one or both loci have codominant alleles or lethal alleles. A summary of these modified phenotypic ratios in adult progeny is shown below.

Allelic Relationships in Dihybrid Parents		Expected Adult Phenotypic Ratio
First Locus	Second Locus	
Dominant-recessive	Codominants	$3:6:3:1:2:1$
Codominants	Codominants	$1:2:1:2:4:2:1:2:1$
Dominant-recessive	Codominant lethal*	$3:1:6:2$
Codominant	Codominant lethal*	$1:2:1:2:4:2$
Lethal*	Codominant lethal*	$4:2:2:1$

* See Example 2.11.

HIGHER COMBINATIONS

The methods for solving two-factor crosses may easily be extended to solve problems involving three or more pairs of independently assorting autosomal factors. Given any number of heterozygous pairs of factors (n) in the F_1, the following general formulas apply:

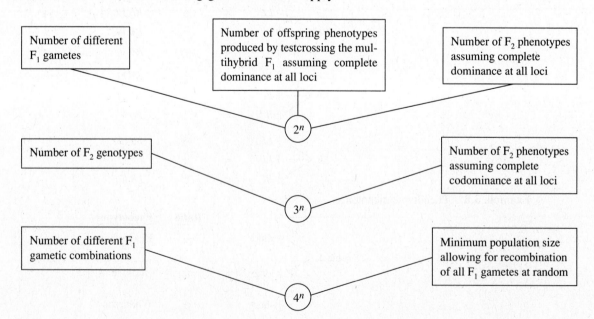

Solved Problems

3.1. Black coat color in Cocker Spaniels is governed by a dominant allele *B* and red coat color by its recessive allele *b*; solid pattern is governed by the dominant allele of an independently assorting locus *S*, and spotted pattern by its recessive allele *s*. A solid-black male is mated to a solid-red female and produces a litter of 6 pups: 2 solid black, 2 solid red, 1 black and white, and 1 red and white. Determine the genotypes of the parents.

Solution:

An unknown portion of a genotype will be indicated by a dash (-).

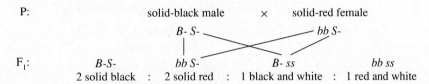

P: solid-black male   ×   solid-red female

F₁: B-S-   bb S-   B- ss   bb ss
2 solid black : 2 solid red : 1 black and white : 1 red and white

Whenever a homozygous double-recessive progeny appears (red and white in this case), each of the parents must have possessed at least one recessive allele at each locus. The black-and-white pup also indicates that both parents were heterozygous at the S locus. The solid-red pups likewise indicate that the male parent must have been heterozygous at the B locus. The solid-black pups fail to be of any help in determining the genotypes of these parents. Complete genotypes may now be written for both parents and for 2 of the pups.

P: solid-black male   ×   solid-red female
                BbSs   *bbSs*

F₁: *BbS-*   *bbS-*   *Bbss*   *bbss*
2 solid black : 2 solid red : 1 black and white : 1 red and white

3.2. How many different crosses may be made (*a*) from a single pair of factors, (*b*) from two pairs of factors, and (*c*) from any given number *n* of pairs of factors?

Solution:

(*a*) All possible matings of the 3 genotypes produced by a single pair of factors may be represented in a genotypic checkerboard.

	AA	*Aa*	*aa*
AA	AA × AA (1)	AA × Aa (2)	AA × aa (3)
Aa	Aa × AA (2)	Aa × Aa (4)	Aa × aa (5)
aa	aa × AA (3)	aa × Aa (5)	aa × aa (6)

The symmetry of matings above and below the squares on the diagonal becomes obvious. The number of different crosses may be counted as follows: 3 in the first column, 2 in the second, and 1 in the third: $3 + 2 + 1 = 6$ different types of matings.

(*b*) There are $3^2 = 9$ different genotypes possible with two pairs of segregating factors. If a 9×9 checkerboard were constructed, the same symmetry would exist above and below the squares on the diagonal as was shown in part (*a*). Again, we may count the different types of matings as an arithmetic progression from 9 to 1; $9 + 8 + 7 + 6 + 5 + 4 + 3 + 2 + 1 = 45$.

(c) The sum of any arithmetic progression of this particular type may be found by the formula $M = \frac{1}{2}(g^2 + g)$ where M = number of different types of matings, and g = number of genotypes possible with n pairs of factors.

3.3. In the garden pea, Mendel found that yellow seed color was dominant to green ($Y > y$) and round seed shape was dominant to shrunken ($S > s$). (a) What phenotypic ratio would be expected in the F_2 from a cross of a pure yellow, round × green, shrunken? (b) What is the F_2 ratio of yellow : green and of round : shrunken?

Solution:

(a)

	P:	*YY SS*	×	*yy ss*
		yellow, round		green, shrunken

	F_1:	*Yy Ss*
		yellow, round

F_2: $\frac{9}{16}$ *Y-S-*   yellow, round
         $\frac{3}{16}$ *Y-ss*   yellow, shrunken
         $\frac{3}{16}$ *yyS-*   green, round
         $\frac{1}{16}$ *yy ss*   green, shrunken

(b) The ratio of yellow : green = ($\frac{9}{16}$ yellow, round + $\frac{3}{16}$ yellow, shrunken) : ($\frac{3}{16}$ green, round + $\frac{1}{16}$ green, shrunken) = 12 : 4 = 3 : 1. The ratio of round : shrunken = ($\frac{9}{16}$ yellow, round + $\frac{3}{16}$ green, round) : ($\frac{3}{16}$ yellow, shrunken + $\frac{1}{16}$ green, shrunken) = 12 : 4 = 3 : 1. Thus at each of the individual loci a 3 : 1 F_2 phenotypic ratio is observed, just as would be expected for a monohybrid cross.

3.4. Tall tomato plants are produced by the action of a dominant allele D, and dwarf plants by its recessive allele d. Hairy stems are produced by a dominant gene H, and hairless stems by its recessive allele h. A dihybrid tall, hairy plant is testcrossed. The F_1 progeny were observed to be 118 tall, hairy : 121 dwarf, hairless : 112 tall, hairless : 109 dwarf, hairy. (a) Diagram this cross. (b) What is the ratio of tall : dwarf; of hairy : hairless? (c) Are these two loci assorting independently of one another?

Solution:

(a)

	Parents:	*Dd Hh*	×	*dd hh*
		tall, hairy		dwarf, hairless

Gametes: (DH) (Dh) (dH) (dh)   (dh)

F_1:

Genotypes	Number	Phenotypes
Dd Hh	118	Tall, hairy
Dd hh	112	Tall, hairless
dd Hh	109	Dwarf, hairy
dd hh	121	Dwarf, hairless

Note that the observed numbers approximate a 1 : 1 : 1 : 1 phenotypic ratio.

(b) The ratio of tall : dwarf = (118 + 112) : (109 + 121) = 230 : 230 or 1 : 1 ratio. The ratio of hairy : hairless = (118 + 109) : (112 + 121) = 227 : 233 or approximately 1 : 1 ratio. Thus the testcross results for each locus individually approximate a 1 : 1 phenotypic ratio.

(c) Whenever the results of a testcross approximate a 1 : 1 : 1 : 1 ratio, it indicates that the two gene loci are assorting independently of each other in the formation of gametes. That is to say, all four types of gametes have an equal opportunity of being produced through the random orientation that non-homologous chromosomes assume on the first meiotic metaphase plate.

3.5. A dominant allele L governs short hair in guinea pigs and its recessive allele l governs long hair. Codominant alleles at an independently assorting locus specify hair color, such that $C^Y C^Y =$ yellow, $C^Y C^W =$ cream, and $C^W C^W =$ white. From matings between dihybrid short, cream pigs ($LlC^Y C^W$), predict the phenotypic ratio expected in the progeny.

Solution:

$$\frac{3}{4} L\text{-} \begin{cases} \frac{1}{4} C^Y C^Y & = & \frac{3}{16} L\text{-}C^Y C^Y & \text{short, yellow} \\ \frac{1}{2} C^Y C^W & = & \frac{6}{16} L\text{-}C^Y C^W & \text{short, cream} \\ \frac{1}{4} C^W C^W & = & \frac{3}{16} L\text{-}C^W C^W & \text{short, white} \end{cases}$$

$$\frac{1}{4} ll \begin{cases} \frac{1}{4} C^Y C^Y & = & \frac{1}{16} llC^Y C^Y & \text{long, yellow} \\ \frac{1}{2} C^Y C^W & = & \frac{2}{16} llC^Y C^W & \text{long, cream} \\ \frac{1}{4} C^W C^W & = & \frac{1}{16} llC^W C^W & \text{long, white} \end{cases}$$

Thus six phenotypes appear in the offspring in the ratio $3:6:3:1:2:1$. The dash (-) in the genotypes L- indicates that either allele L or l may be present, both combinations resulting in a short-haired phenotype.

3.6. Normal leg size, characteristic of the Kerry type of cattle, is produced by the homozygous genotype DD. Short-legged Dexter type cattle possess the heterozygous genotype Dd. The homozygous genotype dd is lethal, producing grossly deformed stillbirths called "bulldog calves." The presence of horns in cattle is governed by the recessive allele of another gene locus p, the polled condition (absence of horns) being produced by its dominant allele P. In matings between polled Dexter cattle of genotype $DdPp$, what phenotypic ratio is expected in the adult progeny?

Solution:

P: $DdPp$ $\times$ $DdPp$
         Dexter, polled   Dexter, polled

F$_1$:

$$\frac{1}{4} DD \begin{cases} \frac{3}{4} P\text{-} & = & \frac{3}{16} DD\, P\text{-} & \text{polled, Kerry} \\ \frac{1}{4} pp & = & \frac{1}{16} DD\, pp & \text{horned, Kerry} \end{cases}$$

$$\frac{1}{2} Dd \begin{cases} \frac{3}{4} P\text{-} & = & \frac{6}{16} Dd\, P\text{-} & \text{polled, Dexter} \\ \frac{1}{4} pp & = & \frac{2}{16} Dd\, pp & \text{horned, Dexter} \end{cases}$$

$$\frac{1}{4} dd \begin{cases} \frac{3}{4} P\text{-} & = & \frac{3}{16} dd\, P\text{-} & \text{lethal} \\ \frac{1}{4} pp & = & \frac{1}{16} dd\, pp & \text{lethal} \end{cases}$$

The phenotypic ratio of viable offspring thus becomes: $\frac{3}{12}$ polled, Kerry; $\frac{1}{12}$ horned, Kerry; $\frac{6}{12}$ polled, Dexter; $\frac{2}{12}$ horned, Dexter.

3.7. Stem color of tomato plants is known to be under the genetic control of at least one pair of alleles such that A- results in the production of anthocyanin pigment (purple stem). The recessive genotype aa lacks this pigment and hence is green. The edge of the tomato leaf may be deeply cut under the influence of a dominant allele C. The recessive genotype cc produces smooth-edged leaves called "potato leaf." The production of two locules in the tomato fruit is a characteristic of the dominant allele M; multiple locules are produced by the recessive genotype mm. A cross is made between two pure lines: purple, potato, biloculed × green, cut, multiloculed. What phenotypic ratio is expected in the F₂?

Solution:

P: *AA cc MM*   ×   *aa CC mm*
       purple, potato, biloculed   green, cut, multiloculed

F₁: *Aa Cc Mm*
          purple, cut, biloculed

F₂:

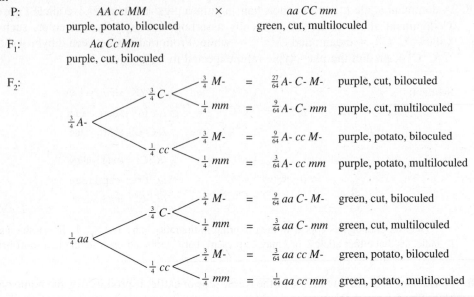

$\frac{3}{4}$ *A*-

$\frac{3}{4}$ *C*- $\frac{3}{4}$ *M*- = $\frac{27}{64}$ *A- C- M-*   purple, cut, biloculed

$\frac{1}{4}$ *mm* = $\frac{9}{64}$ *A- C- mm*   purple, cut, multiloculed

$\frac{1}{4}$ *cc* $\frac{3}{4}$ *M*- = $\frac{9}{64}$ *A- cc M-*   purple, potato, biloculed

$\frac{1}{4}$ *mm* = $\frac{3}{64}$ *A- cc mm*   purple, potato, multiloculed

$\frac{1}{4}$ *aa*

$\frac{3}{4}$ *C*- $\frac{3}{4}$ *M*- = $\frac{9}{64}$ *aa C- M-*   green, cut, biloculed

$\frac{1}{4}$ *mm* = $\frac{3}{64}$ *aa C- mm*   green, cut, multiloculed

$\frac{1}{4}$ *cc* $\frac{3}{4}$ *M*- = $\frac{3}{64}$ *aa cc M-*   green, potato, biloculed

$\frac{1}{4}$ *mm* = $\frac{1}{64}$ *aa cc mm*   green, potato, multiloculed

Supplementary Problems

DIHYBRID CROSSES WITH DOMINANT AND RECESSIVE ALLELES

3.8. The position of the flower on the stem of the garden pea is governed by a pair of alleles. Flowers growing in the axils (upper angle between petiole and stem) are produced by the action of a dominant allele *T*, those growing only at the tip of the stem by its recessive allele *t*. Colored flowers are produced by a dominant gene *C*, and white flowers by its recessive allele *c*. A dihybrid plant with colored flowers in the leaf axils is crossed to a pure strain of the same phenotype. What genotypic and phenotypic ratios are expected in the F₁ progeny?

3.9. In summer squash, white fruit color is governed by a dominant allele (*W*) and yellow fruit color by the recessive (*w*). A dominant allele at another locus (*S*) produces disc-shaped fruit and its recessive allele (*s*) yields sphere-shaped fruit. If a homozygous white disc variety of genotype *WWSS* is crossed with a homozygous yellow sphere variety (*wwss*), the F₁ are all white disc dihybrids of genotype *WwSs*. If the F₁ is allowed to mate at random, what would be the phenotypic ratio expected in the F₂ generation?

3.10. In *Drosophila*, ebony body color is produced by a recessive gene *e* and wild-type (gray) body color by its dominant allele *e⁺*. Vestigial wings are governed by a recessive gene *vg*, and normal wing size (wild type) by its dominant allele *vg⁺*. If wild-type dihybrid flies are crossed and produce 256 progeny, how many of these progeny flies are expected in each phenotypic class?

3.11. Short hair in rabbits is governed by a dominant gene (*L*) and long hair by its recessive allele (*l*). Black hair results from the action of the dominant genotype (*B-*) and brown from the recessive genotype (*bb*). (*a*) In crosses between dihybrid short, black and homozygous short, brown rabbits, what genotypic and phenotypic ratios are expected among their progeny? (*b*) Determine the expected genotypic and phenotypic ratios in progeny from the cross *LlBb* × *Llbb*.

3.12. The genetic information for the following eight parts is found in Problem 3.11. (*a*) What phenotypic ratio is expected among progeny from crosses of *LlBb* × *LlBb*? (*b*) What percentage of the F₁ genotypes in part (*a*) breeds true (i.e., what percentage is of homozygous genotypes)? (*c*) What percentage of the F₁ genotypes is heterozygous for only one pair of genes? (*d*) What percentage of the F_1 genotypes is heterozygous at both loci? (*e*) What percentage of the F_1 genotypes could be used for testcross purposes (i.e., homozygous double recessive)? (*f*) What percentage of the F_1 progeny could be used for testcross purposes at the B locus (i.e., homozygous recessive *bb*)? (*g*) What percentage of all short-haired F_1 individuals is expected to be brown? (*h*) What percentage of all black F_1 individuals will breed true for both black and short hair?

3.13. How many different matings are possible (*a*) when three pairs of factors are considered simultaneously, (*b*) when four pairs of factors are considered simultaneously? *Hint:* See Problem 3.2(*c*).

3.14. (*a*) What percentage of all possible types of matings with two pairs of factors would be represented by matings between identical genotypes? (*b*) What percentage of all the matings possible with three pairs of factors would be represented by matings between nonidentical genotypes?

3.15. The presence of feathers on the legs of chickens is due to a dominant allele (*F*) and clean legs to its recessive allele (*f*). Pea comb shape is produced by another dominant allele (*P*) and single comb by its recessive allele (*p*). In crosses between pure feathered leg, single-combed individuals and pure pea-combed, clean-leg individuals, suppose that only the single-combed, feathered-leg F_2 progeny are saved and allowed to mate at random. What genotypic and phenotypic ratios would be expected among the progeny (F_3)?

3.16. List all the different gametes produced by the following individuals: (*a*) *AA BB Cc*, (*b*) *aa Bb Cc*, (*c*) *Aa Bb cc Dd*, (*d*) *AA Bb Cc dd Ee Ff*.

3.17. The normal cloven-footed condition in swine is produced by the homozygous recessive genotype *mm*. A mule-footed condition is produced by the dominant genotype *M*-. White coat color is governed by the dominant allele of another locus *B* and black by its recessive allele *b*. A white, mule-footed sow (female) is mated to a black, cloven-footed boar (male) and produces several litters. Among 26 offspring produced by this mating, all were found to be white with mule feet. (*a*) What is the most probable genotype of the sow? (*b*) The next litter produced 8 white, mule-footed offspring and 1 white cloven-footed pig. Now, what is the most probable genotype of the sow?

3.18. A white, mule-footed boar (see Problem 3.17) is crossed to a sow of the same phenotype. Among the F_1 offspring there were found 6 white, cloven-footed : 7 black, mule-footed : 15 white, mule-footed : 3 black, cloven-footed pigs. (*a*) If all the black mule-footed F_1 offspring from this type of mating were to be testcrossed, what phenotypic ratio would be expected among the testcross progeny? (*b*) If the sow were to be testcrossed, what phenotypic ratio of progeny would be expected?

3.19. In poultry, a crested head is produced by a dominant gene *C* and plain head by its recessive allele *c*. Black feather color *R*- is dominant to red *rr*. A homozygous black-feathered, plain-headed bird is crossed to a homozygous red-feathered, crested-headed bird. What phenotypic and genotypic ratios are expected from testcrossing only the F_2 black-crested birds? *Hint:* Remember to account for the relative frequencies of the different genotypes in this one phenotypic class.

3.20. Bronze turkeys have at least one dominant allele *R*. Red turkeys are homozygous for its recessive allele *rr*. Another dominant gene *H* produces normal feathers, and the recessive genotype *hh* produces feathers lacking webbing, a condition termed "hairy." In crosses between homozygous bronze, hairy birds and homozygous red, normal-feathered birds, what proportion of the F_2 progeny will be (*a*) genotype *Rrhh*, (*b*) phenotype bronze, hairy, (*c*) genotype *rrHH*, (*d*) phenotype red, normal-feathered, (*e*) genotype *RrHh*, (*f*) phenotype bronze, normal-feathered, (*g*) genotype *rrhh*, (*h*) phenotype red, normal-feathered, (*i*) genotype *RRHh*?

MODIFIED DIHYBRID RATIOS

3.21. In peaches, the homozygous genotype $G^O G^O$ produces oval glands at the base of the leaves, the heterozygous genotype $G^O G^A$ produces round glands, and the homozygous genotype $G^A G^A$ results in the absence of glands. At another locus, a dominant gene *S* produces fuzzy peach skin and its recessive allele *s* produces smooth (nectarine) skin. A homozygous variety with oval glands and smooth skin is crossed to a homozygous variety with fuzzy skin lacking glands at the base of its leaves. What genotypic and phenotypic proportions are expected in the F_2?

3.22. In Shorthorn cattle, coat colors are governed by a codominant pair of alleles C^R and C^W. The homozygous genotype $C^R C^R$ produces red, the other homozygote produces white and the heterozygote produces roan (a mixture of red and white). The presence of horns is produced by the homozygous recessive genotype pp and the polled condition by its dominant allele P. If roan cows heterozygous for the horned gene are mated to a horned, roan bull, what phenotypic ratio is expected in the offspring?

3.23. A gene locus with codominant alleles is known to govern feather color in chickens such that the genotype $F^B F^B$ = black, $F^W F^W$ = splashed white, and $F^B F^W$ = blue. Another locus with codominant alleles governs feather morphology such that $M^N M^N$ = normal-feather shape, $M^N M^F$ = slightly abnormal feathers called "mild frizzle," and $M^F M^F$ = grossly abnormal feathers called "extreme frizzle." If blue, mildly frizzled birds are crossed among themselves, what phenotypic proportions are expected among their offspring?

3.24. In the above problem, if all the blue offspring with normal feathers and all the splashed-white, extremely frizzled offspring are isolated and allowed to mate at random, what phenotypic ratio would be expected among their progeny?

3.25. The shape of radishes may be long (LL), round $(L'L')$, or oval (LL'). Color may be red (RR), white $(R'R')$, or purple (RR'). If a long, white strain is crossed with a round, red strain, what phenotypic proportions are expected in the F_1 and F_2?

3.26. Suppose that two strains of radishes are crossed (see above problem) and produce a progeny consisting of 16 long white, 31 oval purple, 16 oval white, 15 long red, 17 oval red, and 32 long purple. What would be the phenotypes of the parental strains?

3.27. A dominant gene in mice K produces a kinked tail; recessive genotypes at this locus kk have normal tails. The homozygous condition of another locus AA produces a gray color called agouti; the heterozygous condition $A^y A$ produces yellow color; the homozygous genotype $A^y A^y$ is lethal. (a) If yellow mice, heterozygous for kinky tail, are crossed together, what phenotypic proportions are expected in their offspring? (b) What proportion of the offspring is expected to be of genotype $A^y A K k$? (c) If all the yellow offspring were allowed to mate at random, what would be the genotypic and phenotypic ratios among their adult progeny?

3.28. An incompletely dominant gene N in the Romney Marsh breed of sheep causes the fleece of homozygotes to be "hairy," i.e., containing fibers lacking the normal amount of crimp. Normal wool is produced by the homozygous genotype $N'N'$. Heterozygotes NN' can be distinguished at birth by the presence of large, medulated fibers called "halo-hairs" scattered over the body. A gene known as "lethal gray" causes homozygous gray fetuses $(G^l G^l)$ to die before 15 weeks in gestation. The heterozygous genotype $G^l G$ produces gray fleece, and the homozygous genotype GG produces black. If heterozygous halo, gray individuals are mated together, (a) what would be the phenotypic proportions expected in the live progeny, (b) what proportion of the live progeny would carry the lethal gene, (c) what proportion of the live progeny with halo-hairs would carry the lethal gene, (d) what proportion of all the zygotes would be expected to be of genotype $NN'G^l G^l$?

3.29. Infantile amaurotic idiocy (Tay-Sachs disease) is a recessive hereditary abnormality causing death within the first few years of life only when homozygous (ii). The dominant condition at this locus produces a normal phenotype $(I-)$. Abnormally shortened fingers (brachyphalangy) is thought to be due to a genotype heterozygous for a lethal gene (BB^L), the homozygote (BB) being normal, and the other homozygote $(B^L B^L)$ being lethal. What are the phenotypic expectations among teenage children from parents who are both brachyphalangic and heterozygous for infantile amaurotic idiocy?

3.30. In addition to the gene governing infantile amaurotic idiocy in the above problem, the recessive genotype of another locus (jj) results in death before age 18 due to a condition called "juvenile amaurotic idiocy." Only individuals of genotype $I-J-$ will survive to adulthood. (a) What proportion of the children from parents of genotype $IiJj$ would probably not survive to adulthood? (b) What proportion of the adult survivors in part (a) would not be carriers of either hereditary abnormality?

3.31. A genetic condition on chromosome 2 in the fruit fly *Drosophila melanogaster* is lethal when homozygous (Pm/Pm), but when heterozygous (Pm/Pm^+) produces a purplish eye color called "plum." The other homozygous condition (Pm^+/Pm^+) produces wild type eye color. On chromosome 3, a gene called "stubble" produces short, thick bristles when heterozygous (Sb/Sb^+), but is lethal when homozygous (Sb/Sb). The homozygous condition of its alternative allele (Sb^+/Sb^+), produces bristles of normal size (wild type). (a) What phenotypic ratio is expected among progeny from crosses between plum, stubble parents? (b) If the offspring of part (a) are allowed to mate at random to produce an F_2, what phenotypic ratio is expected?

3.32. Feather color in chickens is governed by a pair of codominant alleles such that F^BF^B produces black, F^WF^W produces splashed white, and F^BF^W produces blue. An independently segregating locus governs the length of leg; CC genotypes possess normal leg length, CC^L genotypes produce squatty, shortlegged types called "creepers," but homozygous C^LC^L genotypes are lethal. Determine the kinds of progeny phenotypes and their expected ratios that crosses between dihybrid blue creepers are likely to produce.

3.33. Fat mice can be produced by two independently assorting genes. The recessive genotype ob/ob produces a fat, sterile mouse called "obese." Its dominant allele Ob produces normal growth. The recessive genotype ad/ad also produces a fat, sterile mouse called "adipose" and its dominant allele Ad produces normal growth. What phenotypic proportions of fat versus normal would be expected among the F_1 and F_2 from parents of genotype $Ob/ob, Ad/ad$?

HIGHER COMBINATIONS

3.34. The seeds from Mendel's tall plants were round and yellow, all three characters due to a dominant gene at each of three independently assorting loci. The recessive genotypes $dd, ww,$ and gg produce dwarf plants with wrinkled and green seeds, respectively. (a) If a pure tall, wrinkled, yellow variety is crossed with a pure dwarf, round, green variety, what phenotypic ratio is expected in the F_1 and F_2? (b) What percentage of the F_2 is expected to be of genotype $Dd\ WW\ gg$? (c) If all the dwarf, round, green individuals in the F_2 are isolated and artificially crossed at random, what phenotypic ratio of offspring is expected?

3.35. The coat colors of mice are known to be governed by several genes. The presence of a yellow band of pigment near the tip of the hair is called "agouti" pattern and is produced by the dominant allele A. The recessive condition at this locus (aa) does not have this subapical band and is termed nonagouti. The dominant allele of another locus, B, produces black and the recessive genotype bb produces brown. The homozygous genotype c^hc^h restricts pigment production to the extremities in a pattern called Himalayan, whereas the genotype C- allows pigment to be distributed over the entire body. (a) In crosses between pure brown, agouti, Himalayan and pure black mice, what are the phenotypic expectations of the F_1 and F_2? (b) What proportion of the black-agouti, full-colored F_2 would be expected to be of genotype $AaBBCc$? (c) What percentage of all the Himalayans in the F_2 would be expected to show brown pigment? (d) What percentage of all the agoutis in the F_2 would be expected to exhibit black pigment?

3.36. In addition to the information given in the problem above, a fourth locus in mice is known to govern the density of pigment deposition. The genotype D- produces full color, but the recessive genotype dd produces a dilution of pigment. Another allele at this locus, d^l, is lethal when homozygous, produces a dilution of pigment in the genotype dd^l, and produces full color when in heterozygous condition with the dominant allele Dd^l. (a) What phenotypic ratio would be expected among the live F_2 progeny if the F_1 from the cross $aabbCCDd \times AABBccdd^l$ were allowed to mate at random? (b) What proportion of the live F_2 would be expected to be of genotype $AABbccdd^l$?

3.37. In the parental cross $AABBCCDDEE \times aabbccddee$, (a) how many different F_1 gametes can be formed, (b) how many different genotypes are expected in the F_2, (c) how many squares would be necessary in a gametic checkerboard to accommodate the F_2?

3.38. A pure strain of Mendel's peas, dominant for all seven of his independently assorting genes, was testcrossed. (a) How many different kinds of gametes could each of the parents produce? (b) How many different gametes could the F_1 produce? (c) If the F_1 was testcrossed, how many phenotypes would be expected in the offspring and in what proportions? (d) How many genotypes would be expected in the F_2? (e) How many combinations of F_1 gametes are theoretically possible (considering, e.g., $AABBCCDDEEFFGG$ sperm nucleus $\times$ $aabbccddeeffgg$ egg nucleus a different combination than $AABBCCDDEEFFGG$ egg nucleus $\times$

aabbccddeeffgg sperm nucleus)? (*f*) How many different kinds of matings could theoretically be made among the F$_2$? *Hint:* See solution to Problem 3.2(*c*).

Review Questions

Matching Questions In guinea pigs, black (*B-*) is dominant to white (*bb*). Assorting independently on a different pair of homologues, short hair (*S-*) is dominant to long hair (*ss*). In the parental generation, pure (homozygous) black, short pigs are crossed to white, long pigs. In the F$_2$ we expect the following:

1.	Black, short	A.	$\frac{1}{16}$
2.	Black, long	B.	$\frac{1}{8}$
3.	White, short	C.	$\frac{3}{16}$
4.	White, long	D.	$\frac{1}{2}$
5.	*BbSs*	E.	$\frac{1}{3}$
6.	*BBLL*	F.	$\frac{1}{4}$
7.	*Bbss*	G.	$\frac{3}{4}$
8.	*bbSs*	H.	$\frac{9}{16}$
9.	Short	I.	$\frac{2}{3}$
10.	Homozygous at both loci	J.	None of the above

Multiple-Choice Questions Choose the one best answer.

1. How many genetically different gametes can be made by an individual of genotype *AaBbccDDEe*? (*a*) 5 (*b*) 8 (*c*) 10 (*d*) 32 (*e*) none of the above

2. If an individual of genotype *AaBbCcDd* is testcrossed, how many different phenotypes can appear in the progeny? (*a*) 4 (*b*) 8 (*c*) 12 (*d*) 16 (*e*) none of the above

3. If individuals of genotype *AaBbCc* are intercrossed, how many different phenotypes can appear in their offspring? (*a*) 3 (*b*) 6 (*c*) 8 (*d*) 16 (*e*) none of the above

4. If individuals of genotype *AaBbCc* are intercrossed, how many different genotypes can occur in their progeny? (*a*) 6 (*b*) 8 (*c*) 16 (*d*) 21 (*e*) none of the above

5. If individuals of genotype $G^1G^2H^1H^2J^1J^2$ are intercrossed, how many phenotypes can occur in their offspring? (*a*) 6 (*b*) 12 (*c*) 16 (*d*) 27 (*e*) none of the above

6. The minimum progeny population size allowing for random union of all kinds of gametes from *AaBbCc* parents is (*a*) 9 (*b*) 27 (*c*) 64 (*d*) more than 100 (*e*) none of the above

7. How many different offspring phenotypes can be produced from intercrossing parents of genotype AaB^1B^2? (*a*) 3 (*b*) 4 (*c*) 6 (*d*) more than 6 (*e*) none of the above

Questions 8–10 use the following information. Given that A^1A^1 = lethal, A^1A^2 = gray, A^2A^2 = black, B^1B^1 = long hair, B^1B^2 = short hair, B^2B^2 = very short hair (fuzzy), and parents that are $A^1A^2B^1B^2$:

8. The fraction of the adult offspring that is expected to be gray, fuzzy is (*a*) $\frac{1}{4}$ (*b*) $\frac{1}{2}$ (*c*) $\frac{2}{3}$ (*d*) $\frac{3}{4}$ (*e*) none of the above

9. The fraction of the adult offspring expected to be gray, short is (*a*) $\frac{1}{4}$ (*b*) $\frac{1}{3}$ (*c*) $\frac{1}{2}$ (*d*) $\frac{2}{3}$ (*e*) none of the above

10. If fuzzy is lethal shortly after birth, the fraction of the adult progeny expected to be black, short is
     (a) $\frac{1}{4}$ (b) $\frac{1}{3}$ (c) $\frac{1}{2}$ (d) $\frac{2}{3}$ (e) none of the above

Answers to Supplementary Problems

3.8. $\frac{1}{4}CCTT : \frac{1}{4}CCTt : \frac{1}{4}CcTT : \frac{1}{4}CcTt$; all axial, colored

3.9. $\frac{9}{16}$ white, disc : $\frac{3}{16}$ white, sphere : $\frac{3}{16}$ yellow, disc : $\frac{1}{16}$ yellow, sphere

3.10. 144 wild type : 48 vestigial : 48 ebony : 16 ebony, vestigial

3.11. (a) $\frac{1}{4}LLBb : \frac{1}{4}LlBb : \frac{1}{4}LLbb : \frac{1}{4}Llbb$; $\frac{1}{2}$ short, black : $\frac{1}{2}$ short, brown
     (b) $\frac{1}{8}LLBb : \frac{1}{4}LlBb : \frac{1}{8}LLbb : \frac{1}{4}Llbb : \frac{1}{8}llBb : \frac{1}{8}llbb$;
         $\frac{3}{8}$ short, black : $\frac{3}{8}$ short, brown : $\frac{1}{8}$ long, black : $\frac{1}{8}$ long, brown

3.12. (a) $\frac{9}{16}$ short, black : $\frac{3}{16}$ short, brown : $\frac{3}{16}$ long, black : $\frac{1}{16}$ long, brown (b) 25% (c) 50% (d) 25%
     (e) 6.25% (f) 25% (g) 25% (h) 8.33%

3.13. (a) 378 (b) 3321 **3.14.** (a) 20% (b) 92.86%

3.15. $4FFpp : 4Ffpp : 1ffpp$; 8 feathered leg, single comb : 1 clean leg, single comb

3.16. (a) ABC, ABc (b) aBC, aBc, abC, abc (c) ABcD, ABcd, AbcD, Abcd, aBcD, aBcd, abcD, abcd
     (d) ABCdEF, ABCdEf, ABCdeF, ABCdef, ABcdEF, ABcdEf, ABcdeF, ABcdef, AbCdEF, AbCdEf, AbCdeF,
     AbCdef, AbcdEF, AbcdEf, AbcdeF, Abcdef

3.17. (a) BBMM (b) BBMm

3.18. (a) 2 black, mule-foot : 1 black, cloven-foot (b) $\frac{1}{4}$ white, mule-foot : $\frac{1}{4}$ white, cloven-foot : $\frac{1}{4}$ black,
     mule-foot : $\frac{1}{4}$ black, cloven-foot

3.19. $4RrCc$ = black, crested : $2Rrcc$ = black, plain : $2rrCc$ = red, crested : $1rrcc$ = red, plain

3.20. (a) $\frac{1}{8}$ (b) $\frac{3}{16}$ (c) $\frac{1}{16}$ (d) $\frac{3}{16}$ (e) $\frac{1}{4}$ (f) $\frac{9}{16}$ (g) $\frac{1}{16}$ (h) $\frac{3}{16}$ (i) $\frac{1}{8}$

3.21. $\frac{1}{16}G^AG^ASS : \frac{2}{16}G^AG^ASs : \frac{1}{16}G^AG^Ass : \frac{2}{16}G^AG^OSS : \frac{4}{16}G^AG^OSs : \frac{2}{16}G^AG^Oss : \frac{1}{16}G^OG^OSS : \frac{2}{16}G^OG^OSs : \frac{1}{16}G^OG^Oss$; $\frac{3}{16}$ fuzzy, glandless : $\frac{1}{16}$ smooth, glandless : $\frac{6}{16}$ round gland, fuzzy : $\frac{2}{16}$ round gland, smooth : $\frac{3}{16}$ oval gland, fuzzy : $\frac{1}{16}$ oval gland, smooth

3.22. 1 red, polled : 1 red, horned : 2 roan, polled : 2 roan, horned : 1 white, polled : 1 white, horned

3.23. $\frac{1}{16}$ black : $\frac{1}{8}$ black, mildly frizzled : $\frac{1}{16}$ black, extremely frizzled : $\frac{1}{8}$ blue : $\frac{1}{4}$ blue, mildly frizzled : $\frac{1}{8}$ blue, extremely frizzled : $\frac{1}{16}$ splashed-white : $\frac{1}{8}$ splashed-white, mildly frizzled : $\frac{1}{16}$ splashed-white, extremely frizzled

3.24. 1 black : 2 blue : 1 splashed-white : 2 blue, mildly frizzled : 2 splashed-white, mildly frizzled : 1 splashed-white, extremely frizzled

3.25. F_1 is all oval, purple; F_2 is $\frac{1}{16}$ long, red : $\frac{1}{8}$ long, purple : $\frac{1}{16}$ long, white : $\frac{1}{8}$ oval, red : $\frac{1}{4}$ oval, purple : $\frac{1}{8}$ oval, white : $\frac{1}{16}$ round, red : $\frac{1}{8}$ round, purple : $\frac{1}{16}$ round, white

3.26. Long, purple $\times$ oval, purple

3.27. (*a*) $\frac{1}{2}$ yellow, kinky : $\frac{1}{6}$ yellow : $\frac{1}{4}$ agouti, kinky : $\frac{1}{12}$ agouti, (*b*) $\frac{1}{3}$, (*c*) $\frac{1}{6}A^YAKK$: $\frac{1}{3}A^YAKk$: $\frac{1}{6}A^YAkk$: $\frac{1}{12}AAKK$: $\frac{1}{6}AAKk$: $\frac{1}{12}AAkk$; $\frac{1}{2}$ yellow, kinky : $\frac{1}{6}$ yellow : $\frac{1}{4}$ agouti, kinky : $\frac{1}{12}$ agouti

3.28. (*a*) $\frac{1}{12}$ black, hairy : $\frac{1}{6}$ black, halo-haired : $\frac{1}{12}$ black : $\frac{1}{6}$ gray, hairy : $\frac{1}{3}$ gray, halo-haired : $\frac{1}{6}$ gray (*b*) $\frac{2}{3}$, (*c*) $\frac{2}{3}$, (*d*) $\frac{1}{8}$

3.29. $\frac{1}{3}$ normal : $\frac{2}{3}$ brachyphalangic   **3.30** (*a*) $\frac{7}{16}$ (*b*) $\frac{1}{9}$

3.31. (*a*) $\frac{4}{9}$ plum, stubble : $\frac{2}{9}$ plum : $\frac{2}{9}$ stubble : $\frac{1}{9}$ wild type (*b*) 1 plum, stubble : 1 plum : 1 stubble : 1 wild type

3.32. $\frac{1}{12}$ black : $\frac{1}{6}$ blue : $\frac{1}{12}$ splashed-white : $\frac{1}{6}$ black, creeper : $\frac{1}{3}$ blue, creeper : $\frac{1}{6}$ splashed-white, creeper

3.33. $F_1 = \frac{9}{16}$ normal : $\frac{7}{16}$ fat; $F_2 = \frac{64}{81}$ normal : $\frac{17}{81}$ fat

3.34. (*a*) F_1 is all tall, round, yellow; F_2 is 27 tall, round, yellow : 9 tall, round, green : 9 tall, wrinkled, yellow : 9 dwarf, round, yellow : 3 tall, wrinkled, green : 3 dwarf, round, green : 3 dwarf, wrinkled, yellow : 1 dwarf, wrinkled, green (*b*) 3.12% (*c*) 8 round : 1 wrinkled

3.35. (*a*) F_1 is all agouti, black; F_2 is 27 agouti, black : 9 agouti, black, Himalayan : 9 agouti, brown : 9 black : 3 agouti, brown, Himalayan : 3 black, Himalayan : 3 brown : 1 brown, Himalayan (*b*) $\frac{4}{27}$ (*c*) 25% (*d*) 75%

3.36. (*a*) 189 agouti, black : 216 agouti, black, dilute : 63 agouti, black, Himalayan : 72 agouti, black, Himalayan, dilute : 63 agouti, brown : 72 agouti, brown, dilute : 63 black : 72 black, dilute : 21 agouti, brown, Himalayan : 24 agouti, brown, Himalayan, dilute : 21 black, Himalayan : 24 black, Himalayan, dilute : 21 brown : 24 brown, dilute : 7 brown, Himalayan : 8 brown, Himalayan, dilute, (*b*) $\frac{1}{120}$

3.37. (*a*) 32, (*b*) 243, (*c*) 1024

3.38. (*a*) One each (*b*) 128 (*c*) 128, each with equal frequency (*d*) 2187 (*e*) 16,384 (*f*) 2,392,578

Answers to Review Questions

Matching Questions

1. H   2. C   3. C   4. A   5. F   6. A   7. B   8. B   9. G   10. F

Multiple-Choice Questions

1. *b*   2. *d*   3. *c*   4. *e* (27)   5. *d*   6. *c*   7. *c*   8. *e* ($\frac{1}{6}$)   9. *b*   10. *e* ($\frac{2}{9}$)

Chapter 4

Genetic Interaction

TWO-FACTOR INTERACTIONS

The phenotype is a result of gene products brought to expression in a given environment. The environment includes not only external factors such as temperature and the amount or quality of light but also internal factors such as hormones and enzymes. Genes specify the structure of proteins. Most known enzymes are proteins. **Enzymes** perform catalytic functions, causing the splitting or union of various molecules. **Metabolism** is the sum of all the physical and chemical processes by which living protoplasm is produced and maintained and by which energy is made available for the uses of the organism. These biochemical reactions occur as stepwise conversions of one substance into another, each step being mediated by a specific enzyme. All of the steps that transform a precursor substance to its end product constitute a **biosynthetic pathway.**

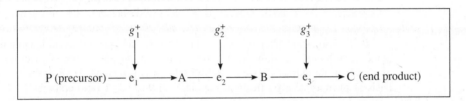

Several genes are usually required to specify the enzymes involved in even the simplest pathways. Each metabolite (A, B, C) is produced by the catalytic action of different enzymes (e_x) specified by different wild-type genes (g_x^+). **Genetic interaction** occurs whenever two or more genes specify enzymes that catalyze steps in a common pathway. If substance C is essential for the production of a normal phenotype, and the recessive mutant alleles g_1, g_2, and g_3 produce defective enzymes, then a mutant (abnormal) phenotype would result from a genotype homozygous recessive at any of the three loci. If g_3 is mutant, the conversion of B to C does not occur and substance B tends to accumulate in excessive quantity; if g_2 is mutant, substance A will accumulate. Thus mutants are said to produce "metabolic blocks." An organism with a mutation in only g_2 could produce a normal phenotype if it were given either substance B or C, but an organism with a mutation in g_3 has a specific requirement for C. Thus gene g_3^+ becomes dependent upon gene g_2^+ for its expression as a normal phenotype. If the genotype is homozygous for the recessive g_2 allele, then the pathway ends with substance A. Neither g_3^+ nor its recessive allele g_3 has any effect on the phenotype. Thus genotype g_2g_2 can hide or mask the phenotypic expression of alleles at the g_3 locus. Originally a gene or locus that suppressed or masked the action of a gene at another locus was termed **epistatic.** The gene or locus suppressed was **hypostatic.** Later it was found that both loci could be mutually epistatic to one another. Now the term "epistasis" has come to be synonymous with almost any type of gene interaction. Dominance involves *intra*allelic gene suppression, or the masking effect that one allele has upon the expression of another allele at the same locus. Epistasis involves *inter*allelic gene suppression, or the masking effect that one gene locus has upon the expression of another. The classical phenotypic ratio of $9:3:3:1$ observed in the progeny of dihybrid parents becomes modified by epistasis into ratios that are various combinations of the $9:3:3:1$ groupings.

Example 4.1. A particularly illuminating example of gene interaction occurs in white clover. Some strains have a high cyanide content; others have a low cyanide content. Crosses between two strains with low cyanide have produced an F_1 with a high concentration of cyanide in their leaves. The F_2 shows a ratio of 9 high cyanide : 7 low cyanide. Cyanide is known to be produced from the substrate cyanogenic glucoside by enzymatic catalysis. One strain of clover has the enzyme but not the substrate. The other strain makes substrate but is unable to convert it to cyanide. The pathway may be diagrammed as follows where G^x produces an enzyme and g^x results in a metabolic block.

$$G^1 \qquad\qquad\qquad\qquad G^2$$

$$A — E_1 \underset{g^1}{\|} \rightarrow B \underset{g^2}{——— E_2 \|} \rightarrow C$$

(unknown   (glucoside)   (cyanide)
precursor)

Tests on leaf extracts have been made for cyanide content before and after the addition of either glucoside or the enzyme E_2.

F_2 Ratio	Genotype	Leaf Extract Alone	Leaf Extract Plus Glucoside	Leaf Extract Plus E_2
9	$G^1\text{-}G^2\text{-}$	+	+	+
3	$G^1\text{-}g^2g^2$	0	0	+
3	$g^1g^1G^2\text{-}$	0	+	0
1	$g^1g^1g^2g^2$	0	0	0

Legend: + = cyanide present, 0 = no cyanide present.

If the leaves are phenotypically classified on the basis of cyanide content of extract alone, a ratio of 9 : 7 results. If the phenotypic classification is based either on extract plus glucoside or on extract plus E_2, a ratio of 12 : 4 is produced. If all of these tests form the basis of phenotypic classification, the classical 9 : 3 : 3 : 1 ratio emerges.

EPISTATIC INTERACTIONS

When epistasis is operative between two gene loci, the number of phenotypes appearing in the offspring from dihybrid parents will be less than 4. There are six types of epistatic ratios commonly recognized, three of which have 3 phenotypes and the other three having only 2 phenotypes.

1. Dominant Epistasis (12 : 3 : 1).

When the dominant allele at one locus, for example, the A allele, produces a certain phenotype regardless of the allelic condition of the other locus, then the A locus is said to be epistatic to the B locus. Furthermore, since the dominant allele A is able to express itself in the presence of either B or b, this is a case of dominant epistasis. Only when the genotype of the individual is homozygous recessive at the epistatic locus (aa) can the alleles of the hypostatic locus (B or b) be expressed. Thus the genotypes A-B- and A-bb produce the same phenotype, where as aaB- and aabb produce 2 additional phenotypes. The classical 9 : 3 : 3 : 1 ratio becomes modified into a 12 : 3 : 1 ratio.

2. Recessive Epistasis (9 : 3 : 4).

If the recessive genotype at one locus (e.g., aa) suppresses the expression of alleles at the B locus, the A locus is said to exhibit recessive epistasis over the B locus. Only if the dominant allele is present at the A locus can the alleles of the hypostatic B locus be expressed. The genotypes A-B- and A-bb produce two additional phenotypes. The 9 : 3 : 3 : 1 ratio becomes a 9 : 3 : 4 ratio.

3. Duplicate Genes with Cumulative Effect (9 : 6 : 1).

If the dominant condition (either homozygous or heterozygous) at either locus (but not both) produces the same phenotype, the F_2 ratio becomes 9 : 6 : 1. For example, where the epistatic genes are involved in producing various amounts of a substance such as pigment, the dominant genotypes of each locus may be considered to produce one unit of pigment independently. Thus genotypes A-bb and aaB- produce one unit of pigment each and therefore have the same phenotype. The genotype *aabb* produces no pigment, but in the genotype *A-B-* the effect is cumulative and two units of pigment are produced.

4. Duplicate Dominant Genes (15 : 1).

The $9:3:3:1$ ratio is modified into a $15:1$ ratio if the dominant alleles of both loci each produce the same phenotype without cumulative effect.

5. Duplicate Recessive Genes (9 : 7).

In the case where identical phenotypes are produced by both homozygous recessive genotypes, the F_2 ratio becomes $9:7$. The genotypes *aaB-*, *A-bb*, and *aabb* produce one phenotype. Both dominant alleles, when present together, complement each other and produce a different phenotype.

6. Dominant-and-Recessive Interaction (13 : 3).

Only two F_2 phenotypes result when a dominant genotype at one locus (e.g., *A-*) and the recessive genotype at the other (*bb*) produce the same phenotypic effect. Thus *A-B-*, *A-bb*, and *aabb* produce one phenotype and *aaB-* produces another in the ratio $13:3$ (see Table 4.1).

Table 4.1. Summary of Epistatic Ratios

Genotypes	*A-B-*	*A-bb*	*aaB-*	*aabb*
Classical ratio	9	3	3	1
Dominant epistasis	12		3	1
Recessive epistasis	9	3	4	
Duplicate genes with cumulative effect	9	6		1
Duplicate dominant genes	15			1
Duplicate recessive genes	9	7		
Dominant and recessive interaction	13		3	

NONEPISTATIC INTERACTIONS

Genetic interaction may also occur without epistasis if the end products of different pathways each contribute to the same trait.

Example 4.2. The dull-red eye color characteristic of wild-type flies is a mixture of two kinds of pigments (B and D) each produced from nonpigmented compounds (A and C) by the action of different enzymes (e_1 and e_2) specified by different wild-type genes (g_1^+ and g_2^+).

$$g_1^+$$
$$\downarrow$$
$$A \longrightarrow e_1 \longrightarrow B$$
$$\left.\begin{array}{c} \\ \\ \end{array}\right\} \text{mixture} = \text{wild-type eye color}$$
$$C \longrightarrow e_2 \longrightarrow D$$
$$\uparrow$$
$$g_2^+$$

The recessive alleles at these two loci (g_1 and g_2) specify enzymatically inactive proteins. Thus a genotype without either dominant allele would not produce any pigmented compounds and the eye color would be white.

Phenotypes	Genotypes	End Products
Wild type	$g_1^+/-,\ g_2^+/-$	B and D
Color B	$g_1^+/-,\ g_2/g_2$	B and C
Color D	$g_1/g_1,\ g_2^+/-$	D and A
White	$g_1/g_1,\ g_2/g_2$	A and C

In the above example, the genes for color B and color D are both dominant to white, but when they occur together they produce a novel phenotype (wild type) by interaction. If the two genes are assorting independently, the classical $9:3:3:1$ ratio will not be disturbed.

Example 4.3. A brown ommochrome pigment is produced in *Drosophila melanogaster* by a dominant gene st^+ on chromosome 3. A scarlet pterin pigment is produced by a dominant gene bw^+ on chromosome 2. The recessive alleles at these 2 loci produce no pigment. When pure scarlet flies are mated to pure brown flies, a novel phenotype (wild type) appears in the progeny.

$$
\begin{array}{lll}
\text{P:} & \text{brown} \times \text{scarlet} \\
& st^+/st^+,\ bw/bw \qquad st/st, bw^+/bw^+ \\
\\
\text{F}_1: & \text{wild type} \\
& st^+/st,\ bw^+/bw \\
\\
\text{F}_2: & 9\ st^+/-,\ bw^+/- \quad \text{wild type} \\
& 3\ st^+/-,\ bw/bw \quad \text{brown} \\
& 3\ st/st,\ bw^+/- \quad \text{scarlet} \\
& 1\ st/st,\ bw/bw \quad \text{white}
\end{array}
$$

INTERACTIONS WITH THREE OR MORE FACTORS

Recall from Chapter 3 that the progeny from trihybrid parents are expected in the phenotypic ratio $27:9:9:9:3:3:3:1$. This classical ratio can also be modified whenever two or all three of the loci interact. Interactions involving four or more loci are also possible. Most genes probably depend to some extent upon other genes in the total genotype. The total phenotype depends upon interactions of the total genotype with the environment.

PLEIOTROPISM

Many and perhaps most of the biochemical pathways in the living organism are interconnected and often interdependent. Products of one reaction chain may be used in several other metabolic schemes. It is not surprising, therefore, that the phenotypic expression of a gene usually involves more than one trait. Sometimes one trait will be clearly evident (major effect) and other, perhaps seemingly unrelated ramifications (secondary effects) will be less evident to the casual observer. In other cases, a number of related changes may be considered together as a **syndrome.** All of the manifold phenotypic expressions of a single gene are spoken of as **pleiotropic** gene effects.

Example 4.4. The syndrome called "sickle-cell anemia" in humans is due to an abnormal hemoglobin. This is the primary effect of the mutant gene. Subsidiary effects of the abnormal hemoglobin include the sickle shape of the cells and their tendency to clump together and clog blood vessels in various organs of the body. As a result, heart, kidney, spleen, and brain damage are common elements of the syndrome. Defective corpuscles are readily destroyed in the body, causing severe anemia.

Solved Problems

TWO-FACTOR INTERACTIONS

4.1. Coat colors of dogs depend upon the action of at least 2 genes. At one locus a dominant epistatic inhibitor of coat color pigment (I-) prevents the expression of color alleles at another independently assorting locus, producing white coat color. When the recessive condition exists at the inhibitor locus (ii), the alleles of the hypostatic locus may be expressed, iiB- producing black and $iibb$ producing brown. When dihybrid white dogs are mated together, determine (a) the phenotypic proportions expected in the progeny, (b) the chance of choosing, from among the white progeny, a genotype homozygous at both loci.

Solution:

(a)

$$\text{P:}\qquad \underset{\text{white}}{IiBb} \times \underset{\text{white}}{IiBb}$$

$$\text{F}_1:\qquad
\left.\begin{array}{l} 9/16\ I\text{-}B\text{-} \\ 3/16\ I\text{-}bb \end{array}\right\} = 12/16\ \text{white}$$

$$3/16\ iiB\text{-} = 3/16\ \text{black}$$
$$1/16\ iibb = 1/16\ \text{brown}$$

(b) The genotypic proportions among the white progeny are as follows:

		Proportion of Total F_1	Proportion of White F_1
$\frac{1}{4}II$	$\frac{1}{4}BB$	1/16 $IIBB$	1/12
	$\frac{1}{2}Bb$	2/16 $IIBb$	2/12
	$\frac{1}{4}bb$	1/16 $IIbb$	1/12
$\frac{1}{2}Ii$	$\frac{1}{4}BB$	2/16 $IiBB$	2/12
	$\frac{1}{2}Bb$	4/16 $IiBb$	4/12
	$\frac{1}{4}bb$	2/16 $Iibb$	2/12
Totals:		12/16	12/12

The only homozygous genotypes at both loci in the above list are $\frac{1}{12}IIBB$ and $\frac{1}{12}IIbb = \frac{2}{12}$ or $\frac{1}{6}$ of all the white progeny. Thus there is 1 chance in 6 of choosing a homozygous genotype from among the white progeny.

4.2. Two white-flowered strains of the sweet pea (*Lathyrus odoratus*) were crossed, producing an F_1 with only purple flowers. Random crossing among the F_1 produced 96 progeny plants, 53 exhibiting purple flowers, and 43 with white flowers. (a) What phenotypic ratio is approximated by the F_2? (b) What type of interaction is involved? (c) What were the probable genotypes of the parental strains?

Solution:

(a) To determine the phenotypic ratio in terms of familiar sixteenths, the following proportion for white flowers may be made: $43/96 = x/16$, from which $x = 7.2$. That is, 7.2 white : 8.8 purple, or approximately a $7:9$ ratio. We might just as well have arrived at the same conclusion by establishing the proportion for purple flowers: $53/96 = x/16$, from which $x = 8.8$ purple.

(b) A $7:9$ ratio is characteristic of duplicate recessive genes where the recessive genotype at either or both of the loci produces the same phenotype.

(c) If aa or bb or both could produce white flowers, then only the genotype A-B- could produce purple. For two white parental strains (pure lines) to be able to produce an all-purple F_1, they must be homozygous for different dominant-recessive combinations. Thus

P: $aaBB \times AAbb$
            white   white

F$_1$: $AaBb$
                    purple

F$_2$:   9/16 $A\text{-}B\text{-}$ = 9/16 purple
               3/16 $A\text{-}bb$ ⎫
               3/16 $aaB\text{-}$ ⎬ = 7/16 white
               1/16 $aabb$ ⎭

4.3. Red color in wheat kernels is produced by the genotype $R\text{-}B\text{-}$, white by the double-recessive genotype ($rrbb$). The genotypes $R\text{-}bb$ and $rrB\text{-}$ produce brown kernels. A homozygous red variety is crossed to a white variety. (*a*) What phenotypic results are expected in the F$_1$ and F$_2$? (*b*) If the brown F$_2$ is artificially crossed at random (wheat is normally self-fertilized), what phenotypic and genotypic proportions are expected in the offspring?

Solution:

(*a*)   P: $RRBB \times rrbb$
                                                   red   white

                                       F$_1$: $RrBb$
                                                           red

                                       F$_2$:   9/16 $R\text{-}B\text{-}$ = 9/16 red
                                                      3/16 $R\text{-}bb$ ⎫
                                                      3/16 $rrB\text{-}$ ⎬ = 6/16 brown
                                                      1/16 $rrbb$ = 1/16 white

(*b*) The proportion of genotypes represented among the brown F$_2$ must first be determined.

	Proportion of Total F$_2$	Proportion of Brown F$_2$
$(\frac{1}{4}RR)(\frac{1}{4}bb)$	1/16 $RRbb$	1/6
$(\frac{1}{2}Rr)(\frac{1}{4}bb)$	2/16 $Rrbb$	2/6
$(\frac{1}{4}rr)(\frac{1}{4}BB)$	1/16 $rrBB$	1/6
$(\frac{1}{4}rr)(\frac{1}{2}Bb)$	2/16 $rrBb$	2/6
Totals:	6/16	6/6

Next, the relative frequencies of the various matings may be calculated in a checkerboard.

	1/6 $RRbb$	2/6 $Rrbb$	1/6 $rrBB$	2/6 $rrBb$
1/6 $RRbb$	1/36 $RRbb \times RRbb$ (1)	2/36 $RRbb \times Rrbb$ (2)	1/36 $RRbb \times rrBB$ (3)	2/36 $RRbb \times rrBb$ (4)
2/6 $Rrbb$	2/36 $Rrbb \times RRbb$ (2)	4/36 $Rrbb \times Rrbb$ (5)	2/36 $Rrbb \times rrBB$ (6)	4/36 $Rrbb \times rrBb$ (7)
1/6 $rrBB$	1/36 $rrBB \times RRbb$ (3)	2/36 $rrBB \times Rrbb$ (6)	1/36 $rrBB \times rrBB$ (8)	2/36 $rrBB \times rrBb$ (9)
2/6 $rrBb$	2/36 $rrBb \times RRbb$ (4)	4/36 $rrBb \times Rrbb$ (7)	2/36 $rrBb \times rrBB$ (9)	4/36 $rrBb \times rrBb$ (10)

Matings	Progeny	Genotypic Proportions (f)	Mating Frequency (m)	m · f
(1) RRbb × RRbb	RRbb	100%	1/36	1/36
(2) RRbb × Rrbb	RRbb	1/2	4/36	4/72
	Rrbb	1/2		4/72
(3) RRbb × rrBB	RrBb	100%	2/36	2/36
(4) RRbb × rrBb	RrBb	1/2	4/36	4/72
	Rrbb	1/2		4/72
(5) Rrbb × Rrbb	RRbb	1/4	4/36	4/144
	Rrbb	1/2		4/72
	rrbb	1/4		4/144
(6) Rrbb × rrBB	RrBb	1/2	4/36	4/72
	rrBb	1/2		4/72
(7) Rrbb × rrBb	RrBb	1/4	8/36	8/144
	rrBb	1/4		8/144
	Rrbb	1/4		8/144
	rrbb	1/4		8/144
(8) rrBB × rrBB	rrBB	100%	1/36	1/36
(9) rrBb × rrBB	rrBB	1/2	4/36	4/72
	rrBb	1/2		4/72
(10) rrBb × rrBb	rrBB	1/4	4/36	4/144
	rrBb	1/2		4/72
	rrbb	1/4		4/144

Summary of progeny genotypes:
1/9 RRbb
2/9 RrBb
2/9 Rrbb
1/9 rrBB
2/9 rrBb
1/9 rrbb

Summary of progeny phenotypes:
2/9 R-B- = 2/9 red
1/3 R-bb ⎫
1/3 rrB- ⎭ = 2/3 brown

1/9 rrbb = 1/9 white

4.4. The following pedigree shows the transmission of swine coat colors through three generations:

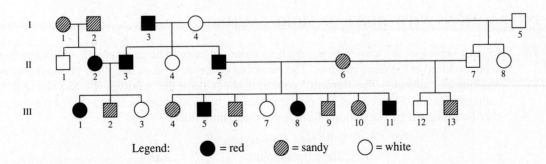

Legend: ● = red   ◩ = sandy   ○ = white

Assume the offspring of II5 × II6 shown in this pedigree occur in the ratio expected from the genotypes represented by their parents. How are these colors most likely inherited?

Solution:

Notice first that 3 phenotypes are expressed in this pedigree. This rules out epistatic combinations producing only 2 phenotypes such as those expressed in dominant and recessive interaction (13 : 3), duplicate dominant genes (15 : 1), and duplicate recessive genes (9 : 7). Epistatic gene interactions producing three phenotypes are those expressed in dominant epistasis ($12:3:1$), recessive epistasis ($9:3:4$), and dominant genes with cumulative action ($9:6:1$). Let us proceed to solve this problem by making an assumption and then applying it to the pedigree to see if the phenotypes shown there can be explained by our hypothesis.

Case 1. Assume dominant epistasis is operative. The genotypes responsible for the 3 phenotypes may be represented as follows: *A-B-* and *A-bb* = first phenotype, *aaB-* = second phenotype, and *aabb* = third phenotype. We must now determine which of the phenotypes represented in this pedigree corresponds to each of the genotypic classes. Obviously the only pure-line phenotype is the third one. Offspring of the mating *aabb* × *aabb* would all be phenotypically identical to the parents. The mating I4 × I5 appears to qualify in this respect and we shall tentatively assume that white coat color is represented by the genotype *aabb*. Certain matings between individuals with the dominant epistatic gene (*A*) could produce three phenotypically different types of offspring (e.g., *AaBb* × *AaBb*). Such a mating is observed between II2 and II3. Therefore we might assume red color to be represented by the genotype *A-*. Sandy color must then be represented by genotype *aaB-*. Matings between sandy individuals could produce only sandy (*aaB-*) or white (*aabb*) progeny. However, sandy parents I1 × I2 produce white and red progeny (II1, II2). Therefore the assumption of dominant interaction must be wrong.

Case 2. Assume recessive epistasis to be operative. The genotypes responsible for the 3 phenotypes in this case may be represented as follows: *A-B-* as first phenotype, *A-bb* as second phenotype, and *aaB-* and *aabb* as third phenotype. As pointed out in Case 1, matings between individuals of genotype *AaBb* are the only kind among identical phenotypes capable of producing all three phenotypes in the progeny. Thus *A-B-* should represent red (e.g., II2 × II3). The *aa* genotypes breed true, producing only white individuals (I4 × I5). Sandy is produced by genotype *A-bb*. Sandy × sandy (I1 × I2) could not produce the red offspring (II2). Therefore the assumption of recessive interaction must be wrong.

Case 3. Assume that duplicate genes with cumulative action are interacting. The genotypes responsible for the 3 phenotypes in this case may be represented as follows: *A-B-* as first phenotype, *A-bb* and *aaB-* as second phenotype, and *aabb* as third phenotype. As explained in the previous two cases, *A-B-* must be red and *aabb* must be white. If we assume that any dominant genotype at either the A locus or B locus contributes one unit of pigment to the phenotype, then either the genotype *aaB-* or *A-bb* could be sandy; we further assume that the presence of both dominant genes (*A-B-*) would contribute two units of pigment to produce a red phenotype. Thus the mating II5 (*AaBb*) red × II6 (*aaBb*) sandy would be expected to produce offspring phenotypes in the following proportions:

$$
\begin{array}{lll}
\text{Red} & A\text{-}B\text{-} & \frac{1}{2}\cdot\frac{3}{4}=\frac{3}{8} \\[4pt]
\text{Sandy} & \begin{cases} A\text{-}bb & \frac{1}{2}\cdot\frac{1}{4}=\frac{1}{8} \\ aaB\text{-} & \frac{1}{2}\cdot\frac{3}{4}=\frac{3}{8} \end{cases} & \Big\}\ \ \tfrac{1}{2} \\[4pt]
\text{White} & aabb & \frac{1}{2}\cdot\frac{1}{4}=\frac{1}{8}
\end{array}
$$

The same phenotypic ratio would be expected if II6 were *Aabb*. These expectations correspond to the ones given in the pedigree (III4–III11) and therefore the hypothesis of dominant genes with cumulative action is consistent with the data.

INTERACTIONS WITH THREE OR MORE FACTORS

4.5. At least three loci are known to govern coat colors in mice. The genotype *C-* will allow pigment to be produced at the other two loci. The recessive genotype *cc* does not allow pigment production, resulting in "albino." The "agouti" pattern depends upon the genotype *A-*, and nonagouti upon the recessive *aa*. The color of the pigment may be black (*B-*) or chocolate (*bb*). Five coat colors may be produced by the action of alleles at these three loci:

Wild type (agouti, black)	*A-B-C-*
Black (nonagouti)	*aaB-C-*
Chocolate (nonagouti)	*aabbC-*
Cinnamon (agouti, chocolate)	*A-bbC-*
Albino	*- - - -cc*

(*a*) What phenotypic frequencies are expected in the F_2 from crosses of pure black with albinos of type *AAbbcc*? (*b*) A cinnamon male is mated to a group of albino females of identical genotype and among their progeny were observed 43 wild type, 40 cinnamon, 39 black, 41 chocolate, and 168 albino. What are the most probable genotypes of the parents?

Solution:

(a) P: $aaBBCC \times AAbbcc$
pure black albino

F_1: $AaBbCc$
wild type

F_2: 27 A-B-C- wild type
9 A-B-cc albino
9 A-bbC- cinnamon
9 aaB-C- black
3 A-$bbcc$ albino
3 aaB-cc albino
3 $aabbC$- chocolate
1 $aabbcc$ albino

Summary of (a): 27/64 wild type
16/64 albino
9/64 cinnamon
9/64 black
3/64 chocolate

(b) P: A-bbC-♂ $\times$ $----cc$♀♀
cinnamon male albino females

F_1: 43 wild type A-B-C-
40 cinnamon A-bbC-

39 black aaB-C-
41 chocolate $aabbC$-

$\underline{168}$ albino $----cc$
331

In part (b), the cinnamon progeny, A-bbC-, indicate b in the female parents. The black progeny, aaB-C-, indicate a in both parents, and B in the female parents. The chocolate progeny, $aabbC$-, indicate a in both parents, and b in the females. The albinos indicate c in the male. The genotype of the male is now known to be $AabbCc$. But the genotype of the albino females is known only to be a-$Bbcc$. They could be either $AaBbcc$ or $aaBbcc$.

Case 1. Assume the females to be $AaBbcc$.

Parents: $AabbCc$♂ $\times$ $AaBbcc$♀♀

The expected phenotypic frequencies among the progeny would be:

A-$BbCc$ wild type $\frac{3}{4} \cdot \frac{1}{2} \cdot \frac{1}{2} = \frac{3}{16}(331) = $ approx. 62
A-$bbCc$ cinnamon $\frac{3}{4} \cdot \frac{1}{2} \cdot \frac{1}{2} = \frac{3}{16}(331) = $ approx. 62
$aaBbCc$ black $\frac{1}{4} \cdot \frac{1}{2} \cdot \frac{1}{2} = \frac{1}{16}(331) = $ approx. 21
$aabbCc$ chocolate $\frac{1}{4} \cdot \frac{1}{2} \cdot \frac{1}{2} = \frac{1}{16}(331) = $ approx. 21
$----cc$ albino $1 \cdot 1 \cdot \frac{1}{2} = \frac{1}{2}(331) = $ approx. 166

Obviously, the expectations deviate considerably from the observations. Therefore, the females are probably not of genotype $AaBbcc$.

Case 2. Assume the females to be of genotype $aaBbcc$.

Parents: $AabbCc$♂ $\times$ $aaBbcc$♀♀

The expected phenotypic frequencies among the progeny would be:

$AaBbCc$ wild type $\frac{1}{2} \cdot \frac{1}{2} \cdot \frac{1}{2} = \frac{1}{8}(331) = $ approx. 41
$AabbCc$ cinnamon $\frac{1}{2} \cdot \frac{1}{2} \cdot \frac{1}{2} = \frac{1}{8}(331) = $ approx. 41
$aaBbCc$ black $\frac{1}{2} \cdot \frac{1}{2} \cdot \frac{1}{2} = \frac{1}{8}(331) = $ approx. 41
$aabbCc$ chocolate $\frac{1}{2} \cdot \frac{1}{2} \cdot \frac{1}{2} = \frac{1}{8}(331) = $ approx. 41
$----cc$ albino $1 \cdot 1 \cdot \frac{1}{2} = \frac{1}{2}(331) = $ approx. 166

Now the expectations correspond very closely to the observations. Hence the genotype of the parental albino females is probably $aaBbcc$.

4.6. Lewis-a blood group substance appears on the human red blood cell when the dominant gene Le is present, but is absent if the dominant gene of the "secretor" locus Se is present. Suppose that from a number of families where both parents are Lewis-a negative of genotype $LeleSese$, we find that most of them have 3 Lewis-a positive : 13 Lewis-a negative children. In a few other families, suppose we find 2 Lewis-a negative : 1 Lewis-a positive. Furthermore, in families where both parents are secretors of genotype $Sese$, we find most of them exhibit a ratio of 3 secretor :

1 nonsecretor, but a few of them show 9 secretor : 7 nonsecretor. Propose a hypothesis to account for these results.

Solution:

If only two loci are interacting, the dominant *Se* gene can suppress the expression of *Le*, resulting in Lewis-a negative blood type. When both parents are dihybrid, we expect a 13 : 3 ratio in the progeny characteristic of dominant and recessive interaction.

P: *LeleSese* × *LeleSese*
              Lewis-a neg.   Lewis-a neg.

F_1:   9 *Le-Se-* ⎫
                3 *leleSe-* ⎬ = 13 Lewis-a negative
                1 *lelesese* ⎭
                3 *Le-sese* = 3 Lewis-a positive

The 9 : 7 ratio found in some families for the secretor trait indicates that two factors are again interacting. This is the ratio produced by duplicate recessive interaction; i.e., whenever the recessive alleles at either of two loci are present, a nonsecretor phenotype results. Let us symbolize the alleles of the second locus by *X* and *x*.

P: *SeseXx* × *SeseXx*
            secretor   secretor

F_1:   9 *Se-X-* = 9 secretors
              3 *Se-xx* ⎫
              3 *seseX-* ⎬ = 7 nonsecretors; the *xx* genotype suppresses the expression of *Se*.
              1 *sesexx* ⎭

If we assume the *x* gene to be relatively rare, then most families will have only the dominant gene *X*, but in a few families both parents will be heterozygous *Xx*. Let us assume that this is the case in those families that produce 2 Lewis-a negative : 1 Lewis-a positive.

P: *LeleSeseXx* × *LeleSeseXx*
             Lewis-a negative   Lewis-a negative

F_1:   27 *Le-Se-X-*
                *9 *Le-Se-xx*
                *9 *Le-seseX-*
                 9 *leleSe-X-*
                *3 *Le-sesexx*
                 3 *leleSe-xx*
                 3 *leleseseX-*
                 1 *lelesesexx*

If *Se* suppresses *Le*, but *xx* suppresses *Se*, then only the genotypes marked with an asterisk (*) will be Lewis-a positive, giving a ratio of 21 Lewis-a positive : 43 Lewis-a negative. This is very close to a 1 : 2 ratio and indeed would appear to be such with limited data.

Supplementary Problems

TWO-FACTOR INTERACTIONS

4.7.   When homozygous yellow rats are crossed to homozygous black rats, the F_1 is all gray. Mating the F_1 among themselves produced an F_2 consisting of 10 yellow, 28 gray, 2 cream-colored, and 8 black. (*a*) How are these colors inherited? (*b*) Show, using appropriate genetic symbols, the genotypes for each color. (*c*) How many of the 48 F_2 rats were expected to be cream-colored? (*d*) How many of the 48 F_2 rats were expected to be homozygous?

4.8. Four comb shapes in poultry are known to be governed by two gene loci. The genotype *R-P-* produces walnut comb, characteristic of the Malay breed; *R-pp* produces rose comb, characteristic of the Wyandotte breed; *rrP-* produces pea comb, characteristic of the Brahma breed; *rrpp* produces single comb, characteristic of the Leghorn breed. (a) If pure Wyandottes are crossed with pure Brahmas, what phenotypic ratios are expected in the F$_1$ and F$_2$? (b) A Malay hen was crossed to a Leghorn cock and produced a dozen eggs, 3 of which grew into birds with rose combs and 9 with walnut combs. What is the probable genotype of the hen? (c) Determine the proportion of comb types that would be expected in offspring from each of the following crosses: (1) *Rrpp* × *RrPP*, (2) *rrPp* × *RrPp*, (3) *rrPP* × *RRPp*, (4) *RrPp* × *rrpp*, (5) *RrPp* × *RRpp*, (6) *RRpp* × *rrpp*, (7) *RRPP* × *rrpp*, (8) *Rrpp* × *Rrpp*, (9) *rrPp* × *Rrpp*, (10) *rrPp* × *rrpp*.

4.9. Listed below are 7 two-factor interaction ratios observed in progeny from various dihybrid parents. Suppose that in each case one of the dihybrid parents is testcrossed (instead of being mated to another dihybrid individual). What phenotypic ratio is expected in the progeny of each testcross? (a) 9 : 6 : 1, (b) 9 : 3 : 4, (c) 9 : 7, (d) 15 : 1, (e) 12 : 3 : 1, (f) 9 : 3 : 3 : 1, (g) 13 : 3.

4.10. White fruit color in summer squash is governed by a dominant gene (*W*) and colored fruit by its recessive allele (*w*). Yellow fruit is governed by an independently assorting hypostatic gene (*G*) and green by its recessive allele (*g*). When dihybrid plants are crossed, the offspring appear in the ratio 12 white : 3 yellow : 1 green. What fruit color ratios are expected from the crosses (a) *Wwgg* × *WwGG*, (b) *WwGg* × green, (c) *Wwgg* × *wwGg*, (d) *WwGg* × *Wwgg*? (e) If 2 plants are crossed producing $\frac{1}{2}$ yellow and $\frac{1}{2}$ green progeny, what are the genotypes and phenotypes of the parents?

4.11. Matings between black rats of identical genotype produced offspring as follows: 14 cream-colored, 47 black, and 19 albino. (a) What epistatic ratio is approximated by these offspring? (b) What type of epistasis is operative? (c) What are the genotypes of the parents and the offspring (use your own symbols)?

4.12. A dominant gene *S* in *Drosophila* produces a peculiar eye condition called "star." Its recessive allele *S$^+$* produces the normal eye of wild type. The expression of *S* can be suppressed by the dominant allele of another locus, *Su-S*. The recessive allele of this locus, *Su-S$^+$*, has no effect on *S$^+$*. (a) What type of interaction is operative? (b) When a normal-eyed male of genotype *Su-S/Su-S, S/S* is crossed to a homozygous wild-type female of genotype *Su-S$^+$/Su-S$^+$, S$^+$/S$^+$*, what phenotypic ratio is expected in the F$_1$ and F$_2$? (c) What percentage of the wild-type F$_2$ is expected to carry the dominant gene for star-eye?

4.13. The Black Langshan breed of chickens has feathered shanks. When Langshans are crossed to the Buff Rock breed with unfeathered shanks, all the F$_1$ have feathered shanks. Out of 360 F$_2$ progeny, 24 were found to have nonfeathered shanks and 336 had feathered shanks. (a) What is the mode of interaction in this trait? (b) What proportion of the feathered F$_2$ would be expected to be heterozygous at one locus and homozygous at the other?

4.14. On chromosome 3 of corn there is a dominant gene (*A$_1$*), which, together with the dominant gene (*A2*) on chromosome 9, produces colored aleurone. All other genetic combinations produce colorless aleurone. Two pure colorless strains are crossed to produce an all-colored F$_1$. (a) What were the genotypes of the parental strains and the F$_1$? (b) What phenotypic proportions are expected among the F$_2$? (c) What genotypic ratio exists among the white F$_2$?

4.15. Two pairs of alleles govern the color of onion bulbs. A pure-red strain crossed to a pure-white strain produces an all-red F$_1$. The F$_2$ was found to consist of 47 white, 38 yellow, and 109 red bulbs. (a) What epistatic ratio is approximated by the data? (b) What is the name of this type of gene interaction? (c) If another F$_2$ is produced by the same kind of a cross, and 8 bulbs of the F$_2$ are found to be of the double-recessive genotype, how many bulbs would be expected in each phenotypic class?

4.16. A plant of the genus *Capsella*, commonly called "shepherd's purse," produces a seed capsule, the shape of which is controlled by two independently assorting genes. When dihybrid plants were interpollinated, 6% of the progeny were found to possess ovoid-shaped seed capsules. The other 94% of the progeny had triangular-shaped seed capsules. (a) What two-factor epistatic ratio is approximated by the progeny? (b) What type of interaction is operative?

4.17. The color of corn aleurone is known to be controlled by several genes; A, C, and R are all necessary for color to be produced. The locus of a dominant inhibitor of aleurone color, I, is very closely linked to that of C. Thus any one or more of the genotypes I-, aa-, cc-, or rr- produces colorless aleurone. (a) What would be the colored : colorless ratio among F_2 progeny from the cross $AAIICCRR \times aaiiCCRR$? (b) What proportion of the colorless F_2 is expected to be homozygous?

4.18. A dominant allele C must be present in order for any pigment to be developed in mice. The kind of pigment produced depends upon another locus such that B- produces black and bb produces brown. Individuals of epistatic genotype cc are incapable of making pigment and are called "albinos." A homozygous black female is testcrossed to an albino male. (a) What phenotypic ratio is expected in the F_1 and F_2? (b) If all the albino F_2 mice are allowed to mate at random, what genotypic ratio is expected in the progeny?

4.19. Suppose that crossing two homozygous lines of white clover, each with a low content of cyanide, produces only progeny with high levels of cyanide. When these F_1 progeny are backcrossed to either parental line, half the progeny has low cyanide content and the other half has high cyanide content. (a) What type of interaction may account for these results? (b) What phenotypic ratio is expected in the F_2? (c) If a 12 : 4 ratio is observed among progeny from parents with high cyanide content, what are the parental genotypes? (d) If the low cyanide F_2, exclusive of the double recessives, are allowed to cross at random among themselves, what proportion of their progeny is expected to contain a high cyanide content?

4.20. In cultivated flowers called "stocks," the recessive genotype of one locus (aa) prevents the development of pigment in the flower, thus producing a white color. In the presence of the dominant allele A, alleles at another locus may be expressed as follows: C- = red, cc = cream. (a) When cream stocks of the genotype $Aacc$ are crossed to red stocks of the genotype $AaCc$, what phenotypic and genotypic proportions are expected in the progeny? (b) If cream stocks crossed to red stocks produce white progeny, what may be the genotypes of the parents? (c) When dihybrid red stocks are crossed together, what phenotypic ratio is expected among the progeny? (d) If red stocks crossed to white stocks produce progeny with red, cream and white flowers, what are the genotypes of the parents?

4.21. An inhibitor of pigment production in onion bulbs (I-) exhibits dominant epistasis over another locus, the genotype iiR- producing red bulbs and $iirr$ producing yellow bulbs. (a) A pure-white strain is crossed to a pure-red strain and produces an all-white F_1 and an F_2 with $\frac{12}{16}$ white, $\frac{3}{16}$ red and $\frac{1}{16}$ yellow. What were the genotypes of the parents? (b) If yellow onions are crossed to a pure-white strain of a genotype different from the parental type in part (a), what phenotypic ratio is expected in the F_1 and F_2? (c) Among the white F_2 of part (a), suppose that 32 were found to be of genotype $IiRR$. How many progeny are expected in each of the three F_2 phenotypic classes?

4.22. For color to be produced in corn kernels, the dominant alleles at three loci must be present (A, C, R). Another locus is hypostatic to these three loci; the dominant allele of this locus (Pr) yields purple pigment and the recessive allele (pr) determines red kernels. (a) What phenotypic proportions are expected in the F_1 and F_2 when a red strain of genotype $AACCRRprpr$ is crossed to a colorless strain of genotype $AACCrrPrPr$? (b) If the red F_2 are crossed among themselves, what genotypic and phenotypic ratios are expected among the progeny?

4.23. Crossing certain genetically identical monohybrid white-bulbed onions produces white and colored progeny in the ratio 3 : 1, respectively. Crossing certain genetically identical monohybrid colored-bulbed onions produces colored and white progeny in the ratio 3 : 1, respectively. White is epistatic to color. (a) What phenotypic ratio is expected among the F_1 and F_2 progeny produced by testcrossing a white variety homozygous for the dominant alleles at two independently assorting loci? (b) What type of interaction is operative? (c) Suppose that the dominant condition (I-) at one locus and/or the recessive condition at the other (cc) could both produce white onion bulbs. White onions of genotype I-C-, in the presence of ammonia fumes, turn yellow. Onions which are white due to the action of cc in their genotype fail to change color in the presence of ammonia fumes. A white plant that turns yellow in ammonia fumes is crossed to a white one that does not change color. The progeny occur in the proportions $\frac{7}{8}$ white : $\frac{1}{8}$ colored. What are the genotypes of the parents? (d) A white plant which changes color in ammonia fumes is crossed to a colored plant. The progeny occur in the ratio 3 colored : 5 white. Determine the genotypes of the parents.

4.24. The color of the flower center in the common yellow daisy may be either purple-centered or yellow-centered. Two genes (*P* and *Y*) are known to interact in this trait. The results of two matings are given below:

(1)

P: $PpYY$ $\times$ $PpYY$
      purple-centered   purple-centered

F₁: $\frac{3}{4}$ P-YY purple-centered
          $\frac{1}{4}$ $ppYY$ yellow-centered

(2)

P: $ppYy$ $\times$ $ppYy$
       yellow-centered   yellow-centered

F₁: $\left.\begin{array}{l}\frac{3}{4}\,ppY\text{-}\\[4pt]\frac{1}{4}\,ppyy\end{array}\right\}$ all yellow-centered

Determine the phenotypic ratios of progeny from the matings (*a*) $PpYy \times PpYy$, (*b*) $PpYy \times ppyy$, (*c*) $PPyy \times ppYY$.

4.25. The aleurone of corn kernels may be either yellow, white, or purple. When pollen from a homozygous purple plant is used to fertilize a homozygous white plant, the aleurone of the resulting kernels are all purple. When homozygous yellow plants are crossed to homozygous white plants, only seeds with yellow aleurone are produced. When homozygous purple plants are crossed to homozygous yellow plants, only purple progeny appear. Some crosses between purple plants produce purple, yellow, and white progeny. Some crosses between yellow plants produce both yellow and white offspring. Crosses between yellow plants never produce purple progeny. Crosses among plants produced from seeds with white aleurone always produce only white progeny. (*a*) Can these results be explained on the basis of the action of a single-gene locus with multiple alleles? (*b*) What is the simplest explanation for the mode of gene action? (*c*) If plants with only dominant alleles at the two loci are crossed to plants grown from white seeds, what phenotypic proportions are expected among their F₂ progeny? (*d*) In part (*c*), how many generations of seeds must be planted in order to obtain an F₂ progeny phenotypically expressing the aleurone genes derived from the adult parent sporophytes? (*e*) What is the advantage of studying the genetics of seed traits rather than traits of the sporophyte?

4.26. Three fruit shapes are recognized in the summer squash (*Cucurbita pepo*): disc-shaped, elongated, and sphere-shaped. A pure disc-shaped variety was crossed to a pure elongated variety. The F₁ were all disc-shaped. Among 80 F₂, there were 30 sphere-shaped, 5 elongated, and 45 disc-shaped. (*a*) Reduce the F₂ numbers to their lowest ratio. (*b*) What types of interaction is operative? (*c*) If the sphere-shaped F₂ cross at random, what phenotypic proportions are expected in the progeny?

4.27. Some crosses between yellow mice produce $\frac{2}{3}$ yellow and $\frac{1}{3}$ agouti offspring. A locus epistatic to the "yellow locus" prevents any pigment formation, resulting in albinos. Some crosses between colored parents produce $\frac{3}{4}$ colored and $\frac{1}{4}$ albino progeny. A cross between a yellow male and an albino female produced $\frac{1}{2}$ albino, $\frac{1}{4}$ yellow, and $\frac{1}{4}$ agouti offspring. (*a*) What are the most likely genotypes of the parents (use your own gene symbols)? (*b*) If the yellow F₁ mice from part (*a*) are crossed among themselves, what phenotypic ratio is expected among their offspring? (*c*) What proportion of the yellow offspring from part (*b*) would be expected to breed true?

4.28. The pedigree on the right illustrates a case of dominant epistasis. (*a*) What symbol represents the genotype *A-B-*? (*b*) What symbol represents the genotype *aaB-*? (*c*) What symbol represents the genotype *aabb*? (*d*) What type of epistasis would be represented if II2 × II3 produced, in addition to ☐ and ◍, an offspring of type ● ? (*e*) What type of interaction would be represented if III5 × III6 produced, in addition to ▨ and ○, an offspring of type ● ?

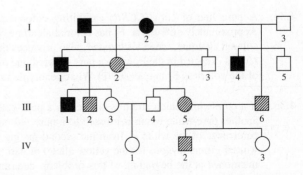

4.29. Given the following pedigree showing three generations of mink breeding, where open symbols represent wild type and solid symbols represent platinum, determine (*a*) the mode of inheritance of these coat colors, (*b*) the most probable genotypes of all individuals in the pedigree (use of familiar symbols such as *A,a* and *B,b* are suitable), (*c*) what phenotypic proportions are expected in progeny from III1 × III2.

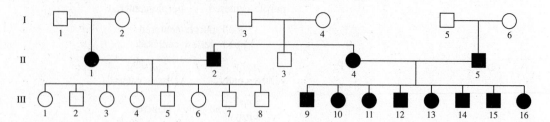

4.30. The pedigree in Fig. (*a*) shows the genetic transmission of feather color in chickens. Open symbols represent white feathers, solid symbols represent colored feathers. Under the assumption of dominant and recessive interaction (given *A-* or *bb* or both = white, *aaB-* = color) assign genotypes to each individual in the pedigree. Indicate by (-) whatever genes cannot be determined.

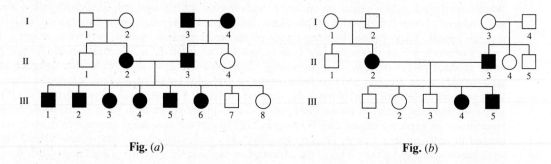

Fig. (*a*)   Fig. (*b*)

4.31. The pedigree in Fig. (*b*) shows the inheritance of deafness in humans. Open symbols represent normal hearing and solid symbols represent deafness. Under the assumption of duplicate recessive interaction (given *A-B-* = normal, *aa* or *bb* or both = deaf) assign genotypes to each individual in the pedigree. Indicate by (-) whatever genes cannot be determined.

INTERACTIONS WITH THREE OR MORE FACTORS

4.32. A wheat variety with colored seeds is crossed to a colorless strain producing an all-colored F_1. In the F_2, $\frac{1}{64}$ of the progeny has colorless seeds. (*a*) How many pairs of genes control seed color? (*b*) What were the genotypes of the parents and the F_1 (use your own symbols)?

4.33. In mice, spotted coat color is due to a recessive gene *s* and solid coat color to its dominant allele *S*. Colored mice possess a dominant allele *C* whereas albinos are homozygous recessive *cc*. Black is produced by a dominant allele *B* and brown by its recessive allele *b*. The *cc* genotype is epistatic to both the B and S loci. What phenotypic ratio is expected among the progeny of trihybrid parents?

4.34. A pure line of corn (*CCRR*) exhibiting colored aleurone is testcrossed to a colorless aleurone strain. Approximately 56% of the F_2 has colored aleurone, the other 44% being colorless. A pure line (*AARR*) with colored aleurone, when testcrossed, also produces the same phenotypic ratio in the F_2. (*a*) What phenotypic ratio is expected in the F_2 when a pure-colored line of genotype *AACCRR* is testcrossed? (*b*) What proportion of the colorless F_2 is *aaccrr*? (*c*) What genotypic ratio exists among the colored F_2?

4.35. If a pure-white onion strain is crossed to a pure-yellow strain, the F_2 ratio is 12 white : 3 red : 1 yellow. If another pure-white onion is crossed to a pure-red onion, the F_2 ratio is 9 red : 3 yellow : 4 white. (*a*) What percentage of the white F_2 from the second mating would be homozygous for the yellow allele? (*b*) If the white F_2 (homozygous for the yellow allele) of part (*a*) is crossed to the pure-white parent of the first mating mentioned at the beginning of this problem, determine the F_1 and F_2 phenotypic expectations.

4.36. For any color to be developed in the aleurone layer of corn kernels, the dominant alleles at two loci plus the recessive condition at a third locus (*A-R-ii*) must be present. Any other genotypes produce colorless aleurone. (*a*) What phenotypic ratio of colored : colorless would be expected in progeny from matings between parental plants of genotype *AaRrIi*? (*b*) What proportion of the colorless progeny in part (*a*) would be expected to be heterozygous at one or more of the three loci? (*c*) What is the probability of picking from among the colored seeds in part (*a*) two that, when grown into adult sporophytes and artificially crossed, would produce some colorless progeny with the triple recessive genotype?

4.37. A dominant gene *V* is known in humans which causes certain areas of the skin to become depigmented, a condition called "vitiligo." Albinism is the complete lack of pigment production and is produced by the recessive genotype *aa*. The albino locus is epistatic to the vitiligo locus. Another gene locus, the action of which is independent of the previously mentioned loci, is known to be involved in a mildly anemic condition called "thalassemia." (*a*) When adult progeny from parents both of whom exhibit vitiligo and a mild anemia is examined, the following phenotypic proportions are observed: $\frac{1}{16}$ normal : $\frac{3}{16}$ vitiligo : $\frac{1}{8}$ mildly anemic : $\frac{1}{12}$ albino : $\frac{3}{8}$ vitiligo and mildly anemic : $\frac{1}{6}$ albino and mildly anemic. What is the mode of genetic action of the gene for thalassemia? (*b*) What percentage of the viable albino offspring in part (*a*) would carry the gene for vitiligo? (*c*) What percentage of viable offspring with symptoms of mild anemia also shows vitiligo?

4.38. When the White Leghorn breed of chickens is crossed to the White Wyandotte breed, all the F_1 birds have white feathers. The F_2 birds appear in the ratio 13 white : 3 colored. When the White Leghorn breed is crossed to the White Silkie breed, the F_1 is white and the F_2 is also 13 white : 3 colored. But when White Wyandottes are crossed to White Silkies, the F_1 is all colored and the F_2 appears in the ratio 9 colored : 7 white. (*a*) How are feather colors inherited in these breeds (use appropriate symbols in your explanation)? (*b*) Show, by use of your own symbols, the genotypes of each of the three breeds (assume the breed is homozygous for all loci under consideration). (*c*) What phenotypic ratio is expected among progeny from trihybrid parents? (*d*) What proportion of the white offspring of part (*c*) is expected to be dihybrid?

4.39. A corn plant which grew from a seed with purple aleurone is self-pollinated. The F_1 produces $\frac{9}{16}$ purple aleurone, $\frac{3}{16}$ yellow and $\frac{4}{16}$ white. Some of the red F_1, when selfed, produce progeny in the ratio 12 red : 3 yellow : 1 white. Some of the purple F_1, when selfed, produce progeny in the ratio of 9 purple : 3 red : 4 white. (*a*) How can these results be explained? Using any appropriate symbols, diagram all three of the crosses mentioned above. (*b*) If, instead of being selfed, each of the above three parental types had been testcrossed, what phenotypic results would be expected? (*c*) What phenotypic proportions are observed in progeny from mating trihybrid purple × dihybrid purple (with the third locus homozygous recessive)?

4.40. For color to be developed in the aleurone layer of corn, the dominant alleles at four loci must be present (A_1, A_2, C, and R). If a line pure for colored aleurone is testcrossed to a noncolored line, find (*a*) the phenotypic ratio expected in the F_1 and F_2, (*b*) the percentage of the colored F_2 expected to be genetically like the F_1, (*c*) the percentage of the colorless F_2 expected to be homozygous for both the A_1 and A_2 alleles. (*d*) If a colored line is testcrossed and 25% of the offspring are colored, how many loci are heterozygous? (*e*) If the colored line in part (*d*) produces $12\frac{1}{2}$% colored offspring, how many loci are heterozygous? (*f*) If all four loci of the colored line in part (*d*) are heterozygous, what percentage of the offspring are expected to be colorless?

Review Questions

Matching Questions   Match the expected phenotypic ratios (right column) in progeny from dihybrid parents under the conditions specified in the left column.

1.	Dominant epistasis	A. 9 : 6 : 1
2.	Recessive epistasis	B. 9 : 3 : 3 : 1
3.	Duplicate genes with cumulative action	C. 9 : 3 : 4
4.	Duplicate dominant interaction	D. 13 : 3
5.	Duplicate recessive interaction	E. 12 : 3 : 1
6.	Dominant and recessive interaction	F. 15 : 1
7.	No interaction	G. 9 : 7

Vocabulary   For each of the following definitions, give the appropriate term and spell it correctly.

1. Biological catalysts that speed the rate of chemical reactions.

2. The material(s) acted upon and changed by the catalyst in question 1.

3. The phenomenon in which a specific genotype(s) at one locus can prevent the phenotypic expression of a genotype(s) at one or more other loci.

4. Adjective describing a locus whose action is suppressed by the phenomenon in question 3.

5. A phenomenon wherein a single gene has more than one phenotypic effect.

6. A collection of phenotypic effects that collectively defines a genetic disease.

Multiple-Choice Questions   Questions 1–5 use the information in the diagram below.

1. The genotype(s) capable of making C is/are   (a) $G^1g^1G^2g^2$ (b) $G^1G^1g^2g^2$ (c) $G^1g^1g^2g^2$
   (d) $g^1g^1G^2G^2$ (e) more than one of the above

2. In a cross between genotypes $g^1g^1G^2G^2 \times G^1G^1g^2g^2$, what fraction of the F_2 is expected to be phenotypically B-positive and C-negative?   (a) $\frac{9}{16}$ (b) $\frac{3}{16}$ (c) $\frac{3}{8}$ (d) $\frac{1}{4}$ (e) none of the above

3. What fraction of the F_2 in the above cross (question 2) is expected to be C-negative?   (a) $\frac{3}{4}$ (b) $\frac{1}{2}$
   (c) $\frac{6}{16}$ (d) $\frac{7}{16}$ (e) none of the above

4. What fraction of the F_2 (in question 2) is expected to be able to make enzyme 2, but not enzyme 1?
   (a) $\frac{3}{4}$ (b) $\frac{3}{16}$ (c) $\frac{9}{16}$ (d) $\frac{3}{8}$ (e) none of the above

5. If a dihybrid is testcrossed, what fraction of the progeny is expected to be able to make C substance?
   (a) $\frac{9}{16}$ (b) $\frac{3}{16}$ (c) $\frac{3}{8}$ (d) $\frac{1}{4}$ (e) none of the above

Questions 6–10 use the information in the following diagram. Enzyme e_3 becomes inactivated by binding to substance P.

6. If the phenotype is determined by the presence or absence of substance N, what type of interaction exists? (*a*) dominant and recessive   (*b*) duplicate recessive   (*c*) duplicate dominant   (*d*) duplicate genes with cumulative action   (*e*) none of the above

7. Approximately (within rounding error) what percentage of the F_1 from $G^3g^3G^4g^4$ parents is expected to be N-positive?   (*a*) 56   (*b*) 19   (*c*) 25   (*d*) 38   (*e*) none of the above

8. When dihybrids are testcrossed, the percentage of their progeny expected to be N-negative is   (*a*) 25   (*b*) 81   (*c*) 75   (*d*) 38   (*e*) none of the above

9. Among the N-positive progeny from dihybrid parents, what fraction is expected to be P-positive? (*a*) $\frac{3}{4}$ (*b*) $\frac{1}{2}$ (*c*) $\frac{2}{3}$ (*d*) $\frac{5}{6}$ (*e*) none of the above

10. What fraction of the progeny from dihybrid parents is expected to be P-positive and N-negative? (*a*) $\frac{9}{16}$ (*b*) $\frac{7}{16}$ (*c*) $\frac{6}{16}$ (*d*) $\frac{3}{4}$ (*e*) none of the above

Answers to Supplementary Problems

4.7. (*a*) Two pairs of nonepistatic genes interact to produce these coat colors.
(*b*) *A-B-* (gray), *A-bb* (yellow), *aaB-* (black), *aabb* (cream)   (*c*) 3   (*d*) 12

4.8. (*a*) F_1: all walnut comb; F_2: $\frac{9}{16}$ walnut : $\frac{3}{16}$ rose : $\frac{3}{16}$ pea : $\frac{1}{16}$ single   (*b*) *RRPp*

(*c*)		*R-P-*	*R-pp*	*rrP-*	*rrpp*
		Walnut	**Rose**	**Pea**	**Single**
	(1)	3/4		1/4	
	(2)	3/8	1/8	3/8	1/8
	(3)	All			
	(4)	1/4	1/4	1/4	1/4
	(5)	1/2	1/2		
	(6)		All		
	(7)	All			
	(8)		3/4		1/4
	(9)	1/4	1/4	1/4	1/4
	(10)			1/2	1/2

4.9. (*a*) $1:2:1$ (*c*) $1:3$ (*e*) $2:1:1$ (*g*) $3:1$
(*b*) $1:1:2$ (*d*) $3:1$ (*f*) $1:1:1:1$

4.10. (*a*) $\frac{3}{4}$ white : $\frac{1}{4}$ yellow   (*d*) $\frac{3}{4}$ white : $\frac{1}{8}$ yellow : $\frac{1}{8}$ green
(*b*) and (*c*) $\frac{1}{2}$ white : $\frac{1}{4}$ yellow : $\frac{1}{4}$ green   (*e*) yellow (*wwGg*) × green (*wwgg*)

4.11. (*a*) $9:3:4$ (*c*) P: *BbCc* (black); F_1: *B-C-* (black), *bbC-* (cream), *B-cc* and *bbcc* (albino)
(*b*) Recessive epistasis

4.12. (*a*) Dominant and recessive interaction   (*b*) F_1: all wild type; F_2: 13 wild type : 3 star   (*c*) 69%

4.13. (*a*) Duplicate dominant genes with only the double-recessive genotype producing nonfeathered shanks   (*b*) 8/15

4.14. (a) P: $A_1A_1a_2a_2 \times a_1a_1A_2A_2$;　F$_1$: $A_1a_1A_2a_2$
(b) $\frac{9}{16}$ colored : $\frac{7}{16}$ colorless　　(c) $\frac{1}{7}A_1A_1a_2a_2 : \frac{2}{7}A_1a_1a_2a_2$:　　$\frac{1}{7}a_1a_1A_2A_2 : \frac{2}{7}a_1a_1A_2a_2 : \frac{1}{7}a_1a_1a_2a_2$

4.15. (a) 9 : 3 : 4　(b) Recessive epistasis　(c) 32 white : 24 yellow : 72 red

4.16. (a) 15 triangular : 1 ovoid　(b) Duplicate dominant interaction

4.17. (a) 13 colorless : 3 colored　(b) $\frac{3}{13}$

4.18. (a) F$_1$: all black;　F$_2$: $\frac{9}{16}$ black : $\frac{3}{16}$ brown : $\frac{4}{16}$ albino　(b) $\frac{1}{4}BBcc : \frac{1}{2}Bbcc : \frac{1}{4}bbcc$

4.19. (a) Duplicate recessive interaction　(b) 9 high cyanide : 7 low cyanide　(c) A-$Bb \times AABb$ or AaB- $\times$ $AaBB$　(d) $\frac{2}{9}$

4.20. (a) $\frac{3}{8}$ red : $\frac{3}{8}$ cream : $\frac{1}{4}$ white;　$\frac{1}{8}AACc : \frac{1}{8}AAcc : \frac{1}{4}AaCc : \frac{1}{4}Aacc : \frac{1}{8}aaCc : \frac{1}{8}aacc$
(b) $Aacc \times AaCc$ (or) $Aacc \times AaCC$
(c) 9 red : 3 cream : 4 white
(d) $AaCc \times aaCc$ (or) $AaCc \times aacc$

4.21. (a) $IIrr \times iiRR$　(b) F$_1$: all white;　F$_2$: $\frac{12}{16}$ white : $\frac{3}{16}$ red : $\frac{1}{16}$ yellow　(c) 16 yellow : 48 red : 192 white

4.22. (a) F$_1$: all purple;　F$_2$: $\frac{9}{16}$ purple : $\frac{3}{16}$ red : $\frac{4}{16}$ white
(b) $\frac{4}{9}AACCprprRR : \frac{4}{9}AACCprprRr : \frac{1}{9}AACCprprrr$;　8 red : 1 white

4.23. (a) F$_1$: all white;　F$_2$: 13 white : 3 colored　　(c) $IiCc \times Iicc$
(b) dominant and recessive interaction　　(d) $IiCc \times iiCc$

4.24. (a) $\frac{9}{16}$ purple-centered : $\frac{7}{16}$ yellow-centered
(b) $\frac{1}{4}$ purple-centered : $\frac{3}{4}$ yellow-centered　　(c) All purple-centered

4.25. (a) No　(b) Dominant epistasis where Y-R- or yyR- produce purple, Y-rr = yellow, and $yyrr$ = white
(c) $\frac{3}{4}$ purple : $\frac{3}{16}$ yellow : $\frac{1}{16}$ white　(d) One　(e) The appearance of seed traits requires one less generation of rearing than that for tissues found in the sporophyte.

4.26. (a) 9 disc : 6 sphere : 1 elongated
(b) Duplicate genes with cumulative effect　　(c) $\frac{2}{3}$ sphere : $\frac{2}{9}$ disc : $\frac{1}{9}$ elongate

4.27. (a) A^yACc ♂ $\times AAcc$♀; for gene symbol meanings, see Problems 2.9 and 4.5　(b) 2 yellow : 1 agouti : 1 albino　(c) Zero

4.28. (a) Solid symbol　(b) Diagonal lines　(c) Open symbol　(d) Recessive epistasis　(e) Duplicate genes with cumulative effect

4.29. (a) Duplicate recessive interaction　(b) A-B- (wild type), aa-- or --bb or $aabb$ (platinum); AaB- (I1, 2), A-Bb (I3, 4), A-B- (I5, 6, II3), $aaBB$ (III1), $AAbb$ (II2), $AaBb$ (III1–III8), either aa or bb or both (II4, 5, III9–III16)　(c) 9 wild type : 7 platinum

4.30. The following set of genotypes is only one of several possible solutions: aaB- (III1, 2, 3, 4, 5, 6), A- or bb or both (III1), a--- (I1, 2), $aaBb$ (I3, 4, II2, 3), $aabb$ (II4, III7, 8).

4.31. The following set of genotypes is only one of several possible solutions: AaB- (I1, 2), A-Bb (I3, 4), A-B- (III, 4, 5), aaB- (II2), $Aabb$ (II3), $AaBb$ (III1, 2, 3), aa or bb or both (III4, 5).

4.32.   (*a*) 3   (*b*) P: *AABBCC* × *aabbcc;*   F$_1$: *AaBbCc*

4.33.   27 solid black : 9 spotted black : 9 solid brown : 3 spotted brown : 16 albino

4.34.   (*a*) 27 colored : 37 colorless   (*b*) $\frac{1}{37}$ (*c*) $\frac{1}{27}AACCRR : \frac{2}{27}AACCRr : \frac{2}{27}AACcRR : \frac{4}{27}AACcRr : \frac{2}{27}AaCCRR : \frac{4}{27}AaCCRr : \frac{4}{27}AaCcRR : \frac{8}{27}AaCcRr$

4.35.   (*a*) 25%   (*b*) F$_1$: all white;   F$_2$: 52 white : 9 red : 3 yellow

4.36.   (*a*) 9 colored : 55 colorless   (*b*) $\frac{48}{55}$ (*c*) $\frac{16}{81}$

4.37.   (*a*) The gene for thalassemia is dominant to its normal allele, causing mild anemia when heterozygous, but is lethal when homozygous   (*b*) 75%   (*c*) 56.25%

4.38.   (*a*) 3 loci involved; one possesses a dominant inhibitor of color (*I*-) and the other two possess different recessive inhibitors of color (*cc* and *oo*). Only the genotype *iiC-O-* produces colored birds; all other genotypes produce white feathers.   (*b*) White Leghorn (*CCOOII*), White Wyandotte (*ccOOii*), White Silkie (*CCooii*)   (*c*) 55 white : 9 colored   (*d*) $\frac{20}{55}$

4.39.   Three allelic pairs assorting independently of one another contribute to seed color: *R* = color, *r* = white (or the color depends on other loci); *P* = purple, *p* = red; *Y* = yellow, *y* = white. The R locus exhibits recessive epistasis over the P locus (hence the 9 : 3 : 4 ratio); i.e., the dominant gene *R* is necessary for any color to be produced by the genotypes at the P locus. The R locus exhibits dominant epistasis over the Y locus (hence the 12 : 3 : 1 ratio); i.e., genotypes at the Y locus can be expressed only when *rr* is also present in the same individual. First cross: *RrPpYy* × *RrPpYy* = 9 : 3 : 3 : 1. Second cross: *RrppYy* × *RrppYy* = 12 : 3 : 1. Third cross: *RrPpyy* × *RrPpyy* = 9 : 3 : 4. (*b*) First cross: 1 purple : 1 red : 1 yellow : 1 white. Second cross: 2 red : 1 yellow : 1 white. Third cross: 2 white : 1 red : 1 purple. (*c*) $\frac{9}{16}$ purple : $\frac{3}{16}$ red : $\frac{1}{8}$ yellow : $\frac{1}{8}$ white.

4.40.   (*a*) F$_1$: all colored;   F$_2$: $\frac{81}{256}$ colored : $\frac{175}{256}$ noncolored   (*b*) 19.75%   (*c*) 4%   (*d*) 2   (*e*) 3   (f) 93.75%

Answers to Review Questions

Matching Questions

1. E   2. C   3. A   4. F   5. G   6. D   7. B

Vocabulary

1. enzymes   2. substrate(s)   3. epistasis   4. hypostatic   5. pleiotropism   6. syndrome

Multiple-Choice Questions

1. *a*   2. *b*   3. *d*   4. *b*   5. *d*   6. *a*   7. *b*   8. *c*   9. *e* (zero)   10. *d*

Chapter 5

The Genetics of Sex

THE IMPORTANCE OF SEX

We are probably too accustomed to thinking of sex in terms of the males and females of our own or domestic species. Plants also have sexes; at least we know that there are male and female portions of a flower. All organisms, however, do not possess only two sexes. Some of the lowest forms of plant and animal life may have several sexes. For example, in one variety of the ciliated protozoan *Paramecium bursaria* there are eight sexes, or "mating types," all morphologically identical. Each mating type is physiologically incapable of conjugating with its own type, but may exchange genetic material with any of the seven other types within the same variety. In most higher organisms, the number of sexes is only two. These sexes may reside in different individuals or within the same individual. An animal possessing both male and female reproductive organs is usually referred to as a **hermaphrodite.** In plants where **staminate** (male) and **pistillate** (female) flowers occur on the same plant, the term of preference is **monoecious.** Moreover, most flowering plants have both male and female parts within the same flower (perfect flower). Relatively few angiosperms are **dioecious,** i.e., having the male and female elements in different individuals. Among the common cultivated crops known to be dioecious are asparagus, date palm, hemp, hops, and spinach.

Whether there are two or more sexes, or whether these sexes reside in the same or different individuals is relatively unimportant. The importance of sex itself is that it is a mechanism that provides for the great amount of genetic variability characterizing most natural populations. The evolutionary process of natural selection depends upon this genetic variability to supply the raw material from which the better adapted types usually survive to reproduce their kind. Many subsidiary mechanisms have evolved to ensure cross-fertilization in most species as a means for generating new genetic combinations in each generation.

SEX-DETERMINING MECHANISMS

Most mechanisms for the determination of sex are under genetic control and may be classified into one of the following categories.

1. Sex Chromosome Mechanisms.

(a) *Heterogametic Males.* In humans, and apparently in all other mammals, the presence of the Y chromosome may determine a tendency to maleness. Normal males are chromosomally XY and females are XX. This produces a $1:1$ sex ratio in each generation. Since the male produces two kinds of gametes as far as the sex chromosomes are concerned, he is said to be the **heterogametic** sex. The female, producing only one kind of gamete, is the **homogametic** sex. This mode of sex determination is commonly referred to as the XY method.

Example 5.1. XY Method of Sex Determination.

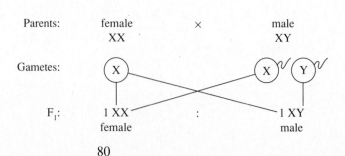

A **testis-determining factor** (TDF) has been delimited to a small segment on the short arm of the human Y chromosome. It is suggested that the gene (or possibly a group of closely linked genes) of the TDF produces a DNA-binding protein that activates one or more other genes (probably on different chromosomes) in a hierarchy or cascade of gene activation that governs the development of the testes. In the absence of TDF, rudimentary gonadal tissue of the embryo would normally develop into an ovary. TDF seems to be highly conserved in mammals. The location of TDF was aided by the discovery of rare exceptions to the rule that XX programs for femaleness and XY programs for maleness. It was found that normal-appearing but sterile XX human males have at least some of the TDF attached to one of their X chromosomes and human XY females have lost a crucial part of the TDF from their Y chromosome.

In some insects, especially those of the orders Hemiptera (true bugs) and Orthoptera (grasshoppers and roaches), males are also heterogametic, but produce either X-bearing sperm or gametes without a sex chromosome. In males of these species, the X chromosome has no homologous pairing partner because there is no Y chromosome present. Thus males exhibit an odd number in their chromosome complement. The one-X and two-X condition determines maleness and femaleness, respectively. If the single X chromosome of the male is always included in one of the two types of gametes formed, then a 1 : 1 sex ratio will be produced in the progeny. This mode of sex determination is commonly referred to as the XO method where the O symbolizes the lack of a chromosome analogous to the Y of the XY system.

Example 5.2. XO Method of Sex Determination.

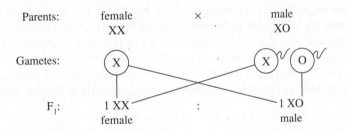

(b) **Heterogametic Females.** This method of sex determination is found in a comparatively large group of insects including the butterflies, moths, caddis flies, and silkworms, and in some birds and fishes. The 1-X and 2-X condition in these species determines femaleness and maleness, respectively. The females of some species (e.g., domestic chickens) have a chromosome similar to that of the Y in humans. In these cases, the chromosomes are sometimes labeled Z and W instead of X and Y, respectively, in order to call attention to the fact that the female (ZW) is the heterogametic sex and the male (ZZ) is the homogametic sex. The females of other species have no homologue to the single sex chromosome as in the case of the XO mechanism discussed previously. To point out this difference, the symbols ZZ and ZO may be used to designate males and females, respectively. A 1 : 1 sex ratio is expected in either case.

Example 5.3. ZO Method of Sex Determination.

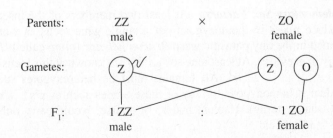

Example 5.4. ZW Method of Sex Determination.

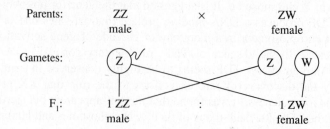

Parents: ZZ   ×   ZW

       male   female

Gametes:

F_1:   1 ZZ   :   1 ZW

    male   female

The W chromosome of the chicken is not a strong female-determining element. Recent studies indicate that sex determination in chickens, and probably birds in general, is similar to that of *Drosophila*, i.e., dependent upon the ratio between the Z chromosomes and the number of autosomal sets of chromosomes (see next section on genic balance).

2. Genic Balance.

The presence of the Y chromosome in *Drosophila*, although it is essential for male fertility, apparently has nothing to do with the determination of sex. Instead, the factors for maleness residing in all of the autosomes are "weighed" against the factors for femaleness residing on the X chromosome(s). If each haploid set of autosomes carries factors with a male-determining value equal to 1, then each X chromosome carries factors with a female-determining value of $1\frac{1}{2}$. Let A represent a haploid set of autosomes. In a normal male (AAXY), the male : female determinants are in the ratio $2 : 1\frac{1}{2}$ and therefore the balance is in favor of maleness. A normal female (AAXX) has a male : female ratio of $2 : 3$ and therefore the balance is in favor of femaleness. Several abnormal combinations of chromosomes have confirmed this hypothesis. For example, an individual with three sets of autosomes and 2 X chromosomes has a ratio of $3 : 3$, which makes its genetic sex neutral, and indeed phenotypically it appears as a sterile intersex.

3. Haplodiploidy.

Male bees are known to develop **parthenogenetically** (without union of gametes) from unfertilized eggs (**arrhenotoky**) and are therefore haploid. Females (both workers and queens) originate from fertilized (diploid) eggs. Sex chromosomes are not involved in this mechanism of sex determination, which is characteristic of the insect order Hymenoptera including the ants, bees, wasps, etc. The quantity and quality of food available to the diploid larva determines whether that female will become a sterile worker or a fertile queen. Thus environment here determines sterility or fertility but does not alter the genetically determined sex. The sex ratio of the offspring is under the control of the queen. Most of the eggs laid in the hive will be fertilized and develop into worker females. Those eggs which the queen chooses not to fertilize (from her store of sperm in the seminal receptacle) will develop into fertile haploid males. Queen bees usually mate only once during their lifetime.

4. Single-Gene Effects.

(*a*) **Complementary Sex Factors.** At least two members of the insect order Hymenoptera are known to produce males by homozygosity at a single-gene locus as well as by haploidy. This has been confirmed in the tiny parasitic wasp *Bracon hebetor* (often called *Habrobracon juglandis*), and more recently in bees also. At least nine sex alleles are known at this locus in *Bracon* and may be represented by $s^a, s^b, s^c, \ldots, s^i$. All females must be heterozygotes such as $s^a s^b, s^a s^c, s^d s^f$, etc. If an individual is homozygous for any of these alleles such as $s^a s^a, s^c s^c$, etc., it develops into a diploid male (usually sterile). Haploid males, of course, would carry only one of the alleles at this locus, e.g., s^a, s^c, s^g, etc.

Example 5.5.

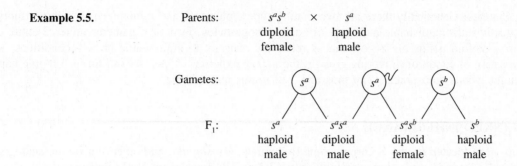

Parents: $s^a s^b$ × s^a
            diploid   haploid
            female   male

Gametes: s^a s^a s^b

F_1: s^a $s^a s^a$ $s^a s^b$ s^b
          haploid   diploid   diploid   haploid
           male   male   female   male

Among the diploid progeny we expect 1 $s^a s^a$ male : 1 $s^a s^b$ female. Among the haploid progeny we expect 1 s^a male : 1 s^b male.

(b) **The "Transformer" Gene of Drosophila.**   A recessive gene (*tra*) on chromosome 3 of *Drosophila*, when homozygous, transforms a diploid female into a sterile male. The X/X, *tra/tra* individuals resemble normal males in external and internal morphology with the exception that the testes are much reduced in size. The gene is without effect in normal males. The presence of this gene can considerably alter the sex ratio (see Problem 5.1). The significance of these kinds of genes resides in the fact that a mechanism of sex determination based on numerous genes throughout the genome can apparently be nullified by a single gene substitution.

(c) **"Mating Type" in Microorganisms.**   In microorganisms such as the alga *Chlamydomonas* and the fungi *Neurospora* and yeast, sex is under control of a single gene. Haploid individuals possessing the same allele of this "mating-type" locus usually cannot fuse with each other to form a zygote, but haploid cells of opposite (complementary) allelic constitution at this locus may fuse. Asexual reproduction in the single-celled motile alga *Chlamydomonas reinhardi* usually involves two mitotic divisions within the old cell wall (Fig. 5-1). Rupture of the sporangium releases the new generation of haploid **zoospores**. If nutritional requirements are satisfied, asexual reproduction may go on indefinitely. In unfavorable conditions where nitrogen balance is upset, daughter cells may be changed

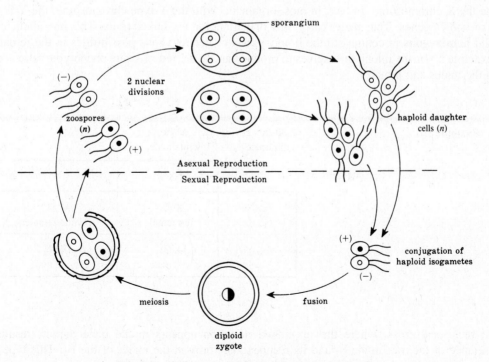

Fig. 5-1.   Life cycle of *Chlamydomonas reinhardi*.

to gametes. Genetically there are two mating types, plus (+) and minus (−), which are morphologically indistinguishable and therefore called **isogametes.** Fusion of gametes unites 2 entire cells
into a diploid nonmotile zygote that is relatively resistant to unfavorable growth conditions. With
the return of conditions favoring growth, the zygote experiences meiosis and forms 4 motile haploid
daughter cells (zoospores), 2 of plus and 2 of minus mating type.

SEX-LINKED INHERITANCE

Any gene located on the X chromosome (mammals, *Drosophila,* and others) or on the analogous Z
chromosome (in birds and other species with the ZO or ZW mechanism of sex determination) is said to
be **sex-linked.** The first sex-linked gene found in *Drosophila* was the recessive white-eye mutation.
Reciprocal crosses involving autosomal traits yield comparable results. This is not true with sex-linked
traits as shown below. When white-eyed females are crossed with wild-type (red-eyed) males, all the
male offspring have white eyes like their mother and all the female offspring have red eyes like their
father.

Example 5.6.

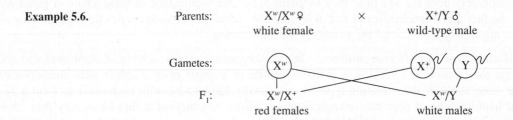

Parents: X^w/X^w ♀   × X^+/Y ♂
          white female   wild-type male

Gametes:

F_1: X^w/X^+ X^w/Y
          red females   white males

This crisscross method of inheritance is characteristic of sex-linked genes. This peculiar type of
inheritance is due to the fact that the Y chromosome carries no alleles homologous to those at the white
locus on the X chromosome. In fact, in most organisms with the Y-type chromosome, the Y is virtually
devoid of known genes. Thus males carry only one allele for sex-linked traits. This one-allelic condition
is termed **hemizygous** in contrast to the homozygous or heterozygous possibilities in the female. If the
F_1 of Example 5.6 mate among themselves to produce an F_2, a 1 red : 1 white phenotypic ratio is expected
in both the males and females.

Example 5.7.

F_1: X^+/X^w × X^w/Y
          red female   white male

F_2:

	X^+	X^w
X^w	X^+/X^w red female	X^w/X^w white female
Y	X^+/Y red male	X^w/Y white male

The reciprocal cross, where the sex-linked mutation appears in the male parent, results in the
disappearance of the trait in the F_1 and its reappearance only in the males of the F_2. This type of skip-
generation inheritance also characterizes sex-linked genes.

Example 5.8.

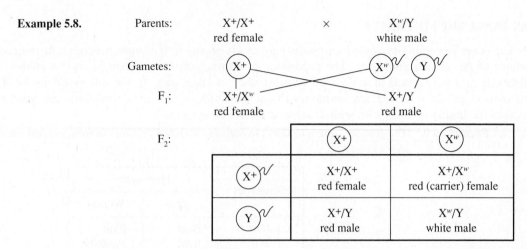

Parents: X⁺/X⁺   ×   Xʷ/Y
           red female   white male

Gametes:

F₁: X⁺/Xʷ   X⁺/Y
           red female   red male

F₂:

	X⁺	Xʷ
X⁺	X⁺/X⁺ red female	X⁺/Xʷ red (carrier) female
Y	X⁺/Y red male	Xʷ/Y white male

Thus a 3 red : 1 white phenotypic ratio is expected in the total F₂ disregarding sex, but only the males show the mutant trait. The phenotypic ratio among the F₂ males is 1 red : 1 white. All F₂ females are phenotypically wild type.

Whenever working with problems involving sex linkage in this book, be sure to list the ratios for males and females separately unless specifically directed by the problem to do otherwise.

In normal diploid organisms with sex-determining mechanisms like that of humans or *Drosophila*, a trait governed by a sex-linked recessive gene usually manifests itself in the following manner: (1) it is usually found more frequently in the male than in the female of the species, (2) it fails to appear in females unless it also appeared in the paternal parent, (3) it seldom appears in both father and son, then only if the maternal parent is heterozygous. On the other hand, a trait governed by a sex-linked dominant gene usually manifests itself by (1) being found more frequently in the female than in the male of the species, (2) being found in all female offspring of a male that shows the trait, (3) failing to be transmitted to any son from a mother that did not exhibit the trait herself.

VARIATIONS OF SEX LINKAGE

The sex chromosomes (X and Y) often are of unequal size, shape, and/or staining qualities. The fact that they pair during meiosis is indication that they contain at least some homologous segments. Genes on the homologous segments are said to be **incompletely sex-linked** or **partially sex-linked** and may recombine by crossing over in both sexes just as do the gene loci on homologous autosomes. Special crosses are required to demonstrate the presence of such genes on the X chromosome, and few examples are known. Genes on the nonhomologous segment of the X chromosome are said to be **completely sex-linked** and exhibit the peculiar mode of inheritance described in the preceding sections. In humans, a few genes are known to reside in the nonhomologous portion of the Y chromosome. In such cases, the trait would be expressed only in males and would always be transmitted from father to son. Such completely Y-linked genes are called **holandric genes** (Fig. 5-2).

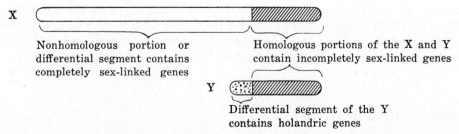

Fig. 5-2. Generalized diagram of X and Y chromosomes. The relative size of these chromosomes and the size of homologous and nonhomologous regions, as well as location of the centromeres (not shown) vary according to the species.

SEX-INFLUENCED TRAITS

The genes governing sex-influenced traits may reside on any of the autosomes or on the homologous portions of the sex chromosomes. The expression of dominance or recessiveness by the alleles of sex-influenced loci is reversed in males and females due, in large part, to the difference in the internal environment provided by the sex hormones. Thus examples of sex-influenced traits are most readily found in the higher animals with well-developed endocrine systems.

Example 5.9. The gene for pattern baldness in humans exhibits dominance in men, but acts recessively in women.

Genotypes	Phenotypes	
	Men	Women
$b'b'$	Bald	Bald
$b'b$	Bald	Nonbald
bb	Nonbald	Nonbald

SEX-LIMITED TRAITS

Some autosomal genes may only come to expression in one of the sexes either because of differences in the internal hormonal environment or because of anatomical dissimilarities. For example, we know that bulls have many genes for milk production that they may transmit to their daughters, but they or their sons are unable to express this trait. The production of milk is therefore limited to variable expression in only the female sex. When the penetrance of a gene in one sex is zero, the trait will be **sex-limited.**

Example 5.10. Chickens have a recessive gene for cock-feathering that is penetrant only in the male environment.

Genotype	Phenotypes	
	Males	Females
HH	Hen-feathering	Hen-feathering
Hh	Hen-feathering	Hen-feathering
hh	Cock-feathering	Hen-feathering

SEX REVERSAL

Female chickens (ZW) that have laid eggs have been known to undergo not only a reversal of the secondary sexual characteristics such as development of cock-feathering, spurs, and crowing, but also the development of testes and even the production of sperm cells (primary sexual characteristics). This may occur when, for example, disease destroys the ovarian tissue, and in the absence of the female sex hormones the rudimentary testicular tissue present in the center of the ovary is allowed to proliferate. In solving problems involving sex reversals, it must be remembered that the functional male derived through sex reversal will still remain genetically female (ZW).

SEXUAL PHENOMENA IN PLANTS

Most flowering plants are monoecious and therefore do not have sex chromosomes. Indeed, the ability of mitotically produced cells with exactly the same genetic endowment to produce tissues with different sexual functions in a perfect flower speaks clearly for the bipotentiality of such plant cells. Well-known examples of dioecism usually are under the genetic control of a single-gene locus. However, at least one well-documented case of chromosomal sexuality is known in plants, i.e., in the genus *Melandrium* (a member of the pink family). Here the Y chromosome determines a tendency to maleness just as it does in humans. Pistillate plants are XX and staminate plants are XY.

The ability of gametes produced by the same individual to unite and produce viable and fertile offspring is common among many families of flowering plants. Self-fertilization is also known to occur in a few of the lower animal groups. The perfect flowers of some monoecious plants fail to open **(cleistogamy)** until after the pollen has matured and accomplished self-fertilization. Self-fertilization is obligatory in barley, beans, oats, peas, soybeans, tobacco, tomato, wheat, and many other crops. In some species, self-fertilization as well as cross-fertilization may occur to varying degrees. For example, cotton and sorghum commonly experience more than 10% cross-fertilization. Still other monoecious species have developed genetic mechanisms that prevent self-fertilization or the development of zygotes produced by the union of identical gametes, making cross-fertilization obligatory. Self-incompatibility in monoecious species can become as efficient in enforcing cross-fertilization as would be exhibited under a dioecious mechanism of sex determination.

Solved Problems

SEX-DETERMINING MECHANISMS

5.1. An autosomal recessive gene (*tra*), when homozygous, transforms a *Drosophila* female (X/X) into a phenotypic male. All such "transformed" males are sterile. The gene is without effect in males (X/Y). A cross is made between a female heterozygous at the *tra* locus and a male homozygous recessive at the same locus. What is the expected sex ratio in the F_1 and F_2?

Solution:

We will use a slash mark (/) to separate alleles or homologous chromosomes, and a comma (,) to separate one gene locus from another.

Parents: X/X, +/*tra*   ×   X/Y, *tra*/*tra*
                        normal female   normal male

Gametes: (X+) (X*tra*)   (X*tra*) (Y*tra*)

F_1:

	X +	X *tra*
X *tra*	X/X, +/*tra* normal females	X/X, *tra*/*tra* "transformed" males
Y *tra*	X/Y, +/*tra* normal males	X/Y, *tra*/*tra* normal males

The F_1 phenotypic proportions thus appear as $\frac{3}{4}$ males : $\frac{1}{4}$ females.

F_2:   The "transformed" F_1 males are sterile and hence do not contribute gametes to the F_2. Two kinds of matings must be considered. First mating = $\frac{1}{2}$ of all possible matings:

$$\begin{array}{ccc} \text{X/X, } +/tra & \times & \text{X/Y, } +/tra \\ \text{females} & & \text{males} \end{array}$$

Offspring:

	X +	X *tra*
X+	X/X, +/+ female	X/X, +/*tra* female
X *tra*	X/X, +/*tra* female	X/X, *tra*/*tra* "transformed" male
Y +	X/Y, +/+ male	X/Y, +/*tra* male
Y *tra*	X/Y, +/*tra* male	X/Y, *tra*/*tra* male

Thus F_2 offspring from this mating type appear in the proportions $\frac{3}{8}$ female : $\frac{5}{8}$ male. But this type of mating constitutes only half of all possible matings. Therefore the contribution to the total F_2 from this mating is $\frac{1}{2} \cdot \frac{3}{8} = \frac{3}{16}$ female : $\frac{1}{2} \cdot \frac{5}{8} = \frac{5}{16}$ male. Second mating $= \frac{1}{2}$ of all possible matings:

$$\begin{array}{ccc} \text{X/X, } +/tra & \times & \text{X/Y, } tra/tra \\ \text{females} & & \text{males} \end{array}$$

This is the same as the original parental mating and hence we expect $\frac{3}{4}$ males : $\frac{1}{4}$ females. Correcting these proportions for the frequency of this mating, we have $\frac{1}{2} \cdot \frac{3}{4} = \frac{3}{8}$ males : $\frac{1}{2} \cdot \frac{1}{4} = \frac{1}{8}$ females. Summary of the F_2 from both matings: males $= \frac{5}{16} + \frac{3}{8} = \frac{11}{16}$; females $= \frac{3}{16} + \frac{1}{8} = \frac{5}{16}$.

SEX-LINKED INHERITANCE

5.2. There is a dominant sex-linked gene B that places white bars on an adult black chicken as in the Barred Plymouth Rock breed. Newly hatched chicks, which will become barred later in life, exhibit a white spot on the top of the head. (*a*) Diagram the cross through the F_2 between a homozygous barred male and a nonbarred female. (*b*) Diagram the reciprocal cross through the F_2 between a homozygous nonbarred male and a barred female. (*c*) Will both of the above crosses be useful in sexing F_1 chicks at hatching?

Solution:

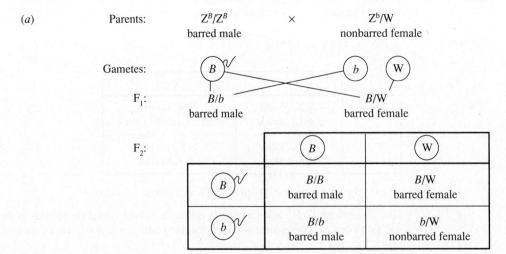

(*a*)   Parents: Z^B/Z^B × Z^b/W
             barred male   nonbarred female

Gametes: B b W

F_1: B/b B/W
    barred male   barred female

F_2:

	B	W
B	B/B barred male	B/W barred female
b	B/b barred male	b/W nonbarred female

(b)

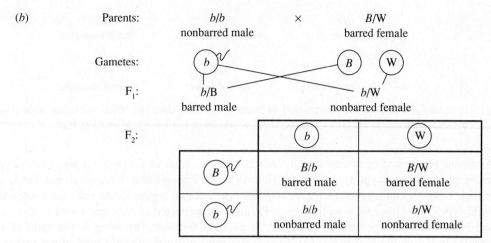

Parents:　　　　b/b　　　　　×　　　　B/W
　　　　　　nonbarred male　　　　　　　barred female

Gametes:　　　b　　　　　　　　B　　W

F_1:　　　b/B　　　　　　　b/W
　　　barred male　　　　nonbarred female

F_2:

	b	W
B	B/b barred male	B/W barred female
b	b/b nonbarred male	b/W nonbarred female

(c)　No. Only the cross shown in (b) would be dignostic in sexing F_1 chicks at birth through the use of this genetic marker. Only male chicks will have a light spot on their heads.

5.3.　A recessive sex-linked gene (h) prolongs the blood-clotting time, resulting in what is commonly called "bleeder's disease" (hemophilia). From the information in the pedigree, answer the following questions. (a) If II2 marries a normal man, what is the chance of her first child being a hemophilic boy? (b) Suppose her first child is actually hemophilic. What is the probability that her second child will be a hemophilic boy? (c) If II3 marries a hemophilic man, what is the probability that her first child will be normal? (d) If the mother of I1 was phenotypically normal, what phenotype was her father? (e) If the mother of I1 was hemophilic, what phenotype was her father?

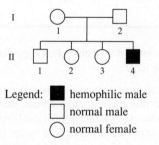

Legend:　■ hemophilic male
　　　　　□ normal male
　　　　　○ normal female

Solution:

(a)　Since II4 is a hemophilic male (hY), the hemophilic allele is on an X chromosome that he received from his mother (I1). But I1 is phenotypically normal and therefore must be heterozygous or a carrier of hemophilia of genotype Hh. I2 and II1 are both normal males (HY). Therefore the chance of II2 being a carrier female (Hh) is $\frac{1}{2}$. When a carrier woman marries a normal man (HY), 25% of their children are expected to be hemophilic boys (hY). The combined probability that she is a carrier *and* will produce a hemophilic boy is $\frac{1}{2} \cdot \frac{1}{4} = \frac{1}{8}$.

(b)　Because her first child was hemophilic, she *must* be a carrier. One-quarter of the children from carrier mothers (Hh) × normal fathers (HY) are expected to be hemophilic boys (hY).

(c)　II3 (like II2) has a 50% chance of being a carrier of hemophilia (Hh). If she marries a hemophilic man (hY), $\frac{1}{2}$ of their children (both boys and girls) are expected to be hemophilic. The combined chance of II3 being a carrier and producing a hemophilic child is $\frac{1}{2} \cdot \frac{1}{2} = \frac{1}{4}$. Therefore the probability that her first child is normal is the complementary fraction, $\frac{3}{4}$.

(d)　It is impossible to deduce the phenotype of the father of I1 from the information given because the father could be either normal or hemophilic and still produce a daughter (I1) which is heterozygous normal (Hh), depending upon the genotype of the normal mother:

$$(1) \quad \begin{array}{ccccc} HH & \times & hY & = & Hh(\text{I1}) \\ \text{normal mother} & & \text{hemophilic father} & & \text{carrier daughter} \end{array}$$

$$(2) \quad \begin{array}{ccccc} Hh & \times & HY & = & Hh(\text{I1}) \\ \text{carrier mother} & & \text{normal father} & & \text{carrier daughter} \end{array}$$

(e) In order for a hemophilic mother (hh) to produce a normal daughter (Hh), her father must possess the dominant normal allele (HY) and therefore would have normal blood clotting time.

5.4. A mutant sex-linked condition called "notch" (N) is lethal in *Drosophila* when hemizygous in males or when homozygous in females. Heterozygous females (Nn) have small notches in the tips of their wings. Homozygous recessive females (nn) or hemizygous males (nY) have normal wings (wild type). (*a*) Other than within sex, calculate the expected phenotypic ratios in the viable F_1 and F_2 when wild-type males are mated to notched females. (*b*) What is the ratio of males : females in the viable F_1 and F_2? (*c*) What is the ratio of notched : wild type in the viable F_1 and F_2?

Solution:

(*a*) Parents: $\quad\quad nY \quad\quad \times \quad\quad Nn$
            wild-type males   notched females

F_1:

	N	n
n	Nn notched females	nn wild-type female
Y	NY lethal	nY wild-type male

The ratio of F_1 viable phenotypes is 1 wild-type female : 1 notched female : 1 wild type male.

F_2: There are two kinds of matings to be considered: (1) $Nn \times nY$, (2) $nn \times nY$. The first mating gives results identical to those of the F_1. The second mating produces equal numbers of wild-type males and females. The two kinds of matings are expected to occur with equal frequency and therefore the contribution which each phenotype makes to the total F_2 must be halved.

First Mating	**Second Mating**
$\frac{1}{4}$ notched females $\times \frac{1}{2} = \frac{1}{8}$	$\frac{1}{2}$ wild females $\times \frac{1}{2} = \frac{1}{4} = \frac{2}{8}$
$\frac{1}{4}$ wild females $\times \frac{1}{2} = \frac{1}{8}$	$\frac{1}{2}$ wild males $\times \frac{1}{2} = \frac{1}{4} = \frac{2}{8}$
$\frac{1}{4}$ wild males $\times \frac{1}{2} = \frac{1}{8}$	
$\frac{1}{4}$ lethal males $\times \frac{1}{2} = \frac{1}{8}$	

The ratio of viable F_2 phenotypes thus becomes 3 wild-type females : 3 wild-type males : 1 notched female.

(*b*) By inspection of the data in part (*a*), it is clear that the sex ratio in the viable F_1 is 2 females : 1 male, and in the F_2 it is 4 females : 3 males.

(*c*) Similarly, the ratio for wing phenotypes in the viable F_1 is 2 wild : 1 notched, and in the F_2 it is 6 wild : 1 notched.

5.5. A recessive sex-linked gene in *Drosophila* (v) produces vermilion eye color when homozygous in females or when hemizygous in males. An autosomal recessive on chromosome 2 (bw) produces brown eye color. Individuals who are homozygous recessive at both the brown and the vermilion loci have white eyes. (*a*) Determine the phenotypic expectations among the F_1 and F_2 when homozygous wild type females are crossed to males that are white-eyed due to the interaction of the brown and vermilion loci. (*b*) Another recessive gene called ''scarlet'' (*st*) on chromosome 3 also produces white eye when homozygous in combination with homozygous recessive brown (*st/st, bw/bw*). Providing at least one bw^+ allele is present, homozygous scarlet, homozygous or hemizygous vermilion, or both produce a nearly identical eye color that we shall call ''orange-red.'' What phenotypic ratio is expected among the F_1 and f_2 progeny from testcrossing wild-type females homozygous at all 3 loci?

Solution:

(*a*)   P: $bw^+/bw^+, v^+/v^+$ × $bw/bw, v/Y$
                           wild-type females   white-eyed females

           F_1: $1/2\ bw^+/bw, v^+/v$ =   wild-type females
                           $1/2\ bw^+/bw, v^+/Y$ =   wild-type males

F_2:

	$bw^+\ v^+$	$bw\ v^+$	$bw^+\ Y$	$bw\ Y$
$bw^+\ v^+$	$bw^+/bw^+, v^+/v^+$ wild type	$bw^+/bw, v^+/v^+$ wild type	$bw^+/bw^+, v^+/Y$ wild type	$bw^+/bw, v^+/Y$ wild type
$bw^+\ v$	$bw^+/bw^+, v^+/v$ wild type	$bw^+/bw, v^+/v$ wild type	$bw^+/bw^+, v/Y$ vermilion	$bw^+/bw, v/Y$ vermilion
$bw\ v^+$	$bw^+/bw, v^+/v^+$ wild type	$bw/bw, v^+/v^+$ brown	$bw^+/bw, v^+/Y$ wild type	$bw/bw, v^+/Y$ brown
$bw\ v$	$bw^+/bw, v^+/v$ wild type	$bw/bw, v^+/v$ brown	$bw^+/bw, v/Y$ vermilion	$bw/bw, v/Y$ white

F_2 summary:

Females	**Males**	
3/4 wild type	3/8 wild type	1/8 brown
1/4 brown	3/8 vermilion	1/8 white

(*b*)   P: $bw^+/bw^+, st^+/st^+, v^+/v^+$ × $bw/bw, st/st, v/Y$
                            wild-type females   white-eyed males

           F_1: $1/2\ bw^+/bw, st^+/st, v^+/v$ =   wild-type females
                           $1/2\ bw^+/bw, st^+/st, v^+/Y$ =   wild-type males

F_2:   **Females:**

$\frac{3}{4}bw^+/-$ ⟨ $\frac{3}{4}st^+/-$ —— $v^+/-$ = wild type 9/16

$\frac{1}{4}st/st$ —— $v^+/-$ = orange-red 3/16

$\frac{1}{4}bw/bw$ ⟨ $\frac{3}{4}st^+/-$ —— $v^+/-$ = brown 3/16

$\frac{1}{4}st/st$ —— $v^+/-$ = white 1/16

Males:

$\frac{3}{4}bw^+/-$ ⟨ $\frac{3}{4}st^+/-$ ⟨ $\frac{1}{2}v^+/Y$ = wild type 9/32

$\frac{1}{2}v/Y$ = orange-red 9/32

$\frac{1}{4}st/st$ ⟨ $\frac{1}{2}v^+/Y$ = orange-red 3/32

$\frac{1}{2}v/Y$ = orange-red 3/32

$\frac{1}{4}bw/bw$ ⟨ $\frac{3}{4}st^+/-$ ⟨ $\frac{1}{2}v^+/Y$ = brown 3/32

$\frac{1}{2}v/Y$ = white 3/32

$\frac{1}{4}st/st$ ⟨ $\frac{1}{2}v^+/Y$ = white 1/32

$\frac{1}{2}v/Y$ = white 1/32

F_2 summary: **Females:**   9/16 wild type, 3/16 orange-red, 3/16 brown, 1/16 white
                  Males: 9/32 wild type, 15/32 orange-red, 3/32 brown, 5/32 white

VARIATIONS OF SEX LINKAGE

5.6. The recessive incompletely sex-linked gene called "bobbed" (*bb*) causes the bristles of *Drosophila* to be shorter and of smaller diameter than the normal bristles produced by its dominant wild-type allele (*bb*$^+$). Determine the phenotypic expectations of the F_1 and F_2 when bobbed females are crossed with each of the 2 possible heterozygous males.

Solution:

Recall that an incompletely sex-linked gene has an allele on the homologous portion of the Y chromosome in a male. The wild-type allele in heterozygous males may be on either the X or the Y, thus making possible two types of crosses.

First Cross:

Parents: $X^{bb}X^{bb}$ × $X^{bb+}Y^{bb}$
                  bobbed females   wild-type males

F_1: $X^{bb}X^{bb+}$ and $X^{bb}Y^{bb}$
          all females wild type   all males bobbed

F_2:

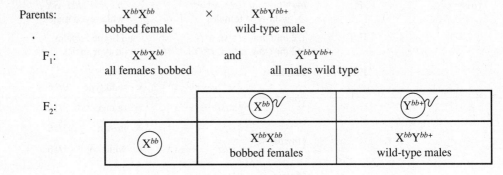

	X^{bb}	X^{bb+}
X^{bb}	$X^{bb}X^{bb}$ bobbed female	$X^{bb}X^{bb+}$ wild-type female
Y^{bb}	$X^{bb}Y^{bb}$ bobbed male	$X^{bb+}Y^{bb}$ wild-type male

Thus $\frac{1}{2}$ of the F_2 females are bobbed and $\frac{1}{2}$ are wild type; $\frac{1}{2}$ of the F_2 males are bobbed and $\frac{1}{2}$ are wild type.

Second Cross:

Parents: $X^{bb}X^{bb}$ × $X^{bb}Y^{bb+}$
                  bobbed female   wild-type male

F_1: $X^{bb}X^{bb}$ and $X^{bb}Y^{bb+}$
          all females bobbed   all males wild type

F_2:

	X^{bb}	Y^{bb+}
X^{bb}	$X^{bb}X^{bb}$ bobbed females	$X^{bb}Y^{bb+}$ wild-type males

Thus all F_2 females are bobbed and all males are wild type.

SEX-INFLUENCED TRAITS

5.7. Let us consider two sex-influenced traits simultaneously, pattern baldness and short index finger, both of which are dominant in men and recessive in women. A heterozygous bald man with long index finger marries a heterozygous long-fingered, bald woman. Determine the phenotypic expectations for their children.

Solution:

Let us first select appropriate symbols and define the phenotypic expression of the 3 genotypes in each sex.

Genotypes	Males	Females	Genotype	Males	Females
B^1B^1	Bald	Bald	F^1F^1	Short-fingered	Short-fingered
B^1B^2	Bald	Nonbald	F^1F^2	Short-fingered	Long-fingered
B^2B^2	Nonbald	Nonbald	F^2F^2	Long-fingered	Long-fingered

P: B^1B^2, F^2F^2 × B^1B^1, F^1F^2
     bald, long-fingered man   bald, long-fingered woman

F$_1$:

$\frac{1}{2}B^1B^1$ < $\frac{1}{2}F^1F^2 = \frac{1}{4}B^1B^1F^1F^2$ bald, short (men) / bald, long (women)
$\frac{1}{2}F^2F^2 = \frac{1}{4}B^1B^1F^2F^2$ bald, long (men) / bald, long (women)

$\frac{1}{2}B^1B^2$ < $\frac{1}{2}F^1F^2 = \frac{1}{4}B^1B^2F^1F^2$ bald, short (men) / nonbald, long (women)
$\frac{1}{2}F^2F^2 = \frac{1}{4}B^1B^2F^2F^2$ bald, long (men) / nonbald, long (women)

F$_1$ summary: **Men:**   1/2 bald, short-fingered : 1/2 bald, long-fingered
          Women: 1/2 bald, long-fingered : 1/2 nonbald, long-fingered

SEX-LIMITED TRAITS

5.8. Cock-feathering in chickens is a trait limited to expression only in males and determined by the autosomal recessive genotype hh. The dominant allele (H) produces hen-feathered males. All females are hen-feathered regardless of genotype. A cock-feathered male is mated to 3 females, each of which produces a dozen chicks. Among the 36 progeny are 15 hen-feathered males, 18 hen-feathered females, and 3 cock-feathered males. What are the most probable genotypes of the 3 parental females?

Solution:

In order for both hen-feathered (H-) and cock-feathered (hh) males to be produced, at least one of the females had to be heterozygous (Hh) or recessive (hh). The following female genotype possibilities must be explored:

(a) 2 HH, 1 Hh	(c) 1 HH, 1 Hh, 1 hh	(e) 2 Hh, 1 hh	(g) 2 HH, 1 hh
(b) 1 HH, 2 Hh	(d) 3 Hh	(f) 1 Hh, 2 hh	(h) 2 hh, 1 HH

Obviously, the more hh or Hh hen genotypes, proportionately more cock-feathered males are expected in the progeny. The ratio of 15 hen-feathered males : 3 cock-feathered males is much greater than the 1 : 1 ratio expected when all 3 females are heterozygous (Hh).

P: hh × Hh
     cock-feathered male   hen-feathered females

F$_1$: $\frac{1}{2}Hh$ hen-feathered males, $\frac{1}{2}hh$ cock-feathered males

Possibility (d) is therefore excluded. Possibilities (e) and (f), which both contain one or more hh genotypes in addition to one or more Hh genotypes, must also be eliminated because these matings would produce even more cock-feathered males than possibility (d). In possibility (g), the 2 HH : 1 hh hens are expected to produce an equivalent ratio of 2 hen-feathered (Hh) : 1 cock-feathered (hh) males. This 2 : 1 ratio should be expressed in the 18 male offspring as 12 hen-feathered : 6 cock-feathered. These numbers compare fairly well with the observed 15 : 3, but possibility (h) would be even less favorable because even more cock-feathered males would be produced. Let us see if one of the remaining three possibilities will give us expected values closer to our observations.

Possibility (c):
                    $\frac{1}{3}HH$ ⎫
     P: hh × $\frac{1}{3}Hh$ ⎬ hen-feathered females
          cock-feathered male $\frac{1}{3}hh$ ⎭

F$_1$: $\frac{1}{3}(hh \times HH) = \frac{1}{3}Hh$ hen-feathered males

$$\tfrac{1}{3}(hh \times Hh) = \begin{cases} \tfrac{1}{3} \cdot \tfrac{1}{2} = \tfrac{1}{6}Hh \text{ hen-feathered males} \\ \tfrac{1}{3} \cdot \tfrac{1}{2} = \tfrac{1}{6}hh \text{ cock-feathered males} \end{cases}$$

$$\tfrac{1}{3}(hh \times hh) = \tfrac{1}{3}hh \text{ cock-feathered males}$$

Summary: Hen-feathered males $= \tfrac{1}{3} + \tfrac{1}{6} = \tfrac{1}{2}$,   Cock-feathered males $= \tfrac{1}{6} + \tfrac{1}{3} = \tfrac{1}{2}$

Again this disagrees with the observations and must be excluded.

Possibility   (b):

P: hh $\times$ $\left.\begin{array}{l}\tfrac{1}{3}HH \\ \tfrac{2}{3}Hh\end{array}\right\}$ hen-feathered females

cock-feathered male

F$_1$: $\tfrac{1}{3}(hh \times HH) = \tfrac{1}{3}Hh$ hen-feathered males

$$\tfrac{2}{3}(hh \times Hh) = \begin{cases} \tfrac{2}{3} \cdot \tfrac{1}{2} = \tfrac{2}{6}Hh \text{ hen-feathered males} \\ \tfrac{2}{3} \cdot \tfrac{1}{2} = \tfrac{2}{6}hh \text{ cock-feathered males} \end{cases}$$

Summary: Hen-feathered males $= \tfrac{1}{3} + \tfrac{2}{6} = \tfrac{2}{3}$,   Cock-feathered males $= \tfrac{2}{6}$ or $\tfrac{1}{3}$

These expectations are no closer to the observations than those of possibility (g).

Possibility   (a):

P: hh $\times$ $\left.\begin{array}{l}\tfrac{2}{3}HH \\ \tfrac{1}{3}Hh\end{array}\right\}$ hen-feathered females

cock-feathered male

F$_1$: $\tfrac{2}{3}(hh \times HH) = \tfrac{2}{3}Hh$ hen-feathered males

$$\tfrac{1}{3}(hh \times Hh) = \begin{cases} \tfrac{1}{3} \cdot \tfrac{1}{2} = \tfrac{1}{6}Hh \text{ hen-feathered males} \\ \tfrac{1}{3} \cdot \tfrac{1}{2} = \tfrac{1}{6}hh \text{ cock-feathered males} \end{cases}$$

Summary: Hen-feathered males $= \tfrac{2}{3} + \tfrac{1}{6} = \tfrac{5}{6}$,   Cock-feathered males $= \tfrac{1}{6}$

Set the observation of 3 cock-feathered males equal to the $\tfrac{1}{6}$, then 5 times 3 or 15 hen-feathered males should represent the $\tfrac{5}{6}$. These expectations agree perfectly with the observations and therefore it is most probable that two of the females were HH and one was Hh.

SEX REVERSAL

5.9.   Suppose that a hen's ovaries are destroyed by disease, allowing its rudimentary testes to develop. Further suppose that this hen was carrying the dominant sex-linked gene B for barred feathers, and upon sex reversal was then crossed to a nonbarred female. What phenotypic proportions are expected in the F$_1$ and F$_2$?

Solution:

Remember that sex determination in chickens is by the ZW method and that sex reversal does not change this chromosomal constitution. Furthermore at least one sex chromosome (Z) is essential for life.

P: BW $\times$ bW

barred female   normal nonbarred female

sex reversed to a

functional male

F$_1$:

	B	W
b	Bb barred male	bW nonbarred female
W	BW barred female	WW lethal

The proportions are thus $\tfrac{1}{3}$ males (all barred) : $\tfrac{2}{3}$ females (half barred and half nonbarred).

F_2:   Two equally frequent kinds of matings are possible among the F_1 birds. First mating $= \frac{1}{2}$ of all matings.

$$Bb \qquad \times \qquad bW$$
barred male   nonbarred female

Progeny Expectations		Correction for Frequency of Mating		Proportion of Total F_2
$\frac{1}{4}Bb$	·	$\frac{1}{2}$	=	$\frac{1}{8}Bb$ barred males
$\frac{1}{4}bb$	·	$\frac{1}{2}$	=	$\frac{1}{8}bb$ nonbarred males
$\frac{1}{4}BW$	·	$\frac{1}{2}$	=	$\frac{1}{8}BW$ barred females
$\frac{1}{4}bW$	·	$\frac{1}{2}$	=	$\frac{1}{8}bW$ nonbarred females

Second mating $= \frac{1}{2}$ of all matings.

$$Bb \qquad \times \qquad BW$$
barred male   barred female

Progeny Expectations		Correction for Frequency of Mating		Proportion of Total F_2	
$\frac{1}{4}BB$	·	$\frac{1}{2}$	=	$\frac{1}{8}BB$	$\Big\}$ $\frac{1}{4}$ barred males
$\frac{1}{4}Bb$	·	$\frac{1}{2}$	=	$\frac{1}{8}Bb$	
$\frac{1}{4}BW$	·	$\frac{1}{2}$	=	$\frac{1}{8}BW$ barred females	
$\frac{1}{4}bW$	·	$\frac{1}{2}$	=	$\frac{1}{8}bW$ nonbarred females	

Summary of the F_2:   Barred males $= \frac{1}{8} + \frac{1}{4} = \frac{3}{8}$ Barred females $= \frac{1}{8} + \frac{1}{8} = \frac{1}{4}$

Nonbarred males $= \frac{1}{8}$ Nonbarred females $= \frac{1}{8} + \frac{1}{8} = \frac{1}{4}$

SEXUAL PHENOMENA IN PLANTS

5.10. A recessive gene in monoecious corn called "tassel-seed" (*ts*), when homozygous, produces only seeds where the staminate inflorescence (tassel) normally appears. No pollen is produced. Thus individuals of genotype *ts/ts* are functionally reduced to a single sex, that of the female. On another chromosome, the recessive gene called "silkless" (*sk*), when homozygous, produces ears with no pistils (silks). Without silks, none of these ears can produce seed and individuals of genotype *sk/sk* are reduced to performing only male functions (production of pollen in the tassel). The recessive gene for tassel-seed is epistatic to the silkless locus. (*a*) What sex ratio is expected in the F_1 and F_2 from the cross *ts/ts, sk^+/sk^+* (female) × *ts^+/ts^+, sk/sk* (male)? (*b*) How could the genes for tassel-seed and silkless be used to establish male and female plants (dioecious) that would continue, generation after generation, to produce progeny in the ratio of 1 male : 1 female?

Solution:

(*a*)   P: *ts/ts, sk^+/sk^+*   ×   *ts^+/ts^+, sk/sk*
                    female   male

     F_1:   *ts^+/ts, sk^+/sk*
                         monoecious
             (both male and female flowers)

     F_2: $\frac{9}{16}$ *$ts^+/-$, $sk^+/-$* $= \frac{9}{16}$ monoecious
             $\frac{3}{16}$ *$ts^+/-$, sk/sk* $= \frac{3}{16}$ male
             $\left.\begin{array}{l} \frac{3}{16} \ ts/ts, sk^+/- \\ \frac{1}{16} \ ts/ts, \ sk/sk \end{array}\right\} = \frac{4}{16}$ female

(*b*)   P: *ts/ts, sk/sk*   ×   *ts^+/ts, sk/sk*
                    female   male

     F_1: $\frac{1}{2}$ *ts^+/ts, sk/sk*   males
             $\frac{1}{2}$ *ts/ts, sk/sk*   females

Subsequent generations would continue to exhibit a 1 : 1 sex ratio for these dioecious plants.

5.11. Pollen tubes containing the same self-incompatibility allele as that found in the diploid tissue of the style grow so slowly that fertilization cannot occur before the flower withers. Pollen produced by a plant of genotype S^1S^3 would be of two types, S^1 and S^3. If this pollen were to land on the stigma of the same plant (S^1S^3), none of the pollen tubes would grow. If these pollen grains (S^1 and S^3) were to alight on a stigma of genotype S^1S^2, then only the tubes containing the S^3 allele would be compatible with the alleles in the tissue of the style. If these pollen grains were to alight on a stigma of genotype S^2S^4, all of the pollen tubes would be functional. Four plant varieties (A, B, C, and D) are crossed, with the results listed in the table below. Notice that two additional varieties (E and F) appear in the progeny. Determine the genotypes for all six varieties in terms of four self-sterility alleles (S^1, S^2, S^3, and S^4).

		Male Parent			
		A	B	C	D
Female parent	A	—	$\frac{1}{4}$C, $\frac{1}{4}$D $\frac{1}{4}$E, $\frac{1}{4}$F	$\frac{1}{2}$C $\frac{1}{2}$D	$\frac{1}{2}$C $\frac{1}{2}$D
	B	$\frac{1}{4}$C, $\frac{1}{4}$D $\frac{1}{4}$E, $\frac{1}{4}$F	—	$\frac{1}{2}$C $\frac{1}{2}$E	$\frac{1}{2}$D $\frac{1}{2}$F
	C	$\frac{1}{2}$A $\frac{1}{4}$D	$\frac{1}{2}$B $\frac{1}{2}$E	—	$\frac{1}{2}$D $\frac{1}{2}$A
	D	$\frac{1}{2}$A $\frac{1}{2}$C	$\frac{1}{2}$B $\frac{1}{2}$F	$\frac{1}{2}$A $\frac{1}{2}$C	—

Solution:

None of the genotypes are expected to be homozygous for the self-incompatibility alleles because pollen containing the same allele present in the maternal tissue is not functional and therefore homozygosity is prevented. Thus 6 genotypes are possible with four self-incompatibility alleles: S^1S^2, S^1S^3, S^1S^4, S^2S^3, S^2S^4, S^3S^4. Crosses between genotypes with both alleles in common produce no progeny (A $\times$ A, B $\times$ B, etc.). Crosses between genotypes with only one allele in common produce offspring in the ratio of 1 : 1 (e.g., $S^1S^2 ♀ \times S^1S^3 ♂ = \frac{1}{2}S^1S^3 : \frac{1}{2}S^2S^3$). Crosses between genotypes with none of their self-incompatibility alleles in common produce progeny in the ratio 1 : 1 : 1 : 1 (e.g., $S^1S^2 \times S^3S^4 = \frac{1}{4}S^1S^3 : \frac{1}{4}S^1S^4 : \frac{1}{4}S^2S^3 : \frac{1}{4}S^2S^4$). Turning now to the table of results, we find the cross B♀ $\times$ A♂ produces offspring in the ratio 1 : 1 : 1 : 1 and therefore neither B nor A contains any alleles in common. If we assume that variety B has the genotype S^1S^4, then variety A must have the genotype S^2S^3 (the student's solution to this problem may differ from the one presented here in the alleles arbitrarily assigned as a starting point). The cross C♀ $\times$ A♂ produces offspring in the ratio 1 : 1, indicating one pair of alleles in common. Since we have already designated variety A to be of genotype S^2SS^3, let us arbitrarily assign the genotype S^1S^2 to variety C. The cross D♀ $\times$ A♂ also indicates that one allele is held in common by these 2 varieties. Let us assign the genotype S^1S^3 to variety D. The genotype for variety E may now be determined from the cross C♀ $\times$ B♂.

P: S^1S^2(C)♀ $\times$ S^1S^4(B)♂

F$_1$: $\frac{1}{2}S^1S^4$ = variety B, $\frac{1}{2}S^2S^4$ = variety E

Likewise, the genotype for variety F may now be determined from the cross D♀ $\times$ B♂.

P: S^1S^3(D)♀ $\times$ S^1S^4(B)♂

F$_1$: $\frac{1}{2}S^1S^4$ = variety B, $\frac{1}{2}S^3S^4$ = variety F

Summary of genotypes for all six varieties:

A = S^2S^3 B = S^1S^4 C = S^1S^2 D = S^1S^3 E = S^2S^4 F = S^3S^4

The student should confirm that the other results shown in the table are compatible with the genotypic assumptions shown above.

Supplementary Problems

SEX DETERMINATION AND SEX-LINKED INHERITANCE

Heterogametic Males (XY and XO Methods)

5.12. A sex-linked recessive gene c produces red-green color blindness in humans. A normal woman whose father was color blind marries a color-blind man. (*a*) What genotypes are possible for the mother of the color-blind man? (*b*) What are the chances that the first child from this marriage will be a color-blind boy? (*c*) Of all the girls produced by these parents, what percentage is expected to be color blind? (*d*) Of all the children (sex unspecified) from these parents, what proportion is expected to be normal?

5.13. The gene for yellow body color y in *Drosophila* is recessive and sex-linked. Its dominant allele y^+ produces wild-type body color. What phenotypic ratios are expected from the crosses (*a*) yellow male $\times$ yellow female, (*b*) yellow female $\times$ wild-type male, (*c*) wild-type female (homozygous) $\times$ yellow male, (*d*) wild-type (carrier) female $\times$ wild-type male, (*e*) wild-type (carrier) female $\times$ yellow male?

5.14. A narrow reduced eye called "bar" is a dominant sex-linked condition (B) in *Drosophila,* and the full wild-type eye is produced by its recessive allele B^+. A homozygous wild-type female is mated to a bar-eyed male. Determine the F_1 and F_2 genotypic and phenotypic expectations.

5.15. Sex determination in the grasshopper is by the XO method. The somatic cells of a grasshopper are analyzed and found to contain 23 chromosomes. (*a*) What sex is this individual? (*b*) Determine the frequency with which different types of gametes (number of autosomes and sex chromosomes) can be formed in this individual. (*c*) What is the diploid number of the opposite sex?

5.16. Male house cats may be black or yellow. Females may be black, tortoise-shell pattern, or yellow. (*a*) If these colors are governed by a sex-linked locus, how can these results be explained? (*b*) Using appropriate symbols, determine the phenotypes expected in the offspring from the cross yellow female $\times$ black male. (*c*) Do the same for the reciprocal cross of part (*b*). (*d*) A certain kind of mating produces females, half of which are tortoise-shell and half are black; half the males are yellow and half are black. What colors are the parental males and females in such crosses? (*e*) Another kind of mating produces offspring, $\frac{1}{4}$ of which are yellow males, $\frac{1}{4}$ yellow females, $\frac{1}{4}$ black males, and $\frac{1}{4}$ tortoise-shell females. What colors are the parental males and females in such crosses?

5.17. In the plant genus *Melandrium,* sex determination is similar to that in humans. A sex-linked gene (l) is known to be lethal when homozygous in females. When present in the hemizygous condition in males (lY), it produces blotchy patches of yellow-green color. The homozygous or heterozygous condition of the wild-type allele (LL or Ll) in females, or the hemizygous condition in males (LY) produces normal dark-green color. From a cross between heterozygous females and yellow-green males, predict the phenotypic ratio expected in the progeny.

5.18. The recessive gene for white eye color in *Drosophila* (w) is sex-linked. Another recessive sex-linked gene governing eye color is vermilion (v), which when homozygous in females or hemizygous in males together with the autosomal gene for brown eye (bw/bw), also produces white eye. White genotypes (wY, ww) are epistatic to the other loci under consideration. (*a*) What phenotypic results are expected among progeny from mating a white-eyed male of genotype (bw/bw, $vw^+/$Y) with a white-eyed female of genotype (bw^+/bw, vw/v^+w)? *Hint:* See Problem 5.5 (*b*) What phenotypic proportions are expected in the progeny from the mating of a vermilion female heterozygous at the brown locus but not carrying the white allele with a male that is white due to the w allele but heterozygous at the brown locus and hemizygous for the vermilion allele? (*c*) Determine the expected phenotypic ratio in the F_1 and F_2 from the reciprocal cross of Problem 5.5(*a*).

Heterogametic Females (ZW and ZO Methods)

5.19. A recessive sex-linked gene (k) influences a slower growth rate of the primary feathers of chickens than its dominant allele (k^+) for fast feathering. This trait can be used for sexing chicks within a few days after hatching. (*a*) If fast-feathering females are crossed to slow-feathering males, what phenotypic ratio is expected among the F_1 and F_2? (*b*) What are the expected F_1 and F_2 phenotypic ratios from crossing fast-feathering males (k^+/k^+) to slow-feathering females? (c) What are the expected F_1 and F_2 phenotypic ratios from crossing fast-feathering males (k^+/k) to slow-feathering females?

5.20. Silver-colored plumage in poultry is due to a dominant sex-linked gene (S) and gold-colored plumage to its recessive allele (s). List the phenotypic and genotypic expectations of the progeny from the matings (a) $s/W♀ \times S/S♂$, (b) $s/W♀ \times S/s♂$, (c) $S/W♀ \times S/s♂$, (d) $S/W♀ \times s/s♂$.

5.21. In the Rosy Gier variety of carrier pigeon, a cross was made between gray-headed females and creamy-headed males. The F_1 ratio was 1 gray-headed female : 1 gray-headed male : 1 creamy-headed male. (a) How may these results be explained? (b) Diagram this cross using appropriate symbols.

5.22. Chickens have an autosomal dominant gene (C) that produces a short-legged phenotype called "creeper" in heterozygotes. Normal legs are produced by the recessive genotype (cc). The homozygous dominant genotype (CC) is lethal. A dominant sex-linked gene (B) produces barred plumage, the recessive allele (b) produces nonbarred plumage. (a) Determine the phenotypic expectations among progeny (of both sexes) from the cross of a barred creeper female and a nonbarred creeper male. (b) Determine the phenotypic ratios within each sex for part (a). (c) Two chickens were mated and produced progeny in the following proportions: $\frac{1}{12}$ nonbarred males, $\frac{1}{6}$ nonbarred creeper females, $\frac{1}{12}$ barred males, $\frac{1}{12}$ nonbarred females, $\frac{1}{6}$ nonbarred creeper males, $\frac{1}{6}$ barred creeper males, $\frac{1}{12}$ barred females, and $\frac{1}{6}$ barred creeper females. What are the genotypes and phenotypes of the parents?

5.23. A dominant autosomal inhibitor (I-) as well as a recessive autosomal inhibitor (cc) prevents any color from being produced in chickens. The genotypes I-C-, I-cc and $iicc$ all produce white chickens; only the genotype iiC- produces colored birds. A recessive sex-linked gene k produces slow growth of the primary wing feathers. Its dominant allele k^+ produces fast feathering. A white ($IICC$) slow-feathering male is mated to a white ($iicc$) fast-feathering female. What are the F_1 and F_2 phenotypic expectations?

5.24. The presence of feathers on the shanks of the Black Langshan breed of chickens is due to the dominant alleles at either or both of two autosomal loci. Nonfeathered shanks are the result of the double-recessive genotype. A dominant sex-linked gene (B) places white bars on a black bird. Its recessive allele (b) produces nonbarred (black) birds. Trihybrid barred males with feathered shanks are mated to dihybrid nonbarred females with feathered shanks. Determine the F_1 phenotypic expectations.

Genic Balance
5.25. In *Drosophila*, the ratio between the number of X chromosomes and the number of sets of autosomes (A) is called the "sex index." Diploid females have a sex index (ratio X/A) $= \frac{2}{2} = 1.0$ Diploid males have a sex ratio of $\frac{1}{2} = 0.5$. Sex index values between 0.5 and 1.0 give rise to intersexes. Values over 1.0 or under 0.5 produce weak and inviable flies called "superfemales" (meta-females) and "supermales" (meta-males), respectively. Calculate the sex index and the sex phenotype in the following individuals: (a) AAX, (b) AAXXY, (c) AAAXX, (d) AAXX, (e) AAXXX, (f) AAAXXX, (g) AAY.

Haplodiploidy
5.26. If the diploid number of the honey bee is 16: (a) how many chromosomes will be found in the somatic cells of the drone (male), (b) how many bivalents will be seen during the process of gametogenesis in the male, (c) how many bivalents will be seen during the process of gametogenesis in the female?

5.27. Seven eye colors are known in the honey bee, each produced by a recessive gene at a different locus: brick (bk), chartreuse (ch), ivory (i), cream (cr), snow (s), pearl (pe), and garnet (g). Suppose that a wild-type queen heterozygous at the brick locus (bk^+/bk) was to be artificially inseminated with a mixture of sperm from seven haploid drones each exhibiting a different one of the seven mutant eye colors. Further assume that the semen contribution of each male contains equal concentrations of sperm, that each sperm has an equal opportunity to enter fertilization, and that each zygote thus formed has an equal opportunity to survive. (a) What percentage of the drone offspring is expected to be brick-eyed? (b) What percentage of worker offspring is expected to be brick-eyed?

Single-Gene Effects
5.28. In the single-celled haploid plant *Chlamydomonas*, there are two mating types, ($+$) and ($-$). There is no morphological distinction between the ($+$) sex and the ($-$) sex in either the spore stage or the gamete stage

(isogametes). The fusion of $(+)$ and $(-)$ gametes produces a $2n$ zygote that immediately undergoes meiosis producing four haploid spores, two of which are $(+)$ and two are $(-)$. (*a*) Could a pair of genes for sex account for the 1:1 sex ratio? (*b*) Does the foregoing information preclude some other form of sex determination? Explain.

5.29. Sex determination in the wasp *Bracon* is either by sex alleles or haplodiploidy. A recessive gene called "veinless" (v) is known to assort independently of the sex alleles; the dominant allele v^+ results in wild type. For each of the 8 crosses listed below, determine the relative frequencies of progeny phenotypes within each of 3 categories: (1) haploid males, (2) diploid males, (3) females. (*a*) v/v, $s^a/s^b \times v^+$, s^a, (*b*) v/v, $s^a/s^b \times v^+$, s^c, (*c*) v/v, $s^a/s^b \times v$, s^b, (*d*) v/v, $s^a/s^b \times v$, s^c, (*e*) v/v^+, $s^a/s^b \times v$, s^a, (*f*) v/v^+, $s^a/s^b \times v$, s^c, (*g*) v^+/v^+, $s^a/s^b \times v$, s^a, (*h*) v^+/v^+, $s^a/s^b \times v$, s^c.

VARIATIONS OF SEX LINKAGE

5.30. An Englishman by the name of Edward Lambert was born in 1717. His skin was like thick bark that had to be shed periodically. The hairs on his body were quill-like and he subsequently has been referred to as the "porcupine man." He had 6 sons, all of whom exhibited the same trait. The trait appeared to be transmitted from father to son through four generations. None of the daughters ever exhibited the trait. In fact, it has never been known to appear in females. (*a*) Could this be an autosomal sex-limited trait? (*b*) How is this trait probably inherited?

5.31. Could a recessive mutant gene in humans be located on the X chromosome if a woman exhibiting the recessive trait and a normal man had a normal son? Explain.

5.32. A holandric gene is known in humans that causes long hair to grow on the external ears. When men with hairy ears marry normal women, (*a*) what percentage of their sons would be expected to have hairy ears, (*b*) what proportion of the daughters is expected to show the trait, (*c*) what ratio of hairy-eared : normal children is expected?

SEX-INFLUENCED TRAITS

5.33. A certain type of white forelock in humans appears to follow the sex-influenced mode of inheritance, being dominant in men and recessive in women. Using the allelic symbols w and w', indicate all possible genotypes and the phenotypes thereby produced in men and women.

5.34. The sex-influenced gene governing the presence of horns in sheep exhibits dominance in males but acts recessively in females. When the Dorset breed (both sexes horned) with genotype hh is crossed to the Suffolk breed (both sexes polled or hornless) with the genotype $h'h'$, what phenotypic ratios are expected in the F_1 and F_2?

5.35. The fourth (ring) finger of humans may be longer or shorter than the second (index) finger. The short index finger is thought to be produced by a gene that is dominant in men and recessive in women. What kinds of children and with what frequency would the following marriages be likely to produce: (*a*) heterozygous short-fingered man × short-fingered woman, (*b*) heterozygous long-fingered woman × homozygous short-fingered man, (*c*) heterozygous short-fingered man × heterozygous long-fingered woman, (*d*) long-fingered man × short-fingered woman?

5.36. In the Ayrshire breed of dairy cattle, mahogany-and-white color is dependent upon a gene C^M which is dominant in males and recessive in females. Its allele for red-and-white (C^R) acts as a dominant in females but recessive in males. (*a*) If a red-and-white male is crossed to a mahogany-and-white female, what phenotypic and genotypic proportions are expected in the F_1 and F_2? (*b*) If a mahogany-and-white cow has a red-and-white calf, what sex is the calf? (*c*) What genotype is *not* possible for the sire of the calf in part (*b*)?

5.37. Long-eared goats mated to short-eared goats produce an ear of intermediate length in the F_1 and an F_2 consisting of $\frac{1}{4}$ long, $\frac{1}{2}$ intermediate, and $\frac{1}{4}$ short in both males and females. Nonbearded male goats mated to bearded female goats produce bearded male progeny and nonbearded female progeny. The F_2 males have

$\frac{3}{4}$ bearded and $\frac{1}{4}$ nonbearded, while the F$_2$ females have $\frac{3}{4}$ nonbearded and $\frac{1}{4}$ bearded. A bearded male with ears of intermediate length whose father and mother were both nonbearded is mated with a nonbearded, intermediate-eared half-sib (sib = sibling = a brother or sister; half-sibs are half-brothers or half-sisters) by the same father but out of a bearded mother. List the phenotypic expectations among the progeny.

5.38. A sex-linked recessive gene in humans produces color-blind men when hemizygous and color-blind women when homozygous. A sex-influenced gene for pattern baldness is dominant in men and recessive in women. A heterozygous bald, color-blind man marries a nonbald woman with normal vision whose father was nonbald and color blind and whose mother was bald with normal vision. List the phenotypic expectations for their children.

SEX-LIMITED TRAITS

5.39. A dominant sex-limited gene is known to affect premature baldness in men but is without effect in women. (a) What proportion of the male offspring from parents, both of whom are heterozygous, is expected to be bald prematurely? (b) What proportion of all their children is expected to be prematurely bald?

5.40. The down of baby junglefowl chicks of genotype S- is darkly striped, whereas the recessive genotype ss produces in both sexes an unstriped yellowish-white down. In the adult plumage, however, the character behaves as a sex-limited trait. Males, regardless of genotype, develop normal junglefowl plumage. Females of genotype S- bear normal junglefowl plumage but the recessive ss is a creamy-buff color. A male bird unstriped at birth is mated to three females, each of which lays 16 eggs. Among the 48 progeny there are 32 unstriped chicks and 16 striped. At maturity there are 16 with creamy-buff and 32 with normal junglefowl plumage. What are the most probable genotypes of the three parental females?

5.41. In the clover butterfly, all males are yellow, but females may be yellow if they are of the homozygous recessive genotype yy or white if they possess the dominant allele (Y-). What phenotypic proportions, exclusive of sex, are expected in the F$_1$ from the cross $Yy \times Yy$?

5.42. The barred plumage pattern in chickens is governed by a dominant sex-linked gene B. The gene for cock-feathering h is recessive in males, its dominant allele H producing hen-feathering. Normal females are hen-feathered regardless of genotype (sex-limited trait). Nonbarred females heterozygous at the hen-feathered locus are crossed to a barred, hen-feathered male whose father was cock-feathered and nonbarred. What phenotypic proportions are expected among the progeny?

5.43. Cock-feathering is a sex-limited trait in chickens (see Example 5.10). In the Leghorn breed, all males are cock-feathered and all females are hen-feathered. In the Sebright bantam breed, both males and females are hen-feathered. In the Hamburg breed, males may be either cock-feathered or hen-feathered, but females are always hen-feathered. (a) How can these results be explained? (b) If the ovaries or testes are removed and the chickens are allowed to molt, they will become cock-feathered regardless of genotype. What kind of chemicals are involved in the expression of genotypes at this locus?

PEDIGREES

5.44. Could the trait represented by the solid symbols in the pedigree below be explained on the basis of (a) a dominant sex-linked gene, (b) a recessive sex-linked gene, (c) a holandric gene, (d) a sex-limited autosomal dominant, (e) a sex-limited autosomal recessive, (f) a sex-influenced autosomal gene dominant in males, (g) a sex-influenced autosomal gene recessive in males?

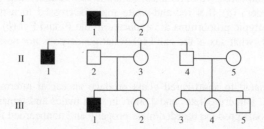

5.45.

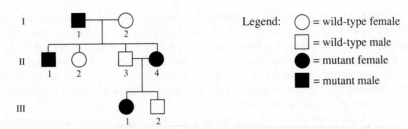

Could the assumption of a sex-linked recessive mutant gene be supported by the above pedigree? Explain

5.46.

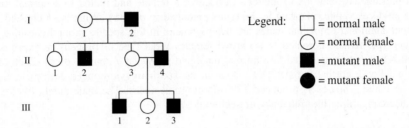

(a)   Could the above pedigree be used as support for a holandric gene?

(b)   Does the above pedigree contradict the assumption of a sex-linked recessive gene for the mutant trait?

(c)   If a mating between III2 and III3 produced a mutant female offspring, which of the above two hypotheses would apply? List the genotype of each individual in the pedigree, using appropriate symbols.

5.47.   Could the trait represented by the solid symbols in the pedigree shown below be produced by (a) an autosomal dominant, (b) an autosomal recessive, (c) a sex-linked dominant, (d) a sex-linked recessive, (e) a sex-limited gene, (f) a holandric gene, (g) a sex-influenced gene?

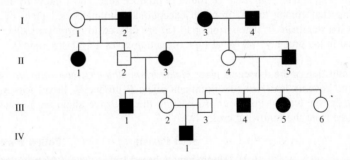

SEX REVERSALS

5.48.   Suppose that a female undergoes sex reversal to become a functional male and is then mated to a normal female. Determine the expected F_1 sex ratios from such matings in species with (a) ZW method of sex determination, (b) XY method of sex determination.

5.49.   The hemp plant is dioecious, probably resulting from an XY mechanism of sex determination. Early plantings (May–June) yield the normal $1:1$ sex ratio. Late plantings in November, however, produce all female plants. If this difference is due to the length of daylight, it should be possible to rear both XY females and XY males under controlled conditions in the greenhouse. What sex ratio would be expected among seedlings grown early in the year from crosses between XY males and XY females?

5.50.   Suppose that a hen carrying the recessive sex-linked allele k for slow feathering underwent a sex reversal and sired chicks from hens carrying the dominant allele k^+ for fast feathering. What genotypic and phenotypic proportions are expected in the F_1 and F_2?

5.51. The developing gonad in young larvae of goldfish (*Carassius auratus*) is ambisexual and subject to differentiate into either an ovary or a testis, irrespective of its sex genotype, by exogenous exposure to heterotypic sex hormones. The sex genes are not the direct cause of sex differentiation, but act indirectly by producing sex-inducing hormones. Female hormones (estrogens) and male hormones (androgens) are usually considered to be responsible for the expression of secondary sexual characteristics and for the maintenance of sexual capacities. However, in the case of this species, estrogens can also act as the *gynotermone* (ovary-inducing agent) and androgens can act as the *androtermone* (testis-inducing agent). (*a*) If females are heterogametic (ZW) and males are homogametic (ZZ), predict the offspring expected from a presumptive male (ZZ) converted by estrone (an estrogenic hormone) treatment into a female and mated to a normal male (ZZ). (*b*) If males are heterogametic (XY) and females are homogametic (XX), predict the zygotic expectations from a presumptive male (XY) induced to become a female and mated to a normal male (XY). (*c*) This species produces viable offspring in the ratios predicted in part (*b*). What is so unusual about this finding? (*d*) As an additional proof that males are heterogametic in this species, a methyltestosterone-induced male of a genotypic female is mated to a normal female. What type of progeny is expected? (*e*) An estrone-induced XY female was mated to a normal male and produced 7 sons (1 died). Each of the 6 viable sons was crossed with normal females (XX). Five of the six matings produced both male and female progeny. The sixth mating, however, produced 198 offspring, all males. The male parent lived 8 years. What does this indicate regarding the frequency of such males?

SEXUAL PHENOMENA IN PLANTS

5.52. A completely pistillate inflorescence (female flower) is produced in the castor bean by the recessive genotype *nn*. Plants of genotype *NN* and *Nn* have mixed pistillate and staminate flowers in the inflorescence. Determine the types of flowers produced in the progeny from the following crosses: (*a*) *NN* ♀ × *Nn* ♂, (*b*) *Nn* ♀ × *Nn* ♂, (*c*) *nn* ♀ × *Nn* ♂.

5.53. Asparagus is a dioecious plant in which maleness (staminate plants) is governed by a dominant gene *P* and femaleness (pistillate plants) by its recessive allele *p*. Sometimes pistillate flowers are found to have small nonfunctional anthers, and then again some staminate flowers may be found to possess immature pistils. Very rarely a staminate plant may be found to produce seed, most likely by self-fertilization. (*a*) What sex ratio is expected among the F_1 from an exceptional staminate-seed plant of genotype *Pp* when selfed? (*b*) When the staminate F_1 plants from part (*a*) are crossed to normal pistillate plants (*pp*), what sex ratio is expected in the progeny? (*c*) What type of mating gives a 1 : 1 sex ratio?

5.54. Sex determination in the dioecious plant *Melandrium album* (*Lychnis dioica*) is by the XY method. A sex-linked gene governs leaf size, the dominant allele *B* producing broad leaves, and the recessive allele *b* producing narrow leaves. Pollen grains bearing the recessive allele are inviable. What phenotypic results are expected from the following crosses?

	Seed Parent		**Pollen Parent**
(*a*)	Homozygous broad-leaf	=	Narrow-leaf
(*b*)	Heterozygous broad-leaf	=	Narrow-leaf
(*c*)	Heterozygous broad-leaf	=	Broad-leaf

5.55. Partial dioecy can be attained in a monoecious plant by the action of a single-gene locus that prevents the production of viable gametes in one of the two types of gametangia (organ-bearing gametes). The male-sterile condition is ordinarily recessive in most plant species where it has been studied. (*a*) Suppose that we artificially cross a pollen parent (*Ss*) onto a male-sterile (egg) parent of genotype *ss*. Determine the phenotypic ratio in the F_1 and F_2 (assuming complete randomness of mating, including selfing, among the F_1 types). (*b*) Determine the F_1 and F_2 expectancies in part (*a*) when the parental cross is *ss* × *SS*. (*c*) If a locus (*A*), assorting independently of the male sterility locus (*S*), is jointly considered in the cross *ssAA* × *Ssaa*, determine the F_1 and F_2 expectancies for the genotypes *S-A-*, *S-aa*, *ssA-*, and *ssaa*. (*d*) Do likewise for part (*c*) where the parental cross is *ssAA* × *SSaa*.

5.56. Two or more genes may cooperate to restrict selfing. An example is known in monoecious sorghum where the action of two complementary genes produces an essentially male plant by making the female structures sterile. Plants heterozygous at both loci (Fs_1/fs_1, Fs_2/fs_2) result in female sterile plants with no effect on their production of pollen. Whenever 3 dominant genes are present (Fs_1/Fs_1, Fs_2/fs_2, or Fs_1/fs_1, Fs_2/Fs_2), dwarf plants are produced that fail to develop a head. Although not yet observed, a genotype with all 4 dominant alleles would presumably also be dwarf and headless. All other genotypes produce normal plants. If these loci assort independently of one another, determine the F_1 phenotypic expectancies from the crosses (a) $Fs_1/fs_1, Fs_2/fs_2 \times Fs_1/fs_1, fs_2/fs_2$, (b) $Fs_1/fs_1, Fs_2/fs_2 \times Fs_1/Fs_1, fs_2/fs_2$.

5.57. In some cases of self-incompatibility, pollen tube growth is so slow that the style withers and dies before fertilization can occur. Sometimes, if pollination is artificially accomplished in the bud stage, the pollen tube can reach the ovary before the style withers. In this case it is possible to produce a genotype homozygous at the self-sterility locus. (a) What would be the expected results from natural pollination of such a homozygote (S^1S^1) by a heterozygote containing one allele in common (S^1S^3)? (b) What would be the result of the reciprocal cross of part (a)? (c) What would be the result of natural pollination of S^1S^1 by S^2S^3? (d) Would the reciprocal cross of part (c) make any difference in the progeny expectations?

5.58. Two heteromorphic types of flowers are produced in many species of the plant genus *Primula*. One type, called "pin," has short anthers and a long style. The other type, called "thrum," has highly placed anthers and a short style. Thrum is produced by a dominant gene (S) and pin by the recessive allele (s). The only pollinations that are compatible are those between styles and anthers of the same height, i.e., between thrum style and pin anther or between thrum anther and pin style. (a) What genotype do all thrum plants possess? (b) If both the pin and thrum are heterozygous for an independently segregating allelic pair (Aa), what genotypic ratio is expected in the next generation?

5.59. The self-incompatibility mechanism of many plants probably involves a series of multiple alleles similar to that found in *Nicotiana*. In this species, pollen tubes grow very slowly or not at all down the style that contains the same allele at the self-incompatibility locus (S). List the genotypic ratio of progeny sporophytes expected from the following crosses:

	Seed Parent		**Pollen Parent**
(a)	S_1S_2	$\times$	S_1S_2
(b)	S_1S_2	$\times$	S_1S_3
(c)	S_1S_2	$\times$	S_3S_4

(d)   How much of the pollen is compatible in each of the above three crosses?

5.60. A cross is made between 2 plants of the self-sterile genotype $S^1S^2 \times S^3S^4$. If all the F_1 progeny are pollinated only by plants of genotype S^2S^3, what genotypic proportions are expected in the F_2?

Review Questions

Vocabulary   For each of the following definitions, give the appropriate term and spell it correctly. Terms are single words unless indicated otherwise.

1. A form of reproduction involving the union of haploid gametes to form a diploid zygote.

2. An animal that has both male and female reproductive organs.

3. A flower having female but no male reproductive parts.

4. An adjective applicable to the sex that produces gametes bearing structurally different sex chromosomes (e.g., half X-bearing and half Y-bearing).

5. The two symbols that represent the sex chromosomes of female chickens, corresponding respectively to the X and Y chromosomes of mammals.

6. The mode of sex determination for *Drosophila*. (Two words.)

7. The mode of sex determination for bees.

8. An adjective applied to genes on the differential (nonhomologous) segment of the Y chromosome.

9. A class of traits governed by autosomal alleles whose dominance relationships are reversed in the two sexes as a consequence of sex hormone differences.

10. A class of autosomal traits having phenotypic variability in a population in only one sex; the other sex exhibits a single phenotype regardless of its genotype.

True-False Questions   Answer each of the following questions either true (T) or false (F).

1. The main function of sex is to produce males and females.

2. Male grasshoppers have only one sex chromosome in each somatic cell.

3. In chickens, the female is the homogametic sex.

4. In *Drosophila,* the Y chromosome does not determine ''maleness,'' but is necessary for fertility.

5. In bees, workers develop from unfertilized eggs.

6. A woman having the sex-linked recessive color-blind trait should have a father who also is color-blind.

7. ''Crisscross'' inheritance for sex-linked human traits occurs when the father has the recessive trait and the mother has the dominant trait.

8. Sex-linked recessive traits in mammalian populations are always expected to be more frequent in males than in females.

9. No genes are common to both the X and Y chromosomes.

10. A holandric gene in humans is not expected to be phenotypically expressed in women.

Multiple-Choice Questions   Choose the one best answer.

1. In an animal with the XO method of sex determination, which of the following could be the normal number of chromosomes in its somatic cells?   (*a*) 26 in males   (*b*) 17 in females   (*c*) 33 in females   (*d*) 13 in males   (*e*) more than one of the above

2. Suppose that in bees the dominant gene b^+ produces wild-type (brown) eyes, and its recessive allele b produces pink eye color. If a pink-eyed queen mates with a brown-eyed drone, their offspring would most likely be   (*a*) only wild-type progeny   (*b*) wild-type workers and pink-eyed drones   (*c*) only pink-eyed progeny   (*d*) workers $= \frac{1}{2}$ wild : $\frac{1}{2}$ pink-eye; all drones wild type   (*e*) insufficient information to allow a definitive answer

3. In the guinea pig pedigree on page 105, supposedly involving sex-linked inheritance: (*a*) II1 could exhibit the dominant trait   (*b*) both I1 and I2 must be carriers of the gene responsible for the trait shown by II1   (*c*) the probability that the next offspring of II2 × II3 has the same phenotype as III1 is 0.5   (*d*) if II1 is crossed to a female genetically like his sister, 75% of his offspring is expected to be phenotypically like their aunt   (*e*) this pedigree is incompatible with a sex-linked explanation

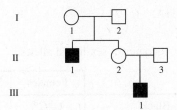

4. The presence of horns in the Dorset breed of sheep is due to a sex-influenced locus with horns dominant in males and recessive in females. Polled (hornless) males are mated to horned females. The fraction of the F_2 expected to be polled is   (a) $\frac{1}{4}$ (b) $\frac{1}{2}$ (c) $\frac{3}{4}$ (d) $\frac{3}{8}$ (e) none of the above

5. In the clover butterfly, all males are yellow, but females may be yellow if they are homozygous (cc) or white if they possess the dominant allele (C-). Matings between heterozygotes are expected to produce an F_1 generation containing   (a) $\frac{1}{2}$ yellow : $\frac{1}{2}$ white   (b) $\frac{3}{4}$ white : $\frac{1}{4}$ yellow   (c) $\frac{3}{8}$ white : $\frac{5}{8}$ yellow   (d) $\frac{9}{16}$ yellow : $\frac{7}{16}$ white   (e) none of the above

6. If sex determination in a species ($2n = 14$) is determined by genic balance (as it is in *Drosophila*), then an intersex could have   (a) 10 autosomes + 2X   (b) 14 chromosomes + 2X   (c) six pairs of autosomes + XY   (d) 21 autosomes + 2X   (e) none of the above

7. The presence of tusks is governed by a holandric gene in a certain mammalian species. When a tusked male is mated to nontusked females, among 100 of their F_2 progeny we would expect to find   (a) 50 tusked males, 50 nontusked females   (b) 25 tusked males, 25 tusked females, 25 nontusked males, 25 nontusked females   (c) 50 nontusked females, 25 tusked males, 25 nontusked males   (d) 50 nontusked males, 25 tusked females, 25 nontusked females   (e) none of the above

8. In a bird species, blue beak is a sex-linked recessive trait; red beak is the alternative dominant trait. If a red-beaked male is mated to blue-beaked females, we would expect to find in the F_1 (a) all progeny red-beaked   (b) all males red-beaked, all females blue-beaked   (c) all males blue-beaked, all females red-beaked   (d) all females red-beaked, $\frac{1}{2}$ of males red-beaked, $\frac{1}{2}$ of males blue-beaked   (e) none of the above.

9. Suppose that the testes of a male (in a species with an XO sex-determination mechanism) experiences a primary sex reversal and begins to produce only eggs. Long tail is a dominant sex-linked trait; short tail is its recessive alternative. If a long-tailed male undergoes a primary sex reversal (to function as a female) and is mated to a short-tailed male, which of the following is expected among the adult progeny?   (a) $\frac{1}{2}$ long-tailed progeny   (b) $\frac{2}{3}$ of males long-tailed   (c) $\frac{1}{4}$ of all progeny long-tailed females   (d) $\frac{1}{3}$ of all progeny long-tailed males   (e) problem is ambiguous; insufficient information

10. A pair of codominant sex-linked alleles in a mammal produce red pigment when homozygous or hemizygous for A^1, colorless when homozygous or hemizygous for A^2 and pink when heterozygous. If a pink female is crossed to a white male, we expect among the progeny   (a) 50% of females are white   (b) 50% of all progeny are pink   (c) 50% of males are pink   (d) 25% of all progeny are white   (e) none of the above

Answers to Supplementary Problems

5.12.   (a) Cc or cc (b) $\frac{1}{4}$ (c) 50%   (d) $\frac{1}{2}$

5.13.   (a) all offspring yellow   (b) All females wild type, all males yellow   (c) all offspring wild type   (d) All females wild type : $\frac{1}{2}$ wild type males : $\frac{1}{2}$ yellow males   (e) Females and males: $\frac{1}{2}$ wild type : $\frac{1}{2}$ yellow

5.14. F_1: B^+/B bar-eyed females, B^+/Y wild type males; F_2 females: $\frac{1}{2}B^+/B^+$ wild type : $\frac{1}{2}B^+/B$ bar eye; F_2 males: $\frac{1}{2}B^+/Y$ wild type : $\frac{1}{2}B/Y$ bar eye

5.15. (*a*) Male (*b*) $\frac{1}{2}(11A + 1X):\frac{1}{2}(11A)$ (*c*) 24

5.16. See Example 10.5. (*a*) A pair of codominant sex-linked alleles.

	Females	Males
Black	$C^B C^B$	$C^B Y$
Tortoise-shell	$C^B C^Y$	—
Yellow	$C^Y C^Y$	$C^Y Y$

(*b*) All males yellow, all females tortoise-shell (*c*) All males black, all females tortoise-shell

(*d*) Tortoise-shell female × black male (*e*) Tortoise-shell female × yellow male

5.17. $\frac{1}{3}$ dark-green females : $\frac{1}{3}$ males with yellow-green patches : $\frac{1}{3}$ males dark green

5.18. (*a*) Males all white-eyed; females: $\frac{1}{4}$ vermilion : $\frac{1}{4}$ wild type : $\frac{1}{4}$ white : $\frac{1}{4}$ brown (*b*) Males and females: $\frac{3}{4}$ vermilion : $\frac{1}{4}$ white (*c*) Males and females: $\frac{3}{8}$ wild type : $\frac{3}{8}$ vermilion : $\frac{1}{8}$ brown : $\frac{1}{8}$ white

5.19. (*a*) F_1: fast males, slow females; F_2: males and females: $\frac{1}{2}$ fast : $\frac{1}{2}$ slow (*b*) F_1: all fast; F_2 males fast; F_2 females: $\frac{1}{2}$ fast : $\frac{1}{2}$ slow (*c*) F_1 both males and females: $\frac{1}{2}$ fast : $\frac{1}{2}$ slow; F_2 males: $\frac{5}{8}$ fast : $\frac{3}{8}$ slow; F_2 females: $\frac{1}{4}$ fast : $\frac{3}{4}$ slow

5.20. (*a*) Silver females (*S*/W), silver males (*S*/*s*) (*b*) Males: $\frac{1}{2}$ silver (*S*/*s*) : $\frac{1}{2}$ gold (*s*/*s*); females: $\frac{1}{2}$ silver (*S*/W) : $\frac{1}{2}$ gold (*s*/W) (*c*) Males: all silver ($\frac{1}{2}$*S*/*S* : $\frac{1}{2}$*S*/*s*); females: $\frac{1}{2}$ silver (*S*/W) : $\frac{1}{2}$ gold (*s*/W) (*d*) All males silver (*S*/*s*), all females gold (*s*/W)

5.21. (*a*) Sex-linked gene with one allele lethal when hemizygous in females or homozygous in males.

	Male	Female
Gray	HH	HW
Cream	HH^1	—
Lethal	$H^1 H^1$	$H^1 W$

(*b*) P: $HW \times HH^1$; F_1: $\frac{1}{3}HH$ gray male : $\frac{1}{3}HH^1$ cream male : $\frac{1}{3}HW$ gray female

5.22. (*a*) $\frac{1}{6}$ nonbar, normal-leg females : $\frac{1}{6}$ bar, normal-leg male : $\frac{1}{3}$ nonbar, creeper female : $\frac{1}{3}$ bar, creeper male

(*b*) Males: $\frac{2}{3}$ bar, creeper : $\frac{1}{3}$ bar, normal leg; females: $\frac{2}{3}$ nonbar, creeper : $\frac{1}{3}$ nonbar, normal leg

(*c*) Bar, creeper male (*CcBb*) × nonbar, creeper female (*CcbW*)

5.23. F_1: males: white, fast; females: white, slow; F_2 males and females: $\frac{13}{32}$ white, fast : $\frac{13}{32}$ white, slow : $\frac{3}{32}$ colored, fast : $\frac{3}{32}$ colored, slow

5.24. Males and females: $\frac{15}{32}$ bar, feathered : $\frac{15}{32}$ nonbar, feathered : $\frac{1}{32}$ bar, nonfeathered : $\frac{1}{32}$ nonbar, nonfeathered

5.25. (*a*) 0.5 male (*c*) 0.67 intersex (*e*) 1.5 superfemale (*g*) lethal

(*b*) 1.0 female (*d*) 1.0 female (*f*) 1.0 female (triploid)

5.26. (*a*) 8 (*b*) None; meiosis cannot occur in haploid males (*c*) 8

5.27.   (a) 50%   (b) 7.14%

5.28.   (a) Yes   (b) No. A sex chromosome mechanism could be operative without a morphological difference in the chromosomes, gametes, or spores.

5.29.

	Haploid Males		Diploid Males		Females	
	Wild Type	Veinless	Wild Type	Veinless	Wild Type	Veinless
(a)	0	All	All	0	All	0
(b)	0	All	0	0	All	0
(c)	0	All	0	All	0	All
(d)	0	All	0	0	0	All
(e)	$\frac{1}{2}$	$\frac{1}{2}$	$\frac{1}{2}$	$\frac{1}{2}$	$\frac{1}{2}$	$\frac{1}{2}$
(f)	$\frac{1}{2}$	$\frac{1}{2}$	0	0	$\frac{1}{2}$	$\frac{1}{2}$
(g)	All	0	All	0	All	0
(h)	All	0	0	0	All	0

5.30.   (a) No. It is highly unlikely that a mutant autosomal sex-limited gene would be transmitted to all his sons through four generations without showing segregation. (b) Holandric gene (Y-linked)

5.31.   Yes, if it was incompletely sex-linked and the father carried the dominant normal gene on the homologous portion of his Y chromosome.

5.32.   (a) 100%   (b) None   (c) 1 hairy : 1 normal

5.33.

Genotypes	Men	Women		Genotypes
w dominant in men:				w' dominant in men:
ww	Forelock	Forelock		$w'w'$
ww'	Forelock	Normal	(or)	$w'w$
$w'w'$	Normal	Normal		ww

5.34. F_1: all males horned, all females polled; F_2 males: $\frac{3}{4}$ horned : $\frac{1}{4}$ polled; F_2 females: $\frac{3}{4}$ polled : $\frac{1}{4}$ horned

5.35.   (a) All males short;   females: $\frac{1}{2}$ short : $\frac{1}{2}$ long   (b) Same as (a)   (c) Males: $\frac{3}{4}$ short : $\frac{1}{4}$ long;   females: $\frac{1}{4}$ short : $\frac{3}{4}$ long   (d) All males short, all females long

5.36.   (a) F_1: $C^M C^R$ mahogany males, $C^M C^R$ red females; F_2 males and females: $\frac{1}{4} C^M C^M : \frac{1}{2} C^M C^R : \frac{1}{4} C^R C^R$; F_2 males: $\frac{3}{4}$ mahogany : $\frac{1}{4}$ red; F_2 females: $\frac{1}{4}$ mahogany : $\frac{3}{4}$ red   (b) Female   (c) $C^M C^M$

5.37.

Phenotype	Males	Females
Bearded, long-eared	3/16	1/16
Bearded, intermediate eared	3/8	1/8
Bearded, short-eared	3/16	1/16
Nonbearded, long-eared	1/16	3/16
Nonbearded, intermediate eared	1/8	3/8
Nonbearded, short-eared	1/16	3/16

5.38.

Phenotype	Daughters	Sons
Bald, normal vision	1/8	3/8
Bald, color blind	1/8	3/8
Nonbald, normal vision	3/8	1/8
Nonbald, color blind	3/8	1/8

5.39. (*a*) $\frac{3}{4}$ (*b*) $\frac{3}{8}$

5.40. ($2ss : 1SS$) or ($2Ss : 1ss$)

5.41. $\frac{5}{8}$ yellow : $\frac{3}{8}$ white

5.42. Males: $\frac{3}{8}$ barred, hen-feathered : $\frac{1}{8}$ barred, cock-feathered : $\frac{3}{8}$ nonbarred, hen-feathered : $\frac{1}{8}$ nonbarred, cock-feathered; females: $\frac{1}{2}$ barred, hen-feathered : $\frac{1}{2}$ nonbarred, hen-feathered

5.43. (*a*) Leghorns are homozygous *hh*. Sebright bantams are homozygous *HH*. Hamburgs are segregating at this locus; one or the other allele has not been "fixed" in the breed. (*b*) Gonads are the source of steroid sex hormones as well as of reproductive cells. The action of these genes is dependent upon the presence or absence of these sex hormones.

5.44. (*a*) No (*b*) Yes (*c*) No (*d*) Yes (*e*) Yes (*f*) Yes (*g*) No

5.45. No. Under the assumption, III1 must be of heterozygous genotype and therefore should be phenotypically normal; III2 must carry the recessive mutant in hemizygous condition and therefore should be phenotypically mutant.

5.46. (*a*) Yes (*b*) No (*c*) Sex-linked recessive gene; *Aa* (I1, II1, 3, III2), *aY* (I2, II2, 4, III1, 3)

5.47. (*a*)–(*f*) No (*g*) Yes (if black is dominant in males and recessive in females)

5.48. (*a*) 2 females : 1 male (*b*) All females

5.49. 2 males : 1 female

5.50. F_1: $\frac{1}{3}k^+/k$ fast males : $\frac{1}{3}k^+/W$ fast females : $\frac{1}{3}k/W$ slow females; F_2: $(\frac{1}{8}k^+/k^+ + \frac{1}{4}k^+/k) = \frac{3}{8}$ fast males : $\frac{1}{8}k/k$ slow males : $\frac{1}{4}k^+/W$ fast females : $\frac{1}{4}k/W$ slow females

5.51. (*a*) All ZZ males (*b*) 1 XX female : 2 XY males : 1 YY male (*c*) In most other organisms with XY sex determination, at least one X chromosome is essential for survival. (*d*) All XX females (*e*) $\frac{1}{6}$ tested sons proved XY; therefore YY males are not rare in this species and they appear to be as viable as normal XY males.

5.52. (*a*) All mixed (*b*) $\frac{3}{4}$ mixed : $\frac{1}{4}$ pistillate (*c*) $\frac{1}{2}$ mixed : $\frac{1}{2}$ pistillate

5.53. (*a*) $\frac{3}{4}$ staminate : $\frac{1}{4}$ pistillate (*b*) $\frac{2}{3}$ staminate : $\frac{1}{3}$ pistillate (*c*) $Pp \times pp$

5.54. (*a*) Only broad-leaved males (*b*) $\frac{1}{2}$ broad-leaved males : $\frac{1}{2}$ narrow-leaved males (*c*) All females broad-leaved; $\frac{1}{2}$ males broad-leaved : $\frac{1}{2}$ males narrow-leaved

5.55. (a) F_1: $\frac{1}{2}$ male sterile : $\frac{1}{2}$ male fertile (normal = monoecious); F_2: $\frac{3}{8}$ male sterile : $\frac{5}{8}$ normal (b) F_1: all normal; F_2: $\frac{1}{4}$ male sterile : $\frac{3}{4}$ normal (c) F_1: $\frac{1}{2}SsAa$ normal : $\frac{1}{2}ssAa$ male sterile; F_2: $\frac{15}{32}S\text{-}A\text{-}$: $\frac{9}{32}ssA\text{-}$: $\frac{5}{32}S\text{-}aa$: $\frac{3}{32}ssaa$ (d) F_1: $SsAa$ normal; F_2: $\frac{9}{16}S\text{-}A\text{-}$: $\frac{3}{16}S\text{-}aa$: $\frac{3}{16}ssA\text{-}$: $\frac{1}{16}ssaa$

5.56. (a) $\frac{1}{8}$ dwarf : $\frac{1}{4}$ female sterile : $\frac{5}{8}$ normal (monoecious) (b) $\frac{1}{2}$ normal : $\frac{1}{4}$ female sterile : $\frac{1}{4}$ dwarf

5.57. (a) All S^1S^3 (b) No progeny (c) $\frac{1}{2}S^1S^2$: $\frac{1}{2}S^1S^3$ (d) No

5.58. (a) Ss (b) $\frac{1}{8}AASs$: $\frac{1}{4}AaSs$: $\frac{1}{8}aaSs$: $\frac{1}{8}AAss$: $\frac{1}{4}Aass$: $\frac{1}{8}aass$

5.59. (a) None (b) $\frac{1}{2}S_1S_3$: $\frac{1}{2}S_2S_3$ (c) $\frac{1}{4}S_1S_3$: $\frac{1}{4}S_1S_4$: $\frac{1}{4}S_2S_3$: $\frac{1}{4}S_2S_4$ (d) a = none, $b = \frac{1}{2}$, c = all

5.60. $\frac{1}{4}S_1S_2$: $\frac{1}{3}S_2S_3$: $\frac{1}{12}S_1S_3$: $\frac{1}{12}S_2S_4$: $\frac{1}{4}S_3S_4$

Answers to Review Questions

Vocabulary

1. sexual
2. hermaphrodite
3. pistillate
4. heterogametic
5. Z, W
6. genic balance
7. haplodiploidy
8. holandric
9. sex-influenced
10. sex-limited

True-False Questions

1. F (sex generates genetic diversity in the population) 2. T 3. F (heterogametic) 4. T 5. F (drones, not workers) 6. T 7. F (mother has recessive trait and father has dominant trait) 8. T 9. F (homologous regions of X and Y chromosomes are necessary for synapsis in meiosis) 10. T

Multiple-Choice Questions

1. *d* 2. *b* 3. *b* 4. *b* 5. *c* 6. *d* 7. *a* 8. *c* 9. *d* 10. *a*

Chapter 6

Linkage and Chromosome Mapping

RECOMBINATION AMONG LINKED GENES

1. Linkage.

When 2 or more genes reside in the same chromosome, they are said to be *linked*. They may be linked together on one of the autosomes or connected together on the sex chromosome (Chapter 5). Genes on different chromosomes are distributed into gametes independently of one another (Mendel's Law of Independent Assortment). Genes on the same chromosome, however, tend to stay together during the formation of gametes. Thus the results of testcrossing dihybrid individuals will yield different results, depending upon whether the genes are linked or on different chromosomes.

Example 6.1. Genes on different chromosomes assort independently, giving a 1 : 1 : 1 : 1 testcross ratio.

Parents: $AaBb$ × $aabb$

Gametes: (AB) (Ab) (aB) (ab)   (ab)

F_1: $\frac{1}{4}AaBb$: $\frac{1}{4}Aabb$: $\frac{1}{4}aaBb$: $\frac{1}{4}aabb$

Example 6.2. Linked genes do not assort independently, but tend to stay together in the same combinations as they were in the parents. Genes to the left of the slash line (/) are on one chromosome and those to the right are on the homologous chromosome.

Parents: AB/ab × ab/ab

Gametes: (AB) (ab)   (ab)

F_1: $\frac{1}{2}AB/ab$: $\frac{1}{2}ab/ab$

Large deviations from a 1 : 1 : 1 : 1 ratio on the testcross progeny of a dihybrid could be used as evidence for linkage. Linked genes do not always stay together, however, because homologous nonsister chromatids may exchange segments of varying length with one another during meiotic prophase. Recall from Chapter 1 that homologous chromosomes pair with one another in a process called "synapsis" and that the points of genetic exchange, called "chiasmata," produce recombinant gametes through crossing over.

2. Crossing Over.

During meiosis each chromosome replicates, forming two identical sister chromatids; homologous chromosomes pair (synapse) and crossing over occurs between nonsister chromatids. This latter process involves the breakage and reunion of only 2 of the 4 strands at any given point on the chromosomes. In the diagram below, a crossover occurs in the region between the A and B loci.

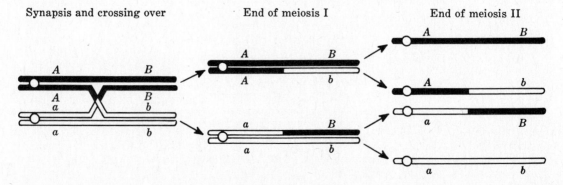

Synapsis and crossing over   End of meiosis I   End of meiosis II

110

Notice that 2 of the meiotic products (*AB* and *ab*) have the genes linked in the same way as they were in the parental chromosomes. These products are produced from chromatids that were not involved in crossing over and are referred to as **noncrossover** or **parental** types. The other 2 meiotic products (*Ab* and *aB*) produced by crossing over have recombined the original linkage relationships of the parent into two new forms called **recombinant** or **crossover** types.

The alleles of double heterozygotes (dihybrids) at two linked loci may appear in either of two positions relative to one another. If the two dominant (or wild-type) alleles are on 1 chromosome and the 2 recessives (or mutants) on the other (*AB/ab*), the linkage relationship is called **coupling phase.** When the dominant allele of one locus and the recessive allele of the other occupy the same chromosome (*Ab/aB*), the relationship is termed **repulsion phase.** Parental and recombinant gametes will be of different types, depending upon how these genes are linked in the parent.

Example 6.3.   Coupling Parent: *AB/ab*

                                        Parental: (AB) (ab)
                        Gametes:
                                    Recombinant: (Ab) (aB)

Example 6.4.   Repulsion Parent: *Ab/aB*

                                    Noncrossover: (Ab) (aB)
                        Gametes:
                                        Crossover: (AB) (ab)

3. Chiasma Frequency.

A pair of synapsed chromosome (bivalent) consists of 4 chromatids called a *tetrad*. Every tetrad usually experiences at least one chiasma somewhere along its length. Generally speaking, the longer the chromosome, the greater the number of chiasmata. Each type of chromosome within a species has a characteristic (or average) number of chiasmata. The frequency with which a chiasma occurs between any two genetic loci also has a characteristic or average probability. The further apart 2 genes are located on a chromosome, the greater the opportunity for a chiasma to occur between them. The closer 2 genes are linked, the smaller the chance for a chiasma occurring between them. These chiasmata probabilities are useful in predicting the proportions of parental and recombinant gametes expected to be formed from a given genotype. The percentage of crossover (recombinant) gametes formed by a given genotype is a direct reflection of the frequency with which a chiasma forms between the genes in question. Only when a crossover forms *between* the gene loci under consideration will recombination be detected.

Example 6.5.   Crossing over outside the A–B region fails to recombine these markers.

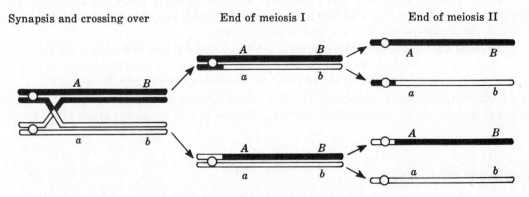

When a chiasma forms between two gene loci, only half of the meiotic products will be of crossover type. Therefore chiasma frequency is twice the frequency of crossover products.

$$\text{Chiasma \%} = 2(\text{crossover \%}) \quad \text{or} \quad \text{Crossover \%} = \tfrac{1}{2}(\text{chiasma \%})$$

Example 6.6. If a chiasma forms between the loci of genes *A* and *B* in 30% of the tetrads of an individual of genotype *AB/ab*, then 15% of the gametes will be recombinant (*Ab* or *aB*) and 85% will be parental (*AB* or *ab*).

Example 6.7. Suppose progeny from the testcross *Ab/aB* × *ab/ab* were found in the proportions 40% *Ab/ab*, 40% *aB/ab*, 10% *AB/ab*, and 10% *ab/ab*. The genotypes *AB/ab* and *ab/ab* were produced from crossover gametes. Thus 20% of all gametes formed by the dihybrid parent were crossover types. This means that a chiasma occurs between these two loci in 40% of all tetrads.

4. Multiple Crossovers.

When 2-strand double crossovers occur between two genetic markets, the products, as detected through the progeny phenotypes, are only parental types.

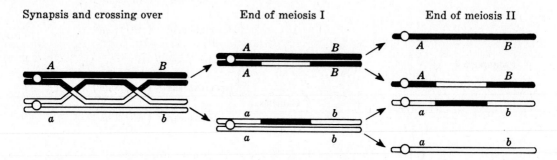

In order to detect these double crossovers, a third gene locus (*C*) between the outside markers must be used.

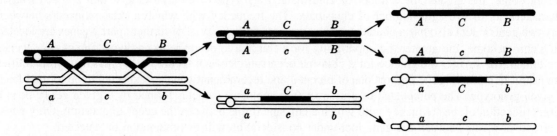

If there is a certain probability that a crossover will form between the *A* and *C* loci and another independent probability of a crossover forming between the *C* and *B* loci, then the probability of a double crossover is the product of the two independent probabilities.

Example 6.8. If a crossover between the *A* and *C* loci occurs in 20% of the tetrads and between *C* and *B* loci in 10% of the tetrads in an individual of genotype *ACB/acb*, then 2% (0.2 × 0.1) of the gametes are expected to be of double-crossover types *AcB* and *aCb*.

Odd numbers of 2-strand crossovers (1, 3, 5, etc.) between two gene loci produce detectable recombinations between the outer markers, but even numbers of two-strand crossovers (2, 4, 6, etc.) do not.

5. Limits of Recombination.

If two gene loci are so far apart in the chromosome that the probability of a chiasma forming between them is 100%, then 50% of the gametes will be parental type (noncrossover) and 50% recombinant (crossover) type. When such dihybrid individuals are testcrossed, they are expected to produce progeny in a 1 : 1 : 1 : 1 ratio as would be expected for genes on different chromosomes. Recombination between 2 linked genes cannot exceed 50% even when multiple crossovers occur between them.

GENETIC MAPPING

1. Map Distance.

The places where genes reside in the chromosome (loci) are positioned in linear order analogous to beads on a string. There are two major aspects to genetic mapping: (i) the determination of the linear order with which the genetic units are arranged with respect to one another (gene order) and (ii) the determination of the relative distances between the genetic units (gene distance). The unit of distance that has the greatest utility in predicting the outcome of certain types of matings is an expression of the probability that crossing over will occur between the 2 genes under consideration. One unit of map distance (**centimorgan**) is therefore equivalent to 1% crossing over.

> **Example 6.9.** If the genotype *Ab/aB* produces 8% each of the crossover gametes *AB* and *ab*, then the distance between *A* and *B* is estimated to be 16 map units.

> **Example 6.10.** If the map distance between the loci *B* and *C* is 12 units, then 12% of the gametes of genotype *BC/bc* should be crossover types; i.e., 6% *Bc* and 6% *bC*.

Each chiasma produces 50% crossover products. Fifty percent crossing over is equivalent to 50 map units. If the average (mean) number of chiasmata is known for a chromosome pair, the total length of the map for that linkage group may be predicted:

$$\text{Total length} = \text{mean number of chiasmata} \times 50$$

2. Two-Point Testcross.

The easiest way to detect crossover gametes in a dihybrid is through the testcross progeny. Suppose we testcross dihybrid individuals in coupling phase (*AC/ac*) and find in the progeny phenotypes 37% dominant at both loci, 37% recessive at both loci, 13% dominant at the first locus and recessive at the second, and 13% dominant at the second locus and recessive at the first. Obviously the last two groups (genotypically *Ac/ac* and *aC/ac*) were produced by crossover gametes from the dihybrid parent. Thus 26% of all gametes (13 + 13) were of crossover types and the distance between the loci *A* and *C* is estimated to be 26 map units.

3. Three-Point Testcross.

Double crossovers usually do not occur between genes less than 5 map units apart. For genes further apart, it is advisable to use a third marker between the other two in order to detect any double crossovers. Suppose that we testcross trihybrid individuals of genotype *ABC/abc* and find in the progeny the following:

36% *ABC/abc*	9% *Abc/abc*	4% *ABc/abc*	1% *AbC/abc*
36% *abc/abc*	9% *aBC/abc*	4% *abC/abc*	1% *aBc/abc*
72% Parental type :	18% Single crossovers	8% Single crossovers :	2% Double crossovers
	between A and B	between B and C	
	(region I)	(region II)	

To find the distance *A–B* we must count all crossovers (both singles and doubles) that occurred in region I = 18% + 2% = 20% or 20 map units between the loci *A* and *B*. To find the distance *B–C* we must again count all crossovers (both singles and doubles) that occurred in region II = 8% + 2% = 10% or 10 map units between the loci *B* and *C*. The *A–C* distance is therefore 30 map units when double crossovers are detected in a three-point linkage experiment and 26 map units when double crossovers are undetected in the two-point linkage experiment above.

Without the middle marker (*B*), double crossovers would appear as parental types and hence we *underestimate* the true map distance (crossover percentage). In this case the 2% double crossovers would appear with the 72% parental types, making a total of 74% parental types and 26% recombinant types. Therefore for any three linked genes whose distances are known, the amount of *detectable* crossovers (recombinants) between the two outer markers *A* and *C* when the middle marker *B* is missing is (*A–B* crossover percentage) plus (*B–C* crossover percentage) minus (2 × double-crossover percentage). This procedure is appropriate only if a crossover in the *A–B* region occurs independently of that in the *B–C* region (see item 8 in this section).

Example 6.11. Given distances $A–B = 20$, $B–C = 10$, $A–C = 30$ map units, the percentage of detectable crossovers from the dihybrid testcross $AC/ac \times ac/ac = 0.20 + 0.10 - 2(0.20)(0.10) = 0.30 - 2(0.02) = 0.30 - 0.04 = 0.26$ or 26% (13% *Ac/ac* and 13% *aC/ac*).

4. Gene Order.

The additivity of map distances allows us to place genes in their proper linear order. Three linked genes may be in any one of three different orders, depending upon which gene is in the middle. We will ignore left and right end alternatives for the present. If double crossovers do not occur, map distances may be treated as completely additive units. When we are given the distances $A–B = 12$, $B–C = 7$, $A–C = 5$, we should be able to determine the correct order.

Case 1. Let us assume that *A* is in the middle.

B	12	A		A	5	C

B	7	C

The distances *B–C* are not equitable. Therefore *A* cannot be in the middle.

Case 2. Let us assume that *B* is in the middle.

A	12	B		B	7	C

A	5	C

The distances *A–C* are not equitable. Therefore *B* cannot be in the middle.

Case 3. Let us assume that *C* is in the middle.

A	5	C		C	7	B

A	12	B

The distances *A–B* are equitable. Therefore *C* must be in the middle. Most students should be able to perceive the proper relationships intuitively.

(a) ***Linkage Relationships from a Two-Point Testcross.*** Parental combinations will tend to stay together in the majority of the progeny and the crossover types will always be the least frequent classes. From this information, the mode of linkage (coupling or repulsion) may be determined for the dihybrid parent.

Example 6.12.

P: Dihybrid Parent   ×   Testcross Parent
            Aa,Bb   *ab/ab*
       (linkage relationships unknown)

F_1:   42% *AaBb* } Parental types   8% *Aabb* } Recombinant types
            42% *aabb*   8% *aaBb*

The testcross parent contributes *ab* to each progeny. The remaining genes come from the dihybrid parent. Thus *A* and *B* must have been on one chromosome of the dihybrid parent and *a* and *b* on the other, i.e., in coupling phase (*AB/ab*), because these were the combinations that appeared with greatest frequency in the progeny.

Example 6.13.

P:	Dihybrid Parent	×	Testcross Parent
	Aa,Bb		*ab/ab*

(linkage relationships unknown)

F₁: 42% *Aabb* } Parental types   8% *AaBb* } Recombinant types
       42% *aaBb* }   8% *aabb* }

By reasoning similar to that in Example 6.12, *A* and *b* must have been on one chromosome of the dihybrid parent and *a* and *B* on the other, i.e., in repulsion phase (*Ab/aB*).

(b) *Linkage Relationships from a Three-Point Testcross.*   In a testcross involving 3 linked genes, the parental types are expected to be most frequent and the double crossovers to be the least frequent. The gene order is determined by manipulating the parental combinations into the proper order for the production of double-crossover types.

Example 6.14.

P:	Trihybrid Parent	×	Testcross Parent
	Aa,Bb,Cc		*abc/abc*

(linkage relationships unknown)

F₁:
36% *Aabbcc*	9% *aabbCc*	4% *AabbCc*	1% *AaBbCc*
36% *aaBbCc*	9% *AaBbcc*	4% *aaBbcc*	1% *aabbcc*
72%	18%	8%	2%

The 72% group is composed of parental types because noncrossover gametes are always produced in the highest frequency. Obviously the only contribution the testcross parent makes to all the progeny is *abc*. Thus the trihybrid parent must have had *A*, *b*, and *c* on one chromosome and *a*, *B*, and *C* on the other. But which locus is in the middle? Again, three cases can be considered.

    Case 1.   Can we produce the least frequent double-crossover types (2% of the F₁) if the *B* locus is in the middle?

$$\underset{a\quad\quad B\quad\quad C}{\overset{A\quad\quad b\quad\quad c}{\Large\times\!\!\times}}\quad \times\ abc/abc\ =\ ABc/abc\ \text{and}\ abC/abc$$

These are not double-crossover types and therefore the *B* locus is not in the middle.

    Case 2.   Can we produce the double-crossover types if the *C* locus is in the middle? Remember to keep *A*, *b*, and *c* on one chromosome and *a*, *B*, and *C* on the other when switching different loci to the middle position.

$$\underset{a\quad\quad C\quad\quad B}{\overset{A\quad\quad c\quad\quad b}{\Large\times\!\!\times}}\quad \times\ acb/acb\ =\ ACb/acb\ \text{and}\ acB/acb$$

These are not double-crossover types and therefore the *C* locus is not in the middle.

    Case 3.   Can we produce the double-crossover types if the *A* locus is in the middle?

$$\underset{B\quad\quad a\quad\quad C}{\overset{b\quad\quad A\quad\quad c}{\Large\times\!\!\times}}\quad \times\ bac/bac\ =\ bac/bac\ \text{and}\ BAC/bac$$

These are the double-crossover types and we conclude that the *A* locus is in the middle.

Now that we know the gene order and the parental linkage relationships, we can deduce the single crossovers. Let us designate the distance *B–A* as region I, and the *A–C* distance as region II. Single crossovers in region I:

$$b \qquad A \qquad c$$
$$\times \; bac/bac \; = \; baC/bac \text{ and } BAc/bac$$
$$B \qquad a \qquad C$$

Single crossovers in region II:

$$b \qquad A \qquad c$$
$$\times \; bac/bac \; = \; bAC/bac \text{ and } Bac/bac$$
$$B \qquad a \qquad C$$

5. Recombination Percentage vs. Map Distance.

In two-point linkage experiments, the chance of double (and other even-numbered) crossovers occurring undetected increases with the unmarked distance (i.e., without segregating loci) between genes. Hence closely linked genes give the best estimate of crossing over. Double crossovers do not occur within 10–12 map units in *Drosophila*. Minimum double-crossover distance varies by species. Within this minimum distance, recombination percentage is equivalent to map distance. Outside it, the relationship becomes nonlinear (Fig. 6-1). True map distance will thus be underestimated by the recombination fraction, with the two becoming virtually independent at large distances.

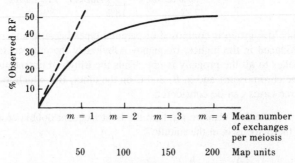

Fig. 6-1. Relationship between observed recombination frequency (RF) and real map units (solid line). Dashed line represents the relationship for very small mean numbers of exchanges per meiosis (*m*). See Problem 7.10 for mapping function. (From *An Introduction to Genetic Analysis,* 2nd ed., by D. T. Suzuki, A. J. F. Griffiths and R. C. Lewontin, W. H. Freeman and Co., San Francisco, 1976.

6. Genetic vs. Physical Maps.

The frequency of crossing over usually varies in different segments of the chromosome, but is a highly predictable event between any two gene loci. Therefore the actual physical distances between linked genes bears no direct relationship to the map distances calculated on the basis of crossover percentages. The linear order, however, is identical in both cases.

7. Combining Map Segments.

Segments of map determined from three-point linkage experiments may be combined whenever 2 of the 3 genes are held in common.

Example 6.15. Consider 3 map segments.

(1) a ——8——b ——10—— c

(2) c ——10—— b ————22———— d

(3) c ——————30—————— e —2— d

Superimpose each of these segments by aligning the genes shared in common.

(1) a —8— b —10— c

(2) d ———22——— b —10— c

(3) d —2— e ——————30—————— c

Then combine the three segments into one map.

The a to d distance $= (d$ to $b) - (a$ to $b) = 22 - 8 = 14$.

The a to e distance $= (a$ to $d) - (d$ to $e) = 14 - 2 = 12$.

d —2— e ————12———— a —8— b ——10—— c

Additional segments of map added in this manner can produce a total linkage map over 100 map units long. However, as explained previously, the maximum recombination between any two linked genes is 50%. That is, genes very far apart on the same chromosome may behave as though they were on different chromosomes (assorting independently).

All other factors being equal, the greater the number of individuals in an experiment, the more accurate the linkage estimates should be. Therefore in averaging the distances from two or more replicate experiments, the linkage estimates may be **weighted** according to the sample size. For each experiment, multiply the sample size by the linkage estimate. Add the products and divide by the total number of individuals from all experiments.

Example 6.16. Let n = number of individuals, d = map distance.

Experiment	n	d	nd
1	239	12.3	2,940
2	652	11.1	7,237
3	966	12.9	12,461
	1857		22,638

$22{,}638/1857 = 12.2$ map units (weighted average)

8. Interference and Coincidence.

In most of the higher organisms, the formation of one chiasma actually reduces the probability of another chiasma forming in an immediately adjacent region of the chromosome. This reduction in chiasma formation may be thought of as being due to a physical inability of the chromatids to bend back upon themselves within certain minimum distances. The net result of this **interference** is the observation of fewer double-crossover types than would be expected according to map distances. The strength of interference varies in different segments of the chromosome and is usually expressed in terms of a **coefficient of coincidence,** or the ratio between the observed and the expected double crossovers.

$$\text{Coefficient of coincidence} = \frac{\%\ \text{observed double crossovers}}{\%\ \text{expected double crossovers}}$$

Coincidence is the complement of interference.

$$\text{Coincidence} + \text{interference} = 1.0$$

When interference is complete (1.0), no double crossovers will be observed and coincidence becomes zero. When we observe all the double crossovers expected, coincidence is unity and interference becomes zero. When interference is 30% operative, coincidence becomes 70%, etc.

Example 6.17. Given the map distances $A–B = 10$ and $B–C = 20$, then $0.1 \times 0.2 = 0.02$ or 2% double crossovers are expected if there is no interference. Suppose we observe 1.6% double crossovers in a testcross experiment.

$$\text{Coincidence} = 1.6/2.0 = 0.8$$

This simply means that we observed only 80% of the double crossovers that were expected on the basis of combining independent probabilities (map distances).

$$\text{Interference} = 1.0 - 0.8 = 0.2$$

Thus 20% of the expected double crossovers did not form due to interference.

The percentage of double crossovers that will probably be observed can be predicted by multiplying the expected double crossovers by the coefficient of coincidence.

Example 6.18. Given a segment of map, $a \quad ^{10} \quad b \quad ^{20} \quad c$, with 40% interference, we expect $0.1 \times 0.2 = 0.02$ or 2% double crossover on the basis of combining independent probabilities. However, we will observe only 60% of those expected because of the interference. Therefore we should observe $0.02 \times 0.6 = 0.012$ or 1.2% double-crossover types.

LINKAGE ESTIMATES FROM F_2 DATA

1. Sex-Linked Traits.

In organisms where the male is XY or XO, the male receives only the Y chromosome from the paternal parent (or no chromosome homologous with the X in the case of XO sex determination). The Y contains, on its differential segment, no alleles homologous to those on the X chromosome received from the maternal parent. Thus for completely sex-linked traits the parental and recombinant gametes formed by the female can be observed directly in the F_2 males, regardless of the genotype of the F_1 males.

Example 6.19. Consider in *Drosophila* the recessive sex-linked bristle mutant scute (*sc*), and on the same chromosome the gene for vermilion eye color (*v*).

P: $\dfrac{+\,+}{+\,+}$ ♀♀ × $\dfrac{sc\ v}{\longrightarrow}$ ♂♂   (→ = Y chromosome)

wild-type females   scute, vermilion males

F_1: $\dfrac{+\,+}{sc\ v}$ ♀♀ and $\dfrac{+\,+}{\longrightarrow}$ ♂♂

wild-type females   wild-type males

F_2:

	♀ \ ♂	+ +	Y
Parental Gametes	+ +	+ +/+ + wild type	+ +/Y wild type
	sc v	+ +/*sc v* wild type	*sc v*/Y scute, vermilion
Crossover Gametes	+ *v*	+ +/+ *v* wild type	+ *v*/Y vermilion
	sc +	+ +/*sc* + wild type	*sc* +/Y scute
		Females	Males

Example 6.20. Let us consider the same two sex-linked genes as in Example 6.19, using acute parental males and vermilion parental females.

P:　　　$\dfrac{+\,v}{+\,v}$ ♀♀　　×　　$\dfrac{sc\,+}{\longrightarrow}$ ♂♂

　　　vermilion females　　　　scute males

F₁:　　　$\dfrac{v}{sc\,+}$ ♀♀　　×　　$\dfrac{+\,v}{\longrightarrow}$ ♂♂

　　wild-type females　　vermilion males

F₂:

	♂	+v	Y
♀			
Parental Gametes	+v	+v/+v vermilion	+v/Y vermilion
	sc +	+v/sc + wild type	sc +/Y scute
Crossover Gametes	++	+v/++ wild type	++/Y wild type
	sc v	+v/sc v vermilion	sc v/Y scute, vermilion
		Females	Males

If the original parental females are double recessive (testcross parent), then both male and female progeny of the F₂ can be used to estimate the percentage of crossing over.

Example 6.21.　　P:　　　$\dfrac{sc\,v}{sc\,v}$ ♀♀　　×　　$\dfrac{+\,+}{\longrightarrow}$ ♂♂

　　　　scute, vermilion females　　　wild-type males

F₁:　　　$\dfrac{sc\,v}{+\,+}$ ♀♀　　×　　$\dfrac{sc\,v}{\longrightarrow}$ ♂♂

　　wild-type females　　scute, vermilion males

F₂:

	♂	sc v	Y
♀			
Parental Gametes	sc v	sc v/sc v scute, vermilion	sc v/Y scute, vermilion
	++	++/sc v wild type	++/Y wild type
Crossover Gametes	sc +	sc +/sc v scute	sc +/Y scute
	+v	+v/sc v vermilion	+v/Y vermilion
		Females	Males

In organisms where the female is the heterogametic sex (ZW or ZO methods of sex determination), the F₂ females can be used for detection of crossing over between sex-linked genes. If the male is used as a testcross parent, both males and females of the F₂ can be used to estimate the strength of the linkage.

2. Autosomal Traits.

A poor alternative to the testcross method for determining linkage and estimating distances is by allowing dihybrid F_1 progeny to produce an F_2 either by random mating among the F_1 or, in the case of plants, by selfing the F_1. Such an F_2 that obviously does not conform to the $9:3:3:1$ ratio expected for genes assorting independently may be considered evidence for linkage. Two methods for estimating the degree of linkage from F_2 data are presented below.

(a) **Square-Root Method.**   The frequency of double-recessive phenotypes in the F_2 may be used as an estimator of the frequency of noncrossover gametes when the F_1 is in coupling phase, and as an estimator of the frequency of crossover gametes when the F_1 is in repulsion phase.

Example 6.22. F_1 in coupling phase.   *AB/ab*

F_2:   The frequency of *ab* gametes $= \frac{1}{2}$ of the frequency of all noncrossover gametes. If the crossover percentage is 20%, we would expect 80% noncrossover gametes (40% *AB* and 40% *ab*). The probability of two *ab* gametes uniting to form the double-recessive *ab/ab* $= (0.4)^2 = 0.16$ or 16%. Now, if we do not know the crossover percentage, but the F_2 data tell us that 16% are double recessive, then the percentage of noncrossover gametes $= 2\sqrt{\text{freq. of double recessives}} = 2\sqrt{0.16} = 2(0.4) = 0.8$ or 80%. If 80% are noncrossovers, the other 20% must be crossover types. Therefore the map distance between *A* and *B* is estimated at 20 units.

Example 6.23. F_1 in repulsion phase.   *Ab/aB*

F_2:   The reasoning is similar to that in Example 6.22. With 20% crossing over we expect 10% of the gametes to be *ab*. The probability of 2 of these gametes uniting to form the double recessive $(ab/ab) = (0.1)^2 = 0.01$ or 1%. Now, if we do not know the crossover percentage, but the F_2 data tell us that 1% are double recessives, then the percentage of crossover gametes $= 2\sqrt{\text{freq. of double recessives}} = 2\sqrt{0.01} = 2(0.1) = 0.2$ or 20%.

(b) **Product-Ratio Method.**   An estimate of the frequency of recombination from double-heterozygous (dihybrid) F_1 parents can be ascertained from F_2 phenotypes *R-S-*, *R-ss*, *rrS-*, and *rrss* appearing in the frequencies *a*, *b*, *c*, and *d*, respectively. The ratio of crossover to parental types, called the **product ratio,** is a function of recombination.

$$\text{For coupling data:} \quad x = bc/ad$$
$$\text{For repulsion data:} \quad x = ad/bc$$

The recombination fraction represented by the value of x may be read directly from a product-ratio table (Table 6.1.). The product-ratio method utilizes all of the F_2 data available and not just the double-recessive class as in the square-root method. The product-ratio method should therefore yield more accurate estimates of recombination than the square-root method.

Example 6.24.   Coupling Data.

P: *RS/RS*   ×   *rs/rs*

F_1:   *RS/rs* (coupling phase)

F_2:
	Phenotypes	Numbers
(a)	R-S-	1221
(b)	R-ss	219
(c)	rrS-	246
(d)	rrss	243

$$x \text{ (for coupling data)} = \frac{bc}{ad} = \frac{(219)(246)}{(1221)(243)} = \frac{53{,}874}{296{,}703} = 0.1816$$

Locating the value of x in the body of the coupling column (Table 6.1), we find that 0.1816 lies between the values 0.1777 and 0.1948, which corresponds to recombination fractions of 0.28 and 0.29, respectively. Therefore, without interpolation, recombination is approximately 28%.

Table 6.1.   Recombination Fraction Estimated by the Product-Ratio Method

Recombination Fraction	Ratio of Products		Recombination Fraction	Ratio of Products	
	ad/bc (Repulsion)	*bc/ad* (Coupling)		*ad/bc* (Repulsion)	*bc/ad* (Coupling)
.00	.000000	.000000	.26	.1608	.1467
.01	.000200	.000136	.27	.1758	.1616
.02	.000801	.000552	.28	.1919	.1777
.03	.001804	.001262	.29	.2089	.1948
.04	.003213	.002283	.30	.2271	.2132
.05	.005031	.003629			
.06	.007265	.005318	.31	.2465	.2328
.07	.009921	.007366	.32	.2672	.2538
.08	.01301	.009793	.33	.2892	.2763
.09	.01653	.01262	.34	.3127	.3003
.10	.02051	.01586	.35	.3377	.3259
.11	.02495	.01954	.36	.3643	.3532
.12	.02986	.02369	.37	.3927	.3823
.13	.03527	.02832	.38	.4230	.4135
.14	.04118	.03347	.39	.4553	.4467
.15	.04763	.03915	.40	.4898	.4821
.16	.05462	.04540	.41	.5266	.5199
.17	.06218	.05225	.42	.5660	.5603
.18	.07033	.05973	.43	.6081	.6034
.19	.07911	.06787	.44	.6531	.6494
.20	.08854	.07671	.45	.7013	.6985
.21	.09865	.08628	.46	.7529	.7510
.22	.1095	.09663	.47	.8082	.8071
.23	.1211	.1078	.48	.8676	.8671
.24	.1334	.1198	.49	.9314	.9313
.25	.1467	.1328	.50	1.0000	1.0000

Source: F. R. Immer and M. T. Henderson, "Linkage studies in barley," *Genetics,* 28: 419–440, 1943.

Example 6.25.   Repulsion Data.

P: Ve/Ve × vE/vE

F_1: Ve/vE (repulsion phase)

	Phenotypes	Numbers
(a)	V-E-	36
(b)	V-ee	12
(c)	vvE-	16
(d)	vvee	2

$$x \text{ (for repulsion data)} = \frac{ad}{bc} = \frac{(36)(2)}{(12)(16)} = \frac{72}{192} = 0.3750$$

Locating the value of x in the body of the repulsion column, we find that 0.3750 lies between the values 0.3643 and 0.3927, which corresponds to recombination fractions of 0.36 and 0.37, respectively. Therefore recombination is approximately 36%.

USE OF GENETIC MAPS

1. Predicting Results of a Dihybrid Cross.

If the map distance between any 2 linked genes is known, the expectations from any type of mating may be predicted by use of the gametic checkerboard.

Example 6.26. Given genes A and B 10 map units apart and parents $AB/AB\,\delta\,\delta \times ab/ab\,♀\,♀$, the F_1 will all be heterozygous in coupling phase (AB/ab). Ten percent of the F_1 gametes are expected to be of crossover types (5% Ab and 5% aB). Ninety percent of the F_1 gametes are expected to be parental types (45% AB and 45% ab). The F_2 can be derived by use of the gametic checkerboard, combining independent probabilities by multiplication.

		Parental Types		Crossover Types	
		0.45 AB	0.45 ab	0.05 Ab	0.05 aB
Parental Types	0.45 AB	0.2025 AB/AB	0.2025 AB/ab	0.0225 AB/Ab	0.0225 AB/aB
	0.45 ab	0.2025 ab/AB	0.2025 ab/ab	0.0225 ab/Ab	0.0225 ab/aB
Crossover Types	0.05 Ab	0.0225 Ab/AB	0.0225 Ab/ab	0.0025 Ab/Ab	0.0025 Ab/aB
	0.05 aB	0.0225 aB/AB	0.0225 aB/ab	0.0025 aB/Ab	0.0025 aB/aB

Summary of Phenotypes: 0.7025 or $70\frac{1}{4}$% $A\text{-}B\text{-}$
0.0475 or $4\frac{3}{4}$% $A\text{-}bb$
0.0475 or $4\frac{3}{4}$% $aaB\text{-}$
0.2025 or $20\frac{1}{4}$% $aabb$

2. Predicting Results of a Trihybrid Testcross.

Map distances or crossover percentages may be treated as any other probability estimates. Given a particular kind of mating, the map distances involved, and either the coincidence or interference for this region of the chromosome, we should be able to predict the results in the offspring generation.

Example 6.27.   Parents: $AbC/aBc \times abc/abc$

Map: $a \overset{10}{\rule{2cm}{0.4pt}} b \overset{20}{\rule{3cm}{0.4pt}} c$

Interference: 40%

Given the above information, the expected kinds and frequencies of progeny genotypes and phenotypes can be determined as follows.

Step 1.   For gametes produced by the trihybrid parent determine the parental types, single crossovers in each of the two regions, and the double-crossover types. Let interval A–B = region I and interval B–C = region II.

F_1:		Step 1	Steps 2–5
Parental Types	AbC aBc	35.6% 35.6%	71.2%
Singles in Region I	ABc abC	4.4% 4.4%	8.8%
Singles in Region II	Abc aBC	9.4% 9.4%	18.8%
Double Crossovers	ABC abc	0.6% 0.6%	1.2%
		100.0%	

Step 2.   The frequency of double crossovers expected to be observed is calculated by multiplying the two decimal equivalents of the map distances by the coefficient of coincidence.

$$0.1 \times 0.2 \times 0.6 = 0.012 \text{ or } 1.2\%$$

This percentage is expected to be equally divided (0.6% each) between the two double-crossover types.

Step 3.   Calculate the single crossovers in region II (between b and c) and correct it for the double crossovers that also occurred in this region:

$$20\% - 1.2\% = 18.8\%$$

equally divided into two classes = 9.4% each.

Step 4.   The single crossovers in region I (between a and b) are calculated in the same manner as step 3:

$$10\% - 1.2\% = 8.8\%$$

divided equally among the two classes = 4.4% each.

Step 5.   Total all the single crossovers and all the double crossovers and subtract from 100% to obtain the percentage of parental types:

$$100 - (8.8 + 18.8 + 1.2) = 71.2\%$$

to be equally divided among the two parental classes = 35.6% each.

For convenience, we need not write out the entire genotype or phenotype of the progeny because, for example, when the gamete AbC from the trihybrid parent unites with the gamete produced by the testcross parent (abc), obviously the genotype is AbC/abc. Phenotypically it will exhibit the dominant trait at the A locus, the recessive trait at the B locus and the dominant trait at the C locus. All this could be predicted directly from the gamete AbC.

An alternative method for predicting F_1 progeny types is by combining the probabilities of crossovers and/or noncrossovers in appropriate combinations. This method can be used only when there is no interference.

Example 6.28.   Parents: $ABC/abc \quad \times \quad abc/abc$

Coincidence: 1.0

	I		II	
Map: a	10	b	20	c

No. of progeny: 2000

Step 1.   Determine the parental, single-crossover and double-crossover progeny types expected.

F_1:		**Step 1**	**Steps 2–5**
Parental Types	ABC	720	
	abc	720	
Singles in Region I	Abc	80	
	aBC	80	
Singles in Region II	ABc	180	
	abC	180	
Double Crossovers	AbC	20	
	aBc	20	
		2000	

Step 2. The number of double crossovers expected to appear in the progeny is $0.1 \times 0.2 \times 2000 = 40$, equally divided between the two double-crossover types (20 each).

Step 3. The probability of a single crossover occurring in region I is 10%. Hence there is a 90% chance that a crossover will not occur in that region. The combined probability that a crossover will not occur in region I and will occur in region II is $(0.9)(0.2) = 0.18$ and the number of region II single-crossover progeny expected is $0.18(2000) = 360$, equally divided between the two classes (180 each).

Step 4. Likewise the probability of a crossover occurring in region I and not in region II is $0.1(0.8) = 0.08$ and the number of region I single-crossover progeny expected is $0.08(2000) = 160$, equally divided among the two classes (80 each).

Step 5. The probability that a crossover will not occur in region I and region II is $0.9(0.8) = 0.72$ and the number of parental-type progeny expected is $0.72(2000) = 1440$, equally divided among the two parental types (720 each).

CROSSOVER SUPPRESSION

Many extrinsic and intrinsic factors are known to contribute to the crossover rate. Among these are the effects of sex, age, temperature, proximity to the centromere or **heterochromatic** regions (darkly staining regions presumed to carry little genetic information), chromosomal aberrations such as inversions, and many more. Two specific cases of crossover suppression are presented in this section: (1) complete absence of crossing over in male *Drosophila* and (2) the maintenance of balanced lethal systems as permanent trans heterozygotes through the prevention of crossing over.

1. Absence of Crossing Over in Male Drosophila.

One of the unusual characteristics of *Drosophila* is the apparent absence of crossing over in males. This fact is shown clearly by the nonequivalent results of reciprocal crosses.

Example 6.29. Testcross of heterozygous females.

Consider 2 genes on the third chromosome of *Drosophila*, hairy (*h*) and scarlet (*st*), approximately 20 map units apart.

P: $h+/+st\,♀♀$ × $h\,st/h\,st\,♂♂$
              wild-type females   hairy, scarlet males

F₁:

♀ \ ♂		$h\,st$	
80% Parental Types	40% $h+$	$h+/h\,st$	= 40% hairy
	40% $+st$	$+st/h\,st$	= 40% scarlet
20% Recombinant Types	10% $h\,st$	$h\,st/h\,st$	= 10% hairy and scarlet
	10% $++$	$++/h\,st$	= 10% wild type

Example 6.30. Testcross of heterozygous males (reciprocal cross of Example 6.29).

P: $h\ st/h\ st$ ♀ ♀ × $h+/+st$ ♂ ♂
  hairy, scarlet females wild-type males

F₁:

♂ \ ♀	$h\ st$
Only Parental Types	$h+$ → $h+/h\ st$ = 50% hairy
	$+st$ → $+st/h\ st$ = 50% scarlet

When dihybrid males are crossed to dihybrid females (both in repulsion phase) the progeny will always appear in the ratio 2:1:1 regardless of the degree of linkage between the genes. The double-recessive class never appears.

Example 6.31. P: $h+/+st$ ♀ ♀ × $h+/+st$ ♂ ♂
  wild-type females wild-type males

F₁:

		50% $h+$	50% $+st$
80% Parental Types	40% $h+$	$h+/h+$ 20% hairy	$h+/+st$ 20% wild type
	40% $+st$	$+st/h+$ 20% wild type	$+st/+st$ 20% scarlet
20% Recombinant Types	10% $h\ st$	$h\ st/h+$ 5% hairy	$h\ st/+st$ 5% scarlet
	10% $++$	$++/h+$ 5% wild type	$++/+st$ 5% wild type

Summary: 50% wild type ⎫
  25% hairy   ⎬ 2:1:1
  25% scarlet ⎭

Drosophila is not unique in this respect. For example, crossing over is completely suppressed in female silkworms. Other examples of complete and partial suppression of crossing over are common in genetic literature.

2. Balanced Lethal Systems.

A gene which is lethal when homozygous and linked to another lethal with the same mode of action can be maintained in permanent dihybrid condition in repulsion phase when associated with a genetic condition that prevents crossing over (see "inversions" in Chapter 8). Balanced lethals breed true and their behavior simulates that of a homozygous genotype. These systems are commonly used to maintain laboratory cultures of lethal, semilethal, or sterile mutants.

Example 6.32. Two dominant genetic conditions, curly wings (Cy) and plum eye color (Pm), are linked on chromosome 2 of *Drosophila* and associated with a chromosomal inversion which prevents crossing over. Cy or Pm are lethal when homozygous. Half the progeny from repulsion heterozygotes die, and the viable half are repulsion heterozygotes just like the parents.

P: $Cy\ Pm^+/Cy^+\ Pm ♀♀$ × $Cy\ Pm^+/Cy^+\ Pm ♂♂$
       curly, plum females   curly, plum males

F₁:

	$Cy\ Pm^+$	$Cy^+\ Pm$
$Cy\ Pm^+$	$Cy\ Pm^+/Cy\ Pm^+$ dies	$Cy\ Pm^+/Cy^+\ Pm$ curly, plum
$Cy^+\ Pm$	$Cy^+\ Pm/Cy\ Pm^+$ curly, plum	$Cy^+\ Pm/Cy^+\ Pm$ dies

Balanced lethals may be used to determine on which chromosome an unknown genetic unit resides (see Problem 6.12). Sex-linked genes make themselves known through the nonequivalence of progeny from reciprocal matings (Chapter 5). Without the aid of a balanced lethal system, the assignment of an autosomal gene to a particular linkage group may be made through observation of the peculiar genetic ratios obtained from abnormal individuals possessing an extra chromosome (trisomic) bearing the gene under study (Chapter 8).

TETRAD ANALYSIS IN ASCOMYCETES

Fungi that produce sexual spores **(ascospores)** housed in a common sac **(ascus)** are called **ascomycetes.** One of the simplest ascomycetes is the unicellular baker's yeast *Saccharomyces cerevisiae* (Fig. 6-2). Asexual reproduction is by budding, a mitotic process usually with unequal cytokinesis. The sexual cycle involves the union of entire cells of opposite mating type, forming a diploid zygote. The diploid cell may reproduce diploid progeny asexually by budding or haploid progeny by meiosis. The 4 haploid nuclei form ascospores enclosed by the ascus. Rupture of the ascus releases the haploid spores, which then germinate into new yeast cells.

Another ascomycete of interest to geneticists is the bread mold *Neurospora crassa* (Fig. 6-3). The fungal mat or **mycelium** is composed of intertwined filaments called **hyphae.** The tips of hyphae may pinch off asexual spores called **conidia,** which germinate into more hyphae. The vegetative hyphae are segmented, with several haploid nuclei in each segment. Hyphae from one mycelium may anastomose

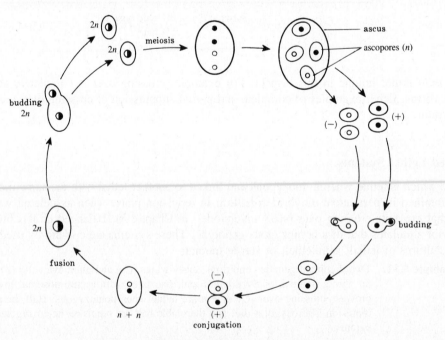

Fig. 6-2.   Life cycle of *Saccharomyces cerevisiae.*

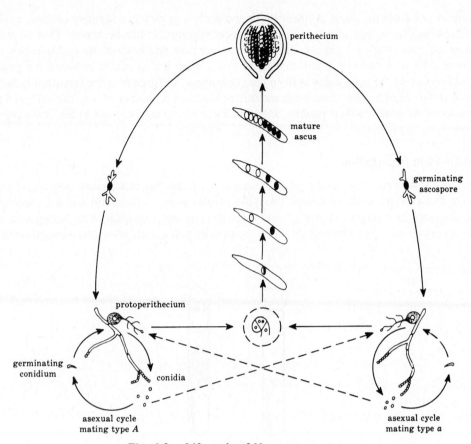

Fig. 6-3. Life cycle of *Neurospora crassa*.

with hyphae of another mycelium to form a mixture of nuclei in a common cytoplasm called a **heterokaryon.** A pair of alleles, *A* and *a*, governs the two mating types. Sexual reproduction occurs only when cells of opposite mating type unite. Specialized regions of the mycelium produce immature female fruiting bodies **(protoperithecia)** from which extrude receptive filaments called **trichogynes.** A conidium or hyphae from the opposite mating type fuses with the trichogyne, undergoes several karyokineses, and fertilizes many female nuclei. Each of the resulting diploid zygotes lies within an elongated sac called the ascus (asci, plural). The zygote divides by meiosis to form 4 nuclei, followed by a mitotic division that yields four pairs of nuclei, maturing into 8 ascospores. A mature fruiting body **(perithecium)** may contain over 100 asci, each containing 8 ascospores. The confines of the ascus force the polar organization of division to orient lengthwise in the ascus and also prevent the meiotic or mitotic products from slipping past each other. Each of the four chromatids of first meiotic prophase are now represented by a pair of ascospores in tandem order within the ascus.

In the case of yeast the ascospores representing the four chromatids of meiosis are in no special order, but in the bread mold *Neurospora* the ascospores are linearly ordered in the ascus in the same sequence as the chromatids were on the meiotic metaphase plate. The recovery and investigation of all of the products from a single meiotic event is called **tetrad analysis.**

Each ascus of *Neurospora*, when analyzed for a segregating pair of alleles, reveals one of two linear ratios: (1) 4 : 4 ratio, attributed to **first-division segregation** and (2) 2 : 2 : 2 : 2 ratio resulting from **second-division segregation.**

1. First-Division Segregation.

A cross between a culture with a wild-type (c^+) spreading form of mycelial growth and one with a restricted form of growth called "colonial" (*c*) is diagrammed in Fig. 6-4(*a*). If the ascospores are removed one by one from the ascus in linear order and each is grown as a separate culture, a linear ratio of 4 colonial : 4 wild type indicates that a first-division segregation has occurred. That is, during first meiotic anaphase both of the c^+ chromatids moved to one pole and both of the c chromatids moved to the other pole. The 4 : 4 ratio indicates that *no crossing over* has occurred between the gene and its centromere. The further the gene locus is from the centromere, the greater is the opportunity for crossing over to occur in this region. Therefore if the meiotic products of a number of asci are analyzed and most of them are found to exhibit a 4 : 4 pattern, then the locus of c must be close to the centromere.

2. Second-Division Segregation.

Let us now investigate the results of a crossover between the centromere and the c locus [Fig. 6-4(b)]. Note that crossing over in meiotic prophase results in a c^+ chromatid and a c chromatid being attached to the same centromere. Hence c^+ and c fail to separate from each other during first anaphase. During second anaphase, sister chromatids move to opposite poles, thus affecting segregation of c^+ from

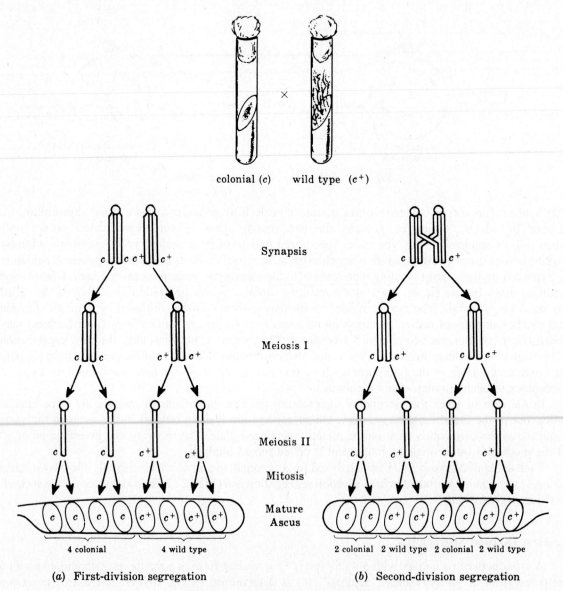

colonial (c)   wild type (c^+)

Synapsis

Meiosis I

Meiosis II

Mitosis

Mature Ascus

4 colonial   4 wild type   2 colonial   2 wild type   2 colonial   2 wild type

(a) First-division segregation   (b) Second-division segregation

Fig. 6-4. *Neurospora* spore patterns.

c. The 2 : 2 : 2 : 2 linear pattern is indicative of a second-division segregation ascus produced by *crossing over* between the gene and its centromere.

RECOMBINATION MAPPING WITH TETRADS

1. Ordered Tetrads.

The frequency of crossing over between the centromere and the gene in question is a reflection of its map distance from the centromere. Thus the percentage of asci showing second-division segregation is a measure of linkage intensity. It must be remembered, however, that one crossover event gives one second-division ascus, but that only half of the ascospores in that ascus are recombinant type. Therefore to convert second-division asci frequency to crossover frequency, we divide the former by two.

2. Unordered Tetrads.

The meiotic products of most ascomycetes seldom are in a linear order as in the ascus of *Neurospora*. Let us analyze unordered tetrads involving 2 linked genes from the cross $+ + \times ab$. The fusion nucleus is diploid ($+ +/ab$) and immediately undergoes meiosis. If a crossover does not occur between these two loci or if a 2-strand double crossover occurs between them, the resulting meiotic products will be of two kinds, equally frequent, resembling the parental combinations. Such a tetrad is referred to as a **parental ditype** (PD).

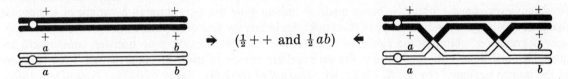

A 4-strand double crossover between the 2 genes results in two kinds of products, neither of which are parental combinations. This tetrad is called a **nonparental ditype** (NPD), and is the rarest of the tetrad double crossovers.

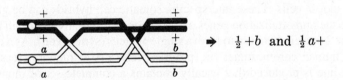

A **tetratype** (TT) is produced by either a single crossover or a 3-strand double crossover (of two types) between the 2 genes.

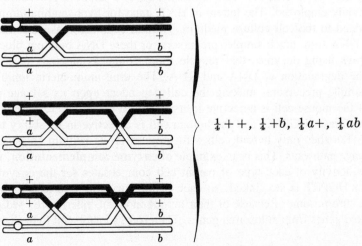

Whenever the number of parental ditypes and nonparental ditypes are statistically nonequivalent, this may be considered evidence for linkage between the 2 genes. To estimate the amount of recombination between the two markers, we use the formula:

$$\text{Recombination frequency} = \frac{\text{NPD} + \frac{1}{2}\text{TT}}{\text{total number of tetrads}}$$

The derivation of the above formula becomes clear when we analyze these diagrams and see that all of the products from an NPD tetrad are recombinant, but only half of the products from a TT tetrad are recombinant. Recombination frequency is not always equivalent to crossover frequency (map distance). If a third genetic marker was present midway between the loci of *a* and *b*, the 3-strand double crossovers could be distinguished from the single crossovers and crossover frequency could thus be determined. Recombination frequency analysis of 2 widely spaced genes thereby can establish only minimum map distances between the 2 genes.

MAPPING THE HUMAN GENOME

Until recently, the only method for mapping human genes was through pedigree analysis. Sex-linked genes are the ones most easily distinguished because of their peculiar inheritance patterns. Assigning autosomal genes to their specific chromosomes was sometimes possible if a chromosomal abnormality (e.g., reciprocal translocation or segmental deletion) was involved. Closely linked genes could occasionally be discovered in large family pedigrees, but loosely linked genes often mimic independent assortment. Now, however, rapid progress is being made in human gene mapping through a variety of techniques (most of which are beyond the scope of this book), including somatic cell hybridization, radiation-induced gene segregation, chromosome-mediated gene transfer, DNS-mediated gene transfer, amino acid sequencing, and linkage disequilibrium. For an excellent review of these procedures, see "The anatomy of the human genome," by V. A. McKusick, *Journal of Heredity,* 71(6): 370–391, Nov.–Dec. 1980.

The technique of **somatic cell hybridization** (SCH) has been very useful in assigning human genes to their respective chromosomes. Typically, human cells (e.g., fibroblasts) are mixed with mouse tumor cells from an established cell line that grows well *in vitro*. Sendai virus or polyethylene glycol (PGE) is added to promote cell fusion. The fusion rate is usually low, but some of the cell fusions will be between human and mouse cells. These interspecific somatic cell hybrids can be grown indefinitively in cell culture, thanks to the immortalization genes of the tumor cell. Initially these cell hybrids are binucleate heterocaryons, but the 2 nuclei often fuse to form a single nucleus **(syncaryon).** As a cell hybrid proliferates by mitosis, various human chromosomes are progressively lost at random (reason unknown) until a surviving stable cell line is produced that usually contains a complete set of mouse chromosomes plus a few human chromosomes. Human chromosomes are easily distinguished from mouse chromosomes, especially when stained with fluorescent dyes that reveal their distinctive banding patterns.

In order to find the hybrid cells among the parental cells, a selective procedure known as the **HAT technique** is commonly employed. The letters in HAT stand for *h*ypoxanthine-*a*minopterin-*t*hymidine, all of which are added to the cell culture medium. Normal cells can make the monomeric nucleotide building blocks of DNA from much simpler precursors, or these DNA building blocks can be produced by **salvage pathways** using enzymes that recycle more complex materials (e.g., hypoxanthine and thymidine) from the degradation of DNA and RNA. The drug aminopterin inhibits the synthesis of nucleotides from simple precursors, making the cell dependent upon its salvage pathways for DNA replication. Now if the mouse cell is defective in its ability to make the enzyme hypoxanthine guanine phosphoribosyl transferase (HGPRT) and the human cell is defective in its ability to make the enzyme thymidine kinase (TK), then only hybrid cells will grow in HAT medium because these enzymes are essential in the salvage pathways. This is an example of **enzyme complementation,** where, in the hybrid cell, the enzymatic activity of each type of parent cell compensates for the enzyme deficiency of the other. The gene for HGPRT is sex-linked, so each of the surviving hybrid cells must also contain at least one human X chromosome. Because of their unique mode of inheritance, pedigree data can easily distinguish sex-linked genes from autosomal genes. Therefore, somatic cell hybridization using the HAT technique would normally be used only to assign markers that exhibit an autosomal pattern of inheritance to their respective autosomes.

Suppose that we wish to assign a human gene for a character to a particular chromosome. The human cell used in the SCH technique must possess a phenotype or marker (such as an enzyme, an antigen, or a drug-resistance factor) that does not exist in the mouse cell. It is then possible to screen multiple stabilized hybrid cell lines for the marker and ascertain which of the human chromosomes remain in each cell line. By correlating presence or absence of the marker with the presence or absence of a particular chromosome in each hybrid cell line, the marker gene can be assigned to its proper chromosome.

Example 6.33. Suppose that we have 20 hybrid cell lines, that our phenotypic marker is human transferrin, and that it is found to be present only in four lines containing (in addition to a human X chromosome) the following human autosomes:

Cell line:	5	9	13	16
Human chromosomes:	1, 7, 16	1, 3	1, 10, 22	1, 5, 11, 16

Since all the cell lines that have the marker also have only chromosome 1 in common, and hybrids lacking the marker never contain chromosome 1, it can be inferred that the gene for transferrin is located on chromosome 1.

Genes that are assigned to the same chromosome by the technique of somatic cell hybridization are said to be **syntenic** (synonymous with ''linked''). It may be possible to determine if the marker gene is on the short or long arm of its chromosome or perhaps to assign it to a limited region of one arm of a chromosome if the chromosome has lost a segment (deletion) or gained a segment belonging to another chromosome (translocation). The loss or addition of a chromosomal segment can then be correlated with the presence or absence of the marker.

Example 6.34. Suppose that one hybrid cell line has the phenotypic marker and contains normal human chromosomes 7 and 13, whereas another hybrid cell line does not have the marker and contains a normal chromosome 13 and a chromosome 7 that is missing the tip of its long arm. It can be inferred that the marker gene is in the segment at the tip of the long arm of chromosome 7.

Solved Problems

RECOMBINATION AMONG LINKED GENES

6.1. In the human pedigree below where the male parent does not appear, it is assumed that he is phenotypically normal. Both hemophilia (h) and color blindness (c) are sex-linked recessives. Insofar as possible, determine the genotypes for each individual in the pedigree.

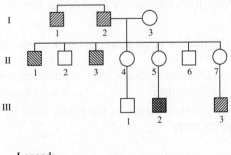

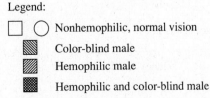

Legend:

☐ ◯ Nonhemophilic, normal vision

▨ Color-blind male

◪ Hemophilic male

◼ Hemophilic and color-blind male

Solution:

Let us begin with males first because, being hemizygous for sex-linked genes, the linkage relationship on their single X chromosome is obvious from their phenotype. Thus I1, I2, and III3 are all hemophilic with normal color vision and therefore must be hC/Y. Nonhemophilic, color-blind males II1 and II3 must be Hc/Y. Normal males II2, II6, and III1 must possess both dominant alleles HC/Y. III2 is both hemophilic and color blind and therefore must possess both recessives hc/Y. Now let us determine the female genotypes. I3 is normal but produces sons, half of which are color blind and half normal. The X chromosome contributed by I3 to her color-blind sons II1 and II3 must have been Hc; the X chromosome she contributed to her normal sons II2 and II6 must have been HC. Therefore the genotype for I3 is Hc/Hc.

Normal females II4, II5, and II7 each receive hC from their father (I2), but could have received either Hc or HC on the X chromosome they received from their mother (I3). II4 has a normal son (III1) to which she gives HC; therefore II4 is probably hC/HC, although it is possible for II4 to be hC/Hc and produce an HC gamete by crossing over. II5, however, could not be hC/HC and produce a son with both hemophilia and color blindness (III2); therefore II5 must be hC/Hc, in order to give the crossover gamete hc to her son.

GENETIC MAPPING

6.2. Two dominant mutants in the first linkage group of the guinea pig govern the traits pollex (Px), which is the ativistic return of thumb and little toe, and rough fur (R). When dihybrid pollex, rough pigs (with identical linkage relationships) were crossed to normal pigs, their progeny fell into 4 phenotypes: 79 rough, 103 normal, 95 rough, pollex, and 75 pollex. (a) Determine the genotypes of the parents. (b) Calculate the amount of recombination between Px and R.

Solution:

(a) The parental gametes always appear with greatest frequency, in this case 103 normal and 95 rough, pollex. This means that the 2 normal genes were on one chromosome of the dihybrid parent and the 2 dominant mutations on the other (i.e., coupling linkage).

$$\text{P:} \qquad \underset{\text{pollex, rough}}{Px\,R/px\,r} \qquad \times \qquad \underset{\text{normal}}{px\,r/px\,r}$$

(b) The 79 rough and 75 pollex types are recombinants, constituting 154 out of 352 individuals = 0.4375 or approximately 43.8% recombination.

6.3. A kidney-bean-shaped eye is produced by a recessive gene k on the third chromosome of *Drosophilia*. Orange eye color, called "cardinal," is produced by the recessive gene cd on the same chromosome. Between these two loci is a third locus with a recessive allele e producing ebony body color. Homozygous kidney, cardinal females are mated to homozygous ebony males. The trihybrid F_1 females are then testcrossed to produce the F_2. Among 4000 F_2 progeny are the following:

1761 kidney, cardinal	97 kidney
1773 ebony	89 ebony, cardinal
128 kidney, ebony	6 kidney, ebony, cardinal
138 cardinal	8 wild type

(a) Determine the linkage relationships in the parents and F_1 trihybrids.
(b) Estimate the map distances.

Solution:

(a) The parents are homozygous lines:

$$\underset{\text{kidney, cardinal}}{k\,e^+\,cd/k\,e^+\,cd\,♀♀} \qquad \times \qquad \underset{\text{ebony}}{k^+\,e\,cd^+/k^+\,e\,cd\,♂♂}$$

The F_1 is then trihybrid:

$$k\,e^+\,cd/k^+\,e\,cd^+$$
wild type

The linkage relationships in the trihybrid F_1 can also be determined directly from the F_2. By far the most frequent F_2 phenotypes are kidney, cardinal (1761) and ebony (1773), indicating that kidney and cardinal were on one chromosome in the F_1 and ebony on the other.

(b) Crossing over between the loci k and e produces the kidney, ebony (128) and cardinal (138) offspring. Double crossovers are the triple mutants (6) and wild type (8). Altogether there are $128 + 138 + 6 + 8 = 280$ crossovers between k and e:

$$280/4000 = 0.07 \text{ or } 7\% \text{ crossing over} = 7 \text{ map units}$$

Crossovers between e and cd produced the single-crossover types kidney (97) and ebony, cardinal (89). Double crossovers again must be counted in this region.

$$97 + 89 + 6 + 8 = 200 \text{ crossovers between } e \text{ and } cd$$
$$200/4000 = 0.05 \text{ or } 5\% \text{ crossing over} = 5 \text{ map units}$$

6.4. The map distances for 6 genes in the second linkage group of the silkworm *Bombyx mori* are shown in the table below. Construct a genetic map which includes all of these genes.

	Gr	Rc	S	Y	P	oa
Gr	—	25	1	19	7	20
Rc	25	—	26	6	32	5
S	1	26	—	20	6	21
Y	19	6	20	—	26	1
P	7	32	6	26	—	27
oa	20	5	21	1	27	—

Solution:

Step 1. It makes little difference where one begins to solve this kind of problem, so we shall begin at the top. The *Gr–Rc* distance is 25 map units, and the *Gr–S* distance is 1 unit. Therefore, the relationship of these three genes may be either

(a) S^1Gr —————————————— ^{25} —————————————— Rc

or

(b) Gr^1S ————————————— ^{24} ————————————— Rc

The table, however, tells us that the distance *S–Rc* is 26 units. Therefore alternative (a) must be correct, i.e., *Gr* is between *S* and *Rc*.

Step 2. The *Gr–Y* distance is 19 units. Again two alternatives are possible:

(c) S^1Gr ———————— ^{19} ———————— Y —— ^{6} —— Rc

or

(d) Y ———————— ^{18} ———————— S^1Gr ———————— ^{25} ———————— Rc

In the table we find that the distance *Y–Rc* = 6. Hence possibility (c) must be correct, i.e., *Y* lies between the loci of *Gr* and *Rc*.

Step 3. The distance *Gr–P* is 7 map units. Two alternatives for these loci are

(e) S^1Gr —— ^{7} —— P ———— ^{12} ———— Y —— ^{6} —— Rc

or

(f) P —— ^{6} —— S^1Gr ———————— ^{19} ———————— Y —— ^{6} —— Rc

The distance *P–S* is read from the table, and thus alternative (f) must be correct.

Step 4. There are 20 units between *Gr* and *oa*. These two genes may be in one of two possible relationships:

(*g*)   *P*   ⁶   *S*ⁱ*Gr*   ¹⁹   *Y*ⁱ*oa*   ⁵   *Rc*

or

(*h*)   *oa*   ¹³   *P*   ⁶   *S*ⁱ*Gr*   ¹⁹   *Y*   ⁶   *Rc*

The table indicates that *Y* and *oa* are 1 map unit apart. Therefore (*g*) is the completed map.

6.5.   Three recessive genes in linkage group V of the tomato are *a* producing absence of anthocyanin pigment, *hl* producing hairless plants, and *j* producing jointless fruit stems (pedicels). Among 3000 progeny from a trihybrid testcross, the following phenotypes were observed:

259 hairless	268 anthocyaninless, jointless, hairless
40 jointless, hairless	941 anthocyaninless, hairless
931 jointless	32 anthocyaninless
260 normal	269 anthocyaninless, jointless

(*a*) How were the genes originally linked in the trihybrid parent? (*b*) Estimate the distance between the genes.

Solution:

(*a*)   The most frequent phenotypes observed among the offspring are the jointless (931) and anthocyaninless, hairless (941). Hence *j* was on one chromosome of the trihybrid parent, *a* and *hl* on the other. The double-crossover (DCO) types are the least frequent phenotypes: jointless, hairless (40) and anthocyaninless (32).

Case 1.   If jointless is in the middle, we could not obtain the double-crossover types as given:

$$\text{P:}\qquad \frac{A\,j\,Hl}{a\,J\,hl}$$

$$\text{F}_1\text{:}\qquad \text{DCO} \begin{cases} A\,J\,Hl = \text{normal} \\ a\,j\,hl \;\; = \text{triple mutant} \end{cases}$$

Case 2.   If *h* is in the middle, the double-crossover types could be formed. Therefore the parental genotype is as shown below:

$$\text{P:}\qquad \frac{J\,hl\,a}{j\,Hl\,A}$$

$$\text{F}_1\text{:}\qquad \text{DCO} \begin{cases} J\,Hl\,a \;\; = \text{anthocyaninless} \\ j\,hl\,A \;\; = \text{jointless, hairless} \end{cases}$$

(*b*)   Now that the genotype of the trihybrid parent is known, we can predict the single-crossover types.

$$\text{P:}\qquad \frac{J\,hl\,a}{j\,Hl\,A}$$

$$\text{F}_1\text{:}\qquad$$ Single crossovers (SCO) between *j* and *hl* (region I) yield:

$$\text{SCO(I)} \begin{cases} J\,Hl\,A = \text{normal (260)} \\ j\,hl\,a \;\; = \text{jointless, hairless, anthocyaninless (268)} \end{cases}$$

Therefore the percentage of *all* crossovers (single and doubles) that occurred between *j* and *hl* is $260 + 268 + 32 + 40 = \frac{600}{3000} = 0.2 = 20\%$ or 20 map units.

Similarly the single crossovers between *hl* and *a* (region II) may be obtained.

P: $\dfrac{J\ hl\ a}{j\ Hl\ A}$

F$_1$:   SCO(II) $\Bigg<$ $J\ hl\ A$ = hairless (259)
$j\ Hl\ a$ = jointless, anthocyaninless (269)

$259 + 269 + 32 + 40 = \frac{600}{3000} = 0.2 = 20\%$ or 20 map units

Note the similarity of numbers between the SCO(II) jointless, anthocyaninless (269) and the SCO(I) triple mutant (268). Attempts to obtain map distances by matching pairs with similar numbers could, as this case proves, lead to erroneous estimates. The single-crossover types in each region must first be determined in order to avoid such errors.

6.6. The recessive mutation called "lemon" (*le*) produces a pale-yellow body color in the parasitic wasp *Bracon hebetor*. This locus exhibits 12% recombination with a recessive eye mutation called "canteloupe" (*c*). Canteloupe shows 14% recombination with a recessive mutation called "long" (*l*), causing antennal and leg segments to elongate. Canteloupe is the locus in the middle. A homozygous lemon female is crossed with a hemizygous long male (males are haploid). The F$_1$ females are then testcrossed to produce the F$_2$. (*a*) Diagram the crosses and the expected F$_1$ and F$_2$ female genotypes and phenotypes. (*b*) Calculate the amount of wild types expected among the F$_2$ females.

Solution:

(*a*)   P: $le\ l^+/le\ l^+$ ♀   × $le^+\ l$ ♂
             lemon   long

F$_1$: $le\ l^+/le^+\ l$ ♀♀   × $le\ l$ ♂♂
             wild type   lemon, long

F$_2$:

		♂ $le\ l$
Parental Types	$le\ l^+$	$le\ l^+/le\ l$ lemon
	$le^+\ l$	$le^+\ l/le\ l$ long
Recombinant Types	$le\ l$	$le\ l/le\ l$ lemon, long
	$le^+\ l^+$	$le^+\ l^+/le\ l$ wild type

(*b*)   Since the canteloupe locus is not segregating in this cross, double crossovers will appear as parental types. The percentage of recombination expected to be observed is $0.12 + 0.14 - 2(0.12)(0.14) = 0.2264 = 22.64\%$. Half of the recombinants are expected to be wild type: $22.64\%/2 = 11.32\%$ wild type.

6.7. Several 3-point testcrosses were made in maize utilizing the genes booster (*B*, a dominant plant color intensifier), liguleless leaf (*lg*$_1$), virescent seedling (*v*$_4$, yellowish-green), silkless (*sk*, abortive pistils), glossy seedling (*gl*$_2$), and tassel-seed (*ts*$_1$, pistillate terminal inflorescence). Using the information from the following testcrosses, map this region of the chromosome.

Testcross 1. Trihybrid parent is heterozygous for booster, liguleless, tassel-seed.

Testcross Progeny

71 booster, liguleless, tassel-seed	17 tassel-seed
111 wild type	24 booster, liguleless
48 liguleless	6 booster
35 booster, tassel-seed	3 liguleless, tassel-seed

Testcross 2. Trihybrid parent is heterozygous for booster, liguleless, tassel-seed.

Testcross Progeny

57 tassel-seed	21 liguleless, tassel-seed
57 booster, liguleless	21 booster, liguleless, tassel-seed
20 wild type	8 booster, tassel-seed
31 booster	7 liguleless

Testcross 3. Trihybrid parent is heterozygous for booster, liguleless, silkless.

Testcross Progeny

52 silkless	56 booster, liguleless
8 booster, silkless	13 liguleless
2 booster, liguleless, silkless	131 liguleless, silkless
148 booster	

Testcross 4. Trihybrid parent is heterozygous for booster, liguleless, silkless.

Testcross Progeny

6 booster	3 liguleless, silkless
137 booster, silkless	30 silkless
291 booster, liguleless, silkless	34 booster, liguleless
142 liguleless	339 wild type

Testcross 5. Trihybrid parent is heterozygous for liguleless, virescent, glossy.

Testcross Progeny

431 wild type	128 virescent, glossy
399 liguleless, virescent, glossy	153 liguelless
256 virescent	44 glossy
310 liguleless, glossy	51 virescent, liguleless

Testcross 6. Trihybrid parent is heterozygous for booster, liguleless, virescent.

Testcross Progeny

60 wild type	18 virescent
37 liguleless, booster, virescent	23 liguleless, booster
32 virescent, booster	11 booster
34 liguleless	12 virescent, liguleless

Testcross 7. Trihybrid parent is heterozygous for virescent, liguleless, booster.

Testcross Progeny

25 booster	8 booster, virescent
11 booster, liguleless	2 liguleless, booster, virescent

Solution:

Following the procedures established in this chapter, we determine from each of the testcrosses the gene order (which gene is in the middle) and the percent crossing over in each region. Note that the results of testcrosses 1 and 2 may be combined, recognizing that the linkage relationships are different in the trihybrid parents. Likewise, the results of 3 and 4 may be combined, as well as testcrosses 6 and 7. The analysis of these seven testcrosses are summarized below in tabular form.

Testcross No.	Trihybrid Parent	Parental Type Progeny	Recombinant Progeny			Total
			Region I	Region II	DCO	
1	$\dfrac{+\ +\ +}{lg_1 B\ ts_1}$	111　71	35　48	17　24	6　3	315
2	$\dfrac{+\ +\ ts_1}{lg_1 B\ +}$	57　57	31　21	20　21	8　7	222
		296	135	82	24	537
			25.1%	15.3%	4.5%	
3*	$\dfrac{+\ B\ +}{lg_1\ +\ sk}$	148　131	52　56	8　13	0　2	410
4	$\dfrac{+\ +\ +}{lg_1 B\ sk}$	339　291	137　142	30　34	6　3	982
		909	387	85	11	1392
			27.8%	6.1%	0.8%	
5	$\dfrac{+\ +\ +}{lg_1 g l_2 v_4}$	431　399	128　153	256　310	44　51	
		830	281	566	95	1772
			15.9%	31.9%	5.4%	
6	$\dfrac{+\ +\ +}{lg_1 B\ v_4}$	60　37	32　34	18　23	11　12	227
7†	$\dfrac{+\ B\ +}{lg_1\ +\ v_4}$	25　0	0　11	8　0	0　2	46
		122	77	49	25	273
			28.2%	17.9%	9.2%	

* Note that in testcross 3, only 7 phenotypes appeared, whereas we expected 8. We suspect that the missing phenotype (wild type) is a double-crossover type because DCO types are expected to be less frequent than the others. The 2 phenotypes with the highest numbers should derive from the parental (noncrossover gametes). Thus, the booster phenotype indicates that the 3 genes B, lg_1^+, and sk^+ were on one parental chromosome; likewise, the other high-frequency progeny phenotype (liguleless and silkless) indicates that the 3 genes lg_1, sk, and B^+ were on the homologous chromosome, but we do not know which of these loci is in the middle. Assuming that the least frequent phenotype (booster, liguleless, silkless) is one of the double-crossover types, we can infer that the booster locus is in the middle; i.e., if parents were lg_1^+, B, sk^+/lg_1, B^+, sk the double crossovers would be $+\ +\ +$ (wild type) and lg_1, B, sk (liguleless, booster, silkless). This inference is confirmed by testcross 4 where all 8 progeny phenotypes are present.

† In testcross 7, only 4 phenotypes appeared in the progeny (no explanation given for the missing phenotypes). One might be tempted to eliminate such bizarre results from a report, but it would be scientifically unethical to do so. Data selection or alteration would be considered fraudulent. A scientist must report all the data or give reasons for failing to do so. However, it is possible to establish the gene order from testcross 6, so that the type of progeny (noncrossovers, single crossovers, and double crossovers) can be identified unambiguously.

To find the map distances between lg_1 and B in the first two testcrosses, we add the double crossovers (4.5%) to the region I single crossovers (25.1%) = 29.6% or 29.6 map units. Likewise, to find the map distance between B and ts_1, we add 4.5% to the region II single crossovers (15.3%) = 19.8% or 19.8 map units. Thus this segment of map becomes

lg_1 ——————29.6—————— B ————19.8———— ts_1

Three other map segments are similarly derived from testcross data:

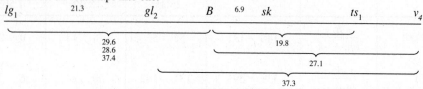

Testcrosses 3 and 4 lg_1 ——————28.6—————— B ——6.9—— sk

Testcross 5 lg_1 ————21.3———— gl_2 ——————————37.3—————————— v_4

Testcrosses 6 and 7 lg_1 ——————————37.4—————————— B ——————27.1—————— v_4

Now let us combine all four maps into one:

lg_1 ————21.3———— gl_2 ———— B ——6.9—— sk ———————— ts_1 ———— v_4

29.6
28.6
37.4

19.8

27.1

37.3

The weighted-average distance lg_1–B is determined next:

Expt.	No. in Expt. x	Distance y	xy
1, 2	537	29.6	15,895.2
3, 4	1392	28.6	39,811.2
6, 7	273	37.4	10,210.2
	2202		65,916.6

65,916.6/2202 = 29.9 map units (weighted average)

The sk–ts_1 distance = $(B\text{–}ts_1) - (B\text{–}sk)$ = 19.8 − 6.9 = 12.9 map units.
The gl_2–B distance has two estimators:

    (1) $(lg_1\text{–}B) - (lg_1 - gl_2)$ = 29.9 − 21.3 = 8.6
    (2) $(gl_2\text{–}v_4) - (B\text{–}v_4)$ = 37.3 − 27.1 = 10.2

All other factors being equal, the second estimate is likely to be less accurate because of the greater distances involved. There is no easy way to accurately average these two values. We will arbitrarily use the estimate of 8.6 map units until more definitive experimental results are obtained.

Likewise, the ts_1–v_4 distance has two estimators:

    (1) $(B\text{–}v_4) - (B\text{–}ts_1)$ = 27.1 − 19.8 = 7.3
    (2) $(gl_2\text{–}v_4) - [(gl_2\text{–}B) + (B\text{–}ts_1)]$ = 37.3 − (8.6 + 19.8) = 8.9

Again, the second estimate is likely to be less accurate because of the distances involved, and we will use 7.3 map units as our estimate of the ts_1–v_4 distance. The unified map now appears as follows:

lg_1 ————21.3———— gl_2 ——8.6—— B ——6.9—— sk ————12.9———— ts_1 ——7.3—— v_4

Additional experimental data may considerably modify certain portions of this genetic map. It should always be remembered that these maps are only estimates, and as such are continually subject to refinements.

LINKAGE ESTIMATES FROM F_2 DATA

6.8. Two dominant sex-linked traits are known in the mouse (*Mus musculus*): bent (*Bn*), appearing as a short crooked tail, and tabby (*Ta*) with dark transverse stripes. Homozygous bent, tabby females are mated to normal (wild-type) males. All of the F_1 offspring are mated together to produce an F_2. Inadvertently, the male-female data from the F_2 were not recorded. Among 200 F_2 offspring were found 141 bent, tabby, 47 wild type, 7 tabby, and 5 bent.

(*a*) Estimate the amount of recombination between bent and tabby assuming that the male : female ratio is 1 : 1.

(*b*) Estimate the amount of recombination when the male : female ratio is variable and unreliable in this colony.

Solution:

(*a*)   P: *Bn Ta/Bn Ta* ♀♀   ×   *bn ta*/Y ♂♂
                  bent, tabby females   normal males

    F_1:   *Bn Ta/bn ta* ♀♀   ×   *Bn Ta*/Y ♂♂
                  bent, tabby females   bent, tabby males

F_2:

♀ \ ♂		*Bn Ta*	Y
Parental Types	*Bn Ta*	*Bn Ta/Bn Ta* bent, tabby	*Bn Ta*/Y bent, tabby
	bn ta	*bn ta/Bn Ta* bent, tabby	*bn ta*/Y wild type (47)
Recombinant Types	*Bn ta*	*Bn ta/Bn Ta* bent, tabby	*Bn ta*/Y bent (5)
	bn Ta	*bn Ta/Bn Ta* bent, tabby	*Bn ta*/Y tabby (7)
		Females	Males

If we assume that the male : female ratio is 1 : 1, then out of 200 offspring, half of them or (100) should have been males. The difference $100 - (47 + 5 + 7) = 41$ estimates the probable number of bent, tabby males. The estimate of recombination from the male data $= (5 + 7)/100 = 0.12$ or 12%.

(*b*) If the male : female ratio is unreliable, then we might better use the 47 wild-type males as an estimator of the number of bent, tabby males. The estimated total number of males $= 47 + 47 + 5 + 7 = 106$. The amount of recombination $= (5 + 7)/106 = 0.113$ or 11.3%.

6.9. White eyes (*w/w* females; *w*/Y males) in *Drosophila* can be produced by the action of a sex-linked recessive gene. White eyes can also be produced through the interaction of 2 other genes; the recessive sex-linked gene *v* for vermilion eye color, and the autosomal recessive gene *bw* for brown eye color (see Problem 5.5). Consider the parental cross: *bw/bw, $w^+v^+/w\,v$* ♀♀ (brown-eyed females) × *bw/bw, w v*/Y ♂♂ (white-eyed males), where the F_1 progeny consists of 70 brown-eyed and 130 white-eyed individuals. Estimate the distance between the sex-linked genes *w* and *v*.

Solution:

F_1:

♀ \ ♂	$bw/, w\ v/$	$bw/, Y/$
Parental Types $bw/, w^+v^+/$	$bw/bw, w^+v^+/w\ v$ brown	$bw/bw, w^+v^+/Y$ brown
$bw/, w\ v/$	$bw/bw, w\ v/w\ v$ white	$bw/bw, w\ v/Y$ white
Recombinant Types $bw/, w^+v/$	$bw/bw, w^+\ v/w\ v$ white	$bw/bw, w^+\ v/Y$ white
$bw/, w\ v^+/$	$bw/bw, w\ v^+\ /w\ v$ white	$bw/bw, w\ v^+/Y$ white

Only the genotypes of the brown offspring are known for certain. The 70 brown offspring constitute only one-half of the offspring produced by noncrossover maternal gametes. Therefore we *estimate* that 70 of the white individuals were also produced by noncrossover maternal gametes. Thus 140 out of 200 F_1 flies are estimated to be parental-type offspring = 70%. The other 30% must be crossover types. The best estimate of linkage between the white and vermilion loci would be 30 map units.

6.10. Elongate tomato fruit is produced by plants homozygous for a recessive gene o, round fruit shape is produced by the dominant allele at this locus (O). A compound inflorescence is the result of another recessive gene s, simple inflorescence is produced by the dominant allele at this locus (S). A Yellow Pear variety (with elongate fruit and simple inflorescence) is crossed to a Grape Cluster variety (with round fruit and compound inflorescence). The F_1 plants are randomly crossed to produce the F_2. Among 259 F_2 are found 126 round, simple: 63 round, compound: 66 long, simple: 4 long, compound. Estimate the amount of recombination by the "square-root method."

Solution:

P: oS/oS × Os/Os
Yellow Pear Variety   Grape Cluster Variety
(long, simple)   (round, compound)

F_1: oS/Os
(round, simple)

F_2:

		Parental Gametes		Crossover Gametes	
		$o\ S$	$O\ s$	$o\ s$	$O\ S$
Parental Gametes	$o\ S$	$o\ S/o\ S$ long, simple	$o\ S/O\ s$ round, simple	$o\ S/o\ s$ long, simple	$o\ S/O\ S$ round, simple
	$O\ s$	$O\ s/o\ S$ round, simple	$O\ s/O\ s$ round, compound	$O\ s/o\ s$ round, compound	$O\ s/O\ S$ round, simple
Crossover Gametes	$o\ s$	$o\ s/o\ S$ long, simple	$o\ s/O\ s$ round, compound	**$o\ s/o\ s$ long, compound**	$o\ s/O\ S$ round, simple
	$O\ S$	$O\ S/o\ S$ round, simple	$O\ S/O\ s$ round, simple	$O\ S/o\ s$ round, simple	$O\ S/O\ S$ round, simple

Notice that the double-recessive phenotype (long, compound) occupies only 1 of the 16 frames in the gametic checkerboard. This genotype is produced by the union of 2 identical double-recessive gametes (o, s). If we let x = the frequency of formation of os gametes, then x^2 = frequency of occurrence of the $o\,s/o\,s$ genotype (long, compound phenotype) = $\frac{4}{259}$ = 0.0154. Thus, $x = \sqrt{0.0154} = 0.124$. But x estimates only half of the crossover gametes. Therefore $2x$ estimates all of the crossover gametes = $2(0.124)$ = 0.248 or 24.8% recombination.

USE OF GENETIC MAPS

6.11. The genes for two nervous disorders, waltzer (v) and jittery (ji) are 18 map units apart on chromosome 10 in mice. A phenotypically normal F_1 group of mice carrying these 2 genes in coupling phase is being maintained by a commercial firm. An order arrives for 24 young mice each of waltzer, jittery, and waltzer plus jittery. Assuming that the average litter size is 7 offspring, and including a 10% safety factor to ensure the recovery of the needed number of offspring, calculate the minimum number of females that need to be bred.

Solution:

F_1:　　　　$v\ ji/+ +$

F_2:　　　　If 18% are crossover types, then 82% should be parental types.

		0.41 v ji	0.41 + +	0.09 v +	0.09 + ji
82% Parental Types	0.41 v ji	0.1681 v ji/v ji waltzer and jittery	0.1681 v ji/+ + wild type	0.0369 v ji/v+ waltzer	0.0369 v ji/+ ji jittery
	0.41 + +	0.1681 + +/v ji wild type	0.1681 + +/+ + wild type	0.0369 + +/v+ wild type	0.0369 + +/+ ji wild type
18% Crossover Types	0.09 v +	0.0369 v +/v ji waltzer	0.0369 v +/+ + wild type	0.0081 v +/v+ waltzer	0.0081 v +/+ ji wild type
	0.09 + ji	0.0369 + ji/v ji jittery	0.0369 + ji/+ + wild type	0.0081 + ji/v+ wild type	0.0081 + ji/+ ji jittery

Summary:　wild type　　　　　= .6681 or 66.81%
　　　　　　waltzer and jittery = .1681 or 16.81%
　　　　　　waltzer　　　　　　= .0819 or 8.19%
　　　　　　jittery　　　　　　= .0819 or 8.19%

Waltzer or jittery phenotypes are least frequent and hence are the limiting factors. If 8.19% of all the progeny are expected to be waltzers, how many offspring need to be raised to produce 24 waltzers? $0.0819x$ = 24, $x = 24/0.0819$ = 293.04 or approximately 293 progeny. Adding the 10% safety factor, 293 + 29.3 = 322.3 or approximately 322 progeny.

If each female has 7 per litter, how many females need to be bred? $\frac{322}{7}$ = 46 females.

CROSSOVER SUPPRESSION

6.12. Suppose you are given a strain of *Drosophila* exhibiting an unknown abnormal genetic trait (mutation). We mate the mutant females to males from a balanced lethal strain ($Cy\ Pm^+/Cy^+\ Pm$, $D\ Sb^+/D^+\ Sb$) where curly wings (Cy) and plum eye (Pm) are on chromosome 2 and dichaete wing (D) and stubble bristles (Sb) are on chromosome 3. Homozygosity for either curly, plum, dichaete, or stubble is lethal. The trait does not appear in the F_1. The F_1 males with curly wings and stubby bristles are then backcrossed to the original mutant females. In the progeny the mutation appears in equal association with curly and stubble. *Drosophila melanogaster* has a haploid number of 4 including an X, 2, 3, and 4 chromosome. (*a*) Determine whether the mutation is a dominant or a recessive. (*b*) To which linkage group (on which chromosome) does the mutation belong?

Solution:

(*a*) If the mutation were a dominant (let us designate it *M*), then each member of the strain (pure line) would be of genotype *MM*. Since the trait does not appear in our balanced lethal stock, they must be homozygous recessive (M^+M^+). Crosses between these two lines would be expected to produce only heterozygous genotypes (M^+M) and would be phenotypically of the mutant type. But since the mutant type did not appear in the F_1, the mutation must be a recessive (now properly redesignated *m*). The dominant wild-type allele may now be designated m^+.

(*b*) Let us assume that this is a sex-linked recessive mutation. The F_1 males receive their single X chromosome from the mutant female (*mm*). Therefore all males of the F_1 should exhibit the mutant trait because males would be hemizygous for all sex-linked genes (*mY*). Since the mutant type did not appear in the F_1, our recessive mutation could not be sex-linked.

Let us assume that our recessive mutation is on the second chromosome. The curly, stubble F_1 males carry the recessive in the heterozygous condition ($Cy\ m^+/Cy^+\ m,\ Sb/Sb^+$). Notice that we omit the designation of loci with which we are not concerned. When these carrier males are then backcrossed to the original mutant females ($Cy^+\ m/Cy^+\ m,\ Sb^+/Sb^+$), the F_2 expectations are as follows:

$Cy\ m^+/Cy^+\ m,\ Sb/Sb^+$ curly, stubble $Cy\ m^+/Cy^+\ m,\ Sb/Sb^+$ *mutant*, stubble
$Cy\ m^+/Cy^+\ m,\ Sb^+/Sb^+$ curly $Cy\ m^+/Cy^+\ m,\ Sb^+/Sb^+$ *mutant*

Note that the mutant cannot appear with curly. Therefore our recessive mutation is not on chromosome 2.

Let us then assume that our mutant gene is on the third chromosome. When F_1 carrier males ($Cy/Cy^+,\ Sb\ m^+/Sb^+\ m$) are backcrossed to the original mutant females ($Cy^+/Cy^+,\ Sb^+\ m/Sb^+\ m$), the F_2 expectations are as follows:

$Cy/Cy^+,\ Sb\ m^+/Sb^+\ m$ curly, stubble $Cy^+/Cy^+,\ Sb\ m^+/Sb^+\ m$ stubble
$Cy/Cy^+,\ Sb^+\ m/Sb^+\ m$ curly, *mutant* $Cy^+/Cy^+,\ Sb^+\ m/Sb^+\ m$ *mutant*

Note that the mutant cannot appear with stubble. Hence our recessive mutation is not on chromosome 3.

If the mutant is not sex-linked, not on 2 nor on 3, then obviously it must be on the fourth chromosome. Let us prove this. When F_1 carrier males ($Cy/Cy^+,\ Sb/Sb^+,\ m^+/m$) are backcrossed to the original mutant females ($Cy^+/Cy^+,\ Sb^+/Sb^+,\ m/m$), the F_2 expectations are as follows:

```
                        ┌── m⁺/m   curly, stubble
              Sb/Sb⁺ ───┤
              /         └── m/m    curly, stubble, mutant
   Cy/Cy⁺ ────┤
              \         ┌── m⁺/m   curly
              Sb⁺/Sb⁺───┤
                        └── m/m    curly, mutant

                        ┌── m⁺/m   stubble
              Sb/Sb⁺ ───┤
              /         └── m/m    stubble, mutant
   Cy⁺/Cy⁺────┤
              \         ┌── m⁺/m   wild type
              Sb⁺/Sb⁺───┤
                        └── m/m    mutant
```

Note that our recessive mutant occurs in equal association with curly and stubble, which satisfied the conditions of the problem. We conclude that this mutation is on the fourth chromosome.

RECOMBINATION MAPPING WITH TETRADS

6.13. A strain of *Neurospora* requiring methionine (*m*) was crossed to a wild-type (m^+) strain with the results shown below. How far is this gene from its centromere?

No. of Asci	Spores			
	1 + 2	3 + 4	5 + 6	7 + 8
6	+	m	+	m
5	m	+	+	m
6	m	+	m	+
7	+	m	m	+
40	m	m	+	+
36	+	+	m	m

Solution:

Noncrossover asci are those that appear with greatest frequency = 40 + 36 = 76 out of 100 total asci. The other 24/100 of these asci are crossover types. While 24% of the asci are crossover types, only half of the spores in these asci are recombinant. Therefore the distance from the gene to the centromere is 12 map units. The origin of each of the crossover type asci is as follows:

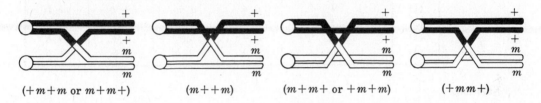

$(+m+m$ or $m+m+)$ $(m++m)$ $(m+m+$ or $+m+m)$ $(+mm+)$

6.14. Two linked genes are involved in a *Neurospora* cross: $(a+) \times (+b)$, where a is closest to the centromere. Diagram the simplest explanation to account for the following spore patterns: (a) $(a\,b)(+\,b)(a\,+)(+\,+)$, (b) $(+\,b)(a\,+)(+\,b)(a\,+)$, (c) $(a\,+)(+\,b)(a\,b)(+\,+)$.

Solution:

(a)   Two kinds of double-crossover events can account for this spore pattern.

(1)   (2)

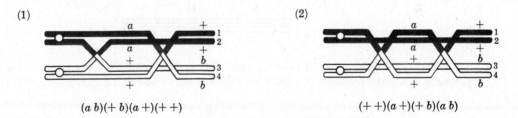

$(a\,b)(+\,b)(a\,+)(+\,+)$ $(+\,+)(a\,+)(+\,b)(a\,b)$

(1) This 4-strand double crossover can be symbolized as $(2, 3)(1, 4)$, which indicates that the first crossover involves strands 2 and 3 and the second crossover involves strands 1 and 4.

(2) This 2-strand double crossover can be symbolized $(1, 4)(1, 4)$. Note that the readings of the two spore patterns are reversed left to right, but otherwise are in the same linear order. Both of these patterns are possible for either kind of crossover depending upon the first meiotic metaphase orientation of the chromosomes.

(b) A single crossover $(2, 3)$ gives the right-to-left pattern; a single crossover $(1, 4)$ gives the left-to-right pattern).

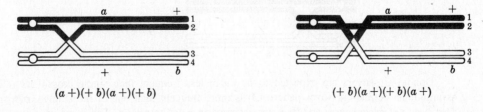

$(a\,+)(+\,b)(a\,+)(+\,b)$ $(+\,b)(a\,+)(+\,b)(a\,+)$

(c) A 3-strand double crossover (2, 3)(2, 4) gives the right-to-left spore pattern; a 3-strand double (1, 4)(2, 4) reverses the pattern.

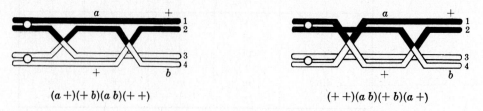

$(a +)(+ b)(a\,b)(+ +)$ $(+ +)(a\,b)(+ b)(a +)$

6.15. Two strains of *Neurospora*, one mutant for gene *a*, the other mutant for gene *b*, are crossed. Results are shown below. Determine the linkage relationships between these 2 genes.

	Percent of Asci	Spores			
		1 + 2	3 + 4	5 + 6	7 + 8
(1)	79	*a +*	*a +*	*+ b*	*+ b*
(2)	14	*a +*	*+ +*	*ab*	*+ b*
(3)	6	*a +*	*ab*	*+ +*	*+ b*
(4)	1	*a +*	*+ b*	*a +*	*+ b*

Solution:

Pattern (1) represents the noncrossover types showing first-division segregation (4 : 4) for both *a* and *b*. Pattern (2) shows second-division segregation (2 : 2 : 2 : 2) for *a*, but first-division segregation for *b*. Genes that show high frequency of second-division segregation are usually further from the centromere than genes with low frequency of second-division segregation. Judging by the relatively high frequency of pattern (2) these are probably single crossovers, and we suspect that *a* is more distal from its centromere than *b*.

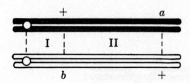

Pattern (3), indicating first-division segregation for *a* and second-division segregation for *b*, cannot be generated by a single crossover if *a* and *b* are linked as shown above, but requires a double crossover.

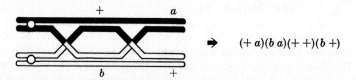 $(+ a)(b\,a)(+ +)(b +)$

Furthermore, pattern (4) could be produced from the linkage relationships as assumed above by a single crossover in region I.

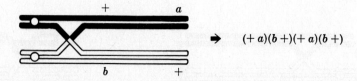 $(+ a)(b +)(+ a)(b +)$

Double crossovers are expected to be much less frequent than single crossovers. Under the above assumptions, double-crossover pattern (3) is more frequent than one of the single-crossover patterns (4). This does not make sense, and thus our assumption must be wrong. The locus of *a* must be further from the centromere than *b*, but it need not be on the same side of the centromere with *b*. Let us place *a* on the other side of the centromere.

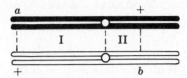

Now a single crossover in region I produces pattern (2), a single crossover in region II produces pattern (3), and a 2-strand double crossover (I, II) produces pattern (4). The percentage of asci are numerically acceptable under this assumption.

The distance *a*–centromere $= \frac{1}{2}(\text{SCO I} + \text{DCO}) = \frac{1}{2}(14 + 1) = 7.5$ map units.
The distance centromere–*b* $= \frac{1}{2}(\text{SCO II} + \text{DCO}) = \frac{1}{2}(6 + 1) = 3.5$ map units.

6.16. The cross $(abc) \times (+++)$ is made in an ascomycete with unordered tetrads. From the analysis of 100 asci, determine the linkage relationships between these 3 loci as completely as the data allow.

(1) 40 $(abc)(abc)(+++)(+++)$ (3) 10 $(a+c)(++c)(ab+)(+b+)$
(2) 42 $(ab+)(ab+)(++c)(++c)$ (4)   8 $(a++)(+++)(abc)(+bc)$

Solution:

Pattern (1) is parental ditype (PD) for *ab*, *ac*, and *bc*. Pattern (2) is PD for *ab*, nonparental ditype (NPD) for *ac* and *bc*. Pattern (3) is tetratype (TT) for *ab* and *ac*, NPD for *bc*. Pattern (4) is TT for *ab* and *ac*, PD for *bc*. For each pair of markers the relative frequencies of each type of tetrad are as follows:

	PD	NPD	TT
ab	40 42 82/100 = 0.82	0	10 8 18/100 = 0.18
ac	40/100 = 0.40	42/100 = 0.42	10 8 18/100 = 0.18
bc	40 8 48/100 = 0.48	42 10 52/100 = 0.52	0

For the *ab* pair, PDs are not equivalent with NPDs. Thus *a* and *b* must be linked. For pairs *ac* and *bc*, PDs are roughly equivalent with NPDs. Thus *c* must be assorting independently on another chromosome. The recombination frequency between *a* and *b* $= \dfrac{\text{NPD} + \frac{1}{2}\text{TT}}{\text{total number of tetrads}} = \dfrac{0 + \frac{1}{2}(18)}{100} = 9\%$ or 9 map units. Single crossovers between either *b* and its centromere or *c* and its centromere or both would produce TTs for *bc*. Since none occurred we can assume that the locus of *b* and *c* are both very near their respective centromeres.

Supplementary Problems

RECOMBINATION AMONG LINKED GENES

6.17. There is 21% crossing over between the locus of *p* and that of *c* in the rat. Suppose that 150 primary oocytes could be scored for chiasmata within this region of the chromosome. How many of these oocytes would be expected to have a chiasma between these 2 genes?

6.18. The longest chromosome in the sweet pea has a minimum uncorrected map length (based on known genetic markers) of 118 units. Cytological observations of the longest chromosome in meiotic cells revealed an average chiasmata frequency of 2.96 per tetrad. Calculate the maximum number of crossover units remaining in this chromosome for the mapping of new genes outside the range already known.

GENETIC MAPPING

6.19. The distances between 8 loci in the second chromosome of *Drosophila* are presented in the following table. Construct a genetic map to include these 8 loci. The table is symmetrical above and below the diagonal.

	d	dp	net	J	ed	ft	cl	ho
d	—	18	31	10	20	19	14.5	27
dp		—	13	28	2	1	3.5	9
net			—	41	11	12	16.5	4
J				—	30	29	24.5	37
ed					—	1	5.5	7
ft						—	4.5	8
cl							—	12.5
ho								—

6.20. The recessive gene *sh* produces shrunken endosperm in corn kernels and its dominant allele *sh*$^+$ produces full, plump kernels. The recessive gene *c* produces colorless endosperm and its dominant allele *c*$^+$ produces colored endosperm. Two homozygous plants are crossed, producing an F_1 all phenotypically plump and colored. The F_1 plants are testcrossed and produce 149 shrunken, colored : 4035 shrunken, colorless : 152 plump, colorless : 4032 plump, colored. (*a*) What were the phenotypes and genotypes of the original parents? (*b*) How are the genes linked in the F_1? (*c*) Estimate the map distance between *sh* and *c*.

6.21. The presence of one of the Rh antigens on the surface of the red blood cells (Rh-positive) in humans is produced by a dominant gene *R*, Rh-negative cells are produced by the recessive genotype *rr*. Oval-shaped erythrocytes (elliptocytosis or ovalocytosis) are caused by a dominant gene *E*, its recessive allele *e* producing normal red blood cells. Both of these genes are linked approximately 20 map units apart on one of the autosomes. A man with elliptocytosis, whose mother had normally shaped erythrocytes and a homozygous Rh-positive genotype and whose father was Rh-negative and heterozygous for elliptocytosis, marries a normal Rh-negative woman. (*a*) What is the probability of their first child being Rh-negative and elliptocytotic? (*b*) If their first child is Rh-positive, what is the chance that it will also be elliptocytotic?

6.22. The Rh genotypes, as discussed in Problem 6.21, are given for each individual in the pedigree shown below. Solid symbols represent elliptocytotic individuals. (*a*) List the *E* locus genotypes for each individual in the pedigree. (*b*) List the *gametic contribution* (for both loci) of the elliptocytotic individuals (of genotype *Rr*) beside each of their offspring in which it can be detected. (*c*) How often in part (*b*) did *R* segregate with *E* and *r* with *e*? (*d*) On the basis of random assortment, in how many of the offspring in part (*b*) would we expect to find *R* segregating with *e* or *r* with *E*? (*e*) If these genes assort independently, calculate the probability of *R* segregating with *E* and *r* with *e* in all 10 cases. (*f*) Is the solution to part (*c*) suggestive of linkage between these two loci? (*g*) Calculate part (*e*) if the siblings III1 and II2 were identical twins (developed from a single egg). (*h*) How are these genes probably linked in I1?

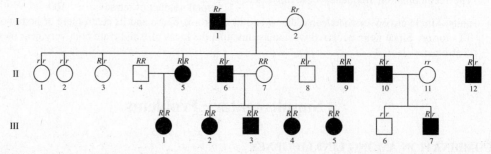

6.23. A hereditary disease called "retinitis pigmentosa" in humans causes excessive pigmentation of the retina with consequent partial or complete blindness. It is caused by a dominant incompletely sex-linked gene *R*. Afflicted individuals appear as solid symbols in the pedigree.

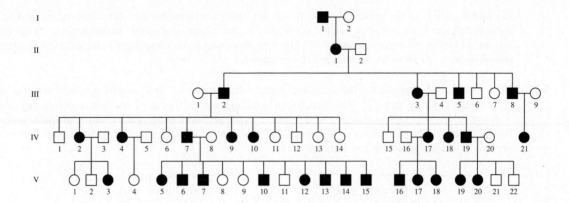

(a) Determine the genotypes, insofar as possible, for each individual in the pedigree, designating the chromosome (X or Y) in which the mutant gene probably resides in the afflicted individuals. Identify each individual that is produced by a crossover gamete. (b) Only in the gametes of afflicted males does the opportunity exist for the mutant gene to cross-over from the X to the Y chromosome. Beginning with afflicted males, wherein the location of the mutant gene is known for certain, determine the number of opportunities (progeny) for the detection of such crossovers. (c) How many crossovers were actually observed? (d) What percentage crossing over does this represent?

6.24. Two recessive genes in *Drosophila* (*b* and *vg*) produce black body and vestigial wings, respectively. When wild-type flies are testcrossed, the F_1 are all dihybrid in coupling phase. Testcrossing the female F_1 produced 1930 wild type : 1888 black and vestigial : 412 black : 370 vestigial. (a) Calculate the distance between *b* and *vg*. (b) Another recessive gene *cn* lies between the loci of *b* and *vg*, producing cinnabar eye color. When wild-type flies are testcrossed, the F_1 are all trihybrid. Testcrossing the F_1 females produced 664 wild type : 652 black, cinnabar, vestigial : 72 black, cinnabar : 68 cinnabar : 70 black : 61 cinnabar, vestigial : 4 black, vestigial : 8 cinnabar. Calculate the map distances. (c) Do the *b–vg* distances calculated in parts (a) and (b) coincide? Explain. (d) What is the coefficient of coincidence?

6.25. In corn, a dominant gene *C* produces colored aleurone; its recessive allele *c* produces colorless. Another dominant gene *Sh* produces full, plump kernels; its recessive allele *sh* produces shrunken kernels due to collapsing of the endosperm. A third dominant gene *Wx* produces normal starchy endosperm and its recessive allele *wx* produces waxy starch. A homozygous plant from a seed with colorless, plump, and waxy endosperm is crossed to a homozygous plant from a seed with colored, shrunken, and starchy endosperm. The F_1 is testcrossed to a colorless, shrunken, waxy strain. The progeny seed exhibits the following phenotypes: 113 colorless, shrunken, starchy : 4 colored, plump, starchy : 2708 colorless, plump, waxy : 626 colorless, plump, starchy : 2 colorless, shrunken, waxy : 116 colored, plump, waxy : : 2538 colored, shrunken, starchy : 601 colored, shrunken, waxy. (a) Construct a genetic map for this region of the chromosome. Round all calculations to the nearest tenth of a percent. (b) Calculate the interference in this region.

6.26. A gene called "forked" (*f*) produces shortened, bent, or split bristles and hairs in *Drosophila*. Another gene called "outstretched" (*od*) results in wings being carried at right angles to the body. A third gene called "garnet" (*g*) produces pinkish eye color in young flies. Wild-type females heterozygous at all three loci were crossed to wild-type males. The F_1 data appear below.

F_1: Females:	all wild type
Males:	57 garnet, outstretched
	419 garnet, forked
	60 forked
	1 outstretched, forked
	2 garnet
	439 outstretched
	13 wild type
	9 outstretched, garnet, forked
	1000

(*a*) Which gene is in the middle? (*b*) What was the linkage relationship between alleles at the forked and outstretched loci in the maternal parent? (*c*) What was the linkage relationship between alleles at the forked and garnet loci in the maternal parent? (*d*) On what chromosome do these 3 genes reside? (*e*) Calculate the map distances. (*f*) How much interference is operative?

6.27. Maize plants homozygous for the recessive gene "variable sterile" (*va*) exhibit irregular distribution of chromosomes during meiosis. Yellowish-green seedlings are the result of another recessive gene called "virescent" (*v*). A third recessive called "glossy" (*gl*) produces shiny leaves. All 3 of these genes are linked. Two homozygous plants were crossed and produced an all normal F_1. When the F_1 was testcrossed, progeny phenotypes appeared as follows:

60 virescent	4 variable sterile, virescent
48 virescent, glossy	40 variable sterile
7 glossy	62 variable sterile, glossy
270 variable sterile, virescent, glossy	235 wild type

(*a*) What were the genotypes and phenotypes of the original parents? (*b*) Diagram the linkage relationships in the F_1. (*c*) Determine the gene order. (*d*) Calculate the amount of recombination observed. (*e*) How much interference is operative?

6.28. Five sex-linked recessive genes of *Drosophila* (*ec, sc, v, cv,* and *ct*) produce traits called echinus, scute, vermilion, crossveinless, and cut, respectively. Echinus is a mutant producing rough eyes with large facets. Scute manifests itself by the absence or reduction in the number of bristles on certain parts of the body. Vermilion is a bright orange-red eye color. Crossveinless prevents the development of supporting structures in the wings. Cut produces scalloped and pointed wings with manifold (pleiotropic) effects in other parts of the body. At the beginning of our experiments we do not know the gene order. From the results of the following three experiments, construct a genetic map for this region of the X chromosome. Whenever possible use weighted averages.

Experiment 1. Echinus females crossed to scute, crossveinless males produced all wild-type females and all echinus males in the F_1. When the F_1 females were testcrossed, the results (including both male and female progeny) were as follows:

810 echinus	89 scute
828 scute, crossveinless	62 echinus, scute
88 crossveinless	103 echinus, crossveinless

Experiment 2. Crossveinless females crossed to echinus, cut males produced all wild-type females and all crossveinless males in the F_1. When the F_1 females were testcrossed, the results (including both male and female progeny) were as follows:

2207 crossveinless	223 crossveinless, cut
2125 echinus, cut	217 echinus
273 echinus, crossveinless	5 wild type
265 cut	3 echinus, crossveinless, cut

Experiment 3. Cut females crossed to vermilion, crossveinless males produced all wild-type females and cut males in the F_1. When the F_1 females were testcrossed, the results (including both male and female progeny) were as follows:

766 vermilion, crossveinless	73 vermilion
759 cut	85 crossveinless, cut
140 vermilion, cut	2 wild type
158 crossveinless	2 vermilion, crossveinless, cut

LINKAGE ESTIMATES FROM F_2 DATA

6.29. Two recessive sex-linked genes are known in chickens (ZW method of sex determination), rapid feathering (*sl*) and gold plumage (*s*). The dominant alleles produce slow feathering (*Sl*) and silver plumage (*S*), respectively. Females of the Silver Penciled Rock breed, with slow feathering and silver plumage, are crossed to males of the Brown Leghorn breed, with rapid feathering and gold plumage. The F_2 progeny data appear below:

	Slow, silver	Rapid, silver	Slow, gold	Rapid, gold
Males	94	40	7	127
Females	117	28	7	156

(a) Determine the F_1 genotypes and phenotypes. (b) In what linkage phase are the F_1 males? (c) Calculate the amount of recombination expected to occur between these two loci in males.

6.30. Assume the genotype AB/AB is testcrossed and produces an F_2 consisting of 37 A-B-, 11 A-bb, 12 aaB-, and 4 aabb. Estimate the percentage recombination between A and B by the square-root method?

6.31. Two recessive genes in the third linkage group of corn produce crinkly leaves and dwarf plants, respectively. A pure crinkly plant is pollinated by a pure dwarf plant. The F_2 progeny consist of 104 normal : 43 dwarf : 51 crinkly : 2 dwarf, crinkly. Using the square-root method, estimate the amount of recombination between these two loci.

6.32. Colored kernel is dominant to colorless in corn; full kernel is dominant to shrunken. A pure-colored, full variety is crossed to a colorless, shrunken variety. In the F_2 there was 73% colored, full : 2% colored, shrunken : 2% colorless, full : 23% colorless, shrunken. Estimate, by the square-root method, the crossover percentage between these 2 genes.

6.33. Several sex-linked genes in chickens are known, among which are the S locus governing plumage color, the K locus controlling the rate of feather development, and the Id locus, which determines whether melanin pigment can develop in the dermis. F_2 data are shown below, where X and Y represent dominant phenotypes and x and y represent recessive phenotypes.

	Coupling				Repulsion			
	XY	*Xy*	*xY*	*xy*	*XY*	*Xy*	*xY*	*xy*
S and *Id*	157	171	145	177	83	108	91	75
K and *S*	603	94	159	648	12	24	26	9

Using the product-ratio method, estimate the amount of recombination between S and Id and between K and S using a weighted average of the estimates derived from coupling and repulsion data.

6.34. The results of selfing dihybrid sweet peas have been reported by several investigators. Let us consider five loci on the "D" chromosome":

$$D_1, d_1 = \text{tendril vs. acacia leaves}$$
$$D_2, d_2 = \text{bright vs. dull flower color}$$
$$D_3, d_3 = \text{presence vs. absence of flake modifier}$$
$$D_4, d_4 = \text{hairy vs. glabrous (smooth)}$$
$$D_5, d_5 = \text{full vs. picotee flower pattern}$$

Ten experiments were carried through the F_2 generation with the following results (let X and Y represent dominant phenotypes and x and y represent recessive phenotypes):

		Coupling Series				Repulsion Series			
		XY	Xy	xY	xy	XY	Xy	xY	xy
(1)	D_1D_2	634	192	163	101	2263	809	882	124
(2)	D_1D_3	286	11	19	79	—	—	—	—
(3)	D_1D_4	3217	790	784	544	692	278	300	58
(4)	D_1D_5	—	—	—	—	3112	1126	1114	277
(5)	D_2D_3	992	273	265	124	296	97	88	20
(6)	D_2D_4	1580	482	421	148	1844	592	603	171
(7)	D_2D_5	1438	443	424	162	1337	465	415	128
(8)	D_3D_4	200	52	44	35	—	—	—	—
(9)	D_3D_5	373	112	103	42	—	—	—	—
(10)	D_4D_5	1076	298	283	188	2537	1003	993	131

(*a*) Using the product-ratio method (Table 6.1) determine the crossover values for each experiment accurate to two decimal places. (*b*) Where the estimates are available in both coupling and repulsion, take a weighted average of the two and express all 10 crossover values to two decimal places on the same map. (*c*) The distance calculated from experiments (D_1D_2) plus (D_1D_3) is not the same as the distance from the experiment involving (D_2D_3). Why? (*d*) What is the total map distance represented by the map in part (*b*)? (*e*) To what average chiasma frequency does the answer to part (*d*) correspond?

6.35. The duplicate recessive genes (r_1 and r_2) produce a short, velvetlike fur called "rex." Two rex rabbits of different homozygous genotypes were mated and produced an F_1 that was then testcrossed to produce 64 rex and 6 normal testcross progeny. (*a*) Assuming independent assortment, how many normal and rex phenotypes would be expected among 70 progeny? (*b*) Do the data indicate linkage? (*c*) What is the genotype and the phenotype of the F_1? (*d*) What is the genotype and phenotype of the testcross individuals? (*e*) Calculate the map distance.

6.36. A dominant gene C is necessary for any pigment to be developed in rabbits. Its recessive allele c produces albino. Black pigment is produced by another dominant gene B and brown pigment by its recessive allele b. The C locus exhibits recessive epistasis over the B locus. Homozygous brown rabbits mated to albinos of genotype $ccBB$ produce an F_1 which is then testcrossed to produce the F_2. Among the F_2 progeny were found 17 black, 33 brown, and 50 albino. (*a*) Assuming independent assortment, what F_2 ratio is expected? (*b*) Do the F_2 results approximate the expectations in part (*a*)? (*c*) What are the genotypes and phenotypes of the F_1? (*d*) What are the genotypes and phenotypes of the testcross individuals? (*e*) Estimate the map distance between these 2 genes.

USE OF GENETIC MAPS

6.37. Two loci are known to be in linkage group IV of the rat. Kinky hairs in the coat and vibrissae (long nose "whiskers") are produced in response to the recessive genotype kk and a short, stubby tail is produced by the recessive genotype st/st. The dominant alleles at these loci produce normal hairs and tails, respectively. Given 30 map units between the loci of k and st, determine the expected F_1 phenotypic proportions from heterozygous parents that are (*a*) both in coupling phase, (*b*) both in repulsion phase, (*c*) one in coupling and the other in repulsion phase.

6.38. In mice, the genes frizzy (*fr*) and albino (*c*) are linked on chromosome 1 at a distance of 20 map units. Dihybrid wild-type females in repulsion phase are mated to dihybrid wild-type males in coupling phase. Predict the offspring phenotypic expectations.

6.39. Deep-yellow hemolymph (blood) in silkworm larvae is the result of a dominant gene Y at locus 25.6 (i.e., 25.6 crossover units from the end of the chromosome). Another dominant mutation Rc, 6.2 map units from the Y locus, produces a yellowish-brown cocoon (rusty). Between these two loci is a recessive mutant oa governing mottled translucency in the larval skin, mapping at locus 26.7. Rc and oa are separated by 5.1 crossover units. An individual that is homozygous for yellow blood, mottled translucent larval skin, and wild-type cocoon color is crossed to an individual of genotype $Y^+ \ oa^+ \ Rc/Y^+ \ oa^+ \ RC$ that spins a rusty cocoon. The F_1 males are then testcrossed to produce 3000 F_2 progeny. Coincidence is assumed to be 10%. (a) Predict the numbers within each phenotypic class that will appear in the F_2 (to the nearest whole numbers). (b) On the basis of probabilities, how many *more* F_2 progeny would need to be produced in order to recover one each of the DCO phenotypes?

6.40. The eyes of certain mutant *Drosophila* have a rough texture due to abnormal facet structure. Three of the mutants that produce approximately the same phenotype (mimics) are sex-linked recessives: roughest (*rst*), rugose (*rg*), and roughex (*rux*). The loci of these genes in terms of their distances from the end of the X chromosome are 2, 11, and 15 map units, respectively. (a) From testcrossing wild-type females of genotype $\dfrac{rst + rux}{+ \; rg \; +}$, predict the number of wild-type and rough-eyed flies expected among 20,000 progeny. Assume no interference. (b) Approximately how many rough-eyed progeny flies are expected for every wild-type individual? (c) If the females of part (a) were of genotype $\dfrac{rst \; rg \; rux}{+ \; + \; +}$, what would be the approximate ratio of wild-type : rough-eyed progeny?

6.41. In Asiatic cotton, a pair of factors (*R* and *r*) controls the presence or absence, respectively, of anthocyanin pigmentation. Another gene, about 10 map units away from the *R* locus, controls chlorophyll production. The homozygous recessive genotype at this locus (*yy*) produces a yellow (chlorophyll deficient) plant that dies early in the seedling stage. The heterozygote *Yy* is phenotypically green and indistinguishable from the dominant homozygote *YY*. Obviously, testcrosses are not possible for the *Y* locus. When dihybrids are crossed together, calculate the expected phenotypic proportions among the seedlings and among the mature F_1 when parents are (a) both in coupling phase, (b) both in repulsion phase, (c) one in coupling and one in repulsion position. (d) Which method [in parts (a), (b) or (c)] is expected to produce the greatest mortality?

6.42. The "agouti" hair pattern, commonly found in many wild animals, is characterized by a small band of light pigment near the tip of the hair. In the rabbit, the agouti locus has a dominant allele *A* that puts the narrow band of light pigment on the hair (agouti pattern). Its recessive allele *a* results in nonagouti (black coat). Approximately 28 map units from the agouti locus is a gene that regulates the size of the agouti band; wide-banded agouti are produced by the recessive allele *w* and normal (narrow) agouti band by the dominant allele *W*. Midway between these two loci is a third locus controlling body size. The dominant allele at this locus (*Dw*) produces normal growth, but the recessive allele *dw* produces a dwarf that dies shortly after birth. Assume the genotype of a group of trihybrid females has the *A* and *Dw* loci in coupling, and the *A* and *W* loci in repulsion. These females are mated to a group of wide-banded agouti males of genotype *A dw w/a Dw w*. (a) Predict the phenotypic percentages (to the nearest decimal) expected in the F_1 at birth. (b) How much genetic death loss is anticipated? (c) Predict the phenotypic percentages expected in the F_1 when mature.

CROSSOVER SUPPRESSION

6.43. A black-bodied *Drosophila* is produced by a recessive gene *b* and vestigial wings by another recessive gene *vg* on the same chromosome. These 2 loci are approximately 20 map units apart. Predict the progeny phenotypic expectations from (a) the mating of repulsion phase females × coupling phase males, (b) the reciprocal cross of part (a), (c) the mating where both parents are in repulsion phase.

6.44. Poorly developed mucous glands in the female silkworm *Bombyx mori* cause eggs to be easily separated from the papers on which they are laid. This is a dominant genetic condition; its wild-type recessive allele Ng^+ produces normally "glued" eggs. Another dominant gene *C*, 14 map units from *Ng*, produces a golden-yellow color on the outside of the cocoon and nearly white inside. Its recessive wild-type allele C^+ produces normally pigmented or wild-type cocoon color. A pure "glueless" strain is crossed to a pure golden strain. The F_1 females are then mated to their brothers to produce the F_2. Predict the number of individuals of different phenotypes expected to be observed in a total of 500 F_2 offspring. *Hint.* Crossing over does not occur in female silkworms.

6.45. Two autosomal recessive genes, "dumpy" (*dp*, a reduction in wing size) and "net" (*net*, extra veins in the wing), are linked on chromosome 2 of *Drosophila*. Homozygous wild-type females are crossed to net, dumpy males. Among 800 F_2 offspring were found: 574 wild type : 174 net, dumpy : 25 dumpy : 27 net. Estimate the map distance.

6.46. Suppose that an abnormal genetic trait (mutation) appeared suddenly in a female of a pure culture of *Drosophila melanogaster*. We mate the mutant female to a male from a balanced lethal strain [*Cy/Pm*, *D/Sb*, where curly (*Cy*) and plum (*Pm*) are on chromosome 2 and dichaete (*D*) and stubble (*Sb*) are on chromosome 3]. About half of the F$_1$ progeny (both males and females) exhibit the mutant phenotype. The F$_1$ mutant males with curly wings and stubble bristles are then mated to unrelated virgin wild-type females. In the F$_2$ the mutant trait never appears with stubble. Recall that this species of *Drosophila* has chromosomes X, 2, 3, and 4. Could the mutation be (*a*) an autosomal recessive, (*b*) a sex-linked recessive, (*c*) an autosomal dominant, (*d*) a sex-linked dominant? (*e*) In which chromosome does the mutant gene reside? (*f*) Suppose the mutant trait in the F$_2$ appeared in equal association with curly and stubble. In which chromosome would the mutant gene reside? (*g*) Suppose the mutant trait in the F$_2$ appeared only in females. In which chromosome would the mutant gene reside? (*h*) Suppose the mutant trait in the F$_2$ never appeared with curly. In which chromosome would the mutant gene reside?

RECOMBINATION MAPPING WITH TETRADS

6.47. Given the adjoining meiotic metaphase orientation in *Neurospora*, determine the simplest explanation to account for the following spore patterns. *Hint.* See Problem 6.14.

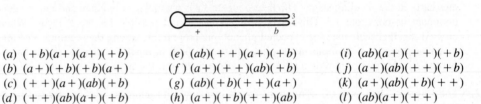

(*a*) (*+b*)(*a+*)(*a+*)(*+b*)	(*e*) (*ab*)(*++*)(*a+*)(*+b*)	(*i*) (*ab*)(*a+*)(*++*)(*+b*)
(*b*) (*a+*)(*+b*)(*+b*)(*a+*)	(*f*) (*a+*)(*++*)(*ab*)(*+b*)	(*j*) (*a+*)(*ab*)(*++*)(*+b*)
(*c*) (*++*)(*a+*)(*ab*)(*+b*)	(*g*) (*ab*)(*+b*)(*++*)(*a+*)	(*k*) (*a+*)(*ab*)(*+b*)(*++*)
(*d*) (*++*)(*ab*)(*a+*)(*+b*)	(*h*) (*a+*)(*+b*)(*++*)(*ab*)	(*l*) (*ab*)(*a+*)(*++*)

6.48. A certain strain of *Neurospora* cannot grow unless adenine is in the culture medium. Adenineless is a recessive mutation (*ad*). Another strain produces yellow conidia (*ylo*). Below are shown the results from crossing these 2 strains. Calculate the map distance between these 2 genes.

No. of Asci	Meiotic Products
106	(*ad+*)(*ad+*)(*+ylo*)(*+ylo*)
14	(*ad+*)(*ad ylo*)(*++*)(*+ylo*)

6.49. A strain of *Neurospora*, unable to synthesize the vitamin thiamine (*t*), is crossed to a strain unable to synthesize the amino acid arginine (*a*).

No. of Asci	Ascospores			
	Pair 1	Pair 2	Pair 3	Pair 4
37	*+ +*	*+ +*	*at*	*at*
33	*+t*	*+t*	*a+*	*a+*
34	*at*	*at*	*+ +*	*+ +*
36	*a+*	*a+*	*+t*	*+t*

What information can be gleaned from these results for use in mapping these two loci?

6.50. Two strains of *Neurospora*, one mutant for gene *x* and the other for gene *y*, were crossed with results as shown below. Determine the gene order and calculate the map distance of each gene from its centromere.

No. of Asci	Meiotic Products
52	(*+y*)(*+y*)(*x+*)(*x+*)
2	(*+ +*)(*xy*)(*+y*)(*x+*)
17	(*x+*)(*+y*)(*x+*)(*+y*)
1	(*xy*)(*x+*)(*+ +*)(*+y*)
6	(*+y*)(*xy*)(*+ +*)(*x+*)
1	(*+y*)(*x+*)(*+ +*)(*xy*)
15	(*x+*)(*+y*)(*+y*)(*x+*)
1	(*+ +*)(*+y*)(*xy*)(*x+*)
5	(*xy*)(*+y*)(*+ +*)(*x+*)

6.51. A riboflavineless strain (r) of *Neurospora* is crossed with a tryptophaneless strain (t) to give

No. of Asci	Meiotic Products	No. of Asci	Meiotic Products
129	$(r+)(r+)(+t)(+t)$	13	$(rt)(r+)(+t)(++)$
1	$(+t)(r+)(r+)(+t)$	17	$(r+)(rt)(++)(+t)$
2	$(r+)(+t)(r+)(+t)$	17	$(r+)(rt)(+t)(++)$
1	$(r+)(+t)(+t)(r+)$	2	$(r+)(++)(rt)(+t)$
15	$(rt)(r+)(++)(+t)$	1	$(rt)(++)(r+)(+t)$

Construct a map that includes these 2 genes.

6.52. Two of the genes *s*, *t*, and *u* are linked; the third assorts independently and is very tightly linked to its centromere. Analyze the unordered tetrads produced by the cross $(stu) \times (+++)$. *Hint:* See Problem 6.16.

No. of Tetrads	Tetrads
59	$(stu)(stu)(+++)(+++)$
53	$(s+u)(s+u)(+t+)(+t+)$
26	$(st+)(+t+)(s+u)(++u)$
30	$(s++)(+++)(stu)(+tu)$
32	$(stu)(+t+)(s+u)(+++)$

Review Questions

Vocabulary   For each of the following definitions, give the appropriate term and spell it correctly. Terms are single words unless indicated otherwise.

1. Adjective applicable to 2 or more human genes inferred to be linked on the same chromosome from somatic cell hybridization experiments.

2. A cross-shaped cytological structure that is observed in paired homologous chromosomes during first meiotic prophase, and that is formed by the reciprocal breaking and rejoining of nonsister chromatids.

3. The genetic event that recombines linked genes. (Two words.)

4. The linkage arrangement in a dihybrid in which the 2 dominant genes are on one chromosome and their corresponding recessive alleles are on the homologous chromosome. (Two words.)

5. The linkage arrangement in a dihybrid in which, on each chromosome of a homologous pair, there is one dominant and one recessive gene. (Two words.)

6. A unit of map distance equivalent to 1% crossing over.

7. The ratio of the double-crossover progeny observed in a three-point testcross relative to the double-crossover progeny expected on the basis of treating map units as if they were independent variables. (One to three words.)

8. The complement of the coefficient of coincidence.

9. A genetic system that can maintain dihybrid genotypes in repulsion phase generation after generation. (Two words.)

10. Investigation of the products of a given meiotic event in ascomycete fungi. (Two words.)

True-False Questions   Answer each of the following questions either true (T) or false (F).

1.   Evidence that genes are linked is most effectively derived from intercrossing dihybrids.

2.   Each chiasma is equivalent to 1% crossing over.

3.   In a dihybrid testcross, progeny produced by 2-strand double crossovers will be indistinguishable from non-crossovers.

4.   The limit of recombination is 50%.

5.   If gene loci A and B are 15 map units apart (x physical units) and if B and C loci are also 15 map units apart, then B and C must also be x physical units apart.

6.   The larger the coincidence, the smaller the interference.

7.   Linkage distance estimates derived from F_2 data depend entirely on the percentage of one phenotypic class in the progeny.

8.   In *Drosophila*, crossing over occurs only in females.

9.   In lines of human–rodent somatic cell hybrids, rodent chromosomes are usually lost faster than human chromosomes.

10.   Conidia are the sexual spores of an ascomycete.

Multiple-Choice Questions   Choose the one best answer.

1.   If a chiasma forms between the loci of genes *A* and *B* in 20% of the tetrads of an individual of genotype *AB/ab*, the percentage of gametes expected to be *Ab* is   (*a*) 40   (*b*) 20   (*c*) 10   (*d*) 5   (*e*) none of the above

2.   The average number of chiasmata that forms in one pair of homologous chromosomes is 1.2. The total length (in map units) for this linkage group is expected to be   (*a*) 120   (*b*) 60   (*c*) 50   (*d*) 30   (*e*) none of the above

For questions 3–7, use the following information. The distances A–B = 15 map units, B–C = 8 map units, and A–C = 23 map units.

3.   In an individual of genotype *AbC/aBc*, the percentage of gametes expected to be *ABC* is   (*a*) 23   (*b*) 11.5   (*c*) 5.75   (*d*) 0.6   (*e*) none of the above

4.   In the cross *Abc/abC* × *abc/abc*, the percentage of *Abc/abc* progeny expected is   (*a*) 39.7   (*b*) 23.4   (*c*) 77.1   (*d*) 48.6   (*e*) none of the above

5.   If from the cross *ABC/abc* × *abc/abc* we observe among 1000 progeny one *AbC/abc* and one *aBc/abc*, then the coefficient of coincidence is estimated to be approximately (within rounding error)   (*a*) 0.054   (*b*) 0.167   (*c*) 0.296   (*d*) 0.333   (*e*) none of the above

6.   The percentage of progeny expected to be *ABC/abc* from the cross *AbC/aBc* × *abc/abc* is   (*a*) 15.0   (*b*) 7.5   (*c*) 6.9   (*d*) 23.0   (*e*) 18.7

7.   If the B–C distance of 8 map units is a weighted average of two experiments (experiment 1 = 7.3 map units based on a sample size of 100; experiment 2 = 8.4 map units), the sample size of experiment 2 was approximately   (*a*) 116   (*b*) 144   (*c*) 167   (*d*) 175   (*e*) 190

8. From the cross $AB/ab \times AB/ab$ we observe 9% of the progeny to be ab/ab. The estimate of the recombination percentage between these two loci is   (*a*) 50   (*b*) 40   (*c*) 35   (*d*) 20   (*e*) none of the above

The following information applies to questions 9 and 10. A trihybrid testcross (order of loci unknown) produced 35 *AbC/abc*, 37 *aBc/abc*, 8 *ABc/abc*, 10 *abC/abc*, 3 *ABC/abc*, 5 *abc/abc*, 1 *Abc/abc*, 1 *aBC/abc*.

9. The gene order   (*a*) is CBA   (*b*) is BAC   (*c*) is BCA   (*d*) cannot be determined from the information provided   (*e*) is none of the above

10. The distance (in map units) between the A and C loci is estimated to be   (*a*) 30   (*b*) 25   (*c*) 20   (*d*) 15   (*e*) none of the above

Answers to Supplementary Problems

6.17.   63

6.18.   30 units

6.19. $net \overset{4}{\rule{1cm}{0.4pt}} ho \overset{7}{\rule{1cm}{0.4pt}} ed^1 ft^1 dp \overset{3.5}{\rule{1cm}{0.4pt}} cl \overset{14.5}{\rule{1.5cm}{0.4pt}} d \overset{10}{\rule{1cm}{0.4pt}} J$

6.20.   (*a*) $sh\ c/sh\ c$ (shrunken, colorless) $\times sh^+\ c^+/sh^+\ c^+$ (plump, colored)   (*c*) 3.6 map units
     (*b*) $sh^+\ c^+/sh\ c$ (coupling phase)

6.21.   (*a*) $\frac{2}{5}$ (*b*) $\frac{1}{5}$

6.22.   (*a*) All open symbols $= ee$, all solid symbols $= Ee$ (*b*) re (III1, II2, III6), RE (II5, 9, III2–5, 7)   (*c*) All 10 cases   (*d*) 5 each   (*e*) $\frac{1}{1024}$ (*f*) Yes   (*g*) $\frac{1}{512}$ (*h*) RE/re (coupling phase)

6.23.   (*a*) all open symbols rr; all afflicted individuals Rr; location of mutant gene is on X chromosome in II1, III2, 3, 5, 8, IV2, 4, 9, 10, 17, 18, 19, 21, V3, 5, 12, 16, 17, 18, 19, 20; location of mutant gene is on Y chromosome in IV7, V6, 7, 10, 13, 14, 15; crossover individuals are IV6, 7, 11, 13, 14, V5, 11, 12; location of mutant gene in I1 is unknown   (*b*) 27 opportunities; they are IV1, 2, 4, 6, 7, 9–14, 21, V5–15, 19–22   (*c*) 8   (*d*) 29.63%

6.24.   (*a*) 17 map units   (*b*) $b\text{-}cn = 8.9$ map units; $cn\text{-}vg = 9.5$ map units   (*c*) No.   In part (*a*), 2-point testcross cannot detect double crossovers that then appear as parental types, thus underestimating the true map distance. (*d*) 0.89

6.25.   (*a*) $c \overset{3.5}{\rule{1cm}{0.4pt}} sh \overset{18.4}{\rule{3cm}{0.4pt}} wx$ (*b*) 86.1%

6.26.   (*a*) f (*b*) Repulsion phase   (*c*) Coupling phase   (*d*) X chromosome (sex-linked)   (*e*) $g\text{-}f = 12.0$, $f\text{-}od = 2.5$ (*f*) None

6.27.   (*a*) $va^+\ gl^+\ v^+/va^+\ gl^+\ v^+$ (wild type) $\times va\ gl\ v/\ va\ gl\ v$ (variable sterile, glossy, virescent)   (*b*) $va^+\ gl^+\ v^+/va\ gl\ v$ (*c*) gl is in the middle   (*d*) $va\text{-}gl = 13.6\%$, $gl\text{-}v = 18.3\%$ (*e*) 39%

6.28.

Experiment 1:	sc	$\overset{7.6}{\rule{2cm}{0.4pt}}$	ec	$\overset{9.7}{\rule{2cm}{0.4pt}}$	cv			
Experiment 2:	ec	$\overset{10.3}{\rule{2cm}{0.4pt}}$	cv	$\overset{8.4}{\rule{2cm}{0.4pt}}$	ct			
Experiment 3:	cv	$\overset{8.2}{\rule{2cm}{0.4pt}}$	ct	$\overset{15.2}{\rule{2cm}{0.4pt}}$	v			
Combined Map:	sc	$\overset{7.6}{\rule{1.5cm}{0.4pt}}$	ec	$\overset{10.1}{\rule{1.5cm}{0.4pt}}$	cv	$\overset{8.3}{\rule{1.5cm}{0.4pt}}$ ct	$\overset{15.2}{\rule{1.5cm}{0.4pt}}$	v

6.29. (*a*) *Sl S/sl s* (slow, silver males) × *sl s*/W (rapid, gold females)   (*b*) Coupling phase   (*c*) 14.2%

6.30. 50%

6.31. 20%

6.32. 4%

6.33.

Genes	Coupling	Repulsion	Weighted Average
S and *Id*	0.48	0.44	0.47
K and *S*	0.15	0.27	0.16

6.34. (*a*)

Genes	D_1D_2	D_1D_3	D_1D_4	D_1D_5	D_2D_3	D_2D_4	D_2D_5	D_3D_4	D_3D_5	D_4D_5
Coupling	0.40	0.08	0.36	—	0.42	0.48	0.47	0.35	0.46	0.38
Repulsion	0.37	—	0.40	0.45	0.45	0.48	0.48	—	—	0.35

(*b*)

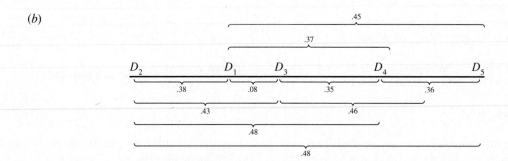

(*c*) (1) Undetected double crossovers underestimate the true distance in the D_2D_3 experiment. (2) Sampling error in different experiments yields slightly different estimates of the true values. (*d*) 117 map units (*e*) 2.34 chiasmata per tetrad

6.35. (*a*) 52.5 rex : 17.5 normal   (*b*) Yes   (*c*) R_1r_2/r_1R_2, normal   (*d*) r_1r_2/r_1r_2, rex   (*e*) 17.14 map units

6.36. (*a*) 2 albino : 1 black : 1 brown   (*b*) No   (*c*) *Cb/cB*, black   (*d*) *cb/cb*, albino   (*e*) 34 map units

6.37.

Phenotype	(*a*)	(*b*)	(*c*)
Normal	0.6225	0.5225	0.5525
Kinky hair	0.1275	0.2275	0.1975
Stub tail	0.1275	0.2275	0.1975
Kinky hair, stub tail	0.1225	0.0225	0.0525

6.38. 54% wild type : 21% frizzy : 21% albino : 4% frizzy, albino

6.39. (*a*) 1408 yellow, mottled : 1408 rusty : 16 yellow, rusty : 16 mottled : 76 yellow, mottled, rusty : 76 wild type. Note: Rounding errors may allow one whole individual difference in each of these phenotypic classes. (*b*) 32,651

6.40. (*a*) 19,964 rough-eyed : 36 wild type   (*b*) Approximately 1 : 555   (*c*) Approximately 1 : 1.289

6.41. $(a)(b)(c)$

	Seedlings			Adult		
	(a)	(b)	(c)	(a)	(b)	(c)
Normal chlorophyll, anthocyanin present	0.7025	0.5025	0.5225	0.9367	0.6700	0.6967
Normal chlorophyll, anthocyanin absent	0.0475	0.2475	0.2275	0.0633	0.3300	0.3033
Yellow, anthocyanin present	0.0475	0.2475	0.2275			
Yellow, anthocyanin absent	0.2025	0.0025	0.0225			

(d) All three crosses = 25% mortality.

6.42. (a) 40.9% wide agouti : 22.0% black : 18.9% narrow agouti, dwarf : 12.1% narrow agouti : 3.1% wide agouti, dwarf : 3.0% black, dwarf (b) 25% (c) 54.5% wide agouti : 29.3% black : 16.1% narrow agouti

6.43. (a) 55% wild type : 20% black : 20% vestigial : 5% black, vestigial
(b), (c) 50% wild type : 25% black : 25% vestigial

6.44. 250 glueless, golden : 125 glueless : 125 golden

6.45. 13 map units

6.46. A dominant trait may appear suddenly in a population by mutation of a recessive wild-type gene to a dominant allelic form. Such a mutant individual would be heterozygous. (a) No (b) No (c) Yes (d) No (e) Chromosome 3 (f) Chromosome 4 (g) X chromosome (sex-linked) (h) Chromosome 2

6.47. (a) (1, 3) (b) (2,4) (c) (1, 3)(1, 3) or (1, 3)(2, 4) (d) (1, 3)(2, 3) or (1, 3)(1, 4) (e) (2, 3)(1, 3) or (1, 4)(1, 3) (f) (2, 3)(2, 3) or (1, 4)(2, 3) (g) (2, 4)(1, 3) or (2, 4)(2, 4) (h) (2, 4)(2, 3) or (2, 4)(1, 4) (i) (1, 3) (j) (2, 3) (k) (2, 4) (l) (1, 4)

6.48. 5.83 map units

6.49. Gene a is segregating independently of t, and both loci are closely linked to their respective centromeres.

6.50. Centromere to y = 18.5 map units; centromere to x = 26.5 map units

6.51.

6.52. Genes u and s are linked on the same side of the centromere with u closest to the centromere. Centromere to u = 16 units, u to s = 14 units. Gene t is on another chromosome and very closely linked to its centromere.

Answers to Review Questions

Vocabulary

1. syntenic
2. chiasma
3. crossing over
4. coupling phase
5. repulsion phase
6. centimorgan
7. coincidence, coincidence coefficient, or coefficient of coincidence
8. interference
9. balanced lethals
10. tetrad analysis

True-False Questions

1. F (testcrossing dihybrids)   2. F (50% crossing over)   3. T   4. T   5. F (crossover distances are not always equal to physical distances; equal lengths of chromosome may experience different amounts of crossing over)   6. T   7. T   8. T   9. F (only human chromosomes are normally lost)   10. F (ascospores)

Multiple-Choice Questions

1. *d*   2. *b*   3. *d*   4. *a*   5. *b*   6. *c*   7. *d*   8. *b*   9. *c*   10. *c*

Chapter 7

Statistical Distributions

THE BINOMIAL EXPANSION

In $(p + q)^n$, the p and q represent the probabilities of alternative independent events, and the power n to which the binomial is raised represents the number of trials. The sum of the factors in the binomial must add to unity; thus

$$p + q = 1$$

Recall from Chapter 2 that when two independent events are occurring with the probabilities p and q, then the probability of their joint occurrence is pq. That is, the combined probability is the product of the independent events. When alternative possibilities exist for the satisfaction of the conditions of the problem, the probabilities are combined by addition.

Example 7.1. In two tosses of a coin, with p = heads = $\frac{1}{2}$ and q = tails = $\frac{1}{2}$, there are four possibilities.

First Toss		Second Toss		Probability
Heads (p)	(and)	Heads (p)	=	p^2
Heads (p)	(and)	Tails (q)	=	pq
Tails (q)	(and)	Heads (p)	=	pq
Tails (q)	(and)	Tails (q)	=	q^2
				1.0

which may be expressed as follows:

$$p^2 \quad + \quad 2pq \quad + \quad q^2 \quad = \quad 1.0$$
$$\text{(2 heads)} \quad \text{(1 head : 1 tail)} \quad \text{(2 tails)}$$

Example 7.2. Expanding the binomial $(p + q)^2$ produces the same expression as in the previous example. Thus $(p + q)^2 = p^2 + 2pq + q^2$.

Example 7.3. When a coin is tossed 3 times, the probabilities for any combination of heads and/or tails can be found from $(p + q)^3 = p^3 + 3p^2q + 3pq^2 + q^3$.
Let p = probability of heads = $\frac{1}{2}$ and q = probability of tails = $\frac{1}{2}$.

No. of Heads	No. of Tails	Term	Probability
3	0	p^3	$(\frac{1}{2})^3 = \frac{1}{8}$
2	1	$3p^2q$	$3(\frac{1}{2})^2(\frac{1}{2}) = \frac{3}{8}$
1	2	$3pq^2$	$3(\frac{1}{2})(\frac{1}{2})^2 = \frac{3}{8}$
0	3	q^3	$(\frac{1}{2})^3 = \frac{1}{8}$

The expansion of $(p + q)^3$ is found by multiplying $(p^2 + 2pq + q^2)$ by $(p + q)$. This process can be extended for higher powers, but obviously becomes increasingly laborious. A short method for expanding $(p + q)$ to any power (n) may be performed by following these rules. (1) The coefficient of the first term is 1. The power of the first factor (p) is n, and that of (q) is 0. (*Note:* Any factor to the zero power is unity.) (2) Thereafter in each term, multiply the coefficient by the power of p and divide by the number of that term in the expansion. The result is the coefficient of the *next* term. (3) Also thereafter, the power of p will decrease by one and the power of q will increase by one in each term of the expansion. (4) The fully expanded binomial will have $(n + 1)$ terms. The coefficients are symmetrical about the middle term(s) of the expansion.

Summary:

Term	Coefficient	Powers	
		p	q
1	1	n	0
2	$n(1)/1$	$n - 1$	1
3	$n(n - 1)/1 \cdot 2$	$n - 2$	2
4	$n(n - 1)(n - 2)/1 \cdot 2 \cdot 3$	$n - 3$	3
.	.	.	.
.	.	.	.
.	.	.	.
$n + 1$	1	0	n

1. Single Terms of the Expansion.

The coefficients of the binomial expansion represent the number of ways in which the conditions of each term may be satisfied. The number of combinations (C) of n different things taken k at a time is expressed by

$$_nC_k = \frac{n!}{(n - k)!k!} \tag{7.1}$$

where $n!$ (called "factorial n") $= n(n - 1)(n - 2) \cdots 1$. ($0! = 1$ by definition.)

Example 7.4. If $n = 4$, then $n! = 4(4 - 1)(4 - 2)(4 - 3) = 4 \cdot 3 \cdot 2 \cdot 1 = 24$.

Example 7.5. The number of ways to obtain 2 heads in three tosses of a coin is

$$_3C_2 = \frac{3!}{(3 - 2)!2!} = \frac{3 \times 2 \times 1}{(1) \times 2 \times 1} = 3$$

These three combinations are HHT, HTH, THH.

Formula (7.1) can be used for calculating the coefficients in a binomial expansion,

$$(p + q)^n = \sum_{k=0}^{n} {_nC_k} p^{n-k} q^k = \sum_{k=0}^{n} \frac{n!}{(n - k)!k!} p^{n-k} q^k \tag{7.2}$$

where $\sum_{k=0}^{n}$ means to sum what follows as k increases by one unit in each term of the expansion from zero to n. This method is obviously much more laborious than the short method presented previously. However, it does have utility in the calculation of one or a few specific terms of a large binomial expansion. To represent this formula in another way, we can let $p = $ probability of the occurrence of one event (e.g., a success) and $q = $ probability of the occurrence of the alternative event (e.g., a failure); then the probability that in n trials a success will occur s times and a failure will occur f times is given by

$$\left(\frac{n!}{s!f!} \right) (p^s)(q^f) \tag{7.3}$$

2. The Multinomial Distribution.

The binomial distribution may be generalized to accommodate any number of variables. If events $e_1, e_2, \ldots, e_k$ can occur with probabilities $p_1, p_2, \ldots, p_k$, respectively, then the probability that $e_1, e_2, \ldots, e_k$ will occur $k_1, k_2, \ldots, k_n$ times, respectively, is

$$\frac{N!}{k_1!k_2! \cdots k_n!} p_1^{k_1} p_2^{k_2} \cdots p_n^{k_n} \tag{7.4}$$

where $k_1 + k_2 + \cdots + k_n = N$.

THE POISSON DISTRIBUTION

When the probability (p) of a rare event (e.g., a specific mutation) is relatively small and the sample size (n) is relatively large, the binomial distribution is essentially the same as a **Poisson distribution,** but is much easier to solve by the latter. Another advantage in using the Poisson distribution instead of the binomial distribution is that it allows analysis of data where pn is known, but neither p nor n alone is known. Under these conditions, any term of the binomial expansion is closely approximated by the point Poisson formula

$$\frac{n!}{k!(n-k)!} p^k q^{(n-k)} = \frac{e^{-np}(np)^k}{k!}$$

where k is the number of the rare events, q is the probability of the common event (e.g., no mutation), and e is the base of the Napierian or natural system of logarithms $\left(\frac{1}{1!} + \frac{1}{2!} + \frac{1}{3!} + \cdots = 2.71828\right.$

$\left. + \cdots \right)$. The mean (μ) of rare events is equivalent to np. The probabilities that such events happen 0, 1, 2, 3, . . . times is given by the series of terms

$$\frac{\mu^0 e^{-\mu}}{0!}, \quad \frac{\mu^1 e^{-\mu}}{1!}, \quad \frac{\mu^2 e^{-\mu}}{2!}, \quad \frac{\mu^3 e^{-\mu}}{3!}, \cdots$$

Table 7.1 displays some values of e^{-np} or $e^{-\mu}$ that can be helpful in solving certain problems.

The variance (see Chapter 9) of the binomial distribution is npq or $np(1-p)$. The Poisson distribution has the same variance, but since p is very small the probability of the common event $(1-p)$ is almost 1.0. Therefore, in a Poisson distribution the mean (np) is essentially the same as the variance.

Knowledge of these aspects of the Poisson distribution will be essential in Chapter 12 for understanding the Luria-Delbrück fluctuation test, a classic experiment that initiated modern bacterial genetics.

Table 7.1.   Values of $e^{-\mu}$
(0 < μ < 1)

μ	0	1	2	3	4	5	6	7	8	9
0.0	1.0000	.9900	.9802	.9704	.9608	.9512	.9418	.9324	.9231	.9139
0.1	.9048	.8958	.8869	.8781	.8694	.8607	.8521	.8437	.8353	.8270
0.2	.8187	.8106	.8025	.7945	.7866	.7788	.7711	.7634	.7558	.7483
0.3	.7408	.7334	.7261	.7189	.7118	.7047	.6977	.6907	.6839	.6771
0.4	.6703	.6636	.6570	.6505	.6440	.6376	.6313	.6250	.6188	.6126
0.5	.6065	.6005	.5945	.5886	.5827	.5770	.5712	.5655	.5599	.5543
0.6	.5488	.5434	.5379	.5326	.5273	.5220	.5169	.5117	.5066	.5016
0.7	.4966	.4916	.4868	.4819	.4771	.4724	.4677	.4630	.4584	.4538
0.8	.4493	.4449	.4404	.4360	.4317	.4274	.4232	.4190	.4148	.4107
0.9	.4066	.4025	.3985	.3946	.3906	.3867	.3829	.3791	.3753	.3716

(μ = 1, 2, 3, . . ., 10)

μ	1	2	3	4	5	6	7	8	9	10
$e^{-\mu}$	.36788	.13534	.04979	.01832	.006738	.002479	.000912	.000335	.000123	.000045

Note: To obtain values of $e^{-\mu}$ for other values of μ use the laws of exponents.
    Example: $e^{-3.48} = (e^{-3.00})(e^{-0.48}) = (.04979)(.6188) = .03081$.

Source: Murray R. Spiegel, *Schaum's Outline of Theory and Problems of Statistics,* McGraw-Hill Book Company, New York, 1961, p. 348.

TESTING GENETIC RATIOS

1. Sampling Theory.

If we toss a coin, we expect that half of the time it will land heads up and half of the time tails up. This hypothesized probability is based upon an infinite number of coin tossings wherein the effects of chance deviations from 0.5 in favor of either heads or tails cancel one another. All actual experiments, however, involve finite numbers of observations and therefore some deviation from the expected numbers (sampling error) is to be anticipated. Let us assume that there is no difference between the observed results of a coin-tossing experiment and the expected results that cannot be accounted for by chance alone (**null hypothesis**). How great a deviation from the expected 50–50 ratio in a given experiment should be allowed before the null hypothesis is rejected? Conventionally, the null hypothesis in most biological experiments is rejected when the deviation is so large that it could be accounted for by chance less than 5% of the time. Such results are said to be **significant.** When the null hypothesis is rejected at the 5% level, we take 1 chance in 20 of discarding a valid hypothesis. It must be remembered that statistics can never render absolute proof of the hypothesis, but merely sets limits to our uncertainty. If we wish to be even more certain that the rejection of the hypothesis is warranted we could use the 1% level, often called **highly significant,** in which case the experimenter would be taking only one chance in a hundred of rejecting a valid hypothesis.

2. Sample Size.

If our coin-tossing experiment is based on small numbers, we might anticipate relatively large deviations from the expected values to occur quite often by chance alone. However, as the sample size increases the deviation should become proportionately less, so that in a sample of infinite size the plus and minus chance deviations cancel each other completely to produce the 50–50 ratio.

3. Degrees of Freedom.

Assume a coin is tossed 100 times. We may arbitrarily assign any number of heads from 0 to 100 as appearing in this hypothetical experiment. However, once the number of heads is established, the remainder is tails and must add to 100. In other words, we have $n - 1$ **degrees of freedom** (df) in assigning numbers at random to the n classes within an experiment.

> **Example 7.6.** In an experiment involving 3 phenotypes ($n = 3$), we can fill 2 of the classes at random, but the number in the third class must constitute the remainder of the total number of individuals observed. Therefore we have $3 - 1 = 2$ degrees of freedom.
>
> **Example 7.7.** A $9 : 3 : 3 : 1$ dihybrid ratio has 4 phenotypes ($n = 4$). There are $4 - 1 = 3$ degrees of freedom.

The number of degrees of freedom in these kinds of problems is the number of variables (n) under consideration minus one. For most genetic problems, the degrees of freedom will be one less than the number of phenotypic classes. Obviously the more variables involved in an experiment the greater the total deviation may be by chance.

4. Chi-Square Test.

In order to evaluate a genetic hypothesis, we need a test that can convert deviations from expected values into the probability of such inequalities occurring by chance. Furthermore, this test must also take into consideration the size of the sample and the number of variables (degrees of freedom). The chi-square test (pronounced ki-; symbolized χ^2) includes all of these factors.

$$\chi^2 = \sum_{i=1}^{n} \frac{(o_i - e_i)^2}{e_i} = \frac{(o_1 - e_1)^2}{e_1} + \frac{(o_2 - e_2)^2}{e_2} + \cdots + \frac{(o_n - e_n)^2}{e_n} \tag{7.5}$$

where $\sum_{i=1}^{n}$ means to sum what follows it as the i classes increase from 1 to n, o represents the number of observations within a class, e represents the number expected in the class according to the hypothesis under test, and n is the number of classes. The value of chi-square may then be converted into the probability that the deviation is due to chance by entering Table 7.2 at the appropriate number of degrees of freedom.

Table 7.2. Chi-Square Distribution

Degrees of Freedom	Probability										
	0.95	0.90	0.80	0.70	0.50	0.30	0.20	0.10	0.05	0.01	0.001
1	0.004	0.02	0.06	0.15	0.46	1.07	1.64	2.71	3.84	6.64	10.83
2	0.10	0.21	0.45	0.71	1.39	2.41	3.22	4.60	5.99	9.21	13.82
3	0.35	0.58	1.01	1.42	2.37	3.66	4.64	6.25	7.82	11.34	16.27
4	0.71	1.06	1.65	2.20	3.36	4.88	5.99	7.78	9.49	13.28	18.47
5	1.14	1.61	2.34	3.00	4.35	6.06	7.29	9.24	11.07	15.09	20.52
6	1.63	2.20	3.07	3.83	5.35	7.23	8.56	10.64	12.59	16.81	22.46
7	2.17	2.83	3.82	4.67	6.35	8.38	9.80	12.02	14.07	18.48	24.32
8	2.73	3.49	4.59	5.53	7.34	9.52	11.03	13.36	15.51	20.09	26.12
9	3.32	4.17	5.38	6.39	8.34	10.66	12.24	14.68	16.92	21.67	27.88
10	3.94	4.86	6.18	7.27	9.34	11.78	13.44	15.99	18.31	23.21	29.59
	Nonsignificant								Significant		

Source: R. A. Fisher and F. Yates, *Statistical Tables for Biological, Agricultural and Medical Research* (6th edition), Table IV, Oliver & Boyd, Ltd., Edinburgh, by permission of the authors and publishers.

An alternative method for computing chi-square in problems involving *only two phenotypes* will give the same result as the conventional method and often makes computation easier,

$$\chi^2 = \frac{(a - rb)^2}{r(a + b)} \tag{7.6}$$

where a and b are the numbers in the two phenotypic classes and r is the expected ratio of a to b.

(a) **Chi-Square Limitations.** The chi-square test as used for analyzing the results of genetic experiments has two important limitations: (1) it must be used only on the numerical data itself, never on percentages or ratios derived from the data; (2) it cannot properly be used for experiments wherein the expected frequency within any phenotypic class is less than 5.

(b) **Correction for Small Samples.** The formula from which the chi-square table is derived is based upon a continuous distribution, namely, that of the "normal" curve (see Chapter 9). Such a distribution might be expected when we plot the heights of a group of people. The most frequent class would be the average height and successively fewer people would be in the taller or shorter phenotypes. All sizes are possible from the shortest to the tallest, i.e., heights form a continuous distribution. However, the kinds of genetic problems in the previous chapters of this book involve separate or discrete phenotypic classes such as blue eyes vs. brown eyes. A correction should therefore be applied in the calculation of chi-square to correct for this lack of continuity. The "Yates Correction for Continuity" is applied as follows:

$$\chi^2 \text{ (corrected)} = \sum_{i=1}^{n} \frac{[|o_i - e_i| - 0.5]^2}{e_i}$$

$$= \frac{[|o_1 - e_1| - 0.5]^2}{e_1} + \frac{[|o_2 - e_2| - 0.5]^2}{e_2} + \cdots + \frac{[|o_n - e_n| - 0.5]^2}{e_n} \tag{7.7}$$

This correction usually makes little difference in the chi-square of most problems, but may become an important factor near the critical values. The Yates correction should be routinely applied whenever only 1 degree of freedom exists, or in small samples where each expected frequency is between 5 and 10. If the corrected and uncorrected methods each lead to the same conclusion, there is no difficulty. However, if these methods do not lead to the same conclusion, then either more data need to be collected or a more sophisticated statistical test should be employed. Most genetic texts make no mention of this correction. Therefore problems in this book requiring the application of Yates's correction will be limited to those in the section entitled "Correction for Small Samples" in both the Solved and Supplementary Problems.

Solved Problems

THE BINOMIAL EXPANSION

7.1. Expand the binomial $(p + q)^5$.

Solution:

1st term: $1p^5q^0$; coefficient of 2nd term $= (5 \cdot 1)/1$
2nd term: $5p^4q^1$; coefficient of 3rd term $= (4 \cdot 5)/2$
3rd term: $10p^3q^2$; coefficient of 4th term $= (3 \cdot 10)/3$
4th term: $10p^2q^3$; coefficient of 5th term $= (2 \cdot 10)/4$
5th term: $5p^1q^4$; coefficient of 6th term $= (1 \cdot 5)/5$
6th term: $1p^0q^5$

Summary: $(p + q)^5 = p^5 + 5p^4q + 10p^3q^2 + 10p^2q^3 + 5pq^4 + q^5$

7.2. Expand $(p + q)^2$ by formula (7.2).

Solution:

$$(p + q)^n = \sum_{k=0}^{n} \frac{n!}{(n - k)!k!} p^{n-k}q^k$$

$$(p + q)^2 = \frac{2!}{(2 - 0)!0!} p^{2-0}q^0 + \frac{2!}{(2 - 1)!1!} p^{2-1}q^1 + \frac{2!}{(2 - 2)!2!} p^{2-2}q^2$$
$$= p^2 + 2pq + q^2$$

Note that $0! = 1$, and $x^0 = 1$ where x is any number.

7.3. Find the middle term of the expansion $(p + q)^{10}$ by application of formula (7.2).

Solution:

The middle term of the expansion $(p + q)^{10}$ is the sixth term since there are $(n + 1)$ terms in the expansion. The power of q starts at zero in the first term and increases by one in each successive term so that the sixth term would have q^5, and so $k = 5$. Then the sixth term is

$$\frac{n!}{(n - k)!k!} p^{n-k}q^k = \frac{10 \cdot 9 \cdot 8 \cdot 7 \cdot 6 \cdot 5!}{(10 - 5)!5!} p^{10-5}q^5 = \frac{10 \cdot 9 \cdot 8 \cdot 7 \cdot 6}{5 \cdot 4 \cdot 3 \cdot 2 \cdot 1} p^5q^5 = 252p^5q^5$$

7.4. A multiple allelic series is known with 7 alleles. How many kinds of matings are possible?

Solution:

$$\begin{array}{ccc} \text{No. of genotypes} \\ \text{possible} \end{array} = \begin{array}{c} \text{No. of different allelic} \\ \text{combinations (heterozygotes)} \end{array} + \begin{array}{c} \text{No. of genotypes with two} \\ \text{of the same alleles (homozygotes)} \end{array}$$

$$= \frac{n!}{(n-k)!k!} + n = \frac{7!}{5!2!} + 7 = \frac{7 \cdot 6 \cdot 5!}{2 \cdot 5!} + 7$$

$$= 21 + 7 = 28 \text{ genotypes}$$

$$\begin{array}{c} \text{No. of different} \\ \text{matings} \end{array} = \begin{array}{c} \text{No. of matings between} \\ \text{unlike genotypes} \end{array} + \begin{array}{c} \text{No. of matings between} \\ \text{identical genotypes} \end{array}$$

$$= \frac{28!}{26!2!} + 28 = \frac{28 \cdot 27 \cdot 26!}{2 \cdot 26!} + 28 = 406$$

7.5. Determine the probability of obtaining 6 heads and 3 tails in nine tosses of a coin by applying formula (*7.3*).

Solution:

In tossing a coin, we may consider heads to be a success (*s*) and tails a failure (*f*). The probability of obtaining 6 successes and 3 failures in 9 trials is

$$\frac{n!}{s!f!}p^s q^f = \frac{9!}{6!3!}p^6 q^3 = \frac{9 \cdot 8 \cdot 7 \cdot 6!}{1 \cdot 2 \cdot 3 \cdot 6!}p^6 q^3 = 84p^6 q^3$$

If the probability of obtaining a head (*p*) is equal to the probability of obtaining a tail (q) $= \frac{1}{2}$, then $84p^6 q^3 = 84(\frac{1}{2})^9 = \frac{84}{512} = \frac{21}{128}$.

7.6. The MN blood types of humans are under the genetic control of a pair of codominant alleles as explained in Example 2.9. In families of size 6 where both parents are blood type MN, what is the chance of finding 3 children of type M, 2 of type MN, and 1 N?

Solution:

$$\text{P:} \qquad L^M L^N \times L^M L^N$$

$$\text{F}_1: \qquad \frac{1}{4}L^M L^M = \text{type M}$$
$$\frac{1}{2}L^M L^N = \text{type MN}$$
$$\frac{1}{4}L^N L^N = \text{type N}$$

Let p_1 = probability of child being type M = $\frac{1}{4}$
$\quad\;\; p_2$ = probability of child being type MN = $\frac{1}{2}$
$\quad\;\; p_3$ = probability of child being type N = $\frac{1}{4}$

Let k_1 = number of children of type M required = 3
$\quad\;\; k_2$ = number of children of type MN required = 2
$\quad\;\; k_3$ = number of children of type N required = $\underline{1}$
$$N = \Sigma k_i \quad= 6$$

$$(p_1 + p_2 + p_3)^N = \frac{N!}{k_1!k_2!k_3!}p_1^{k_1}p_2^{k_2}p_3^{k_3} \qquad\qquad (7.4)$$

$$(p_1 + p_2 + p_3)^6 = \frac{6!}{3!2!1!}\left(\frac{1}{4}\right)^3\left(\frac{1}{2}\right)^2\left(\frac{1}{4}\right) = \frac{6 \cdot 5 \cdot 4 \cdot 3!}{2 \cdot 3!}\left(\frac{1}{4}\right)^4\left(\frac{1}{2}\right)^2 = \frac{15}{256}$$

THE POISSON DISTRIBUTION

7.7. Suppose that only 1 out of 1000 individuals in a population is an albino; all the rest are normally pigmented. If a sample of 100 individuals is drawn at random from this population, calculate, by

Poisson distribution, the probabilities that it contains (*a*) no albinos, (*b*) 1 albino, (*c*) 2 albinos, (*d*) 3 or more albinos.

Solution:

Let n = sample size = 100
   p = probability of albino = 0.001
   np = probable number of albinos in a population of size n = (100)(0.001) = 0.1
   k = number of rare events (albinos) = 1, 2, 3 or more

(*a*) If k = 0, then referring to Table 7.1 we have

$$\frac{e^{-np}(np)^k}{k!} = \frac{e^{-0.1}(0.1)^0}{0!} = \frac{e^{-0.1}(1)}{1} = 0.9048$$

    (Note: any number to the zero power is 1.)

(*b*) If k = 1

$$\frac{e^{-0.1}(0.1)^1}{1!} = (0.9048)(0.1) = 0.09048$$

(*c*) If k = 2

$$\frac{e^{-0.1}(0.1)^2}{2!} = \frac{(0.9048)(0.1)}{2} = 0.004524$$

(*d*) The probability of finding 3 or more albinos is 1 minus the sum of probabilities for 0, 1, and 2 albinos.

$$1 - (0.9048 + 0.09048 + 0.004524) = 1 - 0.999804 = 0.000196$$

Note that trying to solve this problem by applying the binomial distribution

$$1 - [\,_{100}C_0(0.001)^0(0.999)^{100} + \,_{100}C_1(0.001)^1(0.999)^{99} + \,_{100}C_2(0.001)^2(0.999)^{98}]$$

would be a very difficult approach.

7.8. Sex-linked female-sterile mutations can be induced by the chemical mutagen EMS (ethyl methane sulfonate) in *Drosophila melanogaster*. Apparently mutations in many different X-linked genes can result in female sterility. In one experiment involving 131 female-sterile mutations, 58 such EMS-induced genes were each found to have one mutation and 23 genes were found to have two mutations. Estimate the total number of X-linked genes that, if mutated, could produce female sterility.

Solution:

According to the Poisson distribution, we expect x genes to have one mutation with a frequency

$$\frac{(np)e^{-np}}{1!}$$

where n = the total number of female-sterile genes on the X chromosome
   p = the probability of a mutation per such gene
   np = the mean number of mutations per such gene

We expect y genes to have two mutations with a frequency

$$\frac{(np)^2e^{-np}}{2!}$$

We make the ratio

$$\frac{y}{x} = \frac{(np)^2e^{-np}}{2(np)e^{-np}} = \frac{np}{2}$$

From the data given

$$\frac{y}{x} = \frac{23/n}{58/n} = 0.4$$

Thus, $np/2 = 0.4$ or $np = 0.8$.

Since the mean number of mutations per mutable female-sterile gene (np) was observed to be $131/n$, and $np = 0.8$, then

$$0.8 = \frac{131}{n} \qquad \text{or} \qquad n = 164$$

7.9. A bacterial culture susceptible to infection by a virus was inoculated into 20 tubes each containing 0.2 milliliter of broth and allowed to multiply to a concentration of about 10^9 cells per milliliter. After this multiplication, 9 of the tubes were found to contain some cells that had mutated to viral resistance; 11 of the tubes had no resistant cells. Estimate the mutation rate from viral sensitivity to viral resistance in this organism under these experimental conditions.

Solution:

The fraction of cultures with no mutants (x) is $\frac{11}{20} = 0.55$. The zero term of the Poisson distribution is $x = e^{-np}$, where n is the number of cells per culture $= (0.2)(10^9) = 2 \times 10^8$ and p is the probability of mutation from viral sensitivity to viral resistance (mutation rate).

$$0.55 = e^{-p(2 \times 10^8)}$$

From Table 7.1 it is seen that the value of e^{-np} that approximates 0.55 is about 0.6. Therefore,

$$p(2 \times 10^8) = 0.6$$

and

$$p = \frac{0.6}{2 \times 10^8} = 3 \times 10^{-9}$$

Alternatively, taking natural logarithms (obtained from a reference source), from the equation

$$x = e^{-np}$$

we obtain

$$\ln x = -np$$

$$p = \frac{-\ln x}{n} = \frac{-\ln 0.55}{2 \times 10^8} = \frac{0.598}{2 \times 10^8} \approx 3 \times 10^{-9}$$

7.10. In a large population of meioses, 2 tightly linked genes are likely to incur mostly zero crossovers (Poisson distribution). A single crossover is equivalent to 50 map units since only 2 strands in a tetrad are recombined, producing 50% recombinants. For small distances, the observed frequency of recombination (RF) is equivalent to half the actual frequency of crossing over (RF $= \frac{1}{2}$RF'). Because the frequency of multiple crossovers increases with the distance between genes, the RF departs progressively from linearity with the actual map distance (Fig. 6-1). When genes are so far apart that the equivalent of a single crossover occurs in every meiosis, 50% of the meiotic products are expected to be recombinant. Since the expected percentage of recombination among all kinds of double crossovers (2-, 3-, and 4-strand doubles) is also 50%, this is the maximum observed recombination frequency, regardless of the distance between genes. The frequency of meioses with at least one crossover is one minus the fraction with zero crossovers. Hence RF $= \frac{1}{2}(1 - e^{-\mu})$, where $\mu =$ mean number of crossovers per meiosis and $e^{-\mu} =$ zero class frequency expected in a Poisson distribution. RF' $= \mu/2$ because only half the meiotic products from any crossover are expected to be recombinant. If the observed RF between two linked loci is 0.33, estimate the true amount of recombination (map units) and calculate the error of estimate.

Solution:

$$0.33 = \tfrac{1}{2}(1 - e^{-\mu})$$
$$0.66 = 1 - e^{-\mu}$$
$$e^{-\mu} = 1 - 0.66 = 0.34$$

In Table 7.1, $e^{-0.34}$ lies between $\mu = 1$ (0.36788) and $\mu = 2$ (0.13534). Thus, $0.34/0.36788 = 0.9242$, which corresponds to $\mu = 0.08$. Therefore, $\mu = 1.08$, and $RF' = 1.08/2 = 0.54$ or 54 map units. The error of underestimate of the actual distance $= (54 - 33)/54 = \tfrac{21}{54} = 0.39$ or 39%. For use on a calculator, rearrange $RF = \tfrac{1}{2}(1 - e^{-\mu})$ to $e^{-\mu} = 1 - 2RF$; then $\mu = -\ln(1 - 2RF)$.

CHI-SQUARE TEST

7.11. (a) A coin is tossed 10 times and lands heads up 6 times and tails up 4 times. Are these results consistent with the expected 50 : 50 ratio? (b) If the coin is tossed 100 times with the same relative magnitude of deviation from the expected ratio, is the hypothesis still acceptable? (c) What conclusion can be drawn from the results of parts (a) and (b)?

Solution:

(a)

Phenotypic Classes	Observed (o)	Expected (e)	Deviations (o − e)	(o − e)²	(o − e)²/e
Heads	6	$\tfrac{1}{2}(10) = 5$	1	1	$\tfrac{1}{5} = 0.2$
Tails	4	$\tfrac{1}{2}(10) = 5$	−1	1	$\tfrac{1}{5} = 0.2$
	10	10	0		$\chi^2 = 0.4$

Two mathematical check points are always present in the chi-square calculations. (1) The total of the expected column must equal the total observations. (2) The sum of the deviations should equal 0. The squaring of negative deviations converts all values to a positive scale. The number of degrees of freedom is the number of phenotypes minus 1 ($2 - 1 = 1$). We enter Table 7.2 on the first line (df = 1) and find the computed value of 0.4 lying in the body of the table between the values 0.15 and 0.46 corresponding to the probabilities 0.7 and 0.5 shown at the top of the respective columns. This implies that the magnitude of the deviation in our experimental results could be anticipated by chance alone in more than 50% but less than 70% of an infinite number of experiments of comparable size. This range of values is far above the critical probability value of 0.05 or 5%. Therefore we accept the null hypothesis and conclude that our coin is conforming to the expected probabilities of heads = $\tfrac{1}{2}$ and tails = $\tfrac{1}{2}$.

(b) In (a), heads appeared in 60% and tails in 40% of the tosses. The same relative magnitude of deviations will now be considered in a sample of size 100. In problems such as this, where expected values are equivalent in all the phenotypic classes, chi-square may be calculated more rapidly by adding the squared deviations and making a single division by the expected number.

Phenotypes	o	e	o − e	(o − e)²
Heads	60	$\tfrac{1}{2}(100) = 50$	10	100
Tails	40	$\tfrac{1}{2}(100) = 50$	− 10	100
	100	100	0	$\chi^2 = 200/50 = 4.0$

With df = 1, this χ^2 value lies between 6.64 and 3.84, corresponding to the probabilities 0.01 with 0.05, respectively. This means that a deviation as large as or larger than the one observed in this experiment is to be anticipated by chance alone in less than 5% of an infinite number of trials of similar size. This is in the "critical region," and we are therefore obliged to reject the null hypothesis and conclude that our coin is not conforming to the expected 50 : 50 ratio. Either of two explanations may be involved: (1) this is not a normal well-balanced coin or (2) our experiment is among the 1 in 20 (5%) expected to have a large deviation produced by chance alone.

(c) The results of parts (a) and (b) demonstrate the fact that large samples provide a more critical test of a hypothesis than small samples. Proportionately larger deviations have a greater probability of occurring by chance in small samples than in large samples.

7.12. In the garden pea, yellow cotyledon color is dominant to green, and inflated pod shape is dominant to the constricted form. When both of these traits were considered jointly in self-fertilized dihybrids, the progeny appeared in the following numbers: 193 green, inflated: 184 yellow, constricted: 556 yellow, inflated: 61 green, constricted. Test the data for independent assortment.

Solution:

P: $Gg\ Cc$ × $Gg\ Cc$
          yellow, inflated   yellow, inflated

F$_1$:   (expectations) $\frac{9}{16}G\text{-}\ C\text{-}$ yellow, inflated
          $\frac{3}{16}G\text{-}\ cc$ yellow, constricted
          $\frac{3}{16}gg\ C\text{-}$ green, inflated
          $\frac{1}{16}gg\ cc$ green, constricted

Phenotypes	Observed	Expected	Deviation d	d^2	d^2/e
yellow, inflated	556	$\frac{9}{16}(994) = 559.1$	−3.1	9.61	0.017
yellow, constricted	184	$\frac{3}{16}(994) = 186.4$	−2.4	5.76	0.031
green, inflated	193	$\frac{3}{16}(994) = 186.4$	6.6	43.56	0.234
green, constricted	$\underline{61}$	$\frac{1}{16}(994) = \underline{62.1}$	$\underline{-1.1}$	1.21	$\underline{0.019}$
	994	994.0	0		$\chi^2 = 0.301$

$$df = 4 - 1 = 3 \qquad p > 0.95$$

This is not a significant chi-square value, and thus we accept the null hypothesis, i.e., the magnitude of the deviation (o − e) is to be expected by chance alone in greater than 95% of an infinite number of experiments of comparable size. This is far above the critical value of 5% necessary for acceptance of the hypothesis. We may therefore accept the data as being in conformity with a $9:3:3:1$ ratio, indicating that the gene for cotyledon color assorts independently of the gene for pod form.

7.13. Pure red-fleshed tomatoes crossed with yellow-fleshed tomatoes produced an all red F$_1$. Among 400 F$_2$ plants, 90 were yellow. It is hypothesized that a single pair of alleles is involved such that $Y\text{-} =$ red and $yy =$ yellow. Test this hypothesis by use of formula (7.6).

Solution:

P: YY (red)   × yy (yellow)

F$_1$: Yy (red)

F$_2$:   (expectations) $\frac{3}{4}Y\text{-}$ (red)
                              $\frac{1}{4}yy$ (yellow)

Let $a =$ number of yellow-fleshed fruits $= 90$, $b =$ number of red-fleshed fruits $= 400 - 90 = 310$, $r =$ expected ratio of a to $b = \frac{1}{3}$. Then

$$\chi^2 = \frac{(a - rb)^2}{r(a + b)} = \frac{[90 - \frac{1}{3}(310)]^2}{\frac{1}{3}(90 + 310)} = 1.33$$

$$df = 1 \qquad p = 0.2\text{--}0.3$$

This is not a significant value and hence we may accept the hypothesis.

Some work can be saved in this method by always letting the larger number $= a$. Let $a =$ number of red-fleshed fruits $= 310$, $b =$ number of yellow-fleshed fruits $= 90$, $r =$ expected ratio of a to $b = 3$. Then

$$\chi^2 = \frac{[310 - 3(90)]^2}{3(400)} = \frac{(40)^2}{1200} = 1.33$$

7.14. A total of 160 families with 4 children each were surveyed with the following results:

Girls	4	3	2	1	0
Boys	0	1	2	3	4
Families	7	50	55	32	16

Is the family distribution consistent with the hypothesis of equal numbers of boys and girls?

Solution:

Let a = probability of a girl = $\frac{1}{2}$, b = probability of a boy = $\frac{1}{2}$.

$$(a + b)^4 = \quad a^4 \quad + \quad 4a^3b \quad + \quad 6a^2b^2 \quad + \quad 4ab^3 \quad + \quad b^4$$

4 girls 0 boys	3 girls 1 boy	2 girls 2 boys	1 girl 3 boys	0 girls 4 boys

$$= \quad (\tfrac{1}{2})^4 \quad + \quad 4(\tfrac{1}{2})^3(\tfrac{1}{2}) \quad + \quad 6(\tfrac{1}{2})^2(\tfrac{1}{2})^2 \quad + \quad 4(\tfrac{1}{2})(\tfrac{1}{2})^3 \quad + \quad (\tfrac{1}{2})^4$$
$$= \quad \tfrac{1}{16} \quad + \quad \tfrac{4}{16} \quad + \quad \tfrac{6}{16} \quad + \quad \tfrac{4}{16} \quad + \quad \tfrac{1}{16}$$

Expected number with 4 girls and 0 boys = $\frac{1}{16}(160) = 10$

$\qquad\qquad\qquad\quad$ 3 girls and 1 boy $\;= \frac{4}{16}(160) = 40$

$\qquad\qquad\qquad\quad$ 2 girls and 2 boys $= \frac{6}{16}(160) = 60$

$\qquad\qquad\qquad\quad$ 1 girl $\,$ and 3 boys $= \frac{4}{16}(160) = 40$

$\qquad\qquad\qquad\quad$ 0 girls and 4 boys $= \frac{1}{16}(160) = 10$.   Then

$$\chi^2 = \frac{(7 - 10)^2}{10} + \frac{(50 - 40)^2}{40} + \frac{(55 - 60)^2}{60} + \frac{(32 - 40)^2}{40} + \frac{(16 - 10)^2}{10} = 9.02$$

$$\text{df} = 5 - 1 = 4 \quad p = 0.05\text{–}0.10$$

This value is close to, but less than, the critical value 9.49. We may therefore accept the hypothesis, but the test would be more definitive if it could be run on a larger sample. It is a well-known fact that a greater mortality occurs in males than in females and therefore an attempt should be made to ascertain family composition on the basis of sex of *all* children *at birth* including prematures, aborted fetuses, etc.

Correction for Small Samples

7.15. In Problem 7.11(*b*), it was shown that observations of 60 : 40 produced a significant chi-square at the 5% level when uncorrected for continuity. Apply the Yates correction for continuity and retest the data.

Solution:

o	e	[$|o - e| - 0.5$]	[$|o - e| - 0.5$]^2
60	50	$10 - 0.5 = 9.5$	90.25
40	50	$10 - 0.5 = 9.5$	$\underline{90.25}$
			$\chi^2 = 180.50/50 = 3.61$

Notice that the correction 0.5 is always applied to the *absolute value* $|o - e|$ of the deviation of expected from observed numbers. This is not a significant chi-square value. Because the data are discrete (jumping from unit to unit) there is a tendency to underestimate the probability, causing too many rejections of the null hypothesis. The Yates correction removes this bias and produces a more accurate test near the critical values (column headed by a probability of 0.05 in Table 7.2).

Supplementary Problems

THE BINOMIAL EXPANSION

7.16. Black hair in the guinea pig is dominant to white hair. In families of 5 offspring where both parents are heterozygous black, with what frequency would we expect to find (*a*) 3 whites and 2 blacks, (*b*) 2 whites and 3 blacks, (*c*) 1 white and 4 blacks, (*d*) all whites?

7.17. In families of size 3, what is the probability of finding the oldest child to be a girl and the youngest a boy?

7.18. In families of five children, what is the probability of finding (*a*) 3 or more boys, (*b*) 3 or more boys or 3 or more girls?

7.19. A dozen strains of corn are available for a cross-pollination experiment. How many different ways can these strains be paired?

7.20. Five coat colors in mice are agouti, cinnamon, black, chocolate, and albino. (*a*) List all of the possible crosses between different phenotypes. (*b*) Verify the number of different crosses by applying formula (*7.1*).

7.21. In mice litters of size 8, determine (*a*) the most frequently expected number of males and females, (*b*) the term of the binomial part (*a*) represents, (*c*) the percentage of all litters of size 8 expected to have 4 males and 4 females.

7.22. There are at least 12 alleles at the sex-linked "white" locus in *Drosophila*. Find the number of possible (*a*) genotypes, (*b*) types of matings.

7.23. White plumage in chickens can result from the action of a recessive genotype *cc* or from the action of an independently assorting dominant gene *I*. The White Plymouth Rock breed has genotype *ccii* and the White Leghorn breed has genotype *CCII*. The hybrid bird produced by crossing these two breeds is also white. How frequently in clutches (a nest of eggs; a brood of chicks) of 10 chicks produced by hybrid birds would you expect to find 5 colored and 5 white chicks?

7.24. A case of dominant interaction among coat colors has been discovered in the dog: *B*- results in black, *bb* in brown; *I*- inhibits color development, *ii* allows color to be produced. White dogs of genotype *BBII* testcrossed to brown dogs produce all-white puppies in the F_1. In the F_2, determine the fraction of all litters of size 6 that is expected to contain 3 white, 1 black, and 2 brown puppies.

7.25. A pair of alleles in the rat, *C* and *c*, act on coat color in such a way that the genotypes *CC* and *Cc* allow pigment to be produced, but the genotype *cc* prevents any pigment from being produced (albinos). Black rats possess the dominant gene *R* of an independently assorting locus. Cream rats are produced by the recessive genotype *rr*. When black rats of genotype *RRCC* are testcrossed to albino rats, the F_1 is all black. Determine the percentage of F_2 litters of size 7 which is expected to have 4 black, 2 cream, and 1 albino.

7.26. Two independently assorting loci, each with codominant allelic pairs, are involved in the shape and color characteristics of radishes. The shape may be long or round, due to different homozygous genotypes, or oval due to the heterozygous genotype. The color may be red or white due to different homozygous genotypes, or purple due to the heterozygous genotype. A long white variety is crossed to a round red variety. The F_1 is all oval purple. A dozen seeds are saved from each self-pollinated F_1 plant and grown out the next season in sibling groups. Assuming 100% germination, determine the proportion of plants in each group of a dozen progeny expected to exhibit 5 oval, purple: 3 oval, white: 2 round, purple: 1 long, purple: 1 round, red.

THE POISSON DISTRIBUTION

7.27. A bacterial suspension contains 5 million cells per milliliter. This culture is serially diluted tenfold in six successive tubes by adding 1 milliliter from the previous tube into 9 milliliters of diluent fluid. (*a*) How many cells per milliliter are expected in the sixth dilution tube? (b) If $\mu = 5$ and $e^{-5} = 0.006738$ (Table 7.1), calculate the probabilities of finding in the sixth tube 0, 1, 2, 3, 4 cells. (c) Suppose that 5 cells are found in the sixth tube. Give the 95% confidence limits for this estimate of the sixth-tube mean. *Hint:* Confidence limits of 95% are within ± 2 standard deviations of the mean. The variance is the square of the standard deviation. (d) Suppose that each tube contains the expected number of cells. Which tube contains the greatest dilution from which the estimate of the mean number of cells in the tube is accurate to within about 10% of the mean itself?

7.28. Radioactive elements are extensively used in molecular genetic research. Radioactive disintegration of these atoms follow a Poisson distribution. What is the error of estimating the mean number of radioactive disintegrations per minute (dpm) if 100 dpm are actually detected when counted for (a) 1 minute? (b) 100 minutes? *Hint:* The 95% confidence limits are approximated by the mean ± 2 standard deviations. The variance is the square of the standard deviation.

7.29. If two linked genes produce 27.5% recombinants, estimate the probable amount of crossing over that actually occurred between these loci, assuming that the probability of 0, 1, 2, . . . , n exchanges occur during meiosis according to a Poisson distribution.

TESTING GENETIC RATIOS

7.30. Determine the number of degrees of freedom when testing the ratios (a) $3:1$, (b) $9:3:3:1$, (c) $1:2:1$, (d) $9:3:4$. Find the number of degrees of freedom in applying a chi-square test to the results from (e) testcrossing a dihybrid, (f) testcrossing a trihybrid, (g) trihybrid $\times$ trihybrid cross, (h) mating repulsion dihybrid *Drosophila* males and females.

7.31. Two phenotypes appear in an experiment in the numbers $4:16$. (a) How well does this sample fit a $3:1$ ratio? Would a sample with the same proportional deviation fit a $3:1$ ratio if it were (b) 10 times larger than (a), (c) 20 times larger than (a)?

7.32. The flowers of four o'clock plants may be red, pink, or white. Reds crossed to whites produced only pink offspring. When pink flowered plants were crossed they produced 113 red, 129 white, and 242 pink. It is hypothesized that these colors are produced by a single-gene locus with codominant alleles. Is this hypothesis acceptable on the basis of a chi-square test?

7.33. A heterozygous genetic condition called "creeper" in chickens produces shortened and deformed legs and wings, giving the bird a squatty appearance. Matings between creepers produced 775 creeper : 388 normal progeny. (a) Is the hypothesis of a $3:1$ ratio acceptable? (b) Does a $2:1$ ratio fit the data better? (c) What phenotype is probably produced by the gene for creeper when in homozygous condition?

7.34. Among fraternal (nonidentical, dizygotic) twins, the expected sex ratio is 1 MM : 2 MF : 1 FF (M = male, F = female). A sample from a sheep population contained 50 MM, 142 MF, and 61 FF twin pairs. (a) Do the data conform within statistically acceptable limits to the expectations? (b) If identical (monozygotic) twin pairs = total pairs − (2 × MF pairs), what do the data indicate concerning the frequency of monozygotic sheep twins?

7.35. Genetically pure white dogs, when testcrossed to brown dogs, produce an all-white F_1. Data on 190 F_2 progeny: 136 white, 41 black, 13 brown. These coat colors are postulated to be under the genetic control of two loci exhibiting dominant epistasis ($12:3:1$ ratio expected). (a) Test this hypothesis by chi-square. (b) When the F_1 was backcrossed to the brown parental type, the following numbers of phenotypes appeared among 70 progeny: 39 white, 19 black, 12 brown. Are these results consistent with the hypothesis?

7.36. Pure black rats, when testcrossed to albinos, produce only black F_1 offspring. The F_2 in one experiment was found to consist of 43 black, 14 cream, and 22 albino. The genetic control of these coat colors is postulated to involve two gene loci with recessive epistasis ($9:3:4$ ratio expected). Is the genetic hypothesis consistent with the data?

7.37. Colored aleurone in corn is hypothesized to be produced by the interaction of 2 dominant genes in the genotype A-C-; all other genotypes at these two loci produce colorless aleurone. A homozygous colored strain is testcrossed to a pure colorless strain. The F_1 exhibits only kernels with colored aleurone. The F_2 exhibits 3300 colored : 2460 colorless. Analyze the data by chi-square test.

7.38. The results of phenotypic analysis of 96 F_2 progeny in two replicate experiments is shown below.

Experiment	Phenotype 1	Phenotype 2
1	70	26
2	76	20

Calculate chi-square for each experiment assuming a (*a*) 3 : 1 ratio, (*b*) 13 : 3 ratio. (*c*) Which hypothesis is most consistent with the data?

7.39. A total of 320 families with six children each were surveyed with the results shown below. Does this distribution indicate that boys and girls are occurring with equal frequency?

No. of girls	6	5	4	3	2	1	0
No. of boys	0	1	2	3	4	5	6
No. of families	6	33	71	99	69	37	5

7.40. Yellowish-green corn seedlings are produced by a gene called "virescent-4" (v_4). A dark-brown color of the outer seed coat called "chocolate pericarp" is governed by a dominant gene Ch. A virescent-4 strain is crossed to a strain homogyzous for chocolate pericarp. The F_1 is then testcrossed. The resulting progeny are scored for phenotype with the following results: 216 green seedling, light pericarp : 287 green seedling, chocolate pericarp : 293 virescent seedling, light pericarp : 204 virescent seedling, chocolate pericarp. (*a*) Are these results compatible with the hypothesis of independent assortment? (*b*) Perform a genetic analysis of the data in the light of the results of part (*a*).

7.41. Purple anthocyanin pigment in tomato stems is governed by a dominant gene A, and its recessive allele a produces green stem. Hairy stem is governed by a dominant gene Hl, and hairless stem by its recessive allele hl. A dihybrid purple, hairy plant is testcrossed and produces 73 purple, hairy : 12 purple, hairless : 75 green, hairless : 9 green, hairy. (*a*) Is the F_1 purple : green ratio compatible with the expectation for alleles (i.e., a 1 : 1 ratio)? (*b*) Is the F_1 hairy : hairless ratio compatible with the expectation for alleles (i.e., a 1 : 1 ratio)? (*c*) Test the F_1 data for independent assortment (i.e., a 1 : 1 : 1 : 1 ratio). What conclusion do you reach?

7.42. In guinea pigs, it is hypothesized that a dominant allele L governs short hair and its recessive allele l governs long hair. Codominant alleles at an independently assorting locus are assumed to govern hair color, such that $C^y C^y$ = yellow, $C^y C^w$ = cream and $C^w C^w$ = white. From the cross $Ll\,C^y C^w \times Ll\,C^y C^w$, the following progeny were obtained: 50 short cream : 21 short yellow : 23 short white : 21 long cream : 7 long yellow : 6 long white. Are the data consistent with the genetic hypothesis?

Correction for Small Samples

7.43. A dominant gene in corn (Kn) results in the proliferation of vascular tissues in a trait called "knotted leaf." A heterozygous knotted leaf plant is testcrossed to a normal plant producing 153 knotted leaf and 178 normal progeny. Apply Yates' correction in the calculation of chi-square testing a 1 : 1 ratio. Are these results consistent with the hypothesis?

7.44. Observations of 30 : 3 in a genetic experiment are postulated to be in conformity with a 3 : 1 ratio. Is a 3 : 1 ratio acceptable at the 5% level on the basis of (*a*) an uncorrected chi-square test, (*b*) a corrected chi-square test?

Review Questions

Multiple-Choice Questions   Choose the one best answer.

For questions 1–4, use the following information. In guinea pigs, black (*B-*) is a dominant autosomal trait; white (*bb*) is the alternative recessive trait.

1. In families of size 3 from heterozygous parents, the probability of finding 2 black and 1 white progeny is
    (*a*) $\frac{3}{16}$ (*b*) $\frac{27}{64}$ (*c*) $\frac{3}{8}$ (*d*) $\frac{9}{16}$ (*e*) none of the above

2. In families of size 4 from the parental cross *Bb* × *bb*, the probability of finding equal numbers of black and white progeny is   (*a*) $\frac{3}{4}$ (*b*) $\frac{3}{16}$ (*c*) $\frac{1}{4}$ (*d*) $\frac{1}{2}$ (*e*) none of the above

3. In families of size 4 where both parents are heterozygous, the probability of finding the oldest offspring white and all others black is   (*a*) $\frac{27}{256}$ (*b*) $\frac{1}{8}$ (*c*) $\frac{3}{16}$ (*d*) $\frac{3}{64}$ (*e*) none of the above

4. In families of size 5 from heterozygous parents, the probability of finding 2 black males and 3 white females is   (*a*) $\frac{5}{32}$ (*b*) $\frac{64}{1024}$ (*c*) $\frac{8}{4096}$ (*d*) $\frac{64}{16,384}$ (*e*) none of the above

5. Given an autosomal locus with 6 alleles, how many heterozygous genotypes can be formed?   (*a*) 12   (*b*) 15   (*c*) 18   (*d*) 24   (*e*) none of the above

6. With reference to problem 5 above, approximately what percentage of all possible genotypes is represented by homozygotes?   (*a*) 12   (*b*) 18   (*c*) 24   (*d*) 29   (*e*) none of the above

7. Given 5 alleles at a sex-linked locus in humans, the number of different male genotypes possible is
    (*a*) 15   (*b*) 25   (*c*) 32   (*d*) 10   (*e*) none of the above

For questions 8–10, use the following information. In guinea pigs, black coat color is autosomally dominant to white. A heterozygous male is crossed to several heterozygous females and produces 4 white and 16 black progeny.

8. The expected numbers are   (*a*) 10 black and 10 white   (*b*) 17.5 black and 2.5 white   (*c*) 5 white and 15 black   (*d*) 3 black and 1 white   (*e*) none of the above

9. The chi-square value is   (*a*) 0.02   (*b*) 0.27   (*c*) 1.50   (*d*) 2.0   (*e*) none of the above

10. In answering this question, access to a chi-square table (such as Table 7.2) is required. The correct chi-square value for question 9 is
    (*a*) significant, calling for rejection of the null hypothesis
    (*b*) significant, allowing acceptance of the genetic hypothesis
    (*c*) nonsignificant, calling for the rejection of the genetic hypothesis
    (*d*) nonsignificant, allowing the acceptance of the null hypothesis
    (*e*) nonsignificant, invalidating the experimental results

Answers to Supplementary Problems

7.16.   (*a*) 90/1024   (*b*) 270/1024   (*c*) 405/1024   (*d*) 1/1024   **7.18.**   (*a*) $\frac{1}{2}$ (*b*) 1.0

7.17. $\frac{1}{4}$ **7.19.**   66

7.20. (a) (1) agouti × cinnamon (2) agouti × black (3) agouti × chocolate (4) agouti × albino (5) cinnamon × black (6) cinnamon × chocolate (7) cinnamon × albino (8) black × chocolate (9) black × albino (10) chocolate × albino

7.21. (a) 4 males : 4 females (b) 5th (c) 27.34%

7.22. (a) Males = 12; females = 78 (b) 936

7.23. $252(\frac{13}{16})^5(\frac{3}{16})^5 \cong 2.1\%$ by 4-place logarithms   **7.25.** 9.25%

7.24. 1215/65,536   **7.26.** $332,640/4,294,967,296 \cong 7.745 \times 10^{-5}$

7.27. (a) 5 cells in 10 milliliters = 0.5 cell/milliliter
(b) 0 = 0.006738; 1 = 0.033690; 2 = 0.084225; 3 = 0.140375; 4 = 0.175469
(c) 0.03 to 9.97
d) The fourth tube contains 500 cells. The 95% confidence limits = $500 \pm 2\sqrt{500} = 500 \pm 2(22.36) = 500 \pm 44.72$

7.28. (a) $100 \pm 2\sqrt{100} = 100 \pm 2(10) = 100 \pm 20$ or 20% error
(b) $10,000 \pm 2\sqrt{10,000} = 10,000 \pm 2(100) = 10,000 \pm 200 = 2\%$ error

7.29. 40%

7.30. (a) 1 (b) 3 (c) 2 (d) 2 (e) 3 (f) 7 (g) 7 (h) 2 (2 : 1 : 1 ratio expected; see "crossover suppression" in Chapter 6)

7.31. (a) $\chi^2 = 0.27$; $p = 0.5$–0.7; acceptable (b) $\chi^2 = 2.67$; $p = 0.1$–0.2; acceptable (c) $\chi^2 = 5.33$; $p = 0.01$–0.05; not acceptable.

7.32. Yes. $\chi^2 = 1.06$; $p = 0.5$–0.7; acceptable

7.33. (a) $\chi^2 = 43.37$; $p < 0.001$; not acceptable (b) $\chi^2 = 0.000421$; $p > 0.95$; a 2 : 1 ratio fits the data almost perfectly (c) Lethal

7.34. (a) $\chi^2 = 4.76$; $0.10 > p > 0.05$; hypothesis acceptable (b) Monozygotic twins are estimated to be -31; the negative estimate indicates that identical sheep twins are rare provided that unlike-sex twins do not have a survival advantage over like-sex twins.

7.35. (a) $\chi^2 = 1.22$; $p = 0.5$–0.7; acceptable (b) Yes; expected 2 : 1 : 1 ratio; $\chi^2 = 2.32$; $p = 0.3$–0.5

7.36. Yes; $\chi^2 = 0.35$; $p = 0.8$–0.9

7.37. 9 : 7 ratio expected; $\chi^2 = 2.54$; $p = 0.1$–0.2; genetic hypothesis is acceptable.

7.38. (a) *Experiment 1:* $\chi^2 = 0.22$; $p = 0.5$–0.7.   *Experiment 2:* $\chi^2 = 0.88$; $p = 0.3$–0.5.
(b) *Experiment 1:* $\chi^2 = 4.38$; $p = 0.05$–0.01.   *Experiment 2:* $\chi^2 = 0.27$; $p = 0.5$–0.7.
(c) 3 : 1 ratio

7.39. Yes. $\chi^2 = 2.83$; $p = 0.8$–0.9; the distribution is consistent with the assumption that boys and girls occur with equal frequency.

7.40. (a) No. $\chi^2 = 25.96$; $p < 0.001$ (b) v_4 is linked to Ch, exhibiting approximately 42% recombination

7.41. (a) Yes. $\chi^2 = 0.006$; $p = 0.90$–0.95 (b) Yes. $\chi^2 = 0.148$; $p =$ approx. 0.7 (c) $\chi^2 = 95.6$; $p < 0.001$; the observations do not conform to a 1 : 1 : 1 : 1 ratio, therefore genes a and hl are probably linked.

7.42.   Yes; $\chi^2 = 2.69$; $p = 0.7$–0.8

7.43.   Yes; $\chi^2 = 1.74$; $p = 0.1$–0.2

7.44.   (a) No. $\chi^2 = 4.45$; $p < 0.05$ (b) Yes. $\chi^2 = 3.64$; $p > 0.05$

Answers to Review Questions

1. *b*   2. *e* $\left(\frac{3}{8}\right)$ 3. *a*   4. *e* $\left(\frac{90}{1024}\right)$ 5. *b*   6. *d*   7. *e* (5)   8. *c*   9. *b*   10. *d*

Chapter 8

Cytogenetics

THE UNION OF CYTOLOGY WITH GENETICS

Perhaps one reason Mendel's discoveries were not appreciated by the scientific community of his day (1865) was that the mechanics of mitosis and meiosis had not yet been discovered. During the years 1870–1900 rapid advances were made in the study of cells (**cytology**). At the turn of the century, when Mendel's laws were rediscovered, the cytological basis was available to render the statistical laws of genetics intelligible in terms of physical units. **Cytogenetics** is the hybrid science which attempts to correlate cellular events, especially those of the chromosomes, with genetic phenomena.

VARIATION IN CHROMOSOME NUMBER

Each species has a characteristic number of chromosomes. Most higher organisms are diploid, with two sets of homologous chromosomes: one set donated by the father, the other set by the mother. Variation in the number of sets of chromosomes (**ploidy**) is commonly encountered in nature. It is estimated that one-third of the angiosperms (flowering plants) have more than two sets of chromosomes (polyploid). The term **euploidy** is applied by organisms with chromosomes that are multiples of some basic number (n).

1. Euploidy.

(*a*) *Monoploid.* One set of chromosomes (n) is characteristically found in the nuclei of some lower organisms such as fungi. Monoploids in higher organisms are usually smaller and less vigorous than the normal diploids. Few monoploid animals survive. A notable exception exists in male bees and wasps. Monoploid plants are known but are usually sterile.

(*b*) *Triploid.* Three sets of chromosomes ($3n$) can originate by the union of a monoploid gamete (n) with a diploid gamete ($2n$). The extra set of chromosomes of the triploid is distributed in various combinations to the germ cells, resulting in genetically unbalanced gametes. Because of the sterility that characterizes triploids, they are not commonly found in natural populations.

(*c*) *Tetraploid.* Four sets of chromosomes ($4n$) can arise in body cells by the somatic doubling of the chromosome number. Doubling is accomplished either spontaneously or it can be induced in high frequency by exposure to chemicals such as the alkaloid colchicine. Tetraploids are also produced by the union of unreduced diploid ($2n$) gametes.

    (i) **Autotetraploid.** The prefix "auto" indicates that the ploidy involves only homologous chromosome sets. Somatic doubling of a diploid produces four sets of homologous chromosomes (autotetraploid). Union of unreduced diploid gametes from the same species would accomplish the same result. Meiotic chromosome pairing usually produces quadrivalents (4 synapsing chromosomes) that can produce genetically balanced gametes if **disjunction** is by 2s, i.e., 2 chromosomes of the quadrivalent going to one pole and the other 2 to the opposite pole. If disjunction is not stabilized in this fashion for all quadrivalents, the gametes will be genetically unbalanced. Sterility will be expressed in proportion to the production of unbalanced gametes.

    (ii) **Allotetraploid.** The prefix "allo" indicates that nonhomologous sets of chromosomes are involved. The union of unreduced ($2n$) gametes from different diploid species could produce, in one step, an allotetraploid that appears and behaves like a new species. Alternatively, two diploid plant species may hybridize to produce a sterile diploid F_1. The sterility results from the failure of each set of chromosomes to provide sufficient genetic homology to affect pairing. The sterile diploid can become fertile if it undergoes doubling of the chromosome number. The allotetraploid thus produced has two matched sets of chromosomes that can pair just as effectively as in the diploid. Double diploids of this kind, found only in plants, are called **amphidiploids.**

Example 8.1. Let the diploid set of chromosomes of one species be *AA* and that of the other species be *BB*.

$$P: \qquad AA \quad \times \quad BB$$

$$F_1: \qquad AB \quad \text{(sterile hybrid)}$$
$$\downarrow \quad \text{(chromosome doubling)}$$

$$\text{Amphidiploid:} \qquad AABB \quad \text{(fertile)}$$

(d) **Polyploid.** This term can be applied to any cell with more than $2n$ chromosomes. Ploidy levels higher than tetraploid are not commonly encountered in natural populations, but some of our most important crops are polyploid. For example, common bread wheat is hexaploid ($6n$), some strawberries are octaploid ($8n$), etc. Some triploids as well as tetraploids exhibit a more robust phenotype than their diploid counterparts, often having larger leaves, flowers, and fruits **(gigantism).** Many commercial fruits and ornamentals are polyploids. Sometimes a specialized tissue within a diploid organism will be polyploid. For example, some liver cells of humans are polyploid. A common polyploid with which the reader should already be familiar is the triploid endosperm tissue of corn and other grains. Polyploids offer an opportunity for studying **dosage effects,** i.e., how two or more alleles of one locus behave in the presence of a single dose of an alternative allele. "Dominance" refers to the masking effect that one allele has over another allele. When one allele in the pollen is able to mask the effect of a double dose of another allele in the resulting endosperm, the former is said to exhibit **xenia** over the latter.

Example 8.2. In corn, starchy endosperm is governed by a gene *S* that shows xenia with respect to its allele for sugary endosperm (*s*). Four genotypes are possible for these triploid cells: starchy = *SSS, SSs, Sss*; sugary = *sss*.

The term *haploid*, strictly applied, refers to the gametic chromosome number. For diploids ($2n$) the haploid number is n; for an allotetraploid ($4n$) the haploid (reduced) number is $2n$; for an allohexaploid ($6n$) the haploid number is $3n$; etc. Lower organisms such as bacteria and viruses are called haploids because they have a single set of genetic elements. However, since they do not form gametes comparable to those of higher organisms, the term "monoploid" would seem to be more appropriate.

2. Aneuploidy.

Variations in chromosome number may occur that do not involve whole sets of chromosomes, but only parts of a set. The term **aneuploidy** is given to variations of this nature, and the suffix "-somic" is a part of their nomenclature.

(a) **Monosomic.** Diploid organisms that are missing one chromosome of a single pair are monosomics with the genomic formula $2n - 1$. The single chromosome without a pairing partner may go to either pole during meiosis, but more frequently will lag at anaphase and fails to be included in either nucleus. Monosomics can thus form two kinds of gametes, (n) and ($n - 1$). In plants, the $n - 1$ gametes seldom function. In animals, loss of one whole chromosome often results in genetic unbalance, which is manifested by high mortality or reduced fertility.

(b) **Trisomic.** Diploids which have one extra chromosome are represented by the chromosomal formula $2n + 1$. One of the pairs of chromosomes has an extra member, so that a trivalent structure may be formed during meiotic prophase. If 2 chromosomes of the trivalent go to one pole and the third goes to the opposite pole, then gametes will be ($n + 1$) and (n), respectively. Trisomy can produce different phenotypes, depending upon which chromosome of the complement is present in triplicate. In humans, the presence of one small extra chromosome (autosome 21) has a very deleterious effect resulting in Down syndrome, formerly called "mongolism."

(c) **Tetrasomic.** When one chromosome of an otherwise diploid organism is present in quadruplicate, this is expressed as $2n + 2$. A quadrivalent may form for this particular chromosome during meiosis which then has the same problem as that discussed for autotetraploids.

(d) **Double Trisomic.** If 2 different chromosomes are each represented in triplicate, the double trisomic can be symbolized as $2n + 1 + 1$.

(e) **Nullosomic.** An organism that has lost a chromosome pair is a nullosomic. The result is usually lethal to diploids $(2n - 2)$. Some polyploids, however, can lose 2 homologues of a set and still survive. For example, several nullosomics of hexaploid wheat $(6n - 2)$ exhibit reduced vigor and fertility but can survive to maturity because of the genetic redundancy in polyploids.

VARIATION IN CHROMOSOME SIZE

In general, chromosomes of most organisms are too small and too numerous to be considered as good subjects for cytological investigation. *Drosophila* was considered to be a favorable organism for genetic studies because it produces large numbers of progeny within the confines of a small bottle in a short interval of time. Many distinctive phenotypes can be recognized in laboratory strains. It was soon discovered that crossing over does not occur in male fruit flies, thereby making it especially useful for genetic analyses. Later, its unusual sex mechanism was found to be a balance between male determiners on the autosomes and female determiners on the sex chromosomes. Although it had been known for over 30 years that some species of dipterans had extra large chromosomes in certain organs of the body, their utility in cytogenetic studies of *Drosophila* was not recognized until about 1934. There are only four pairs of chromosomes in the diploid complement of *D. melanogaster,* but their size in reproductive cells and most body cells is quite small. Unusually large chromosomes, 100 times as large as those in other parts of the body, are found in the larval salivary gland cells. Each giant **polytene** chromosome (Fig. 8-1) is composed of hundreds of chromatids paired along their identical DNA sequences throughout their length. Furthermore, each pair of homologous polytene chromosomes is also constantly synapsed in these somatic cells. Distinctive crossbandings (appearing when chromosomes are stained) represent regions (called **chromomeres**) of the chromatid bundle containing highly coiled or condensed DNA that is interspersed between regions of less condensation. The crossbanding pattern of each chromosome is characteristic of each species, but the pattern may change in a precise sequence at various stages of development. Chromosomal aberrations (translocations, inversions, duplications, deletions, etc.) can often be easily recognized in these polytene chromosomes under the light microscope.

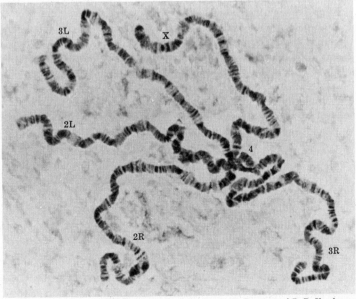

Courtesy of B. P. Kaufmann

Fig. 8-1.   Salivary gland chromosomes of *Drosophila melanogaster*

VARIATION IN THE ARRANGEMENT OF CHROMOSOME SEGMENTS

1. Translocations.

Chromosomes occasionally undergo spontaneous rupture, or can be induced to rupture in high frequency by ionizing radiation. The broken ends of such chromosomes behave as though they were "sticky" and may rejoin into nonhomologous combinations (**translocations**). A reciprocal translocation involves the exchange of segments between 2 nonhomologous chromosomes. During meiosis, an individual that is structurally heterozygous for a reciprocal translocation (i.e., 2 structually normal chromosomes and 2 chromosomes that are attached to nonhomologous pieces, as shown in Example 8.3) must form a cross-shaped configuration in order to affect pairing or synapsis of all homologous segments. A structural heterozygote may or may not be genetically heterozygous at one or more loci, but this is of no concern for the present purpose. In many of the following diagrams, only chromosomes (not chromatids) are shown and centromeres are omitted for the sake of simplicity.

Example 8.3.   Assume that a reciprocal translocation occurs between chromosomes 1-2 and 3-4.

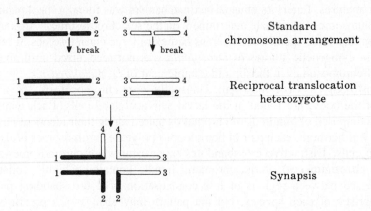

The only way that functional gametes can be formed from a translocation heterozygote is by the alternate disjunction of chromosomes.

Example 8.4.   At the end of the meiotic prophase begun in Example 8.3, a ring of 4 chromosomes is formed. If the adjacent chromosomes move to the poles as indicated in the diagram below, all of the gametes will contain some extra segments (duplications) and some pieces will be missing (deficiencies).

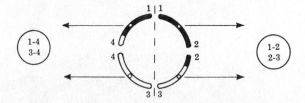

Example 8.5.   By forming a "figure-8," alternate disjunction produces functional gametes.

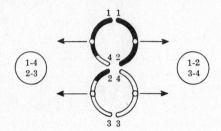

Translocation heterozygotes have several distinctive manifestations. (1) If an organism produces gametes with equal facility by either segregation of adjacent chromosomes (Example 8.4) or by alternate chromosomes (Example 8.5), semisterility occurs because only the latter mechanism produces functional gametes. (2) Some genes that formerly were on nonhomologous chromosomes will no longer appear to be assorting independently. (3) The phenotypic expression of a gene may be modified when it is translocated to a new position in the genome. **Position effects** are particularly evident when genes in euchromatin (lightly staining areas usually containing genetic elements) are shifted near heterochromatic regions (darker staining areas presumably devoid of active genes).

(a) ***Translocation Complexes.***   In the evening primrose of the genus *Oenothera,* an unusual series of reciprocal translocations has occurred involving all 7 of its chromosome pairs. If we label each chromosome end with a different number, the normal set of 7 chromosomes would be 1-2, 3-4, 5-6, 7-8, 9-10, 11-12, and 13-14; a translocation set would be 2-3, 4-5, 6-7, 8-9, 10-11, 12-13, and 14-1. A multiple translocation heterozygote like this would form a ring of 14 chromosomes during meiosis. Different lethals in each of the two haploid sets of 7 chromosomes enforces structural heterozygosity. Since only alternate segregation from the ring can form viable gametes, each group of 7 chromosomes behaves as though it were a single large linkage group with recombination confined to the pairing ends of each chromosome. Each set of 7 chromosomes that is inherited as a single unit is called a **Renner complex.**

> **Example 8.6.**   In *Oenothera lamarckiana,* one of the Renner complexes is called *gaudens* and the other is called *velans*. This species is largely self-pollinated. The lethals become effective in the zygotic stage so that only the *gaudens-velans* (G-V) zygotes are viable. *Gaudens-gaudens* (G-G) or *velans-velans* (V-V) zygotes are lethal.

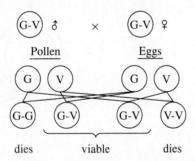

> **Example 8.7.**   The two complexes in *O. muricata* are called *rigens* (R) and *curvans* (C). Gametic lethals in each complex act differentially in the gametophytes. Pollen with the *rigens* complex are inactive; eggs with the *curvans* complex are inhibited. Only the *curvans* pollen and the *rigens* eggs are functional to give the *rigens-curvans* complex in the zygote.

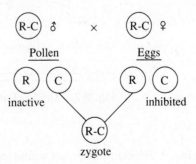

2. Inversions.

Assume that the normal order of segments within a chromosome is (1-2-3-4-5-6) and that breaks occur in regions 2-3 and 5-6, and that the broken piece is reinserted in reverse order. The inverted chromosome now has segments (1-2-5-4-3-6). One way in which inversions might arise is shown in Fig. 8-2. An inversion heterozygote has one chromosome in the inverted order and its homologue in the normal order. During meiosis the synaptic configuration attempts to maximize the pairing between homologous regions in the 2 chromosomes. This is usually accomplished by a loop in one of the chromosomes. Crossing over within the inverted segment gives rise to crossover gametes which are inviable because of duplications and deficiencies. Chromatids that are not involved in crossing over will be viable. Thus as we have seen with translocations, inversions produce semisterility and altered linkage relationships. Inversions are sometimes called "crossover suppressors." Actually they do not prevent crossovers from occurring but they do prevent the crossover products from functioning. Genes within the inverted segment are thus held together and transmitted as one large linked group. Balanced lethal systems (Chapter 6) involve either a translocation or an inversion to prevent the recovery of crossover products and thus maintain heterozygosity generation after generation. In some organisms, these "inversions" have a selective advantage under certain environmental conditions and become more prevalent in the population than the standard chromosome order. Two types of inversion heterozygotes will be considered in which crossing over occurs within the inverted segment.

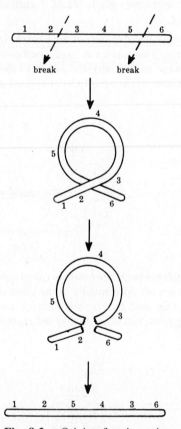

Fig. 8-2. Origin of an inversion.

(a) *Pericentric Inversion.* The centromere lies within the inverted region. First meiotic anaphase figures appear normal unless crossing over occurs within the inversion. If a single 2-strand crossover occurs within the inversion, the 2 chromatids of each chromosome will usually have arms of unequal length (unless there are chromosome segments of equal length on opposite sides of the inversion). Half of the meiotic products in this case (resulting from crossing over) are expected to contain duplications and deficiencies and would most likely be nonfunctional. The other half of the gametes (noncrossovers) are functional; one-quarter have the normal segmental order, one-quarter have the inverted arrangement.

Example 8.8. Assume an inversion heterozygote as shown below with crossing over in region 3-4.

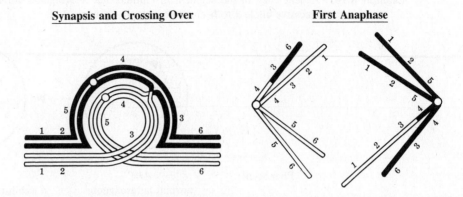

Synapsis and Crossing Over	First Anaphase

(b) *Paracentric Inversion.* The centromere lies outside the inverted segment. Crossing over within the inverted segment produces a **dicentric** chromosome (possessing 2 centromeres) that forms a **bridge** from one pole to the other during first anaphase. The bridge will rupture somewhere along its length and the resulting fragments will contain duplications and/or deficiencies. Also, an **acentric** fragment (without a centromere) will be formed; and since it usually fails to move to either pole, it will not be included in the meiotic products. Again, half of the products are nonfunctional, one-quarter are functional with a normal chromosome, and one-quarter are functional with an inverted chromosome.

Example 8.9. Assume an inversion heterozygote as shown below with crossing over in region 4-5.

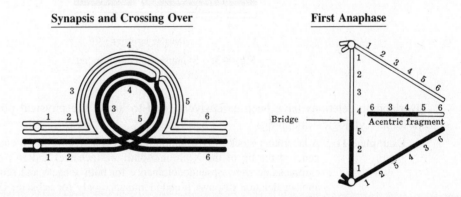

Synapsis and Crossing Over	First Anaphase

VARIATION IN THE NUMBER OF CHROMOSOMAL SEGMENTS

1. Deletions (Deficiencies).

Loss of a chromosomal segment may be so small that it includes only a single gene or part of a gene. In this case the phenotypic effects may resemble those of a mutant allele at that locus. For example, the "notch" phenotype of *Drosophila* discussed in Problem 5.4, is a sex-linked deletion which acts like a dominant mutation; a deletion at another sex-linked locus behaves as a recessive mutation, producing yellow body color when homozygous. Deletions never backmutate to the normal condition, because a lost piece of chromosome cannot be replaced. In this way, as well as others to be explained in subsequent chapters, a deletion can be distinguished from a gene mutation. A loss of any considerable portion of a chromosome is usually lethal to a diploid organism because of genetic unbalance. When an organism heterozygous for a pair of alleles, *A* and *a*, loses a small portion of the chromosome bearing the dominant allele, the recessive allele on the other chromosome will become expressed phenotypically. This is called **pseudodominance,** but it is a misnomer because the condition is hemizygous rather than dizygous at this locus.

> **Example 8.10.**   A deficiency in the segment of chromosome bearing the dominant gene *A* allows the recessive allele *a* to become phenotypically expressed.

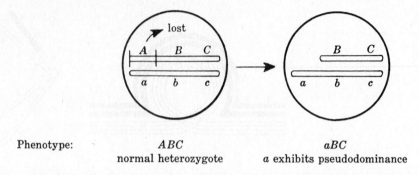

Phenotype: *ABC*   *aBC*
                 normal heterozygote   *a* exhibits pseudodominance

A deletion heterozygote may be detected cytologically during meiotic prophase when the forces of pairing cause the normal chromosome segment to bulge away from the region in which the deletion occurs (Fig. 8-3).

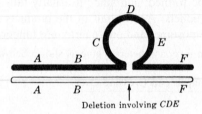

Fig. 8-3.   Synapsis in a deletion heterozygote.

Overlapping deletions have been extensively used to locate the physical position of genes in the chromosome (cytological mapping).

> **Example 8.11.**   A laboratory stock of *Drosophila* females is heterozygous in coupling phase for 2 linked genes at the tip of the X chromosome, *ac* (achaete) and *sc* (scute). A deletion in one chromosome shows pseudodominance for both achaete and scute. In other individuals, another deletion displays pseudodominance only for achaete. Obviously, these two deletions overlap. In the giant chromosomes of *Drosophila*, the absence of these segments of chromosome is easily seen. The actual location of the scute gene resides in the band or bands which differentiate the two overlapping deletions.

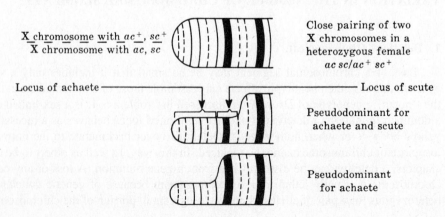

2. Duplications (Additions).

Extra segments in a chromosome may arise in a variety of ways. Generally speaking, their presence is not as deleterious to the organism as a deficiency. It is assumed that some duplications are useful in the evolution of new genetic material. Because the old genes can continue to provide for the present requirements of the organism, the superfluous genes may be free to mutate to new forms without a loss in immediate adaptability. Genetic redundancy, of which this is one type, may protect the organism from the effects of a deleterious recessive gene or from an otherwise lethal deletion. During meiotic pairing the chromosome bearing the duplicated segment bulges away from its normal homologue to maximize the juxtaposition of homologous regions. In some cases, extra genetic material is known to cause a distinct phenotypic effect. Relocation of chromosomal material without altering its quantity may result in an altered phenotype (position effect).

Example 8.12. A reduced eye size in *Drosophila*, called ''bar eye,'' is known to be associated with a duplicated region on the X chromosome. Genetically the duplication behaves as a dominant factor. Wild-type flies arise in homozygous bar-eye cultures with a frequency of about 1 in 1600. With approximately the same frequency, a very small eye called ''double-bar'' is also produced. These unusual phenotypes apparently arise in a pure bar culture by improper synapsis and unequal crossing over as shown below, where the region (*a-b-c-d*) is a duplication.

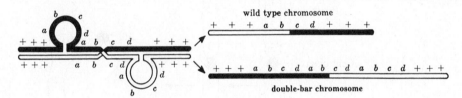

VARIATION IN CHROMOSOME MORPHOLOGY

1. Isochromosomes.

It has already been shown that a translocation can change the structure of the chromosome both genetically and morphologically. The length of the chromosome may be longer or shorter, depending upon the size of the translocated piece. An inversion does not normally change the length of the chromosome, but if the inversion includes the centromere (pericentric), the position of the centromere may be changed considerably. Deletions or duplications, if viable, may sometimes be detected cytologically by a change in the size of the chromosome (or banding pattern in the case of the giant chromosomes of *Drosophila*), or by the presence of ''bulges'' in the pairing figure. Chromosomes with unequal arm lengths may be changed to **isochromosomes** having arms of equal length and genetically homologous with each other, by an abnormal transverse division of the centromere. The telocentric X chromosome of *Drosophila* may be changed to an ''attached-X'' form by a misdivision of the centromere (Fig. 8-4).

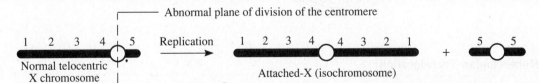

Fig. 8-4. Origin of attached-X chromosome. Segment 5 is nonessential heterochromatin.

2. Bridge-Breakage-Fusion-Bridge Cycles.

The shape of a chromosome may change at each division once it has broken. Following replication of a broken chromosome, the broken ends of the sister chromatids may be fused by DNA repair mechanisms. Such broken ends are said to be ''sticky.'' When the chromatids move to opposite poles, a bridge is formed. The bridge will break somewhere along its length and the cycle repeats at the next division. This sequence of events is called the **bridge-breakage-fusion-bridge cycle.** Mosaic tissue appearing as irregular patches of an unexpected phenotype on a background of normal tissue **(variegation)** can be produced by such a cycle. The size of the unusual tissue generally bears an inverse relationship to the period of development at which the original break occurred; i.e., the earlier the break occurs, the larger will be the size of the abnormal tissue.

3. Ring Chromosomes.

Chromosomes are not always rod-shaped. Occasionally **ring chromosomes** are encountered in plants or animals. If breaks occur at each end of a chromosome, the broken ends may become joined to form a ring chromosome (Fig. 8-5). If an acentric fragment is formed by union of the end pieces, it will soon be lost. The phenotypic consequences of these deletions vary, depending on the specific genes involved. Crossing over between ring chromosomes can lead to bizarre anaphase figures.

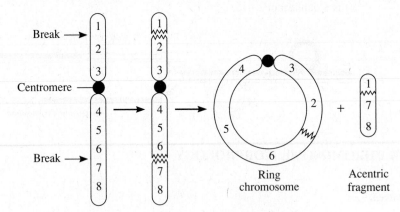

Fig. 8-5.   Formation of a ring chromosome.

Example 8.13.   A single exchange in a ring homozygote produces a double bridge at first anaphase.

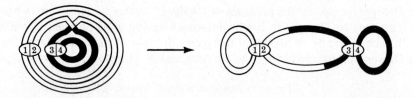

4. Robertsonian Translocation.

A whole arm fusion **(Robertsonian translocation)** is an eucentric, reciprocal translocation between 2 acrocentric chromosomes where the break in one chromosome is near the front of the centromere and the break in the other chromosome is immediately behind its centromere. The smaller chromosome thus formed consists of largely inert heterochromatic material near the centromeres; it usually carries no essential genes and tends to become lost. A Robertsonian translocation thus results in a reduction of the chromosome number (Fig. 8-6).

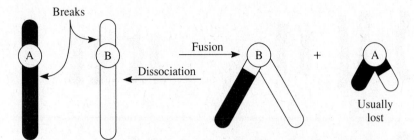

Fig. 8-6. Formation of a metacentric chromosome by fusion of two acrocentric chromosomes (Robertsonian translocation). Dissociation is
not possible if the small chromosome is lost.

Example 8.14. Humans have 46 chromosomes whereas the great apes (chimpanzees, gorillas, and orang-
utans) have 48. It seems likely that humans evolved from a common human/ape ancestor
by (among other structural changes) centric fusion of two acrocentrics to produce a single
large chromosome (2) containing the combined genetic content of the two acrocentrics.
Structural rearrangements of chromosomes may lead to reproductive isolation and the
formation of new species. The mule is a hybrid from crossing the horse ($2n = 64$) and
the ass or donkey ($2n = 62$). The mule is sterile because there is insufficient homology
between the two sets of chromosomes to pair successfully at meiosis.

HUMAN CYTOGENETICS

The diploid human chromosome number of 46 (23 pairs) was established by Tjio and Levan in 1956.
When grouped as homologous pairs, the somatic chromosome complement **(karyotype)** of a cell becomes
an **idiogram.** Formerly, a chromosome could be distinguished only by its length and the position of its
centromere at the time of maximum condensation (late prophase). No single autosome could be easily
identified, but a chromosome could be assigned to one of seven groups (A–G) according to the "Denver
system" of classification (Fig. 8-7). Group A consists of large, metacentric chromosomes (1-3); group
B contains submedian chromosomes (4-5); group C has medium-sized chromosomes with submedian
centromeres (pairs 6-12); group D consists of medium-sized chromosomes (pairs 13-15) with one very
short arm (acrocentric); chromosomes in group E (16-18) are a little shorter than in group D with median
or submedian centromeres; group F (19-20) contains short, metacentric chromosomes; and group G has
the smallest acrocentric chromosomes (21, 22). The X and Y sex chromosomes are not members of the
autosome groups, and are usually placed together in one part of the idiogram. The Y chromosome may
vary in size from one individual to another but usually has the appearance of G-group autosomes. The
X chromosome has the appearance of a group C autosome.

More recently, special staining techniques (e.g., Giemsa, quinacrine) have revealed specific banding
patterns (G bands, Q bands, etc.) for each chromosome, allowing individual identification of each
chromosome in the karyotype (Fig. 8-8).

The X chromosome can be identified in many nondividing (interphase) cells of females as a dark-
staining mass called **sex chromatin** or **Barr body** (after Dr. Murray L. Barr) attached to the nuclear
membrane. The analogue of sex chromatin in certain white blood cells is a "drumstick" appendage
attached to the multilobed nucleus of neutrophilic leukocytes. Dr. Mary Lyon theorizes that sex chromatin
results from condensation [**heterochromatinization** (darkly stained)] and inactivation of any X chromosomes in excess of one per cell. Sex-linked traits are not expressed more intensely in females with
two doses of X-linked genes than in males with only 1 X chromosome. At a particular stage early in
development of females, 1 of the 2 X chromosomes in a cell becomes inactivated as a **dosage compensation**
mechanism. Different cells inactivate 1 of the 2 chromosomes in an apparently random manner, but
subsequently all derived cells retain the same functional chromosome. Females are thus a mixture of two

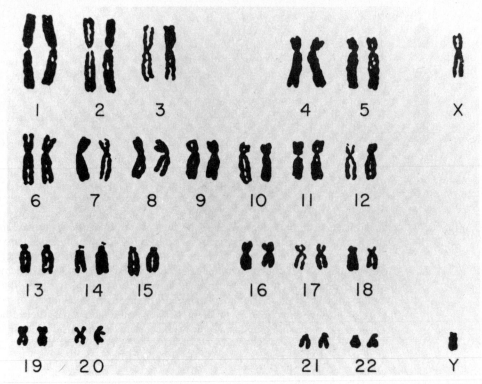

Fig. 8-7. Karyotype of the chromosomes of a normal human male. [From L. P. Wisniewski and K. Hirschhorn (eds.), *A Guide to Human Chromosome Defects,* 2nd ed., The March of Dimes Birth Defects Foundation, White Plains, N.Y.; BD:OAS XVI(6), 1980, with permission.]

kinds of cells; in some cells 1 X chromosome is active, and in different cells the other X chromosome is active. The same principle applied to mammals other than humans.

Prenatal screening of babies for gross chromosomal aberrations (polyploidy, aneuploidy, deletions, translocations, etc.), as well as sex prediction, is now possible. A fluid sample can be taken from the "bag of water" (**amnion**) surrounding the fetus *in utero,* a process termed **amniocentesis.** The cells found in amniotic fluid are of fetal origin. Such cells can be cultured *in vitro* in a highly nutritive solution,

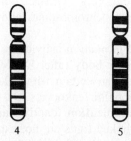

Fig. 8-8. Diagrams of the banding patterns that distinguish human chromosomes 4 and 5.

treated with colchicine to stop division at metaphase, subjected to a hypotonic salt solution to cause the cells to swell and scatter the chromosomes, placed on a slide, stained, and photographed under a microscope. Individual chromosomes are then cut from the resulting photograph and matched as homologous pairs to form an idiogram.

Example 8.15. Aneuploid females with only one X chromosome (XO) have a karyotype with $2n - 1 = 45$. They are called **Turner females** (after Henry Turner, who first described them), and they exhibit a group of characteristics that together define **Turner syndrome:** short stature, webbing of neck skin, underdeveloped gonads, shieldlike chest, and impaired intelligence. Turner females are sex-chromatin-negative.

Example 8.16. Abnormal males possessing an extra X chromosome (XXY) have a karyotype with $2n + 1 = 47$. They are called **Klinefelter males** (after Harry Klinefelter, who first described them), and they exhibit **Klinefelter syndrome:** sterility, long limbs, feminine breast development (gynecomastia), sparse body hair, and mental deficiency. Klinefelter males are sex-chromatin-positive. If some portion of the extra X chromosome is not inactivated, this could account for the phenotypic differences not only between XXY Klinefelter males and XY normal males but also between XO Turner females and XX normal females.

Example 8.17. XXX "superfemales" **(metafemales)** are karyotyped as $2n + 1 = 47$ trisomics and exhibit two Barr bodies. These individuals may range phenotypically from normal fertile females to nearly like those with **Turner syndrome.** They have a high incidence of mental retardation.

Example 8.18. Tall, trisomic XYY males were first discovered in relatively high frequencies in penal and mental institutions. The presence of an extra Y chromosome was thought to predispose such a male to antisocial behavior, hence the name "tall-aggressive syndrome." Subsequently, more XYY males have been found among the noninstitutionalized population, casting doubt upon the validity of the above hypothesis. XYY males do tend to have subnormal IQs, however, and this may contribute to impulsive behavior.

Example 8.19. **Down syndrome** (named after the physician Langdon Down and formerly called mongolism or mongolian idiocy) is usually associated with a trisomic condition for one of the smallest human autosomes (21). It is the most common chromosomal abnormality in live births (1/600 births). These unfortunate individuals are mentally retarded, short, possessing eye folds resembling those of Mongolian races, have stubby fingers and a swollen tongue. Women over 45 years of age are about 20 times more likely to give birth to a child with Down syndrome than are women aged 20. Nondisjunction of chromosome pair 21 during spermatogenesis can also produce a child with Down syndrome, but paternal age does not seem to be associated with its incidence. In about 2–5% of the cases, the normal chromosome number is present ($2n = 46$), but the extra chromosome 21 is attached (translocated) to one of the larger autosomes.

Example 8.20. Human autosomal monosomics are rarer than trisomics, possibly because harmful recessive mutants on the remaining homologue are hemizygous and can be expressed. Most cases of autosomal monosomy are mosaics of normal diploid ($2n$) and monosomic ($2n - 1$) cells resulting from *mitotic* nondisjunctions. Mosaics involving sex chromosomes are also known: e.g., XO:XX, XO:XY, XXY:XX, as well as autosomal mosaics such as 21-21:21-21-21, etc.

Example 8.21. Babies missing a portion of the short arm of chromosome 5 have a distinctive catlike cry; hence the French name *cri du chat* ("cry of the cat") syndrome. They also are mentally retarded, have moon faces, saddle noses, small mandibles (micrognathia), and malformed, low-set ears.

Example 8.22. Deletion of part of the long arm of chromosome 22 produces an abnormality known as a **Philadelphia chromosome** (so named because it was discovered in that city). It is found only in the bone marrow (along with chromosomally normal cells) in approximately 90% of patients with chronic myelocytic leukemia (a kind of cancer). Usually the missing piece of chromosome 22 can be found translocated to one of the larger autosomes (most frequently chromosome 9). See Example 14.34.

Solved Problems

Variation in Chromosome Numbers

8.1. Suppose that an autotetraploid of genotype *AAaa* forms only diploid gametes by random assortment from the quadrivalents (formed by synapsis of 4 chromosomes) during meiosis. Recall that chromosomes separate during the first meiotic division; sister chromatids separate during the second meiotic division. The A locus is so close to the centromere that crossing over in this region is negligible. (*a*) Determine the expected frequencies of zygotic genotypes produced by selfing the autotetraploid. (*b*) Calculate the expected reduction in the frequency of progeny with a recessive phenotype in comparison with that of a selfed diploid of genotype *Aa*.

Solution:

(*a*) Let us identify each of the 4 genes as follows: A^1, A^2, a^1, a^2 (A^1 and A^2 represent identical dominant alleles; a^1 and a^2 represent identical recessive alleles at the A locus).

For genes that are tightly linked to their centromeres, the distribution of alleles into gametes follows the same pattern as chromosomal assortment. Let us first use a checkerboard to determine the kinds and frequencies of different combinations of alleles in pairs expected in the diploid gametes of the autotetraploid.

	A^1	A^2	a^1	a^2
A^1	—	A^1A^2	A^1a^1	A^1a^2
A^2		—	A^2a^1	A^2a^2
a^1			—	a^1a^2
a^2				—

Because sister chromotids separate at meiosis II, the diagonal of the above table represents the nonexistent possibility of a given chromosome (or identical allele) with itself in a gamete. The table is symmetrical on either side of the diagonal. Ignoring the superscript identification of alleles, the expected ratio of possible diploid gametes is 1 *AA* : 4 *Aa* : 1 *aa* = 1/6 *AA* : 2/3 *Aa* : 1/6 *aa*. Using these diploid gametic expectations, let us now construct a zygotic checkerboard for the prediction of tetraploid progeny genotypes.

	1/6 *AA*	2/3 *Aa*	1/6 *aa*
1/6 *AA*	1/36 *AAAA*	2/18 *AAAa*	1/36 *AAaa*
2/3 *Aa*	2/18 *AAAa*	4/9 *AAaa*	2/18 *Aaaa*
1/6 *aa*	1/36 *AAaa*	2/18 *Aaaa*	1/36 *aaaa*

Ratio of offspring genotypes: 1/36 *AAAA* (quadruplex) : 8/36 *AAAa* (triplex) : 18/36 *AAaa* (duplex) : 8/36 *Aaaa* (simplex) : 1/36 *aaaa* (nulliplex).

(*b*) If one dose of the dominant allele is sufficient to phenotypically mask one or more doses of the recessive allele, then the phenotypic ratio is expected to be 35*A* : 1*a*. One-quarter of the offspring of a selfed diploid heterozygote (*Aa*) is expected to be of the recessive phenotype. The reduction in the frequency of the recessive trait is from 1/4 to 1/36, or ninefold. When homozygous genotypes produce a less desirable phenotype than heterozygotes, polyploidy can act as a buffer to reduce the incidence of homozygotes.

8.2.   Assume that an autotetraploid of genotype $AAaa$ has the A locus 50 or more map units from the centromere, so that the equivalent of a single crossover always occurs between the centromere and the A locus. In this case, the *chromatids* will assort independently. Further assume that random assortment of chromatids to the gametes occurs by 2s. Determine (*a*) the expected genotypic ratio of the progeny that results from selfing this autotetraploid, and (*b*) the expected increase in the incidence of heterozygous genotypes compared with selfed diploids of genotype Aa.

Solution:

(*a*)   Let each of the genes of the duplex tetraploid be labeled as shown in the illustration below. All capital letters represent identical dominant genes; all lowercase letters represent identical recessive alleles. As

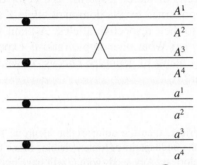

in Problem 8.1, let us first use a checkerboard to determine the kinds and frequencies of different combinations of alleles (in pairs) expected in the gametes of the autotetraploid. Note in the illustration that (for example) alleles A^1 and A^2, originally on sister chromatids, can enter the same gamete if crossing over occurs between the centromere and the A locus. Likewise, any other pair of alleles could enter a gamete by the same mechanism (chromatid assortment). Random assortment (by 2s) of 8 chromatids of the autotetraploid during meiosis is shown in the following table. Note that the diagonal of the table represents the nonsense union of any given allele with itself (e.g., A^1 with A^1). The table is symmetrical on either side of the diagonal.

	A^1	A^2	A^3	A^4	a^1	a^2	a^3	a^4
A^1	—	A^1A^2	A^1A^3	A^1A^4	A^1a^1	A^1a^2	A^1a^3	A^1a^4
A^2		—	A^2A^3	A^2A^4	A^2a^1	A^2a^2	A^2a^3	A^2a^4
A^3			—	A^3A^4	A^3a^1	A^3a^2	A^3a^3	A^3a^4
A^4				—	A^4a^1	A^4a^2	A^4a^3	A^4a^4
a^1					—	a^1a^2	a^1a^3	a^1a^4
a^2						—	a^2a^3	a^2a^4
a^3							—	a^3a^4
a^4								—

Ignoring the superscript identification of alleles, the expected ratio of possible diploid gametes is 6 AA : 16 Aa : 6 aa or 3 : 8 : 3. Using these gametic expectations, we can now construct a zygotic checkerboard to generate the expected progeny.

	3 AA	8 Aa	3 aa
3 AA	9 $AAAA$	24 $AAAa$	9 $AAaa$
8 Aa	24 $AAAa$	64 $AAaa$	24 $Aaaa$
3 aa	9 $AAaa$	24 $Aaaa$	9 $aaaa$

Summary of progeny genotypes: 9 *AAAA* (quadruplex) : 48 *AAAa* (triplex) : 82 *AAaa* (duplex) : 48 *Aaaa* (simplex) : 9 *aaaa* (nulliplex).

(b)   The total of the numbers $(3 + 8 + 3)$ along the top or side of the preceding table is 14. Thus the total of all crossproducts in the table is $14 \times 14 = 196$. Nine genotypes are homozygous *AAAA*, and another nine are homozygous *aaaa*. .Thus, all other genotypes $(196 - 18 = 178)$ are heterozygotes. Selfing the autotetraploid produces $\frac{178}{196} = 91\%$ heterozygous progeny. Selfing a diploid of genotype *Aa* produces 50% heterozygous progeny. The increase from 50 to 91% is $\frac{41}{50} = 82\%$.

8.3.   Pericarp is the outermost layer of the corn kernel and is maternal in origin. A dominant gene (*B*) produces brown pericarp, and its recessive allele (*b*) produces colorless pericarp. Tissue adjacent to the pericarp is aleurone (triploid). Purple pigment is deposited in the aleurone when the dominant gene *C* is present; its recessive allele *c* results in colorless aleurone. Aleurone is actually a single specialized layer of cells of the endosperm. The color of endosperm itself is modified by a pair of alleles. Yellow is governed by the dominant allele *Y* and white by the recessive allele *y*. Both *C* and *Y* show xenia to their respective alleles. A plant which is *bbCcYy* is pollinated by a plant of genotype *BbCcYy*. (*a*) What phenotypic ratio is expected among the progeny kernels? (*b*) If the F$_1$ is pollinated by plants of genotype *bbccyy*, in what color ratio will the resulting F$_2$ kernels be expected to appear?

Solution:

(*a*)   If pericarp is colorless, then the color of the aleurone shows through. If aleurone is also colorless, then the color of the endosperm becomes visible. Since the maternal parent is *bb*, the pericarp on all F$_1$ seeds will be colorless. Any seeds with *C* will have purple aleurone. Only if the aleurone is colorless (*ccc*) can the color of the endosperm be seen.

$$\text{Parents:} \quad bbCcYy\female \quad \times \quad BbCcYy\male$$

$$\text{F}_1: \qquad \tfrac{3}{4}\,C\text{-}\text{-} \qquad = \qquad \tfrac{3}{4} \text{ purple}$$

$$\tfrac{1}{4}\,ccc \begin{cases} \tfrac{3}{4}\,Y\text{-}\text{-} & = & \tfrac{3}{16} \text{ yellow} \\[4pt] \tfrac{1}{4}\,yyy & = & \tfrac{1}{16} \text{ white (colorless)} \end{cases}$$

(*b*)   Half of the F$_1$ embryos is expected to be *Bb* and will thus lay down a brown pericarp around their seeds (F$_2$); the other half is expected to be *bb* and will envelop its seeds with a colorless pericarp. Thus half of the seeds on the F$_1$ plants will be brown. Of the remaining half that has colorless pericarp, we need show only as much of the genotype as is necessary to establish the phenotype.

bb F$_1$		Diploid Fusion Nucleus		Sperm Nucleus		Triploid Tissue
$\tfrac{1}{2} \times \tfrac{1}{4}\,CC$	$=$	$\tfrac{1}{8}\,CC$	$+$	c	$=$	$\tfrac{1}{8}\,CCc$ purple
$\tfrac{1}{2} \times \tfrac{1}{2}\,Cc$	$=$	$\tfrac{1}{4}\begin{cases}\tfrac{1}{8}\,CC \\ \tfrac{1}{8}\,cc\begin{cases}\tfrac{1}{16}\,YY \\ \tfrac{1}{16}\,yy\end{cases}\end{cases}$	$\begin{matrix}+\\+\\+\end{matrix}$	$\begin{matrix}c\\cy\\cy\end{matrix}$	$\begin{matrix}=\\=\\=\end{matrix}$	$\begin{matrix}\tfrac{1}{8}\,CCc \text{ } purple\\\tfrac{1}{16}\,cccYYy \text{ yellow}\\\tfrac{1}{16}\,cccyyy \text{ white}\end{matrix}$
$\tfrac{1}{2} \times \tfrac{1}{4}\,cc$	$=$	$\tfrac{1}{8}\begin{cases}\tfrac{1}{16}\,ccYY \\ \tfrac{1}{16}\,ccyy\end{cases}$	$\begin{matrix}+\\+\end{matrix}$	$\begin{matrix}cy\\cy\end{matrix}$	$\begin{matrix}=\\=\end{matrix}$	$\begin{matrix}\tfrac{1}{16}\,cccYYy \text{ yellow}\\\tfrac{1}{16}\,cccyyy \text{ white}\end{matrix}$

Summary of F$_2$ seed colors: $\tfrac{1}{2}$ brown : $\tfrac{1}{4}$ purple : $\tfrac{1}{8}$ yellow : $\tfrac{1}{8}$ white.

8.4.   "Eyeless" is a recessive gene (*ey*) on the tiny fourth chromosome of *Drosophila*. A male trisomic for chromosome 4 with the genotype $+ + ey$ is crossed to a disomic eyeless female of genotype *ey ey*. Determine the genotypic and phenotypic ratios expected among the progeny by random assortment of the chromosomes to the gametes.

Solution:

Three types of segregation are possible in the formation of gametes in the triploid.

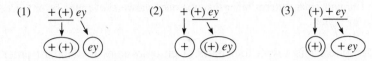

(1) + (+) *ey*   (2) + (+) *ey*   (3) (+) + *ey*

Summary of sperm genotypes: 1 + + : 2 = *ey* : 2 + : 1 *ey*.

The union of these sperms with eggs of genotype *ey* results in the following progeny:

$$
\left.\begin{array}{l}
1 + + \ ey \\
2 + ey \ ey \\
2 + ey
\end{array}\right\} = 5 \ \text{wild type}
$$

$$1 \ ey \ ey \qquad = 1 \ \text{eyeless}$$

VARIATION IN THE ARRANGEMENT OF CHROMOSOME SEGMENTS

8.5. In 1931 Stern found two different translocations in *Drosophila* from which he developed females possessing heteromorphic X chromosomes. One X chromosome had a piece of the Y chromosome attached to it; the other X was shorter and had a piece of chromosome IV attached to it. Two sex-linked genes were used as markers for detecting crossovers, the recessive trait carnation eye color (*car*) and the dominant trait bar eye (*B*). Dihybrid bar females with heteromorphic chromosomes (both mutant alleles on the X portion of the X-IV chromosome) were crossed to hemizygous carnation males with normal chromosomes. The results of this experiment provided cytological proof that genetic crossing over involves an actual physical exchange between homologous chromosome segments. Diagram the expected cytogenetic results of this cross showing all genotypes and phenotypes.

Solution:

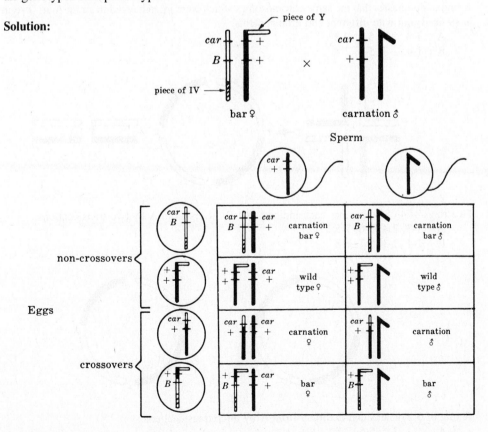

The existence of a morphologically normal X chromosome in recombinant male progeny with carnation eyes provides cytological proof that genetic crossing over is correlated with physical exchange between homologous chromosomes in the parents. Similarly, all other phenotypes correlate with the cytological picture. Chromosomal patterns other than the ones shown above may be produced by crossing over outside the inverted region.

8.6. Consider an organism with four pairs of chromosomes in standard order, the ends of which we shall label, 1-2, 3-4, 5-6, 7-8. Strain A crossed to the standard strain gives a ring of 4 plus 2 bivalents during meiotic prophase in the progeny. Strain B crossed to the standard strain also gives a ring of 4 plus 2 bivalents. In each of the four situations that follow, explain how a cross of strain A × strain B could produce (*a*) 4 bivalents, (*b*) ring of 4 plus 2 bivalents, (*c*) 2 rings of 4, (*d*) ring of 6 plus 1 bivalent.

Solution:

A ring of 4 indicates a reciprocal translocation involving 2 nonhomologous chromosomes. As a starting point, let us assume that strain A has experienced a single reciprocal translocation so that the order is 1-3, 2-4, 5-6, 7-8. Strain B also shows a ring of 4 with the standard, but we do not know whether the translocation involves the same chromosome as strain A or different chromosomes. The results of crossing A × B will indicate which of the B chromosomes have undergone translocations.

(*a*) Formation of only bivalents indicates that complete homology exists between the chromosomes in strains A and B. Therefore strain B has the same translocation as that in strain A. During prophase I of meiosis, each chromosome consists of 2 identical sister chromatids. To simplify the following diagrams, neither chromatids nor centromeres are shown.

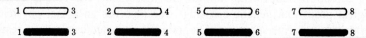

(*b*) A ring of 4 indicates that the same chromosomes which were interchanged in strain A are also involved in strain B, but with different end arrangements.

     A: 1-3, 2-4, 5-6, 7-8
     B: 1-4, 2-3, 5-6, 7-8

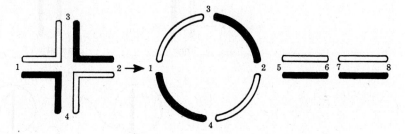

(*c*) Two rings of 4 chromosomes each indicate that B differs from A by two translocations.

     A: 1-3, 2-4, 5-6, 7-8
     B: 1-4, 2-3, 5-7, 6-8

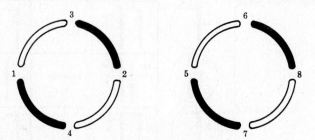

(*d*) A ring of 6 indicates that B differs from A by three translocations.

     A: 1-3, 2-4, 5-6, 7-8
     B: 1-2, 3-5, 4-6, 7-8

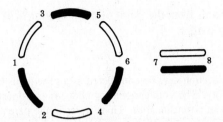

8.7. The centromere of chromosome V in corn is about 7 map units from the end. The gene for light-yellow (virescent) seedling (*v*) is 10 map units from this end, and a gene that shortens internode length called brevis (*bv*) is 12 map units from this end. The break point of a translocation (*T*) is 20 map units from this end. A translocation heterozygote involving chromosomes V and VIII of genotype + *bv t/v* + *T* is pollinated by a normal (nontranslocated, *t*) plant of genotype *v bv t/v bv t*. If gametes are formed exclusively by alternate segregation from the ring of chromosomes formed by the translocation heterozygote, predict the ratio of progeny genotypes and phenotypes from this cross (considering multiple crossovers to be negligible).

Solution:

First let us diagram the effect that crossing over will have between the centromere and the point of translocation. We will label the ends of chromosome V with 1-2, and of chromosome VIII with 3-4. A cross-shaped pairing figure is formed during meiosis.

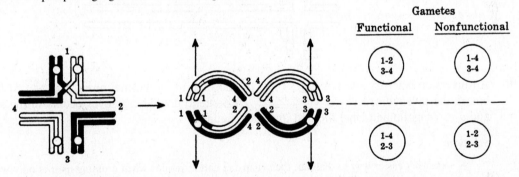

Alternate segregation produces half functional and half nonfunctional (duplication-deficiency) gametes. Note that the nonfunctional gametes derive only from the crossover chromatids. Thus recovery of chromatids that experience a crossover between the centromere and the point of translocation is prevented. The combination of genes in this region of the chromosome is prevented from being broken up by crossing over and are thus transmitted as a unit. This situation is analogous to the block of genes within an inversion that are similarly held together as a genetic unit. Noncrossover chromatids will form two types of functional gametes with equal frequency: + *bv t* and *v* + *T*. Expected zygotes are: $\frac{1}{2}$ + *bv t/v bv t* = brevis, homozygous for the normal chromosome order and $\frac{1}{2}$ *v* + *T/v bv t* = virescent, heterozygous for the translocation.

8.8. Shrunken endosperm of corn is governed by a recessive gene *sh* and waxy endosperm by another recessive *wx*. Both of these loci are linked on chromosome 9. A plant that is heterozygous for a translocation involving chromosomes 8 and 9 and that developed from a plump, starchy kernel is pollinated by a plant from a shrunken, waxy kernel with normal chromosomes. The progeny are

171 shrunken, starchy, normal ear
205 plump, waxy, semisterile ear
82 plump, starchy, normal ear
49 shrunken, waxy, semisterile ear
17 shrunken, starchy, semisterile ear
40 plump, waxy, normal ear
6 plump, starchy, semisterile ear
3 shrunken, waxy, normal ear.

(*a*) How far is each locus from the point of translocation? (*b*) Diagram and label the pairing figure in the plump, starchy parent.

Solution:

(*a*) The point of translocation may be considered as a gene locus because it produces a phenotypic effect, namely, semisterility. The conventional symbol for translocation is *T*, and *t* is used for the normal chromosome without a translocation. Gene order in the parents must be

$$\frac{+\ wx\ T}{sh\ +\ t} \times \frac{sh\ wx\ t}{sh\ wx\ t}$$

in order for double crossovers to produce the least frequent phenotypes

$$+\ +\ T = \text{plump, starchy, semisterile ear}$$
$$sh\ wx\ t = \text{shrunken, waxy, normal ear}$$

The map distances are calculated in the usual way for a 3-point testcross.

Distance *sh–wx* = (82 + 49 + 6 + 3)/573 = 24.4 map units
Distance *wx–T* = (17 + 40 + 6 + 3)/573 = 11.5 map units
Distance *sh–T* = 24.4 + 11.5 = 35.9 map units

(*b*)

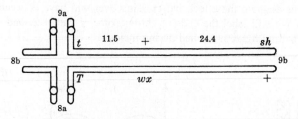

8.9. An inversion heterozygote possesses one chromosome in the normal order ●————*a b c d e f g h* and one in the inverted order ●————*a b f e d c g h*. A 4-strand double crossover occurs in the areas *f-e* and *d-c*. Diagram and label the first anaphase figures.

Solution:

A somewhat easier way to diagram the synapsing chromosomes when crossing over is only within the inversion as shown below. This is obviously not representative of the actual pairing figure. Let the crossover in the *c-d* region involve strands 2 and 3, and the crossover in the *e-f* region involve strands 1 and 4.

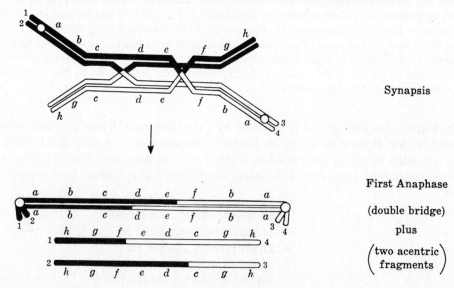

8.10. Eight regions of a dipteran chromosome are easily recognized cytologically and labeled *a–h*. Four different races within this species have the chromosomal orders as listed:

(1) *ahbdcfeg*,   (2) *aedcfbhg*,   (3) *ahbdgefc*,   (4) *aefcdbhg*

Assuming that each race evolved by a single inversion from another race, show how the four races could have originated.

Solution:

An inversion in (1) involving *cfeg* produces the order for (3).

$$(1)\ a\ h\ b\ d\ \underline{c\ f\ e\ g} \rightarrow (3)\ a\ h\ b\ d\ g\ e\ f\ c$$

No single inversion in (3) can produce any of the other chromosomal orders. However, a different inversion in (1) can produce an order for (4).

$$(1)\ a\ \underline{h\ b\ d\ c\ f\ e}\ g \rightarrow (4)\ a\ e\ f\ c\ d\ b\ h\ g$$

Race 4, in turn, can give rise to (2) by a single inversion.

$$(4)\ a\ e\ \underline{f\ c\ d}\ b\ h\ g \rightarrow (2)\ a\ e\ d\ c\ f\ b\ h\ g$$

If (1) were the original ancestor, the evolutionary pattern would be $2 \leftarrow 4 \leftarrow 1 \rightarrow 3$. If (2) were the original ancestor, the evolutionary pattern would be $2 \rightarrow 4 \rightarrow 1 \rightarrow 3$. If (3) were the original ancestor, the evolutionary pattern would be $3 \rightarrow 1 \rightarrow 4 \rightarrow 2$. If (4) were the original ancestor, the evolutionary pattern would be $2 \leftarrow 4 \rightarrow 1 \rightarrow 3$. Since we do not know which of the four was the original ancestor, we can briefly indicate all of these possibilities by using doubled-headed arrows: $2 \leftrightarrow 4 \leftrightarrow 1 \leftrightarrow 3$.

VARIATION IN CHROMOSOME MORPHOLOGY

8.11. Yellow body color in *Drosophila* is produced by a recessive gene *y* at the end of the X chromosome. A yellow male is mated to an attached-X female ($\widehat{XX}$) heterozygous for the *y* allele. Progeny are of two types: yellow females and wild-type females. What insight does this experiment offer concerning the stage (2 strand or 4 strand) at which crossing over occurs?

Solution:

Let us assume that crossing over occurs in the 2-strand stage, i.e., before the chromosome replicates into 2 chromatids.

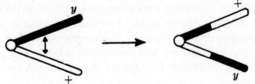

The yellow male produces gametes with either a *y*-bearing X chromosome or one with the Y chromosome that is devoid of genetic markers. Trisonomic X ($\widehat{XX}X$) flies seldom survive (superfemales). Those with $\widehat{XX}$ will be viable heterozygous wild-type attached-X females. Crossing over fails to produce yellow progeny when it occurs in the 2-strand stage.

Let us assume that crossing over occurs after replication of the chromosome, i.e., in the 4-strand stage:

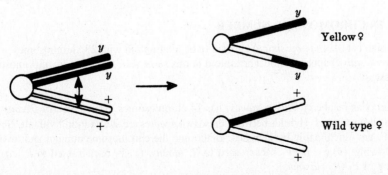

The appearance of yellow females in the progeny is proof that crossing over occurs in the 4-strand stage.

8.12. Data from *Drosophila* studies indicate that noncrossover (NCO) rings are recovered in equal frequencies with NCO rods from ring-rod heterozygotes. What light does this information shed on the occurrence of sister-strand crossing over?

Solution:

Let us diagram the results of a sister-strand crossover in a rod and in a ring chromosome.

(*a*)   Rod Chromosome

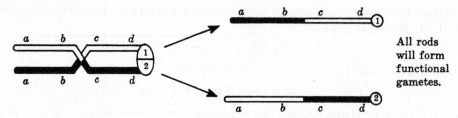

(*b*)   Ring Chromosome

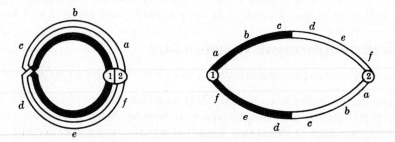

The double bridge at anaphase will rupture and produce nonfunctional gametes with duplications or deficiencies. These would fail to be recovered in viable offspring. The fact that both rings and rods are recovered with equal frequency argues against the occurrence of sister-strand crossing over.

Modern techniques (involving autoradiography with labeled thymidine or fluorescence microscopy of cultured cells that have incorporated 5-bromodeoxyuridine in place of thymine) reveal that some sister-strand exchanges occur by a repair mechanism when DNA is damaged. One of the initiating steps that transforms a normal cell to a cancer cell is DNA damage. Hence, screening chemicals for their ability to induce sister-strand exchanges is one method for detecting potential cancer-inducing agents (carcinogens).

Supplementary Problems

VARIATION IN CHROMOSOME NUMBER

8.13. Abyssinian oat (*Avena abyssinica*) appears to be a tetraploid with 28 chromosomes. The common cultivated oat (*Avena sativa*) appears to be a hexaploid in this same series. How many chromosomes does the common oat possess?

8.14. The European raspberry (*Rubus idaeus*) has 14 chromosomes. The dewberry (*Rubus caesius*) is a tetraploid with 28 chromosomes. Hybrids between these two species are sterile F_1 individuals. Some unreduced gametes of the F_1 are functional in backcrosses. Determine the chromosome number and level of ploidy for each of the following: (*a*) F_1, (*b*) F_1 backcrossed to *R. idaeus*, (*c*) F_1 backcrossed to *R. caesius*, (*d*) chromosome doubling of F_1 (*R. maximus*).

8.15. There are 13 pairs of chromosomes in Asiatic cotton (*Gossypium arboreum*) and also 13 pairs in an American species *G. thurberi*. Interspecific crosses between *arboreum* and *thurberi* are sterile because of highly irregular chromosome pairing during meiosis. The American cultivated cotton (*Gossypium hirsutum*) has 26 pairs of chromosomes. Crosses of *arboreum* × *hirsutum* or *thurberi* × *hirsutum* produce triploids with 13 bivalents (pairs of chromosomes) and 13 univalents (single unpaired chromosomes). How can this cytological information be used to interpret the evolution of *hirsutum*?

8.16. If two alleles, *A* and *a*, exist at a locus, 5 genotypic combinations can be formed in an autotetraploid: quadruplex (*AAAA*), triplex (*AAAa*), duplex (*AAaa*), simplex (*Aaaa*), nulliplex (*aaaa*). Assume *A* exhibits xenia over *a*. For each of these five genotypes determine the expected phenotypic ratio (*A* : *a*) when (*a*) the locus is tightly linked to its centromere (chromosomal assortment) and the genotype is selfed, (*b*) the locus is assorting chromosomally and the genotype is testcrossed, (*c*) the locus is far from its centromere so that chromatids assort independently and the genotype is selfed, (*d*) the locus assorts by chromatids and the genotype is testcrossed.

8.17. The loci of genes *A* and *B* are on different chromosomes. A dihybrid autotetraploid plant of genotype *AAaaBBbb* is self-pollinated. Assume that only diploid gametes are formed and that the loci of *A* and *B* are very close to their respective centromeres (chromosomal segregation). Find the phenotypic expectations of the progeny.

8.18. The flinty endosperm character in maize is produced whenever 2 or all 3 of the alleles in this triploid tissue are *F*. In the presence of its alternative allele *F'* in double or triple dose, a floury endosperm is produced. White endosperm color is produced by a triple dose of a recessive allele *y*, its dominant allele *Y* exhibiting xenia and producing yellow endosperm. The loci of *F* and *Y* assort independently. (*a*) In crosses between parents of genotype *FF'Yy*, what phenotypic ratio is expected in the progeny seed? (*b*) Pollen from a plant of genotype *FF'Yy* is crossed onto a plant of genotype *FFyy*. Compare the phenotypic ratios produced by this cross with its reciprocal cross.

8.19. The diploid number of the garden pea is $2n = 14$. (*a*) How many different trisomics could be formed? (*b*) How many different double trisomics could be formed?

8.20. The diploid number of an organism is 12. How many chromosomes would be expected in (*a*) a monosomic, (*b*) a trisomic, (*c*) a tetrasomic, (*d*) a double trisomic, (*e*) a nullisomic, (*f*) a monoploid, (*g*) a triploid, (*h*) an autotetraploid?

8.21. Sugary endosperm of corn is regulated by a recessive gene *s* on chromosome IV and starchy endosperm by its dominant allele *S*. Assuming $n + 1$ pollen grains are nonfunctional, predict the genotypic and phenotypic ratios of endosperm expected in the progeny from the cross of (*a*) diploid *ss* pollinated by trisomic-IV of genotype *SSs*, (*b*) diploid *Ss* pollinated by trisomic-IV of genotype *SSs*.

8.22. A dominant gene w^+ produces yellow flowers in a certain plant species and its recessive allele *w* produces white flowers. Plants trisomic for the chromosome bearing the color locus will produce *n* and $n + 1$ functional female gametes, but viable pollen has only the *n* number. Find the phenotypic ratio expected from each of the following crosses:

	Seed Parent		Pollen Parent
(*a*)	+ + *w*	×	+ + *w*
(*b*)	+ *w* *w*	×	+ + *w*
(*c*)	+ + *w*	×	+ *w*
(*d*)	+ *w* *w*	×	+ *w*

8.23. Shrunken endosperm is the product of a recessive gene *sh* on chromosome III of corn; its dominant allele *Sh* produces full, plump kernels. Another recessive gene *pr* on chromosome V gives red color to the aleurone, and its dominant allele *Pr* gives purple. A diploid plant of genotype *Sh/sh,Pr/pr* was pollinated by a plant trisomic for chromosome III of genotype *Sh/Sh/sh,Pr/pr*. If $n + 1$ pollen grains are nonfunctional, determine the phenotypic ratio expected in the progeny endosperms.

8.24. Normal women possess 2 sex chromosomes (XX) and normal men have a single X chromosome plus a Y chromosome that carries male determiners. Rarely a woman is found with marked abnormalities of primary and secondary sexual characteristics, having only 1 X chromosome (XO). The phenotypic expressions of this monosomic-X state is called Turner syndrome. Likewise, men are occasionally discovered with an XXY constitution exhibiting corresponding abnormalities called Klinefelter syndrome. Color blindness is a sex-linked recessive trait. (*a*) A husband and wife both had normal vision, but one of their children was a color-blind Turner girl. Diagram this cross, including the gametes that produced this child. (*b*) In another family the mother is color blind and the father has normal vision. Their child is a Klinefelter with normal vision. What gametes produced this child? (*c*) Suppose the same parents in part (*b*) produced a color-blind Klinefelter. What gametes produced this child? (*d*) The normal diploid number for humans is 46. A trisomic condition for chromosome 21 results in Down syndrome. At least one case of Down-Klinefelter has been recorded. How many chromosomes would this individual be expected to possess?

VARIATION IN ARRANGEMENT OF CHROMOSOME SEGMENTS

8.25. Colorless aleurone of corn kernels is a trait governed by a recessive gene *c* and is in the same linkage group (IX) with another recessive gene *wx* governing waxy endosperm. In 1931 Creighton and McClintock found a plant with one normal IX chromosome, but its homologue had a knob on one end and a translocated piece from another chromosome on the other end. A dihybrid colored, starchy plant with the heteromorphic IX chromosome shown below was testcrossed to a colorless, waxy plant with normal chromosomes. The results of this experiment provided cytological proof that genetic crossing over involves an actual physical exchange between homologous chromosome segments. Diagram the results of this cross, showing all genotypes and phenotypes.

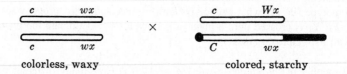

colorless, waxy   colored, starchy

8.26. Nipple-shaped tips on tomato fruit is the phenotypic expression of a recessive gene *nt* on chromosome V. A heterozygous plant (*Nt/nt*) that is also heterozygous for a reciprocal translocation involving chromosomes V and VIII is testcrossed to a plant with normal chromosomes. The progeny were 48 normal fruit, fertile : 19 nipple fruit, fertile : 11 normal fruit, semisterile : 37 nipple fruit, semisterile. What is the genetic position of the locus of gene *Nt* with respect to the point of translocation?

8.27. Given a pericentric inversion heterozygote with 1 chromosome in normal order (1 2 3 4.5 6 7 8) and the other in the inverted order (1 5.4 3 2 6 7 8), diagram the first anaphase figure after a 4-strand double crossover occurs: one crossover involves the regions between 4 and the centromere (.); the other crossover occurs between the centromere and 5.

8.28. A 4-strand double crossover occurs in an inversion heterozygote. The normal chromosome order is (.1 2 3 4 5 6 7 8); the inverted chromosome order is (.1 2 7 6 5 4 3 8). One crossover is between 1 and 2 and the other is between 5 and 6. Diagram and label the first anaphase figures.

8.29. Diagram and label the first anaphase figure produced by an inversion heterozygote whose normal chromosome is (.*a b c d e f g h*) and with the inverted order (.*a b f e d c g h*). Assume that a 2-strand double crossover occurs in the regions *c-d* and *e-f*.

8.30. A chromosome with segments in the normal order is (.*a b c d e f g h*). An inversion heterozygote has the abnormal order (.*a b f e d c g h*). A 3-strand double crossover occurs involving the regions between *a* and *b* and between *d* and *e*. Diagram and label the first and second anaphase figures.

8.31. Given the pairing figure for an inversion heterozygote with 3 crossovers as indicated on page 201, diagram the first anaphase.

8.32. Four races of a species are characterized by variation in the segmental order (*a–h*) of a certain chromosome.

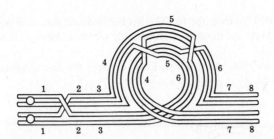

Race 1: *a b c d e f g h*   Race 3: *g f e a c d b h*
Race 2: *g f e b d c a h*   Race 4: *a c b d e f g h*

A fifth race, with still a different chromosomal order, is postulated to have existed in the past but is now extinct. Explain the evolutionary origin of these races in terms of single inversion differences. *Hint:* See Problem 8.10.

8.33. A species of the fruit fly is differentiated into five races on the basis of differences in the banding patterns of one of its giant chromosomes. Eight regions of the chromosome are designated *a–h*. If each of these races is separated by a single overlapping inversion, devise a scheme to account for the evolution of the five races: (1) *a d g h f c b e*, (2) *f h g d a c b e*, (3) *f h c a d g b e*, (4) *f h g b c a d e*, (5) *f a d g h c b e*

VARIATION IN THE NUMBER OF CHROMOSOME SEGMENTS

8.34. In higher animals, even very small deficiencies, when homozygous, are usually lethal. A recessive gene *w* in mice results in an abnormal gait called "waltzing." A waltzing male was crossed to several homozygous normal females. Among several hundred offspring one was found to be a waltzer female. Presumably, a deficiency in the chromosome carrying the w^+ allele caused the waltzing trait to appear as pseudodominant. The pseudodominant waltzer female was then crossed to a homozygous normal male and produced only normal offspring. (*a*) List 2 possible genotypes for the normal progeny from the above cross. (*b*) Suppose that 2 males, one of each genotype produced in part (*a*), were backcrossed to their pseudodominant mother and each produced 12 zygotes. Assuming that homozygosity for the deletion is lethal, calculate the expected combined number of waltzer and normal progeny.

VARIATION IN CHROMOSOME MORPHOLOGY

8.35. Vermilion eye color in *Drosophila* is a sex-linked recessive condition; bar eye is a sex-linked dominant condition. An attached-X female with vermilion eyes, also having a Y chromosome (XXY), is mated to a bar-eyed male. (*a*) Predict the phenotypic ratio that is expected in the F_1 flies. (*b*) How much death loss is anticipated in the F_1 generation? (Hint: see Problem 5.25) (*c*) What phenotypic ratio is expected in the F_2?

8.36. Two recessive sex-linked traits in *Drosophila* are garnet eye (*g*) and forked bristle (*f*). The attached-X chromosomes of females heterozygous for these genes are diagrammed below.

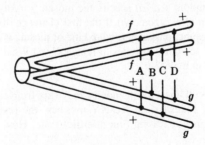

A crossover between two chromatids attached to the same centromere is called a reciprocal exchange; a crossover between 2 chromatids attached to different centromeres is a nonreciprocal exchange. Approximately 7% of the daughters from these attached-X females were + + /*f g*, 7% were *f* + /+ +, 7% were *f g*/+ *g* and the remainder were *f* + /+ *g*. (*a*) Which of the single exchanges (A, B, C, or D in the diagram) could produce the daughters (1) + + /*f g* and *f* + /+ *g*, (2) *f* + /+ + and *f g*/+ *g*? (*b*) Are chromatids attached to the same centromere more likely to be involved in an exchange than chromatids attached to different centromeres? (*c*) Does the fact that neither homozygous wild type nor garnet-forked progeny were found shed any light on the number of chromatids which undergo exchange at any one locus?

8.37. Given the ring homozygote at the left (below), diagram the first anaphase figure when crossovers occur at position (*a*) A and B, (*b*) A and C, (*c*) A and D.

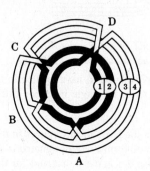 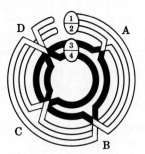

8.38. Given the ring-rod heterozygote at the right (above), diagram the first anaphase figure when crossovers occur at positions (*a*) A and B, (*b*) A and C, (*c*) A and D.

HUMAN CYTOGENETICS

8.39. Meiotic non-disjunction of the sex chromosomes in either parent can produce a child with Klinefelter syndrome (XXY) or Turner syndrome (XO). Color blindness is due to a sex-linked recessive gene. (*a*) If a color-blind woman and man with normal vision produce a color-blind Klinefelter child, in which parent did the non-disjunctional event occur? (*b*) If a heterozygous woman with normal vision and a man with normal vision produce a color-blind Klinefelter child, how can this be explained?

8.40. Explain what type of abnormal sperm unites with a normal egg to produce an XYY offspring. Specifically, how does such an abnormal gamete arise?

8.41. **Mosaicism** is the presence in an individual of two or more cell lines of different chromosomal constitution, each cell line being derived from the same zygote. In contrast, fusion of cell lines from different zygotes produces a **chimera.** Mosaicism results from abnormal postzygotic (mitotic) divisions of three kinds: (1) nondisjunction during the first cleavage division of the zygote, (2) nondisjunction during later mitotic divisions, and (3) anaphase lag, in which one member of a chromosome pair fails to segregate chomatids from the metaphase plate, and that chromatid fails to be included in the daughter cell nuclei (the entire chromosome is thus lost). Assuming that nondisjunction of chromatids affects only one member of a pair of chromosomes of the diploid set, (*a*) specify the mosaic karyotypes expected from nondisjunction during the first cleavage division of a zygote. (*b*) If the first cleavage division is normal, but the second cleavage division involves a nondisjunctional event, what kind of mosaic is expected? (*c*) What kind of mosaic results from anaphase lag of the sex chromosomes in females? (*d*) What kind of mosaic results from anaphase lag of the sex chromosomes in males?

8.42. In mosaics of XX and XO cell lines, the phenotype may vary from complete Turner syndrome to a completely normal appearing female. Likewise, in XO/XY mosaics, the phenotypic variation ranges from complete Turner syndrome to a normal appearing (but infertile) male. How can these variations be explained?

8.43. Suppose that part of the short arm of one chromosome 5 becomes nonreciprocally attached to the long-arm end of one chromosome 13 in the diploid set. This is considered to be a ''balanced translocation'' because essentially all of the genetic material is present and the phenotype is normal. One copy of the short arm of chromosome 5 produces *cri du chat* syndrome; three copies lead to early postnatal death. If such a translocation individual has children by a chromosomally normal partner, predict the (*a*) chromosomal and (*b*) phenotypic expectations.

8.44. About 2% of patients with Down syndrome have a normal chromosome number of 46. The extra chromosome 21 has been nonreciprocally translocated onto another autosome of the D or G group. These individuals are referred to as *translocation mongols,* and because this condition tends to be hereditary, it is also called *familial mongolism.* (*a*) Suppose that one phenotypically normal parent has 45 chromosomes, one of which is a translocation of the centromere and long arm of a D-group chromosome (either 14 or 15) and the long arm minus the centromere of a G-group chromosome (21). The short arms of each chromosome (presumably carrying no vital genes) are lost in previous cell divisions. If gametes from this translocated parent unite with those from a normal diploid individual, predict the chromosomal and phenotypic expectations in their progeny. (*b*) Assuming that in one parent the translocation is between chromosomes 21 and 22, that the centromere of the translocation is that of chromosome 22 (*like* centromeres go to opposite poles), and that the other parent is a normal diploid, predict the chromosomal and phenotypic expectations in their children. (*c*) Make the same analysis as in part (*b*), assuming that the centromere of the 21/22 translocation chromosome is that of chromosome 21. (*d*) Assuming that in one parent the translocation involves 21/21 and the other parent is a normal diploid, predict the chromosomal and phenotypic expectations in their children. (*e*) Among the live offspring of parts (*c*) and (*d*), what are the risks of having a Down child?

8.45. The photograph accompanying this problem is at the back of the book. It shows the chromosomes from a human cell. Cut out the chromosomes and construct an idiogram. Do not look at the answer until you have solutions to the following questions. (*a*) Is the specimen from a male or a female? (*b*) What possible kinds of chromosomal abnormalities may be present in this patient?

REVIEW QUESTIONS

Matching Questions   Choose the one best match of each numbered item with one of the lettered items.

1. Monoploid	A. *Cri du chat* syndrome
2. Chromosome 5 deletion	B. Salivary gland cell chromosome
3. Monosomic	C. $2n + 1 + 1$
4. Double trisomic	D. Prenatal sex identification
5. Somatic chromosome pairing	E. Trisomy 21
6. Renner complex	F. Chronic myelocytic leukemia
7. Double-bar eye	G. *Oenothera*
8. Philadelphia chromosome	H. Drone bee
9. Barr body	I. Unequal crossing over
10. Down syndrome	J. Turner syndrome

Vocabulary   For each of the following definitions, give the appropriate term and spell it correctly. Terms are single words unless indicated otherwise.

1. A cell or organism containing three sets of chromosomes.

2. A cell or organism produced by doubling the chromosome number of an interspecific hybrid.

3. Any variation in chromosome number that does not involve whole sets of chromosomes.

4. A cell or organism having a genomic formula $2n - 1$.

5. An adjective applicable to a giant chromosome consisting of hundreds of chromatid strands.

6. Exchange of pieces between 2 nonhomologous chromosomes. (Two words.)

7. Altered phenotypic expression of a gene as a consequence of movement from its normal location. (Two words.)

8. A chromosomal aberration that, with the help of crossing over within the aberration, can lead to "bridge and fragment" formation. (Two words.)

9. Phenotypic expression of a recessive gene as a consequence of loss of a chromosomal segment bearing the corresponding dominant allele.

10. The arrangement of the somatic chromosome complement (karyotype) of a cell in groups of homologous pairs.

True-False Questions   Answer each of the following statements either true (T) or false (F).

1. The discipline of biology that attempts to correlate cellular events with genetic phenomena is cryogenetics.

2. Triploids and autotetraploids are usually sterile.

3. Interspecific diploid hybrids are usually fertile.

4. The genomic formula for a trisomic is $3n$.

5. Balanced lethal systems require either a translocation or an inversion to maintain heterozygosity generation after generation.

6. Overlapping inversions have been used to locate the physical positions of linked genes.

7. Production of viable recombination progeny resulting from crossing over within an inversion structural heterozygote is not possible.

8. Normal human males are sex-chromatin negative.

9. Normal human females heterozygous for a pair of sex-linked alleles have only one such allele expressed in a given cell.

10. The phenomenon called gigantism is associated with the large polytene chromosomes in certain cells of *Drosophila* larvae.

Multiple-Choice Questions   Choose the one best answer.

1. A treatment often used to induce polyploidy experimentally in plants is   (*a*) X-rays   (*b*) gibberellic acid   (*c*) colchicine   (*d*) acridine dyes   (*e*) azothioprene

2. A mechanism that can cause a gene to move from one linkage group to another is   (*a*) translocation   (*b*) inversion   (*c*) crossing over   (*d*) duplication   (*e*) dosage compensation

3. If during synapsis a certain kind of abnormal chromosome is always forced to bulge away from its normal homologue, the abnormality is classified as   (*a*) an inversion   (*b*) a duplication   (*c*) an isochromosome   (*d*) a deficiency   (*e*) none of the above

4. If 4 chromosomes synapse into a cross-shaped configuration during meiotic prophase, the organism is heterozygous for a   (*a*) pericentric inversion   (*b*) deletion   (*c*) translocation   (*d*) paracentric inversion   (*e*) none of the above

5. A segment of chromosome may be protected from recombination by   (*a*) an inversion   (*b*) a translocation   (*c*) balanced lethals   (*d*) more than one of the above   (*e*) all of the above

6. A person with Klinefelter syndrome is considered a   (*a*) monosomic   (*b*) triploid   (*c*) trisomic   (*d*) deletion heterozygote   (*e*) none of the above

7. Given a normal chromosome with segments labeled C123456 (C = centromere), a homologue containing an inversion including regions 3–5, and a single 2-strand crossover between regions 4 and 5; then the acentric fragment present during first meiotic anaphase is　　(*a*) 63456　(*b*) 12344321　(*c*) 65521　(*d*) 654321　(*e*) none of the above

8. Pseudodominance may be observed in heterozygotes for　　(*a*) a deletion　(*b*) a duplication　(*c*) a paracentric inversion　(*d*) a reciprocal translocation　(*e*) more than one of the above

9. The most easily recognized characteristic of an inversion heterozygote in plants is (*a*) gigantism　(*b*) semisterility　(*c*) a cross-shaped chromosome configuration during meiosis　(*d*) pseudodominance　(*e*) none of the above

10. If the garden pea has 14 chromosomes in its diploid complement, how many double trisomics could theoretically exist?　　(*a*) 6　(*b*) 9　(*c*) 16　(*d*) 21　(*e*) none of the above

Answers to Supplementary Problems

8.13. 42

8.14. (*a*) 21, triploid　(*b*) 28, tetraploid　(*c*) 35, pentaploid　(*d*) 42, hexaploid

8.15. Half of the chromosomes of *hirsutum* have homology with *arboreum,* and the other half with *thurberi.* Doubling the chromosome number of the sterile hybrid (*thurberi* × *arboreum*) could produce an amphidiploid with the cytological characteristics of *hirsutum.*

8.16.

Genotype	(*a*)	(*b*)	(*c*)	(*d*)
Quadruplex	All *A*	All *A*	All *A*	All *A*
Triplex	All *A*	All *A*	783 *A* : 1 *a*	27 *A* : 1 *a*
Duplex	35 *A* : 1 *a*	5 *A* : 1 *a*	20.8 *A* : 1 *a*	3.7 *A* : 1 *a*
Simplex	3 *A* : 1 *a*	1 *A* : 1 *a*	2.48 *A* : 1 *a*	0.87 *A* : 1 *a*
Nulliplex	All *a*	All *a*	All *a*	All *a*

8.17. 1225 *AB* : 35 *Ab* : 35 *aB* : 1 *ab*

8.18. (*a*) $\frac{3}{8}$ flinty, yellow : $\frac{1}{8}$ flinty, white : $\frac{3}{8}$ floury, yellow : $\frac{1}{8}$ floury, white

(*b*)

	Original Cross	Reciprocal Cross
Flinty, white	$\frac{1}{2}$	$\frac{1}{4}$
Flinty, yellow	$\frac{1}{2}$	$\frac{1}{4}$
Floury, white		$\frac{1}{4}$
Floury, yellow		$\frac{1}{4}$

8.19. (*a*) 7　(*b*) 21

8.20. (*a*) 11　(*b*) 13　(*c*) 14　(*d*) 14　(*e*) 10　(*f*) 6　(*g*) 18　(*h*) 24

8.21. (*a*) 2 *Sss* (starchy) : 1 *sss* (sugary)　(*b*) $\frac{1}{3}$ *SSS* : $\frac{1}{6}$ *SSs* : $\frac{1}{3}$ *Sss* : $\frac{1}{6}$ *sss* : $\frac{5}{6}$ starchy : $\frac{1}{6}$ sugary

8.22.   (*a*) 17 yellow : 1 white   (*b*) 5 yellow : 1 white   (*c*) 11 yellow : 1 white   (*d*) 3 yellow : 1 white

8.23. $\frac{15}{24}$ plump, purple : $\frac{5}{24}$ plump, red : $\frac{3}{24}$ shrunken, purple : $\frac{1}{24}$ shrunken, red

8.24.   (*a*) P: X^{C}X^c × X^{C}Y; gametes: (X^c) (O) ; F$_1$: X^{c}O   (*b*) (X^c) (X^{C}Y)   (*c*) (X^{c}X^c) (Y)   (*d*) 48

8.25.

	Noncrossovers		Crossovers	
	c ——— *Wx* / *C* ——— *wx*		*c* ——— *wx* / *C* ——— *Wx*	
c ——— *wx*	*c* ——— *Wx* / *C* ——— *wx*		*c* ——— *wx* / *C* ——— *Wx*	
	c ——— *wx* / *c* ——— *wx*		*c* ——— *wx* / *c* ——— *wx*	
	colorless, starchy	colored, waxy	colorless, waxy	colored, starchy

8.26.   26.1 map units from the point of translocation.

8.27.   **8.28.**   **8.29.**

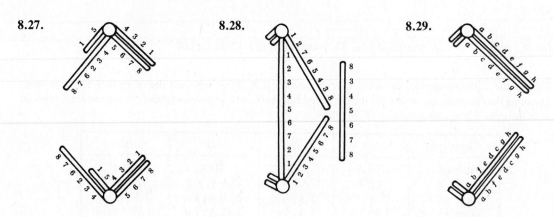

8.30.   First anaphase: a diad, a loop chromatid, and an acentric fragment; second anaphase: the diad splits into 2 monads and the loop forms a bridge. The acentric fragment formed during meiosis I would not be expected to be present at meiosis II.

8.31.   Two loop chromatids and two acentric fragments.

8.32.   If the order of the extinct race (5) was *g f e d b c a h* or *a c d b e f g h,* then: $1 \leftrightarrow 4 \leftrightarrow 5 \leftrightarrow 2 \leftrightarrow 3$.

8.33.   4 ↘   ↗ 1
            2
       5 ↗   ↘ 3

8.34.   (*a*) $+/w$ and $+/(-)$ (heterozygous deficiency)   (*b*) 9 waltzers : 12 normals

8.35.   (*a*) All daughters have vermilion eyes (X͡XY); all sons have bar eyes (XY).   (*b*) 50% death loss; nullo-X is lethal (YY); superfemales (X͡XX) usually die.   (*c*) Same as part (*a*).

8.36. (*a*) (1) D or C (2) B or A   (*b*) No. Reciprocal vs. nonreciprocal exchanges are occurring in a 1 : 1 ratio, indicating that chromatids attached to the same centromere are involved in an exchange with the same frequency as chromatids attached to different centromeres. Daughters with genotype $f + / + g$ resulting from single crossovers of type C cannot be distinguished from nonexchange chromatids.   (*c*) Two exchanges in the garnet-forked region involving all 4 strands, as well as one nonreciprocal exchange between f and the centromere, are required to give homozygous wild-type and garnet-forked daughters. Their absence is support for the assumption that only 2 of the 4 chromatids undergo exchange at any one locus.

8.37. (*a*)   **8.38.** (*a*)

(*b*)   (*b*)

(*c*)   (*c*)

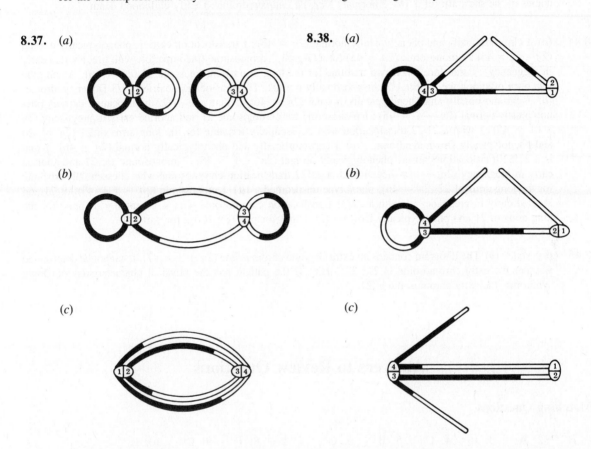

8.39. (*a*) Either nondisjunction of the 2 X chromosomes occurred in the mother in the first meiotic division or nondisjunction of the 2 sister chromatids occurred in the second meiotic division.   (*b*) Nondisjunction during the second meiotic division of the sister chromatids of the X chromosome bearing the recessive color-blind gene would produce an egg with 2 X chromosomes bearing only the color-blind alleles. Alternatively, if crossing over occurs between the centromere and the color-blind locus and is followed by nondisjunction of the X chromosomes at the first meiotic division, one of the four meiotic products would be expected to contain 2 recessive color-blind alleles.

8.40. A sperm bearing 2 Y chromosomes is produced by nondisjunction of the Y sister chromatids during the second meiotic division. The other product of that same nondisjunctional second meiotic division would contain no sex chromosome; when united with a normal egg, an XO Turner female would be expected.

8.41. (*a*) Half of the individual's cells should be trisomic ($2n + 1 = 47$); the other half should be monosomic ($2n - 1 = 45$).   (*b*) Three cell lines are established (45/46/47). Each line should "breed true," barring further mitotic abnormalities.   (*c*) XX/XO; sex-chromatin-positive, Turner syndrome.   (*d*) XY/XO; may resemble Turner's syndrome or be a hermaphrodite with physical characteristics of both sexes.

8.42. If mitotic nondisjunction occurs early in embryogenesis, mosaicism is likely to be widespread throughout the body. If it occurs late in embryogenesis, mosaicism may be limited to only one organ or to one patch of tissue. If chromosomally abnormal cells are extensive in reproductive tissue or in endocrine tissues responsible for gamete and/or sex hormone production, the effects on sterility are likely to be more intensively expressed.

8.43. (a) 1 normal karyotype : 1 balanced translocation : 1 deficient for short arm of chromosome 5 : 1 with three copies of the short arm of 5 (b) 2 normal : 1 *cri-du-chat* syndrome : 1 early childhood death

8.44. (a) 1 chromosomally and phenotypically normal ($2n = 46$) : 1 translocation carrier, phenotypically normal ($2n - 1 = 45$) : 1 monosomic ($2n = 45$) for a G-group chromosome (incompatible with life; aborted early in pregnancy) : 1 translocation Down trisomic for the long arm of chromosome 21 ($2n = 46$). Among the live born offspring we expect 1/3 chromosomally normal : 1/3 translocation carriers: 1/3 Down syndrome. (b) 1 chromosomally and phenotypically normal ($2n = 46$) : 1 that is a 21/22 translocation carrier, phenotypically normal ($2n - 1 = 45$) : 1 monosomic for chromosome 21 and aborted early in pregnancy ($2n - 1 = 45$) : 1 with a 21/22 translocation who is essentially trisomic for the long arms of 21 ($2n = 46$) and phenotypically Down syndrome. (c) 1 chromosomally and phenotypically normal ($2n = 46$) : 1 that is a 21/22 translocation carrier, phenotypically normal ($2n - 1 = 45$) : 1 monosomic for 22 and aborted early in pregnancy ($2n - 1 = 45$) : 1 with a 21/22 translocation chromosome who is essentially trisomic for the long arms of 22 ($2n = 46$), phenotype unspecified. (d) 1 monosomic ($2n - 1 = 45$) for 21 and aborted early in pregnancy : 1 with a 21/21 translocation chromosome who is essentially trisomic for the long arms of 21 and phenotypically Down. (e) 1 in 3 for part (c); 100% for part (d).

8.45. (a) Male (b) The idiogram contains an extra G-group chromosome ($2n + 1 = 47$). It cannot be determined whether the extra chromosome is 21, 22, or Y. If the patient has the physical characteristics of Down syndrome, the extra chromosome is 21.

Answers to Review Questions

Matching Questions

1. H   2. A   3. J   4. C   5. B   6. G   7. I   8. F   9. D   10. E

Vocabulary

1. triploid
2. allotetraploid (amphidiploid)
3. aneuploidy
4. monosomic
5. polytene
6. reciprocal translocation
7. position effect
8. paracentric inversion
9. pseudodominance
10. idiogram

True-False Questions

1. F (cytogenetics)   2. T   3. F (sterile)   4. F ($2n + 1$)   5. T   6. F (overlapping deletions)   7. T   8. T   9. T   10. F (some kinds of polyploidy are associated with phenotypic exaggeration)

Multiple-Choice Questions

1. *c*   2. *a*   3. *b*   4. *c*   5. *e*   6. *c*   7. *a*   8. *a*   9. *b*   10. *d*

Chapter 9

Quantitative Genetics and Breeding Principles

QUALITATIVE VS. QUANTITATIVE TRAITS

The classical Mendelian traits encountered in the previous chapters have been qualitative in nature, i.e., traits that are easily classified into distinct phenotypic categories. These discrete phenotypes are under the genetic control of only one or a very few genes with little or no environmental modification to obscure the gene effects. In contrast to this, the variability exhibited by many agriculturally important traits fails to fit into separate phenotypic classes (discontinuous variability), but instead forms a spectrum of phenotypes that blend imperceptively from one type to another (continuous variability). Economically important traits such as body weight gains, mature plant heights, egg or milk production records, and yield of grain per acre are **quantitative,** or **metric,** traits with continuous variability. The basic difference between qualitative and quantitative traits involves the number of genes contributing to the phenotypic variability and the degree to which the phenotype can be modified by environmental factors. Quantitative traits may be governed by many genes (perhaps 10–100 or more), each contributing such a small amount to the phenotype that their individual effects cannot be detected by Mendelian methods. Genes of this nature are called **polygenes.** All genes act in concert with other genes. Thus, more than one gene may contribute to a given trait. Furthermore, each gene usually has effects on more than one trait (pleiotropy). The idea that each character is controlled by a single gene (the one-gene–one-trait hypothesis) has often been falsely attributed to Mendel. But even he recognized that a single factor (or gene) might have manifold effects on more than one trait. For example, he observed that purple flowers are correlated with brown seeds and a dark spot on the axils of leaves; similarly, white flowers are correlated with light-colored seeds and no axillary spots on the leaves. In *Drosophila,* many geneic loci (e.g., genes named *dumpy, cut, vestigial, apterous*) are known to contribute to a complex character such as wing development. Each of these genes also has pleiotropic effects on other traits. For example, the gene for vestigial wings also effects the halteres (balancers), bristles, egg production in females, and longevity.

Structural genes produce products such as enzymes that participate in multistep biochemical pathways (Chapter 4) or proteins that regulate the activity of one or more other genes in metabolic or developmental pathways. Because of the complex interactions within these pathways, a gene product acting at any one step might have phenotypic effects (either positively or negatively) on the development of two or more characters. For a given gene, some of its pleiotropic effects may be relatively strong for certain traits, whereas its effects on other traits may be so weak that they are difficult or impossible to identify by Mendelian techniques. It is the totality of these pleiotropic effects of numerous loci (polygenes) that constitutes the genetic base of a quantitative character. In addition to this genetic component, the phenotypic variability of a quantitative trait in a population usually has an environmental component. It is the task of the geneticist to determine the magnitude of the genetic and environmental components of the total phenotypic variability of each quantitative trait in a population. In order to accomplish this task, use is made of some rather sophisticated mathematics, especially of statistics. Only some of the more easily understood rudiments of this branch of genetics will be presented in this chapter. Below are summarized some of the major differences between quantitative and qualitative genetics.

the shepherd or herdsman other than keeping the flock or herd together, warding off predators, etc. This mating method is most likely to generate the greatest genetic diversity among the progeny.

2. Positive Assortative Mating.

This method involves mating individuals that are more alike, either phenotypically or genotypically, than the average of the selected group.

(a) Based on Genetic Relatedness.

Inbreeding is the mating of individuals more closely related than the average of the population to which they belong. Figure 9-9(a) shows a pedigree in which no inbreeding is evident because there is no common ancestral pathway from B to C (D, E, F, and G all being unrelated). In the inbred pedigree of Fig. 9-9(b), B and C have the same parents and thus are full sibs (brothers and/or sisters). In the standard pedigree form shown in Fig. 9-9(b), sires appear on the upper lines and dams on the lower lines. Thus B and D are males; C and E are females. It is desirable to convert a standard pedigree into an arrow diagram for analysis [Fig. 9-9(c)]. The **coefficient of relationship** (R) estimates the percentage of genes held in common by two individuals because of their common ancestry. Since one transmits only a sample half of one's genotype to one's offspring, each arrow in the diagram represents a probability of $\frac{1}{2}$. The sum (Σ) of all pathways between two individuals through common ancestors is the coefficient of relationship.

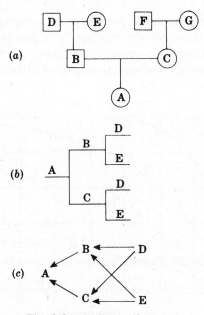

Fig. 9-9.   Pedigree diagrams.

Example 9.22.   In the arrow diagram of Fig. 9-9(c), there are two pathways connecting B and C. The coefficient of relationship between individuals B and C (R_{BC}) = $\Sigma(\frac{1}{2})^s$, where s is the number of steps (arrows) from B to the common ancestor and back to C.

B and C probably contain $(\frac{1}{2})(\frac{1}{2}) = \frac{1}{4}$ of their genes in common through ancestor D.

Similarly, B and C probably contain $\frac{1}{4}$ of their genes in common through ancestor E.

The sum of these two pathways is the coefficient of relationship between the full sibs B and C; $R_{BC} = \frac{1}{4} + \frac{1}{4} = \frac{1}{2}$ or 50%.

When matings occur only between closely related individuals (inbreeding) the genetic effect is an increase in homozygosity. The most intense form of inbreeding is self-fertilization. If we start with a population containing 100 heterozygous individuals (*Aa*) as shown in Table 9.1, the expected number of homozygous genotypes is increased by 50% due to selfing in each generation.

Table 9.1. Expected Increase in Homozygosity Due to Selfing

Generation	AA	Aa	aa	Percent Heterozygosity	Percent Homozygosity
0		100		100	0
1	25	50	25	50	50
2	25	12.5	25	12.5	25	25	75
3	37.5	6.25	12.5	6.25	37.5	12.5	87.5
4	43.75	3.125	6.25	3.125	43.75	6.25	93.75

Other less intense forms of inbreeding produce a less rapid approach to homozygosity, shown graphically in Fig. 9-10. As homozygosity increases in a population, due to either inbreeding or selection, the genetic variability of the population decreases. Since heritability depends upon the relative amount of genetic variability, it also decreases so that in the limiting case (pure line) heritability becomes zero.

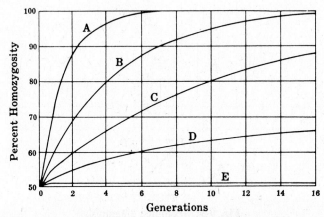

Fig. 9-10. Increase in percentage of homozygosity under various systems of inbreeding. (A) self-fertilization, (B) full sibs, (C) double first cousins, (D) single first cousins, (E) second cousins.

When population size is reduced to a small isolated unit containing less than about 50 individuals, inbreeding very likely will result in a detectable increase in genetic uniformity. The **coefficient of inbreeding** (symbolized by F) is a useful indicator of the probable effect that inbreeding has had at two levels.

(1) On an *individual basis,* the coefficient of inbreeding indicates the probability that the 2 alleles at any locus are identical by descent, i.e., they are both replication products of a gene present in a common ancestor.

(2) On a *population basis,* the coefficient of inbreeding indicates the percentage of all loci that were heterozygous in the base population that now have probably become homozygous due to the effects of inbreeding. The base population is that point in the history of the population from which we desire to begin a calculation of the effects of inbreeding. Many loci are probably homozygous at the time we establish our base population. The inbreeding coefficient then measures the *additional* increase in homozygosity due to matings between closely related individuals.

The coefficient of inbreeding (F) can be determined for an individual in a pedigree by several similar methods.

(1) If the common ancestor is not inbred, the inbreeding coefficient of an individual (F_x) is half the coefficient of relationship between the sire and dam (R_{SD}):

$$F_x = \tfrac{1}{2}R_{SD} \tag{9.23}$$

(2) If the common ancestors are not inbred, the inbreeding coefficient is given by

$$F_x = \Sigma(\tfrac{1}{2})^{p_1+p_2+1} \tag{9.24}$$

where p_1 is the number of generations (arrows) from one parent back to the common ancestor and p_2 is the number of generations from the other parent back to the same ancestor.

(3) If the common ancestors are inbred (F_A), the inbreeding coefficient of the individual must be corrected for this factor:

$$F_x = \Sigma[(\tfrac{1}{2})^{p_1+p_2+1}(1 + F_A)] \tag{9.25}$$

(4) The coefficient of inbreeding of an individual may be calculated by counting the number of arrows (n) that connect the individual through one parent back to the common ancestor and back again to the other parent, and applying the formula

$$F_x = \Sigma(\tfrac{1}{2})^n(1 + F_A) \tag{9.26}$$

The following table will be helpful in calculating F.

n	1	2	3	4	5	6	7	8	9
$(\tfrac{1}{2})^n$	0.5000	0.2500	0.1250	0.0625	0.0312	0.0156	0.0078	0.0039	0.0019

Linebreeding is a special form of inbreeding utilized for the purpose of maintaining a high genetic relationship to a desirable ancestor. Fig. 9-11 shows a pedigree in which close linebreeding to B has been practiced so that A possesses more than 50% of B's genes. D possesses 50% of B's genes and transmits 25% to C. B also contributes 50% of his genes to C. Hence C contains 50% + 25% = 75% B genes and transmits half of them (37.5%) to A. B also contributes 50% of his genes to A. Therefore A has 50% + 37.5% = 87.5% of B's genes.

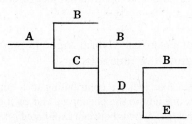

Fig. 9-11. Pedigree exemplifying close linebreeding.

(b) *Based on Phenotypic Similarity*.

Positive phenotypic assortative mating is seldom practiced in its purest form among the selected individuals, i.e., mating only "look-alikes" or those with nearly the same selection indices. However, it can be used in conjunction with random mating; a few of the best among the selected group are "hand coupled," artificially cross-pollinated, or otherwise forced to breed.

Example 9.23. A beef cattle rancher may maintain a small "show string" in addition to a commercial herd. The few show animals would be closest to the ideal breed type (conformation of body parts, size for age, color markings, shape of horns, etc.) and would be mated like-to-like in hopes of generating more of the same for displaying at fairs and livestock expositions. The rest of the herd would be randomly mated to produce slaughter beef. Some of the cows from the commercial herd might eventually be selected for the show string; some of the young bulls or cows of the show string might not prove to be good enough to save for show and yet perform adequately as members of the commercial herd.

Both inbreeding and positive phenotypic assortative mating tend to reduce genetic heterozygosity, but the theoretical end results are quite different.

Example 9.24. As a model consider a metric trait governed by two loci, each with a pair of alleles both additive and equal in effect. Inbreeding among the five phenotypes would ultimately fix four homozygous lines (*AABB, AAbb, aaBB, aabb*). Positive phenotypic assortative mating would only fix two lines (*AABB* and *aabb*).

The rate at which heterozygous loci can be fixed (brought to homozygosity) in a population can be greatly accelerated by combining a system of close inbreeding with the additional restriction of positive phenotypic assortative mating; in other words, they must also "look" alike.

3. Negative Assortative Mating.

(a) *Based on Genetic Relatedness*.

When a mating involves individuals that are more distantly related than the average of the selected group it is classified as a negative genetic assortative mating. This may involve crossing individuals belonging to different families or crossing different inbred varieties of plants or crossing different breeds of livestock. It may occasionally involve crossing closely related species such as the horse and ass (donkey, burro) to produce the hybrid mule. The usual purpose of these "outcrosses" is an attempt to produce offspring of superior phenotypic quality (but not necessarily in breeding value) to that normally found in the parental populations.

Many recessives remain hidden in heterozygous conditions in noninbred populations, but as homozygosity increases in an inbred population there is a greater probability that recessive traits, many of which are deleterious, will begin to appear. One of the consequences of inbreeding is a loss in vigor (i.e., less productive vegetatively and reproductively) that commonly accompanies an increase in homozygosity **(inbreeding depression)**. Crosses between inbred lines usually produce a vigorous hybrid F_1 generation. This increased "fitness" of heterozygous individuals has been termed **heterosis.** The genetic basis of heterosis is still a subject of controversy, largely centered about two theories.

(1) The *dominance theory* of heterosis. Hybrid vigor is presumed to result from the action and interaction of dominant growth or fitness factors.

Example 9.25. Assume that four loci are contributing to a quantitative trait. Each recessive genotype contributes one unit to the phenotype and each dominant genotype contributes two units to the phenotype. A cross between two inbred lines could produce a more highly productive (heterotic) F_1 than either parental line.

P:	$AA\ bb\ CC\ d$	$\times$	$aa\ BB\ cc\ DD$
Phenotypic Value:	$2 + 1 + 2 + 1 = 6$		$1 + 2 + 1 + 2 = 6$
F_1:		$Aa\ Bb\ Cc\ Dd$	
		$2 + 2 + 2 + 2 = 8$	

(2) The *overdominance theory* of heterosis. Heterozygosity per se is assumed to produce hybrid vigor.

Example 9.26. Assume that 4 loci are contributing to a quantitative trait, recessive genotypes contribute 1 unit to the phenotype, heterozygous genotypes contribute 2 units, and homozygous dominant genotypes contribute $1\frac{1}{2}$ units.

P:	$aa\ bb\ CC\ DD$	$\times$	$AA\ BB\ cc\ dd$
Phenotypic Value:	$1 + 1 + 1\frac{1}{2} + 1\frac{1}{2} = 5$		$1\frac{1}{2} + 1\frac{1}{2} + 1 + 1 = 5$
F_1:		$Aa\ Bb\ Cc\ Dd$	
		$2 + 2 + 2 + 2 = 8$	

Phenotypic variability in the hybrid generation is generally much less than that exhibited by the inbred parental lines (Fig. 9-12). This indicates that the heterozygotes are less subject to environmental influences than the homozygotes. Geneticists use the term "buffering" to indicate that the organism's development is highly regulated genetically ("canalized"). Another term often used in this connection is **homeostasis,** which signifies the maintenance of a "steady state" in the development and physiology of the organism within the normal range of environmental fluctuations.

A rough guide to the estimation of heterotic effects (H) is obtained by noting the average excess in vigor that F_1 hybrids exhibit over the midpoint between the means of the inbred parental lines (Fig. 9-12).

$$H_{F_1} = \overline{X}_{F_1} - \tfrac{1}{2}(\overline{X}_{P_1} + \overline{X}_{P_2}) \tag{9.27}$$

The heterosis exhibited by an F_2 population is commonly observed to be half of that manifested by the F_1 hybrids.

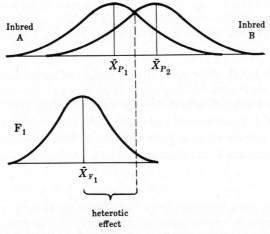

Fig. 9-12. Heterosis in the progeny from crossing inbred lines.

(b) Based on Phenotypic Dissimilarity.

When intermediate phenotypes are preferred, they are more likely to be produced by mating opposite phenotypes. For example, general-purpose cattle can be produced by crossing a beef type with a dairy type. The offspring commonly produce an intermediate yield of milk and hang up a fair carcass when slaughtered (although generally not as good in either respect as the parental types). The same is true of the offspring from crossing an egg type (such as the Leghorn breed of chicken) with a meat type (such as the Cornish). Crossing phenotypic opposites may also be made to correct specific defects.

Example 9.27. Brahman cattle have more heat tolerance and resistance to certain insects than European cattle breeds. Brahmans are often crossed to these other breeds in order to create hybrids with the desirable qualities of both parental populations.

Example 9.28. Sometimes "weedy" relatives of agriculturally important crops may carry genes for resistance to specific diseases. Hybrids from such crosses may acquire disease resistance, and successive rounds of selection combined with backcrossing to the crop variety can eventually fix the gene or genes for disease resistance on a background that is essentially totally that of the cultivated species.

Solved Problems

QUASI-QUANTITATIVE TRAITS

9.1. Two homozygous varieties of *Nicotiana longiflora* have mean corolla lengths of 40.5 and 93.3 millimeters. The average of the F_1 hybrids from these two varieties was of intermediate length. Among 444 F_2 plants, none was found to have flowers either as long as or as short as the average of the parental varieties. Estimate the minimal number of pairs of alleles segregating from the F_1.

Solution:

If four pairs of alleles were segregating from the F_1, we expect $(\frac{1}{4})^4 = \frac{1}{256}$ of the F_2 to be as extreme as one or the other parental average. Likewise, if five pairs of alleles were segregating, we expect $(\frac{1}{4})^5 = \frac{1}{1024}$ of the F_2 to be as extreme as one parent or the other. Since none of the 444 F_2 plants had flowers this extreme, more than four loci (minimum of five loci) are probably segregating from the F_1.

9.2. The mean internode length of the Abed Binder variety of barley was found to be 3.20 millimeters. The mean length in the Asplund variety was 2.10 millimeters. Crossing these two varieties produced an F_1 and F_2 with average internode lengths of 2.65 millimeters. About 6% of the F_2 had an internode length of 3.2 millimeters, and another 6% had a length of 2.1 millimeters. Determine the most probable number of gene pairs involved in internode length and the approximate contribution each gene makes to the phenotype.

Solution:

With one pair of genes we expect about $\frac{1}{4}$ or 25% of the F_2 to be as extreme as one of the parents. With two pairs of genes we expect approximately $\frac{1}{16}$ or 6.25% as extreme as one parent. Thus we may postulate two pairs of genes. Let A and B represent growth factors and a and b represent null genes.

P: *AA BB*   ×   *aa bb*
                   Abed Binder   Asplund
        4 growth genes = 3.2 millimeters   0 growth genes = 2.1 millimeters

F_1:   *Aa Bb*
                        2 growth genes = 2.65 millimeters

The difference $2.65 - 2.10 = 0.55$ millimeter is the result of 2 growth genes. Therefore each growth gene contributes 0.275 millimeter to the phenotype.

F_2:

No. of Growth Genes	Mean Internode Length (millimeters)	Frequency	Genotypes
4	3.200	1/16	AABB
3	2.925	1/4	AaBB, AABb
2	2.650	3/8	AAbb, AaBb, aaBB
1	2.375	1/4	aaBb, Aabb
0	2.100	1/16	aabb (physiological minimum due to residual genotype)

9.3. A large breed of chicken, the Golden Hamburg, was crossed to small Sebright Bantams. The F_1 was intermediate in size. The mean size of the F_2 was about the same as that of the F_1, but the variability of the F_2 was so great that a few individuals were found to exceed the size of either parental type (**transgressive variation**). If all of the alleles contributing to size act with equal and cumulative effects, and if the parents are considered to be homozygous, how can these results be explained?

Solution:

Let capital letters stand for growth genes (active alleles) and small letters stand for alleles that do not contribute to growth (null alleles). For simplicity we will consider only four loci.

P: *aa BB CC DD*   ×   *AA bb cc dd*
          large Golden Hamburg   small Sebright Bantam
          6 active alleles   2 active alleles

F_1:   *Aa Bb Cc Dd*
                    intermediate-sized hybrid
                        4 active alleles

F_2:   Some genotypes could segregate out in the F_2 with phenotypic values that exceed that of the parents. For example:

AA BB CC DD   8 active alleles⎱ larger than
Aa BB CC DD   7 active alleles⎰ Golden Hamburg

Aa bb cc dd   1 active allele ⎱ smaller than
aa bb cc dd   0 active alleles⎰ Sebright Bantams
                 (physiological minimum)

THE NORMAL DISTRIBUTION

9.4. A representative sample of lamb weaning weights is shown below. Determine the weight limits within which 95% of all lambs from this population are expected to be found at weaning time.

81	81	83	101	86
65	68	77	66	92
94	85	105	60	90
94	90	81	63	58

Solution:

The standard deviation is calculated as follows.

$$\overline{X} = \frac{\Sigma X}{N} = \frac{1620}{20} = 81.0$$

X	$X - \overline{X}$	$(X - \overline{X})^2$
81	0	0
65	-16	256
94	$+13$	169
94	$+13$	169
81	0	0
68	-13	169
85	$+4$	16
90	$+9$	81
83	$+2$	4
77	-4	16
105	$+24$	576
81	0	0
101	$+20$	400
66	-15	225
60	-21	441
63	-18	324
86	$+5$	25
92	$+11$	121
90	$+9$	81
58	-23	529
$\Sigma X = 1620$	$\Sigma(X - \overline{X}) = 0$	$\Sigma(X - \overline{X})^2 = 3602$

$$s = \sqrt{\frac{\Sigma(X - \overline{X})^2}{N - 1}} = \sqrt{\frac{3602}{19}} = 13.77$$

95% of all weaning weights are expected to lie within $\pm 2s$ of the mean. Thus $\overline{X} \pm 2s = 81.0 \pm 2(13.77) = 81.0 \pm 27.54$. The upper limit is 108.54 and the lower limit is 53.46.

9.5. The average fleece weight in a large band of sheep together with its standard deviation was calculated to be 10.3 ± 1.5 pounds. The statistics for fleece grade (on a scale from 0 to 10) was 5.1 ± 0.7 units. Which trait is relatively more variable?

Solution:

Relative variability may be determined from a comparison of their coefficients of variation (CV).

$$\text{CV (fleece weight)} = s/\overline{X} = 1.5/10.3 = 0.146$$
$$\text{CV (fleece grade)} \;\; = 0.7/5.1 = 0.137$$

Fleece weight has a slightly higher coefficient of variation and thus is relatively more variable than fleece grade.

9.6. The Flemish breed of rabbits has an average body weight of 3600 grams. The Himalayan breed has a mean of 1875 grams. Matings between these two breeds produce an intermediate F_1 with a standard deviation of ± 162 grams. The variability of the F_2 is greater as indicated by a standard deviation of ± 230 grams. (*a*) Estimate the number of pairs of factors contributing to mature body weight in rabbits. (*b*) Estimate the average metric contribution of each active allele.

Solution:

(*a*) From equation (*9.6*),

$$N = \frac{D^2}{8(\sigma_{PF2}^2 - \sigma_{PF1}^2)} = \frac{(3600 - 1875)^2}{8(230^2 - 162^2)} = 13.95 \text{ or approximately 14 pairs}$$

(*b*) The difference $3600 - 1875 = 1725$ grams is attributed to 14 *pairs* of factors or 28 active alleles. The average contribution of each active allele is $\frac{1725}{28} = 61.61$ grams.

9.7. In a population having a phenotypic mean of 55 units, a total genetic variance for the trait of 35 units^2, and an environmental variance of 14 units^2, between what two phenotypic values will approximately 68% of the population be found?

Solution:

$$\sigma_P^2 = \sigma_G^2 + \sigma_E^2 = 35 + 14 = 49, \quad \sigma_P = 7.$$

68% of a normally distributed population is expected to be found within the limits $\mu \pm \sigma = 55 \pm 7$, or between 48 units and 62 units.

TYPES OF GENE ACTION

9.8. The F_1 produced by crossing two varieties of tomatoes has a mean fruit weight of 50 grams and a phenotypic variance of 225 gram^2. The F_1 is backcrossed to one of the parental varieties having a mean of 150 grams. Assuming that tomato fruit weight is governed by multiplicative gene action, predict the variance of the backcross progeny.

Solution:

The expected mean of the backcross progeny is the geometric mean of 150 and 50, or $\sqrt{150 \times 50} = \sqrt{7500} = 86.6$. If multiplicative gene action is operative the variance is dependent upon the mean, thus producing a constant coefficient of variation in segregating populations.

F_1 coefficient of variation = $s/\overline{X} = \sqrt{225}/50 = 0.3$, and so the coefficient of variation in the backcross generation is also expected to be 0.3.

Standard deviation of backcross = $0.3(86.6) = 25.98$.

Variance of backcross = $(25.98)^2 = 675$ gram^2.

HERITABILITY

9.9. Identical twins are derived from a single fertilized egg (monozygotic). Fraternal twins develop from different fertilized eggs (dizygotic) and are expected to have about half of their genes in common. Left-hand middle-finger-length measurements were taken on the fifth birthday in samples (all of the same sex) of identical twins, fraternal twins, and unrelated individuals from a population of California Caucasians. Using only variances between twins and between unrelated members of the total population, devise a formula for estimating the heritability of left-hand middle-finger length at 5 years of age in this population.

Solution:

Let V_i = phenotypic variance between identical twins, V_f = phenotypic variance between fraternal twins, and V_t = phenotypic variance between randomly chosen pairs from the total population of which these twins are a part. All of the phenotypic variance between identical twins is nongenetic (environmental); thus $V_i = V_e$. The phenotypic variance between fraternal twins is partly genetic and partly environmental. Since fraternal twins are 50% related, their genetic variance is expected to be only half that of unrelated individuals; thus $V_f = \frac{1}{4}V_g + V_e$. The difference $(V_f - V_i)$ estimates half of the genetic variance.

$$V_f - V_i = \underbrace{\tfrac{1}{2}V_g + V_e}_{V_f} - \underbrace{V_e}_{V_i} = \tfrac{1}{2}V_g$$

Therefore, heritability is twice that difference divided by the total phenotypic variance.

$$h^2 = \frac{2(V_f - V_i)}{V_t}$$

9.10. Two homozygous varieties of *Nicotiana longiflora* were crossed to produce F_1 hybrids. The average variance of corolla length for all three populations was 8.76. The variance of the F_2 was 40.96. Estimate the heritability of flower length in the F_2 population.

Solution:

Since the two parental varieties and the F_1 are all genetically uniform, their average phenotypic variance is an estimate of the environmental variance (V_e). The phenotypic variance of the F_2 (V_t) is partly genetic and partly environmental. The difference ($V_t - V_e$) is the genetic variance (V_g).

$$h^2 = \frac{V_g}{V_t} = \frac{V_t - V_e}{V_t} = \frac{40.96 - 8.76}{40.96} = 0.79$$

9.11. Given the phenotypic variances of a quantitative trait in two pure lines (V_{P1} and V_{P2}), in their F_1 and F_2 progenies (V_{F1} and V_{F2}), in the backcross progeny $F_1 \times P_1(V_{B1})$ and in the backcross progeny $F_1 \times P_2(V_{B2})$, show how estimates of additive genetic variance (V_A), dominance genetic variance (V_D), and environmental variance (V_E) can be derived.

Solution:

Since all of the phenotypic variance within pure lines and their genetically uniform F_1 progeny is environmental,

$$V_E = \frac{V_{P1} + V_{P2} + V_{F1}}{3}$$

Therefore (from page 218),
$$V_{F2} - V_E = (\tfrac{1}{2}A + \tfrac{1}{4}D + E) - E \qquad (1)$$
$$= \tfrac{1}{2}A + \tfrac{1}{4}D$$

Likewise (from page 218),
$$V_{B1} + V_{B2} = \tfrac{1}{2}A + \tfrac{1}{2}D + 2E \qquad (2)$$
$$(V_{B1} + V_{B2}) - 2V_E = \tfrac{1}{4}A + \tfrac{1}{2}D$$

By multiplying equation (1) by 2 and subtracting equation (2) from the result, we can solve for A.

$$A + \tfrac{1}{2}D = 2(V_{F2} - V_E)$$
$$\tfrac{1}{2}A + \tfrac{1}{2}D = (V_{B1} + V_{B2}) - 2V_E$$
$$\overline{\tfrac{1}{2}A \qquad\quad = V_A}$$

By substituting $\tfrac{1}{2}A$ into equation (1), we can solve for $\tfrac{1}{4}D = V_D$.

9.12. The pounds of grease fleece weight was measured in a sample from a sheep population. The data listed below is for the average of both parents (X, midparent) and their offspring (Y).

X	11.8	8.4	9.5	10.0	10.9	7.6	10.8	8.5	11.8	10.5
Y	7.7	5.7	5.8	7.2	7.3	5.4	7.2	5.6	8.4	7.0

(*a*) Calculate the regression coefficient of offspring on midparent and estimate the heritability of grease fleece weight in this population. (*b*) Plot the data and draw the regression line. (*c*) Calculate the correlation coefficient and from that estimate the heritability.

Solution:

(a)

X	Y	X^2	Y^2	XY
11.8	7.7	139.24	59.29	90.86
8.4	5.7	70.56	32.49	47.88
9.5	5.8	90.25	33.64	55.10
10.0	7.2	100.00	51.84	72.00
10.9	7.3	118.81	53.29	79.57
7.6	5.4	57.76	29.16	41.04
10.8	7.2	116.64	51.84	77.76
8.5	5.6	72.25	31.36	47.60
11.8	8.4	139.24	70.56	99.12
10.5	7.0	110.25	49.00	73.50
$\Sigma X = 99.8$	$\Sigma Y = 67.3$	$\Sigma X^2 = 1015.00$	$\Sigma Y^2 = 462.47$	$\Sigma XY = 684.43$

$$n = 10$$

$$\frac{(\Sigma X)^2}{n} = \frac{(99.8)^2}{10} = \frac{9960.04}{10} = 996.0$$

$$\frac{\Sigma X \Sigma Y}{n} = \frac{(99.8)(67.3)}{10} = \frac{6716.54}{10} = 671.65$$

$$b = \frac{\Sigma XY - [(\Sigma X \Sigma Y)/n]}{\Sigma X^3 - [(\Sigma X)^2/n]} = \frac{684.43 - 671.65}{1015 - 996} = \frac{12.78}{19} = 0.6726$$

The regression of offspring on midparent is an estimate of heritability:

$$h^2 = 0.67$$

(b) Data plot and regression line:

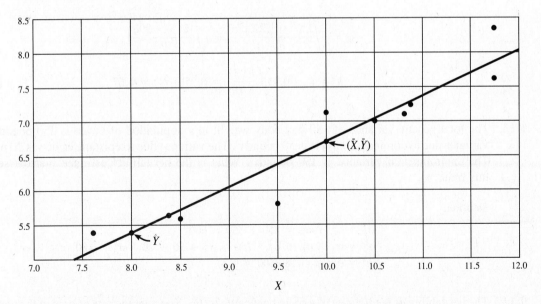

The regression line goes through the intersection of the two means $(\overline{X}, \overline{Y})$; $\overline{X} = 99.8/10 = 9.98$; $\overline{Y} = 67.3/10 = 6.73$. The regression line intersects the Y axis at the Y intercept (a).

$$a = \overline{Y} - b\overline{X}$$
$$= 6.73 - 0.673(9.98) = 0.01$$

Now let us choose a value of X that is distant from $(\overline{X}, \overline{Y})$ but easily plotted on the graph (e.g., $X = 8.0$). The corresponding value of Y is estimated to be

$$\hat{Y} = a + bX = 0.01 + 0.673(8.0) = 5.39$$

These two points $[(\overline{X}, \overline{Y})$ and $\hat{Y}]$ establish the regression line with slope $b = 0.67$. For every 1-pound increase in midparent values, offspring tend to produce 0.67 pound.

same numerator as b

$$r = \frac{\overbrace{\Sigma XY - [(\Sigma X \Sigma Y)/n]}}{\underbrace{\sqrt{\{\Sigma X^2 - [(\Sigma X)^2/n]\} \{\Sigma Y^2 - [(\Sigma Y)^2/n]\}}}}$$

same denominator as b

$$\Sigma Y^2 = 462.47$$
$$\frac{(\Sigma Y)^2}{n} = \frac{4529.29}{10} = 452.93$$

$$r = \frac{12.78}{\sqrt{(19)(462.47 - 452.93)}} = \frac{12.78}{\sqrt{181.26}} = \frac{12.78}{13.46} = 0.95$$

Therefore, the X and Y values are very highly positively correlated. Note that two variables can be highly correlated without also being nearly equal. Two variables are perfectly correlated if for one unit change in one variable there is a constant change (either plus or minus) in the other. Negative correlations for heritability estimates are biologically meaningless. Different traits, however, may have negative genetic correlations (e.g., total milk production vs. butterfat percentage in dairy cattle); many of the same genes that contribute positively to milk yield also contribute negatively to butterfat content.

$$h^2 = b = r\left(\frac{s_Y}{s_X}\right)$$

$$s_Y = \sqrt{\frac{\Sigma Y^2 - [(\Sigma Y)^2/n]}{n - 1}} = \sqrt{\frac{462.47 - 452.93}{9}} = 1.03$$

$$s_X = \sqrt{\frac{\Sigma X^2 - [(\Sigma X)^2/n]}{n - 1}} = \sqrt{\frac{1015 - 996}{9}} = 1.45$$

$$h^2 = b = 0.95\left(\frac{1.03}{1.45}\right) = 0.95(0.71) = 0.67$$

9.13. The total genetic variance of 180-day body weight in a population of swine is 250 pounds^2. The variance due to dominance effects is 50 pounds^2. The variance due to epistatic effects is 20 pounds^2. The environmental variance is 350 pounds^2. What is the heritability estimate (narrow sense) of this trait?

Solution:

$$\sigma_P^2 = \sigma_G^2 + \sigma_E^2 = 250 + 350 = 600$$
$$\sigma_G^2 = \sigma_A^2 + \sigma_D^2 + \sigma_I^2, \quad 250 = \sigma_A^2 + 50 + 20, \quad \sigma_A^2 = 180$$
$$h^2 = \sigma_A^2/\sigma_P^2 = 180/600 = 0.3$$

9.14. The heritability of feedlot rate of gain in beef cattle is 0.6. The average rate of gain in the population is 1.7 pounds/day. The average rate of gain of the individuals selected from this population to be the parents of the next generation is 2.8 pounds/day. What is the expected average daily gain of the progeny in the next generation?

Solution:

$$\Delta P = \overline{P}_p - \overline{P} = 2.8 - 1.7 = 1.1. \quad \Delta G = h^2(\Delta P) = 0.6(1.1) = 0.66. \quad \overline{P}_2 = \overline{P}_1 + \Delta G = 2.36$$
pounds/day.

SELECTION METHODS

9.15. Fifty gilts (female pigs) born each year in a given herd can be used for proving sires. Average litter size at birth is 10 with 10% mortality to maturity. Only the 5 boars (males) with the highest sire index will be saved for further use in the herd. If each test requires 18 mature progeny, how much culling can be practiced among the progeny tested boars, i.e., what proportion of those tested will not be saved?

Solution:

Each gilt will produce an average of $10 - (0.1)(10) = 9$ progeny raised to maturity. If 18 mature progeny are required to prove a sire, then each boar should be mated to 2 gilts. (50 gilts)/(2 gilts per boar) = 25 boars can be proved. $20/25 = 4/5 = 80\%$ of these boars will be culled.

9.16. Given the following pedigree with butterfat records on the cows and equal-parent indices on the bulls, estimate the index for young bull X (*a*) using information from A and B, (*b*) when the record made by B is only one lactation, and that made in another herd.

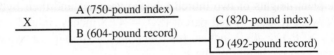

Solution:

(*a*) The midparent index (estimate of transmitting ability) for X is $(750 + 604)/2 = 677$.

(*b*) Since we cannot rely on B's record, we should use information from C and D, recalling that X is separated by two Mendelian segregations from the grandparents. Then $X = \frac{750}{2} + \frac{820}{4} + \frac{492}{4} = 703$.

MATING METHODS

9.17. Calculate the inbreeding coefficient for A in the following pedigree.

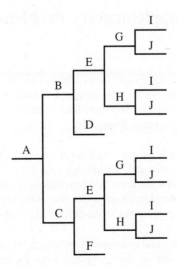

Solution:

First we must convert the pedigree to an arrow diagram.

There is only one pathway from B to C and that goes through ancestor E. However, ancestor E is himself inbred. Note that the parents of E are full sibs, i.e., G and H are 50% related (see Example 9.22). By formula (9.23),

$$F_E = \tfrac{1}{2}R_{GH} = \tfrac{1}{2}(0.5) = 0.25$$

The inbreeding coefficient of A is given by equation (9.26),

$$F_A = \Sigma \left(\tfrac{1}{2}\right)^n (1 + F_{ancestor}) = \left(\tfrac{1}{2}\right)^3(1 + 0.25) = 0.156$$

where n is the number of arrows connecting the individual (A) through one parent (B) back to the common ancestor (E) and back again to the other parent (C).

9.18. The average plant heights of two inbred tobacco varieties and their hybrids have been measured with the following results: inbred parent (P_1) = 47.8 inches, inbred parent (P_2) = 28.7 inches, F_1 hybrid $(P_1 \times P_2)$ = 43.2 inches. (a) Calculate the amount of heterosis exhibited by the F_1. (b) Predict the average height of the F_2.

Solution:

(a) The amount of heterosis is expressed by the excess of the F_1 average over the midpoint between the two parental means.

$$\text{Heterosis of } F_1 = \overline{X}_{F_1} - \tfrac{1}{2}(\overline{X}_{F_1} + \overline{X}_{P_2}) = 43.2 - \tfrac{1}{2}(47.8 + 28.7) = 43.2 - 38.25 = 4.95 \text{ inches}$$

(b) As a general rule the F_2 shows only about half the heterosis of the F_1: $\tfrac{1}{2}(4.95)$ = 2.48. Hence the expected height of F_2 plants = 38.25 + 2.48 = 40.73 inches.

Supplementary Problems

QUASI-QUANTITATIVE TRAITS

9.19. Beginning at some arbitrary date, two varieties of wheat were scored for the length of time (in days) to heading, from which the following means were obtained: variety X = 13.0 days, variety Y = 27.6 days. From a survey of 5,504,000 F_2 progeny, 86 were found to head out in 13 days or less. How many pairs of factors are probably contributing to early flowering?

9.20. Suppose that the average skin color on one racial population is 0.43 (measured by the reflectance of skin to red light of 685-nanometer wavelength); the average skin color of a population racially distinct from the first is 0.23; and racial hybrids between these two populations average 0.33. If about 1/150 offspring from hybrid (racially mixed) parents have skin colors as extreme as the average of either race, estimate the number of segregating loci in the hybrid parents that contribute to skin color variability in their offspring.

9.21. Suppose that 5 pairs of genes with equal and cumulative effects are contributing to body weight in laboratory albino rats. Two highly inbred strains (homozygous) have the extreme high and low mature weights, respectively. A hybrid F_1 generation is produced by crossing these two lines. The average cost of raising a rat to maturity is $2.00. What will it probably cost the breeder to recover in the F_2 a rat that is as extreme as the high parental line?

THE NORMAL DISTRIBUTION

9.22. From a sample of 10 pig body weights determine (a) mean body weight, (b) sample standard deviation (s), (c) the weight that will probably be exceeded by $2\frac{1}{2}\%$ of this population. Pig weights: 210, 215, 220, 225, 215, 205, 220, 210, 215, 225.

VARIANCE

9.23. Suppose 6 pairs of genes were contributing to a metric trait in a cultivated crop. Two parental lines with averages of 13,000 pounds/acre and 7000 pounds/acre produced an intermediate hybrid F_1 with a variance of 250,000 pounds^2. Estimate the standard deviation of the F_2 by formula (9.6).

9.24. Two strains of mice were tested for susceptibility to a carcinogenic drug. The susceptible strain had an average of 75.4 tumorous lung nodules, whereas the resistant strain failed to develop nodules. The F_1 from crossing these two strains had an average of 12.5 nodules with a standard deviation of ± 5.3; the F_2 had 10.0 ± 14.1 nodules. Estimate the number of gene pairs contributing to tumor susceptibility by use of formula (9.6).

TYPES OF GENE ACTION

9.25. Calculate the metric values of the parents and their F_1 hybrids in the cross $AA\ B'B'\ CC\ D'D' \times A'A'\ BB\ C'C'\ DD$ assuming (a) additive gene action where unprimed alleles contribute 3 units each to the phenotype and primed alleles contribute 6 units each, (b) primed alleles are fully dominant to unprimed alleles; at a given locus, genotypes with one or two primed alleles produce 12 units and the recessive genotype produces 6 units.

9.26. Several generations of selection and inbreeding in a laboratory strain of mice produced a giant strain with a mean of 40 grams at 2 months of age and a midget strain with an average of 12 grams. The phenotypic variance of the giant strain is 26.01 and of the midget strain is 2.92. (a) Calculate the coefficient of variation for the giant and the midget strains. (b) On the basis of your findings in part (a), calculate the expected mean of the F_1 produced by crossing these two lines.

9.27. Several examples of multiplicative gene action are known in crosses between tomato varieties. Calculate the arithmetic mean and geometric mean for each F_1 and compare each of their absolute deviations from the F_1 mean. The mean fruit weight in grams for each group is given in parentheses.

	Variety 1	Variety 2	F_1
(a)	Yellow Pear (12.4)	Honor Bright (150.0)	(47.5)
(b)	Yellow Pear (12.4)	Peach (42.6)	(23.1)
(c)	Dwarf Aristocrat (112.4)	Peach (42.6)	(67.1)
(d)	Tangerine (173.6)	Red Currant (1.1)	(8.3)

HERITABILITY

9.28. Let V_i = phenotypic variance between identical twins, V_f = phenotypic variance between fraternal twins, and heritability $(h^2) = (V_f - V_i)/V_f$. Given the following differences in intelligence quotients (IQ) of 20 pairs of twins (all females, reared together, and identically tested at the same age), estimate the heritability of IQ.

Identical twins	6	2	7	2	4	4	3	5	5	2
Fraternal twins	10	7	13	15	12	11	14	9	12	17

9.29. Suppose that population A has a mean IQ of 85 and that of population B is 100. Estimates of heritability of IQ in both populations are relatively high (0.4 to 0.8). Explain why each of the following statements is false.

(a) Heritability estimates measure the degree to which a trait is determined by genes.

(b) Since the heritability of IQ is relatively high, the average differences between the two populations must be largely due to genetic differences.

(c) Since population B has a higher average IQ than population A, population B is genetically superior to A.

9.30. Flower lengths were measured in two pure lines, their F_1 and F_2 and backcross progenies. To eliminate multiplicative effects, logarithms of the measurements were used. The phenotypic variances were $P_1 = 48$, $P_2 = 32$, $F_1 = 46$, $F_2 = 130.5$, $B_1(F_1 \times P_1) = 85.5$, and $B_2(F_1 \times P_2) = 98.5$. (a) Estimate the environmental variance (V_E), the additive genetic variance (V_A), and the dominance genetic variance (V_D). (b) Calculate the degree of dominance. (c) Estimate the narrow heritability of flower length in the F_2. *Hint:* See Problem 9.11.

9.31. Let r_1 = phenotypic correlation of full sibs, r_2 = phenotypic correlation of half sibs, r_3 = correlation of offspring with one parent, r_4 = correlation of monozygotic twins, and r_5 = correlation of dizygotic twins. In the following formulas, determine the values of x and/or y:

$$(a)\ h^2 = x(r_1 - r_2) \qquad (b)\ h^2 = xr_1 - yr_3 \qquad (c)\ h^2 = x(r_4 - r_5)$$

9.32. In the following table, Y represents the average number of bristles on a specific thoracic segment of *Drosophila melanogaster* in four female offspring and X represents the number of bristles in the mother (dam) of each set of 4 daughters.

Family	1	2	3	4	5	6	7	8	9	10
X	9	6	9	6	7	8	7	7	8	9
Y	8	6	7	8	8	7	7	9	9	8

(a) Calculate the daughter-dam regression. (b) Estimate the heritability of bristle number in this population assuming $s_X = s_Y$.

9.33. The regression coefficient (b) represents how much one variable is expected to change per unit change in some other variable. The correlation coefficient (r) reflects how closely the data points are to the regression line (perfect correlation = ± 1). Using only these definitions (no formulas), determine the regression of X_1 on X_2 and their correlation from the following pairs of measurements:

X_1	11	12	13	14	15
X_2	13	15	17	19	21

9.34. Around 1903, Pearson and Lee collected measurements of brother and sister heights from more than 1000 British families. A sample of 11 of such families is shown below.

Family No.	1	2	3	4	5	6	7	8	9	10	11
Brother	71	68	66	67	70	71	70	73	72	65	66
Sister	69	64	65	63	65	62	65	64	66	59	62

(a) Calculate the regression coefficient of sisters' height on brothers' height. (b) Calculate the regression coefficient of brothers' height on sisters' height. (c) The correlation coefficient (r) is the geometric mean of the above two regression coefficients; determine r. (d) If the variance of brothers' heights $s_B^2 = 74$ and that of sisters' $s_S^2 = 66$, calculate the heritability of body height from r. Does the answer make biological sense? Explain.

9.35. A flock of chickens has an average mature body weight of 6.6 pounds. Individuals saved for breeding purposes have a mean of 7.2 pounds. The offspring generation has a mean of 6.81 pounds. Estimate the heritability of mature body weight in this flock.

9.36. Yearly wool records (in pounds) are taken from a sample of 10 sheep: 11.8, 8.4, 9.5, 10.0, 10.9, 7.8, 10.8, 8.5, 11.8, 10.5. (a) Calculate the range within which approximately 95% of the sheep in this population are expected to be found. (b) If the additive genetic variance is 0.60, what is the heritability estimate of wool production in this breed?

9.37. Determine (a) the dominance variance and (b) the environmental variance from the following information: heritability [formula (9.9)] = 0.3, phenotypic variance = 200 pounds^2, total genetic variance = 100 pounds^2, and epistatic variance is absent.

9.38. Thickness of backfat in a certain breed of swine has been estimated to have a heritability of 80%. Suppose the average backfat thickness of this breed is 1.2 inches and the average of individuals selected from this population to be the parents of the next generation is 0.8 inch. What is the expected average of the next generation?

9.39. The average yearly milk production of a herd of cows is 18,000 pounds. The average milk production of the individuals selected to be parents of the next generation is 20,000 pounds. The average milk production of the offspring generation is 18,440 pounds. (a) Estimate the heritability of milk production in this population. (b) If the phenotypic variance of this population is 4,000,000 pounds^2, estimate the additive genetic variance. (c) Between what two values is the central 68% of the original (18,000 pound average) population expected to be found?

9.40. The average weight at 140 days in a swine population is 180 pounds. The average weight of individuals selected from this population for breeding purposes is 195 pounds. Heritability of 140-day weight in swine is 30%. Calculate (a) selection differential, (b) expected genetic gain in the progeny, (c) predicted average 140-day weight of the progeny.

9.41. About 1903 Johannsen, a Danish botanist, measured the weight of seeds in the Princess Variety of bean. Beans are self fertilizing and therefore this variety is a pure line. The weights in centigrams of a small but representative sample of beans are listed below.

19	31	18	24	27	28	25	30	29
22	29	26	23	20	24	21	25	29

(a) Calculate the mean and standard deviation for bean weight in this sample. (b) Calculate the environmental variance. (c) Estimate the heritability of bean weight in this variety. (d) If the average bean weight of individuals selected to be parents from this population is 30 centigrams, predict the average bean weight of the next generation.

SELECTION METHODS

9.42. The length of an individual beetle is 10.3 millimeters or 0.5 when expressed in "standardized" form. The average measurement for this trait in the beetle population is 10.0 millimeters. What is the variance of this trait?

9.43. Given the swine selection index I = 0.14W − 0.27S, where W is the pig's own 180-day weight and S is its market score. (a) Rank the following three animals according to index merit:

Animal	Weight	Score
X	220	48
Y	240	38
Z	200	30

(b) If differences in index score are 20% heritable, and parents score 3.55 points higher than the average of the population, how much increase in the average score of the progeny is expected?

9.44. A beef cattle index (I) for selecting replacement heifers takes the form $I = 6 + 2WW' + WG'$, where WW' is weaning weight in standardized form and WG' is weaning grade in standardized form. The average weaning weight of the herd = 505 pounds with a standard deviation of ±34.5 pounds. The average weaning grade (a numerical score) is 88.6 with a standard deviation of ±2.1. Which of the following animals has the best overall merit?

Animal	Actual Weaning Weight	Actual Weaning Grade
A	519	88
B	486	91

9.45. Suppose 360 ewes (female sheep) are available for proving sires. All ewes lamb; 50% of ewes lambing have twins. The 10 rams with the highest progeny test scores will be kept as flock sires. How much selection can be practiced among the progeny-tested individuals, i.e., what proportion of those tested can be saved if a test requires (a) 18 progeny, (b) 12 progeny, (c) 6 progeny?

9.46. During the same year 3 dairy bulls were each mated to a random group of cows. The number of pounds of butterfat produced by the dams and their daughters (corrected to a 305-day lactation at maturity with twice daily milking) was recorded as shown below.

Bull	Dam	Dam's Record	Daughter's Record
A	1	600	605
	2	595	640
	3	615	625
	4	610	600
B	5	585	610
	6	590	620
	7	620	605
	8	605	595
C	9	590	590
	10	590	595
	11	610	600
	12	600	605

(a) Calculate the sire index for each of the 3 sires. (b) Which sire would you save for extensive use in your herd?

MATING METHODS

9.47. A is linebred to B in the following pedigree. Calculate the inbreeding coefficient of A.

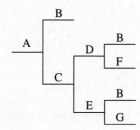

9.48. Given the following arrow diagram, calculate the inbreeding coefficient of A.

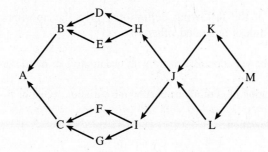

9.49. Calculate the inbreeding of A in the following. *Hint:* There are nine pathways between B and C.

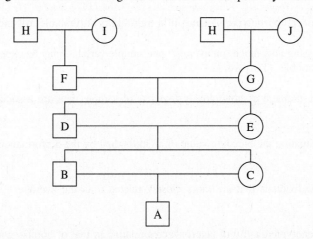

9.50. The yield of seed (in bushels per acre) and plant height (in centimeters) was measured on several generations of corn. Calculate by equation (9.27), (a) the amount of heterosis in the F_1 resulting from crossing the parental varieties with the inbreds, (b) the yield and height expectations of the F_2.

	Seed Yield	Plant Height
Parental varieties	73.3	265
Inbreds	25.0	193
F_1 hybrids	71.4	257

Review Questions

Matching Questions   Choose the one best match of each numbered item with one of the lettered items. Each letter may be used only once.

1. σ^2 A. σ_G^2/σ_P^2
2. h^2 B. Sample standard deviation
3. b C. Inbreeding coefficient
4. r D. Standardized variable
5. F E. Regression coefficient
6. $s/\bar{X}$ F. Coefficient of genetic relationship
7. $(X - \bar{X})/s$ G. Sample coefficient of variation
8. R H. Population variance
9. ΔG I. Correlation coefficient
10. $\sqrt{\Sigma(X - \bar{X})^2/(n - 1)}$ J. None of the above

Vocabulary For each of the following definitions, give the appropriate term and spell it correctly. Terms are single words unless indicated otherwise.

1. The kind of phenotypic variation associated with quantitative or metric traits. (One or two words.)

2. A bell-shaped distribution of continuous phenotypic variation. (One or two words.)

3. A squared standard deviation.

4. A type of allelic interaction in which the phenotype of a heterozygote is outside the phenotypic limits of the corresponding homozygotes.

5. The proportion of the phenotypic variance of a trait that is attributable to gene effects.

6. A statistic expressing how much (on average) one sample variable may be expected to change per unit change in some other variable. (Two words.)

7. A statistical measurement of how closely two sets of sample data are associated, having limits ± 1. (Two words.)

8. A method of estimating the breeding value of an individual by the performance or phenotype of its offspring. (Two words.)

9. The mating of individuals that are more closely related than the average of the population to which they belong.

10. The superior phenotypic quality of heterozygotes relative to that of homozygotes, commonly called "hybrid vigor."

True-False Questions Answer each of the following statements either true (T) or false (F).

1. Quantitative traits are commonly studied by making counts and ratios of progeny phenotypes from parents of contrasting phenotypes.

2. A parameter is a measurement derived from a sample.

3. Most metric traits of economic importance have high heritabilities (h^2 greater than 0.5).

4. Mass selection is the best method for improving metric traits with low heritabilities (h^2 less than 0.2).

5. Family selection is based upon the merits of ancestors.

6. Matings between siblings are the most extreme form of inbreeding possible among sexually reproducing species.

7. Linebreeding is a special form of inbreeding used to maintain a high genetic relationship to a desired ancestor.

8. Both inbreeding and positive assortative mating tend to reduce genetic heterozygosity, but the theoretical end results are quite different.

9. Loss of vigor (vegetative and/or reproductive) commonly accompanies an increase in polygenic homozygosity.

10. Most of our food is produced by mating methods that are essentially panmictic.

Multiple-Choice Questions   Choose the one best answer.

For problems 1–3, use the following information. Two pure lines of corn have mean cob lengths of 9 and 3 inches, respectively. The polygenes involved in this trait all exhibit additive gene action.

1. Crossing these two lines is expected to produce a progeny with mean cob length (in inches) of   (a) 12.0   (b) 7.5   (c) 6.0   (d) 2.75   (e) none of the above

2. If the variation in F_1 cob length ranges from 5.5 to 6.5 inches, this variation is estimated to be due to segregation at   (a) two loci   (b) three loci   (c) four loci   (d) five loci   (e) none of the above

3. If only 2 segregating loci contribute to cob length, and we represent the parental cross as *AABB* (9-inch average cob length) × *aabb* (3-inch average), the fraction of the F_2 expected to be 4.5 inches is   (a) $\frac{1}{8}$ (b) $\frac{1}{16}$ (c) $\frac{3}{32}$ (d) $\frac{3}{16}$ (e) none of the above

4. If a mouse population has an average adult body weight of 25 grams with a standard deviation of ± 3 grams, the percentage of the population expected to weigh less than 22 grams is approximately   (a) 16   (b) 33   (c) 68   (d) 50   (e) 25

5. With reference to problem 4, if the genetic variance in mouse body weight is 2.7, the environmental variance is approximately   (a) 22.3   (b) 6.3   (c) 0.3   (d) 3.3   (e) none of the above

6. In another population of mice, the total genetic variance of adult body weight is 4 grams^2 and the environmental variance is 12 grams^2. The broad estimate of heritability for this trait in this population is approximately   (a) 0.15   (b) 0.20   (c) 0.25   (d) 0.33   (e) none of the above

7. If the correlation coefficient between body weight of full sibs is 0.15, then the heritability of this trait in this population is   (a) less than 0.15   (b) 0.25   (c) 0.3   (d) 0.6   (e) none of the above

For problems 8–10, use the following information. A population of adult mice has a mean body weight of 30 grams. The average weight of mice selected for breeding purposes is 34 grams. The progeny produced by random mating among the selected parents average 30.5 grams.

8. The selection differential (in grams) is   (a) 0.5   (b) 4   (c) 3.5   (d) 2   (e) none of the above

9. The genetic gain (in grams) is   (a) 0.5   (b) 4   (c) 3.5   (d) 2   (e) none of the above

10. The heritability estimate for adult body weight in this population is   (a) 0.050   (b) 0.625   (c) 0.125   (d) 0.250   (e) none of the above

Answers to Supplementary Problems

9.19. Eight pairs of factors

9.20. Three or four loci (pairs of alleles)

9.21. $2048

9.22. (*a*) 216 pounds   (*b*) ±6.58 pounds   (*c*) 229.16 pounds

9.23. ±1000 pounds/acre

9.24. 4.16 or approximately 4 gene pairs

9.25. (*a*) Both parents, F_1 = 36 units   (*b*) Both parents = 36 units, F_1 = 48 units

9.26. (*a*) Giant strain = 0.13, midget strain = 0.14   (*b*) Multiplicative gene action is indicated by the similarity of the two coefficients of variation; $\overline{X}_{F_1}$ = 21.9 grams.

9.27.

	Arithmetic Mean	Absolute Deviation from F_1 Mean	Geometric Mean	Absolute Deviation from F_1 Mean
(*a*)	81.2	33.7	43.1	4.4
(*b*)	27.5	4.4	23.0	0.1
(*c*)	77.5	10.4	69.2	2.1
(*d*)	87.3	79.0	13.8	5.5

9.28. 0.64

9.29. (*a*) Heritability estimates measure the proportion of the total phenotypic variation for a trait among individuals of a population that is due to genetic variation. There is no genetic variation in a pure line (heritability = 0), but blood groups (for example) would still be 100% determined by genes.   (*b*) Suppose that a group of identical twins were divided, one member of each pair to the two populations A and B. Each population would then have the same genetic constitution. If population A is not given equal social, educational, and vocational opportunities with population B, then A might be expected to show lower average IQ. In other words, the average IQs of these populations would be reflective solely of nongenetic (environmental) differences regardless of the heritability estimates made in each population.   (*c*) The answer to part (*b*) demonstrates that the difference between phenotypic averages of two populations does not necessarily imply that one population is genetically superior to the other. Important environmental differences may be largely responsible for such deviations. We could imagine that a pure line (heritability = 0) would be very well suited to a particular environment, whereas a highly genetically heterogeneous population with a high heritability for the same trait might be relatively poorly adapted to that same environment. In other words, the high heritabilities for IQ within populations A and B reveal nothing about the causes of the average phenotypic differences between them.

9.30. (*a*) V_E = 42.0, V_A = 77.0, V_D = 11.5   (*b*) 0.55 (*c*) 0.59

9.31. (*a*) $x = 4$ (*b*) $x = 4, y = 2$ (*c*) $x = 2$

9.32. (*a*) $b = 0.22$ (*b*) $h^2 = 2b = 0.49$

9.33. $b = 0.5, r = 1.0$

9.34. (*a*) 0.527   (*b*) 0.591   (*c*) 0.558   (*d*) Since neither sister nor brother can be considered dependent variables, two solutions are possible; $h^2 = 2r(s_S/s_B) = 1.054$ or $h^2 = 2r(s_B/s_S) = 1.182$. Heritability cannot be greater than 1.0. Since human siblings are usually reared together, their common environments have probably made them more alike than they would have been had they been reared in randomly chosen environments. Heritability estimates made from regression or correlation calculations assume that the populations are normally distributed and there are no environmental correlations between relatives. If either or both of these assumptions are invalid, so is the corresponding heritability elements.

9.35. 0.35

9.36. (*a*) 7.17–12.83 pounds   (*b*) 0.3

9.37. (*a*) 40 pounds^2 (*b*) 100 pounds^2

9.38. 0.88 inch

9.39. (*a*) 0.22   (*b*) 880,000 pounds^2 (*c*) 16,000–20,000 pounds

9.40. (*a*) 15 pounds   (*b*) 4.5 pounds   (*c*) 184.5 pounds

9.41. (*a*) $\bar{X} = 25$ centigrams, $s = \pm 3.94$ centigrams   (*b*) 15.53 centigrams^2; note that this is the square of the phenotypic standard deviation in part (*a*). In pure lines, all of the variance is environmentally induced. (*c*) $h^2 = 0$, since a pure line is homozygous; there is no genetic variability.   (*d*) $\bar{X} = 25$ centigrams; no genetic gain can be made by selecting in the absence of genetic variability.

9.42. 0.36 millimeter^2

9.43. (*a*) Y = 23.34, Z = 19.90, X = 17.84   (*b*) 0.71 point

9.44. $I_A = 6.526$, $I_B = 6.041$; A excels in overall merit.

9.45. (*a*) 1/3 (*b*) 22.2%   (*c*) 1/9

9.46. (*a*) A = 630.0, B = 615.0, C = 597.5   (*b*) Sire A

9.47. 0.25

9.48. 0.0351

9.49. 0.4375

9.50. (*a*) Heterosis for seed yield = 22.2 bushels/acre, for plant height = 28 centimeters   (*b*) 60.3 bushels/acre, 243 centimeters

Answers to Review Questions

Matching Questions

1. H   2. A   3. E   4. I   5. C   6. G   7. D   8. F   9. J (genetic gain)   10. B

Vocabulary

1. continuous variation
2. normal (or Gaussian) distribution
3. variance
4. overdominance
5. heritability (broad definition)

6. regression coefficient
7. correlation coefficient
8. progeny test
9. inbreeding
10. heterosis

True-False Questions

1. F (qualitative traits)   2. F (statistic, not parameter)   3. F (moderate to low; $< 50\%$)   4. F (high heritabilities)   5. F (merits of contemporary relatives; e.g., full sibs)   6. F (selfing is possible in many plant species)   7. T   8. T   9. T   10. T

Multiple-Choice Questions

1. *c*   2. *e* (environmental)   3. *e* ($\frac{1}{4}$)   4. *a*   5. *b*   6. *c*   7. *c*   8. *b*   9. *a*   10. *c*

Chapter 10

Population Genetics

HARDY-WEINBERG EQUILIBRIUM

A **Mendelian population** may be considered to be a group of sexually reproducing organisms with a relatively close degree of genetic relationship (such as a species, subspecies, breed, variety, strain) residing within defined geographic boundaries wherein interbreeding occurs. If all the gametes produced by a Mendelian population are considered as a hypothetical mixture of genetic units from which the next generation will arise, we have the concept of a **gene pool.**

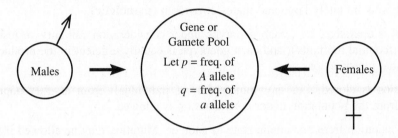

If we consider a pair of alleles (*A* and *a*), we will find that the percentage of gametes in the gene pool bearing *A* or *a* will depend upon the genotypic frequencies of the parental generation whose gametes form the pool. For example, if most of the population were of the recessive genotype *aa,* then the frequency of the recessive allele in the gene pool would be relatively high, and the percentage of gametes bearing the dominant (*A*) allele would be correspondingly low.

When matings between members of a population are completely at random, i.e., when every male gamete in the gene pool has an equal opportunity of uniting with every female gamete, then the zygotic frequencies expected in the next generation may be predicted from a knowledge of the gene (allelic) frequencies in the gene pool of the parental population. That is, given the relative frequencies of *A* and *a* gametes in the gene pool, we can calculate (on the basis of the chance union of gametes) the expected frequencies of progeny genotypes and phenotypes. If *p* = percentage of *A* alleles in the gene pool and *q* = percentage of *a* alleles, then we can use the checkerboard method to produce all the possible chance combinations of these gametes.

♀ \ ♂	p Ⓐ	q ⓐ
p Ⓐ	p^2 *AA*	pq *Aa*
q ⓐ	pq *Aa*	q^2 *aa*

Note that $p + q = 1$, i.e., the percentage of *A* and *a* gametes must add to 100% in order to account for all of the gametes in the gene pool. The expected genotypic (zygotic) frequencies in the next generation then may be summarized as follows:

$$(p + q)^2 = p^2 + 2pq + q^2 = 1.0$$
$$AA \quad Aa \quad aa$$

249

Thus p^2 is the fraction of the next generation expected to be homozygous dominant (AA), $2pq$ is the fraction expected to be heterozygous (Aa), and q^2 is the fraction expected to be recessive (aa). All of these genotypic fractions must add to unity to account for all genotypes in the progeny population.

This formula, expressing the genotypic expectations of progeny in terms of the gametic (allelic) frequencies of the parental gene pool, is called the **Hardy-Weinberg law.** If a population conforms to the conditions on which this formula is based, there should be no change in the gametic or the zygotic frequencies from generation to generation. Should a population initially be in disequilibrium, one generation of random mating is sufficient to bring it into genetic equilibrium and thereafter the population will remain in equilibrium (unchanging in gametic and zygotic frequencies) as long as the Hardy-Weinberg conditions persist.

Several assumptions underlie the attainment of genetic equilibrium as expressed in the Hardy-Weinberg equation.

(1) The population is infinitely large and mates at random **(panmictic).**

(2) No selection is operative, i.e., each genotype under consideration can survive just as well as any other (no differential mortality), and each genotype is equally efficient in the production of progeny (no differential reproduction).

(3) The population is closed, i.e., no immigration of individuals from another population into nor emigration from the population under consideration is allowed.

(4) There is no mutation from one allelic state to another. Mutation may be allowed if the forward and back mutation rates are equivalent, i.e., A mutates to a with the same frequency that a mutates to A.

(5) Meiosis is normal so that chance is the only factor operative in gametogenesis.

If we define **evolution** as any change in a population from the Hardy-Weinberg equilibrium conditions, then a violation of one or more of the Hardy-Weinberg restrictions could cause the population to move away from the gametic and zygotic equilibrium frequencies. Changes in gene frequencies can be produced by a reduction in population size; by selection, migration, or mutation pressures; or by **meiotic drive** (nonrandom assortment of chromosomes). No population is infinitely large, spontaneous mutations cannot be prevented, selection and migration pressures usually exist in most natural populations, etc., so it may be surprising to learn that despite these violations of Hardy-Weinberg restrictions many genes do conform, within statistically acceptable limits, to equilibrium conditions between two successive generations. Changes too small to be statistically significant deviations from equilibrium expectations between any two generations can nonetheless accumulate over many generations to produce considerable alterations in the genetic structure of a population.

A **race** is a genetically (and usually geographically) distinctive interbreeding population of a species. The number of races one wishes to recognize generally depends on the purpose of the investigation. Populations that differ significantly in gene frequencies at one or more loci may be considered as different races. Human races are defined on the basis of gene frequency differences in qualitative traits such as blood groups, hair texture, eye color, etc., as well as by mean and standard deviation differences in quantitative traits such as skin color, body build, shapes of noses, lips, eyes, etc. Races of a given species can freely interbreed with one another. Members of different species, however, are reproductively isolated to a recognizable degree. **Subspecies** are races that have been given distinctive taxonomic names. Varieties, breeds, strains, etc. of cultivated plants or domesticated animals may also be equated with the racial concept. Geographic isolation is usually required for populations of a species to become distinctive races. Race formation is a prerequisite to the splitting of one species into two or more species **(speciation).** Differentiation at many loci over many generations is generally required to reproductively isolate these groups by time of breeding, behavioral differences, ecological requirements, hybrid inviability, hybrid sterility and other such mechanisms.

Equilibrium at an autosomal genetic locus becomes fully established in a nonequilibrium population after one generation of random mating under Hardy-Weinberg conditions regardless of the number of alleles at that locus. However, when autosomal allelic frequencies are dissimilar in the sexes, they become equilibrated after one generation of random mating, but the genotypic frequencies do not become equilibrated until the second generation of random mating. If the frequencies of sex-linked alleles are unequal in the sexes, the equilibrium value is approached rapidly during successive generations of random mating in an oscillatory manner by the two sexes. This phenomenon derives from the fact that females (XX) carry twice as many sex-linked alleles as do males (XY). Females receive their sex-linked heredity equally from both parents, but males receive their sex-linked heredity only from their mothers. The difference between the allelic frequencies in males and females is halved in each generation under random mating. Within each sex, the deviation from equilibrium is halved in each generation, with sign reversed. The average frequency of one allele ($\bar{p}$) in the entire population is also the equilibrium approached by each sex during successive generations of random mating.

$$\bar{p} = \tfrac{2}{3}p_f + \tfrac{1}{3}p_m$$

Although alleles at a single autosomal locus reach equilibrium following one generation of random mating, gametic equilibrium involving two independently assorting genes is approached rapidly over a number of generations. At equilibrium, the product of coupling gametes equals the product of repulsion gametes.

> **Example 10.1.** Consider one locus with alleles A and a at frequencies represented by p and q, respectively. A second locus has alleles B and b at frequencies r and s, respectively. The expected frequencies of coupling gametes AB and ab are pr and qs, respectively. The expected frequencies of repulsion gametes Ab and aB are ps and qr, respectively. At equilibrium, $(pr)(qs) = (ps)(qr)$. Also at equilibrium, the disequilibrium coefficient (d) is $d = (pr)(qs) - (ps)(qr) = 0$.

For independently assorting loci under random mating, the disequilibrium value of d is halved in each generation during the approach to equilibrium because unlinked genes experience 50% recombination. The approach to equilibrium by linked genes, however, is slowed by comparison because they recombine less frequently than unlinked genes (i.e., less than 50% recombination). The closer the linkage, the longer it takes to reach equilibrium. The disequilibrium (d_t) that exists at any generation (t) is expressed as

$$d_t = (1 - r)d_{t-1}$$

where r = frequency of recombination and d_{t-1} = disequilibrium in the previous generation.

> **Example 10.2.** If $d = 0.25$ initially and the 2 loci experience 20% recombination (i.e., the loci are 20 map units apart), the disequilibrium that would be expected after one generation of random mating is $d_t = (1 - 0.2)(0.25) = 0.2$. This represents $0.20/0.25 = 0.8$ or 80% of the maximum disequilibrium that could exist for a pair of linked loci.

CALCULATING GENE FREQUENCIES

1. Autosomal Loci with Two Alleles.

(a) Codominant Autosomal Alleles.

When codominant alleles are present in a 2-allele system, each genotype has a distinctive phenotype. The numbers of each allele in both homozygous and heterozygous conditions may be counted in a sample of individuals from the population and expressed as a percentage of the total number of alleles in the sample. If the sample is representative of the entire population (containing proportionately the same numbers of genotypes as found in the entire population) then we can obtain an estimate of the allelic frequencies in the gene pool. Given a sample of N individuals of which D are homozygous for one allele (A^1A^1), H are heterozygous (A^1A^2), and R are homozygous for the other allele (A^2A^2), then N = D + H + R. Since each of the N individuals are diploid at this locus, there are 2N alleles represented in the sample. Each A^1A^1 genotype has two A^1 alleles. Heterozygotes have only one A^1 allele. Letting p represent the frequency of the A^1 allele and q the frequency of the A^2 allele, we have

$$p = \frac{2D + H}{2N} = \frac{D + \tfrac{1}{2}H}{N} \qquad q = \frac{H + 2R}{2N} = \frac{\tfrac{1}{2}H + R}{N}$$

(b) **Dominant and Recessive Autosomal Alleles.**

Determining the gene frequencies for alleles that exhibit dominance and recessive relationships requires a different approach from that used with codominant alleles. A dominant phenotype may have either of 2 genotypes, AA or Aa, but we have no way (other than by laboriously testcrossing each dominant phenotype) of distinguishing how many are homozygous or heterozygous in our sample. The only phenotype whose genotype is known for certain is the recessive (aa). If the population is in equilibrium, then we can obtain an estimate of q (the frequency of the recessive allele) from q^2 (the frequency of the recessive genotype or phenotype).

> **Example 10.3.** If 75% of a population was of the dominant phenotype (A-), then 25% would have the recessive phenotype (aa). If the population is in equilibrium with respect to this locus, we expect q^2 = frequency of aa.
>
> Then $q^2 = 0.25$, $q = 0.5$, $p = 1 - q = 0.5$.

(c) **Sex-Influenced Traits.**

The expression of dominance and recessive relationships may be markedly changed in some genes when exposed to different environmental conditions, most notable of which are the sex hormones. In sex-influenced traits (Chapter 5), the heterozygous genotype usually will produce different phenotypes in the two sexes, making the dominance and recessive relationships of the alleles appear to reverse themselves. We shall consider only those sex-influenced traits whose controlling genes are on autosomes. Determination of allelic frequencies must be indirectly made in one sex by taking the square root of the frequency of the recessive phenotype ($q = \sqrt{q^2}$). A similar approach in the opposite sex should give an estimate of p. Corroboration of sex influence is obtained if these estimates of p and q made in different sexes add close to unity.

2. Autosomal Loci with Multiple Alleles.

If we consider three alleles, A, a', and a, with the dominance hierarchy $A > a' > a$, occurring in the gene pool with respective frequencies p, q, and r, then random mating will generate zygotes with the following frequencies:

$$(p + q + r)^2 = p^2 + 2pq + 2pr + q^2 + 2qr + r^2 = 1$$

Genotypes:	$\underbrace{AA \quad Aa' \quad Aa}$	$\underbrace{a'a' \quad a'a}$	$\underbrace{aa}$
Phenotypes:	A	a'	a

For ease in calculation of a given allelic frequency, it may be possible to group the phenotypes of the population into just two types.

> **Example 10.4.** In a multiple allelic system where $A > a' > a$, we could calculate the frequency of the top dominant allele A by considering the dominant phenotype (A) in contrast to all other phenotypes produced by alleles at this locus. The latter group may be considered to be produced by an allele a_x, which is recessive to A.
>
> Let p = frequency of allele A, q = frequency of allele a_x.
> q^2 = frequency of phenotypes other than A.
> $q = \sqrt{q^2}$
> $p = 1 - q$ = frequency of gene A.

Many multiple allelic series involve codominant relationships such as $(A^1 = A^2) > a$, with respective frequencies p, q, and r. More genotypes can be phenotypically recognized in codominant systems than in systems without codominance.

$$(p + q + r)^2 = p^2 + 2pr + 2pq + q^2 + 2qr + r^2 = 1$$

Genotypes:	$\underbrace{A^1A^1 \quad A^1a}$	$\underbrace{A^1A^2}$	$\underbrace{A^2A^2 \quad A^2a}$	$\underbrace{aa}$
Phenotypes:	A^1	A^1A^2	A^2	a

The use of this formula in calculating multiple allelic frequencies is presented in Problems 10.9 and 10.10. Similar methods may be utilized to derive other formulas for calculating gene frequencies in multiple allelic systems with more than 3 alleles, but their computation becomes too involved for our purposes at the introductory level. Therefore multiple allelic problems in this chapter will be mainly concerned with 3 alleles.

3. Sex-Linked Loci.

(a) *Codominant Sex-Linked Alleles.*

Data from both males and females can be used in the direct computation of sex-linked codominant allelic frequencies. Bear in mind that in organisms with an X-Y mechanism of sex determination, the heterozygous condition can only appear in females. Males are hemizygous for sex-linked genes.

Example 10.5. In domestic cats, black melanin pigment is deposited in the hair by a sex-linked gene; its alternative allele produces yellow hair. Random inactivation of one of the X chromosomes occurs in each cell of female embryos. Heterozygous females are thus genetic mosaics, having patches of all-black and all-yellow hairs called tortoise-shell pattern. Since only one sex-linked allele is active in any cell, the inheritance is not really codominant, but the genetic symbolism used is the same as that for codominant alleles.

	Phenotypes		
	Black	Tortoise-Shell	Yellow
Females	C^bC^b	C^bC^y	C^yC^y
Males	C^bY	—	C^yY

Let p = frequency of C^b, q = frequency of C^y.

$$p = \frac{2\left(\begin{array}{c}\text{no. of black}\\\text{females}\end{array}\right) + \left(\begin{array}{c}\text{no. of tortoise-}\\\text{shell females}\end{array}\right) + \left(\begin{array}{c}\text{no. of black}\\\text{males}\end{array}\right)}{2(\text{no. females}) + \text{no. males}}$$

$$q = \frac{2\left(\begin{array}{c}\text{no. of yellow}\\\text{females}\end{array}\right) + \left(\begin{array}{c}\text{no. of tortoise-}\\\text{shell females}\end{array}\right) + \left(\begin{array}{c}\text{no. of yellow}\\\text{males}\end{array}\right)}{2(\text{no. females}) + \text{no. males}}$$

(b) *Dominant and Recessive Sex-Linked Alleles.*

Since each male possesses only one sex-linked allele, the frequency of a sex-linked trait among males is a direct measure of the allelic frequency in the population, assuming, of course, that the allelic frequencies thus determined are representative of the allelic frequencies among females as well.

TESTING A LOCUS FOR EQUILIBRIUM

In cases where dominance is involved, the heterozygous class is indistinguishable phenotypically from the homozygous dominant class. Hence there is no way of checking the Hardy-Weinberg expectations against observed sample data unless the dominant phenotypes have been genetically analyzed by observation of their progeny from testcrosses. Only when codominant alleles are involved can we easily check our observations against the expected equilibrium values through the chi-square test (Chapter 7).

Degrees of Freedom.

The number of variables in chi-square tests of Hardy-Weinberg equilibrium is not simply the number of phenotypes minus 1 (as in chi-square tests of classical Mendelian ratios). The number of observed variables (number of phenotypes $= k$) is further restricted by testing their conformity to an expected Hardy-Weinberg frequency ratio generated by a number of additional variables (number of alleles, or allelic frequencies $= r$). We have $(k - 1)$ degrees of freedom in the number of phenotypes, $(r - 1)$ degrees of freedom in establishing the frequencies for the r alleles. The combined number of degrees of freedom is $(k - 1) - (r - 1) = k - r$. Even in most chi-square tests for equilibrium involving multiple alleles, the number of degrees of freedom is the number of phenotypes minus the number of alleles.

Solved Problems

HARDY-WEINBERG EQUILIBRIUM

10.1. In a population gene pool, the alleles A and a are at initial frequencies p and q, respectively. Prove that the gene frequencies and the zygotic frequencies do not change from generation to generation as long as the Hardy-Weinberg conditions are maintained.

Solution:

Zygotic frequencies generated by random mating are

$$p^2(AA) + 2pq(Aa) + q^2(aa) = 1$$

All of the gametes of AA individuals and half of the gametes of heterozygotes will bear the dominant allele (A). Then the frequency of A in the gene pool of the next generation is

$$p^2 + pq = p^2 + p(1 - p) = p^2 + p - p^2 = p$$

Thus each generation of random mating under Hardy-Weinberg conditions fails to change either the allelic or zygotic frequencies.

10.2. Prove the Hardy-Weinberg law by finding the frequencies of all possible kinds of matings and from these generating the frequencies of genotypes among the progeny using the symbols shown below.

	Alleles		Genotypes		
	A	a	AA	Aa	aa
Frequency:	p	q	p^2	$2pq$	q^2

Solution:

There are six kinds of matings (ignoring male-female differences) that are easily generated in a mating table.

		Male Parent		
		$AA\ p^2$	$Aa\ 2pq$	$aa\ q^2$
Female Parent	$AA\ p^2$	p^4	$2p^3q$	p^2q^2
	$Aa\ 2pq$	$2p^3q$	$4p^2q^2$	$2pq^3$
	$aa\ q^2$	p^2q^2	$2pq^3$	q^4

The matings $AA \times Aa$ occur with the frequency $4p^3q$. Half the offspring from this mating are expected to be $AA\ [\frac{1}{2}(4p^3q) = 2p^3q]$, and half are expected to be Aa (again with the frequency $2p^3q$). Similar reasoning generates the frequencies of genotypes among the progeny shown in the following table.

	Mating	Frequency	Genotypic Frequencies among Progeny		
			AA	Aa	aa
(1)	$AA \times AA$	p^4	p^4	—	—
(2)	$AA \times Aa$	$4p^3q$	$2p^3q$	$2p^3q$	—
(3)	$AA \times aa$	$2p^2q^2$	—	$2p^2q^2$	—
(4)	$Aa \times Aa$	$4p^2q^2$	p^2q^2	$2p^2q^2$	p^2q^2
(5)	$Aa \times aa$	$4pq^3$	—	$2pq^3$	$2pq^3$
(6)	$aa \times aa$	q^4	—	—	q^4

$$\text{Sums:} \quad (AA) = p^4 + 2p^3q + p^2q^2 = p^2(p^2 + 2pq + q^2) \quad = p^2$$
$$(Aa) = 2p^3q + 4p^2q^2 + 2pq^3 = 2pq(p^2 + 2pq + q^2) = 2pq$$
$$(aa) = p^2q + 2pq^3 + q^4 = q^2(p^2 + 2pq + q^2) \quad = \underline{q^2}$$
$$\text{Total} = 1.00$$

10.3. At what allelic frequency does the homozygous recessive genotype (aa) become twice as frequent as the heterozygous genotype (Aa) in a Hardy-Weinberg population?

Solution:

Let q = frequency of recessive allele, p = frequency of dominant allele.
The frequency of homozygous recessives (q^2) is twice as frequent at heterozygotes ($2pq$) when

$$q^2 = 2(2pq)$$
$$= 4pq$$
$$= 4q(1 - q)$$
$$= 4q - 4q^2$$
$$0 = 4q - 5q^2$$
$$0 = q(4 - 5q)$$

Therefore, either $q = 0$ (which is obviously an incorrect solution), or

$$4 - 5q = 0$$
$$5q = 4$$
$$q = \tfrac{4}{5} \text{ or } 0.8$$

Proof:

$$q^2 = 2(2pq)$$
$$(0.8)^2 = 4(0.2)(0.8)$$
$$0.64 = 0.64$$

CALCULATING GENE FREQUENCIES

Autosomal Loci with Two Alleles.

Codominant Autosomal Alleles.

10.4. In Shorthorn cattle, the genotype C^RC^R is phenotypically red, C^RC^W is roan (a mixture of red and white), and C^WC^W is white. (a) If 108 red, 48 white and 144 roan animals were found in a sample of Shorthorns from the central valley of California, calculate the estimated frequencies of the C^R allele and the C^W allele in the gene pool of the population. (b) If this population is completely panmictic, what zygotic frequencies would be expected in the next generation? (c) How does the sample data in part (a) compare with the expectations for the next generation in part (b)? Is the population represented in part (a) in equilibrium?

Solution:

(a)

Numbers	Phenotypes	Genotypes
108	Red	$C^R C^R$
144	Roan	$C^R C^W$
48	White	$C^W C^W$
300		

First, let us calculate the frequency of the C^R allele. There are 108 red individuals each carrying 2 C^R alleles; $2 \times 108 = 216$ C^R alleles. There are 144 roan individuals each carrying only 1 C^R allele; $1 \times 144 = 144$ C^R alleles. Thus the total number of C^R alleles in our sample is $216 + 144 = 360$. Since each individual is a diploid (possessing two sets of chromosomes, each bearing one of the alleles at the locus under consideration), the total number of alleles represented in this sample is $300 \times 2 = 600$. The fraction of all alleles in our sample of type C^R becomes $\frac{360}{600} = 0.6$ or 60%. The other 40% of the alleles in the gene pool must be of type C^W. We can arrive at this estimate for C^W by following the same procedure as above. There are $48 \times 2 = 96$ C^W alleles represented in the homozygotes and 144 in the heterozygotes; $96 + 144 = 240$; $240/600 = 0.4$ or 40% C^W alleles.

(b) Recall that panmixis is synonymous with random mating. We will let the frequency of the C^R allele be represented by $p = 0.6$, and the frequency of the C^W allele be represented by $q = 0.4$. Then according to the Hardy-Weinberg law, we would expect as genotypic frequencies in the next generation

$$p^2 = (0.6)^2 = 0.36 \ C^R C^R \ : \ 2pq = 2(0.6)(0.4) = 0.48 \ C^R C^W \ : \ q^2 = (0.4)^2 = 0.16 \ C^W C^W$$

(c) In a sample of size 300 we would expect $0.36(300) = 108 \ C^R C^R$ (red), $0.48(300) = 144 \ C^R C^W$ (roan), and $0.16(300) = 48 \ C^W C^W$ (white). Note that these figures correspond exactly to those of our sample. Since the genotypic and gametic frequencies are not expected to change in the next generation, the original population must already be in equilibrium.

Dominant and Recessive Autosomal Alleles.

10.5. White wool is dependent upon a dominant allele B and black wool upon its recessive allele b. Suppose that a sample of 900 sheep of the Rambouillet breed in Idaho gave the following data: 891 white and 9 black. Estimate the allelic frequencies.

Solution:

$$p^2(BB) + 2pq(Bb) + q^2(bb) = 1.0$$

If we assume the population is in equilibrium, we can take the square root of that percentage of the population that is of the recessive genotype (phenotype) as our estimator for the frequency of the recessive allele.

$$q = \sqrt{q^2} = \sqrt{9/900} = 0.1 = \text{frequency of allele } b$$

Since $p + q = 1$, the frequency of allele B is 0.9.

10.6. It is suspected that the excretion of the strongly odorous substance methanethiol is controlled by a recessive gene m in humans; nonexcretion is governed by the dominant allele M. If the frequency of m is 0.4 in a population, what is the probability of finding 2 nonexcretor boys and 1 excretor girl in families of size 3 in this population where both parents are nonexcretors?

Solution:

In order that 2 nonexcretor parents produce an excretor child, they must both be heterozygous Mm, in which case $\frac{1}{4}$ of their children would be expected to be excretors (mm). Girls are expected with a frequency of 0.5. Therefore the probability of $Mm \times Mm$ parents producing an excretor girl is $(\frac{1}{4})(\frac{1}{2}) = \frac{1}{8}$. The probability of having a nonexcretor boy $= (\frac{3}{4})(\frac{1}{2}) = \frac{3}{8}$. The probability of a nonexcretor individual in this population being heterozygous can be estimated from the equilibrium expectations. Let $q = 0.4$, then $p = 0.6$.

$$
\begin{array}{ccccccc}
p^2\,MM & + & 2pq\,Mm & + & q^2\,mm & = & 1.0 \\
(0.6)^2 & + & 2(0.6)(0.4) & + & (0.4)^2 & = & 1.0 \\
\underbrace{0.36 \qquad + \qquad 0.48}_{\text{nonexcretor}} & & & + & \underbrace{0.16}_{\text{excretor}} & = & 1.0
\end{array}
$$

The probability of a nonexcretor individual being heterozygous is $48/(36 + 48) = 0.57$. The probability of both parents being heterozygous $= (0.57)^2 = 0.325$.

Let $a =$ probability of heterozygous parents producing a nonexcretor boy $= \frac{3}{8}$,
  $b =$ probability of heterozygous parents producing an excretor girl $= \frac{1}{8}$.

The probability of heterozygous parents producing 2 nonexcretor boys and 1 excretor girl is found in the second term of the expansion $(a + b)^3 = a^3 + 3a^2b + \cdots$; thus $3(\frac{3}{8})^2(\frac{1}{8}) = 0.053$. The probability that both nonexcretor parents are heterozygous *and* produce 2 nonexcretor boys and 1 excretor girl is $(0.325)(0.053) = 0.017$ or 1.7%.

10.7. Two independently assorting recessive genes govern production of salmon silks (*sm*) and shrunken endosperm (*sh*) of maize. A sample from a population that is mating at random yielded the following data: 6 shrunken : 10 salmon, shrunken : 30 wild type : 54 salmon. Determine the frequencies of the salmon allele q and shrunken allele t.

Solution:

6 *Sm-sh sh*	shrunken
10 *sm sm sh sh*	salmon, shrunken
30 *Sm-Sh-*	wild type
54 *sm sm Sh-*	salmon
100	

Let $q^2 =$ frequency of the recessive trait, salmon silks $= (10 + 54)/100 = 0.64$; $q = 0.8$.
Let $t^2 =$ frequency of the recessive trait, shrunken endosperm $= (6 + 10)/100 = 0.16$; $t = 0.4$.

Sex-Influenced Traits.

10.8. In the human population, an index finger shorter than the ring finger is thought to be governed by a sex-influenced gene that appears to be dominant in males and recessive in females. A sample of the males in this population was found to contain 120 short and 210 long index fingers. Calculate the expected frequencies of long and short index fingers in females of this population.

Solution:

Since the dominance relationships are reversed in the two sexes, let us use all lowercase letters with superscripts to avoid confusion with either dominance or codominance symbolism.

Genotype	Phenotypes	
	Males	Females
s^1s^1	Short	Short
s^1s^2	Short	Long
s^2s^2	Long	Long

Let $p =$ frequency of s^1 allele, $q =$ frequency of s^2 allele. $p^2(s^1s^1) + 2pq(s^1s^2) + q^2(s^2s^2) = 1.0$.
In males, the allele for long finger s^2 is recessive. Then $q = \sqrt{q^2} = \sqrt{210/(120 + 210)} = \sqrt{0.64} = 0.8$; $p = 1 - 0.8 = 0.2$.

In females, short index finger is recessive. Then $p^2 = (0.2)^2 = 0.04$ or 4% of the females of this population will probably be short fingered. The other 96% should possess long index fingers.

Autosomal Loci with Multiple Alleles.

10.9. A multiple allelic system governs the coat colors of rabbits; C = full color, c^h = Himalayan, c = albino, with dominance expressed as $C > c^h > c$ and occurring with the frequencies p, q, and r, respectively. (a) If a population of rabbits containing full-colored individuals, Himalayans, and albinos, is mating at random, what is the expected genotypic ratio in the next generation in terms of p, q, and r? (b) Derive a formula for the calculation of allelic frequencies from the expected phenotypic frequencies. (c) A sample from a rabbit population contains 168 full-color, 30 Himalayan, and 2 albino. Calculate the allelic frequencies p, q, and r. (d) Given the allelic frequencies $p = 0.5$, $q = 0.1$, and $r = 0.4$, calculate the expected genotypic ratios among the full-colored rabbits.

Solution:

(a) The zygotic expectations from a population mating at random with allelic frequencies p, q, and r can be found by expanding $(p + q + r)^2$.

	p (C)	q (c^h)	r (c)
p (C)	p^2 CC	pq Cc^h	pr Cc
q (c^h)	pq Cc^h	q^2 c^hc^h	qr c^hc
r (c)	pr Cc	qr c^hc	r^2 cc

Summary:

Genotypic Frequencies	Genotypes	Phenotypes
p^2	CC	
$2pq$	Cc^h	Full color
$2pr$	Cc	
q^2	c^hc^h	Himalayan
$2qr$	c^hc	
r^2	cc	Albino

(b) r = frequency of allele $c = \sqrt{\text{frequency of albinos}} = \sqrt{r^2}$

q = frequency of allele c^h; let H = frequency of the Himalayan phenotype.

$$q^2 + 2qr = H$$

Completing the square,

$$q^2 + 2qr + r^2 = H + r^2 \quad (q + r)^2 = H + r^2 \quad q + r = \sqrt{H + r^2} \quad q = \sqrt{H + r^2} - r$$

p = frequency of allele $C = 1 - q - r$.

(c) The frequency of allele $c = r = \sqrt{2/(168 + 30 + 2)} = \sqrt{\frac{2}{200}} = 0.1$. To calculate the frequency of the allele c^h, let H represent the frequency of the Himalayan phenotype in the population; then $q = \sqrt{H + r^2} - r = \sqrt{\frac{30}{200} + 0.01} - 0.1 = 0.3$. The frequency of the allele $C = p = 1 - q - r = 1 - 0.1 - 0.3 = 0.6$.

(d)

$$
\begin{aligned}
p^2CC &= (0.5)^2 &= 0.25 \\
2pq\ Cc^h &= 2(0.5)(0.1) &= 0.10 \\
2pr\ Cc &= 2(0.5)(0.4) &= \underline{0.40}
\end{aligned}
\right\} \text{full color}
$$

$$0.75$$

Therefore considering only the full-colored rabbits, we expect

$$25/75\ CC = 33\tfrac{1}{3}\%$$
$$10/75\ Cc^h = 13\tfrac{1}{3}\%$$
$$40/75\ Cc = \underline{53\tfrac{1}{3}\%}$$

100% of the full-colored rabbits

10.10. The ABO blood group system is governed by a multiple allelic system in which some codominant relationships exist. Three alleles, I^A, I^B, and i, form the dominance hierarchy $(I^A = I^B) > i$. (a) Determine the genotypic and phenotypic expectations for this blood group locus from a population in genetic equilibrium. (b) Derive a formula for use in finding the allelic frequencies at the ABO blood group locus. (c) Among New York Caucasians, the frequencies of the ABO blood groups were found to be approximately 49% type O, 36% type A, 12% type B, and 3% type AB. What are the allelic frequencies in this population? (d) Given the population in part (c) above, what percentage of type A individuals is probably homozygous?

Solution:

(a) Let p = frequency of I^A allele, q = frequency of I^B allele, r = frequency of i allele. The expansion of $(p + q + r)^2$ yields the zygotic ratio expected under random mating.

Genotypic Frequencies	Genotypes	Phenotypes (Blood Groups)
p^2	$I^A I^A$	A
$2pr$	$I^A i$	A
q^2	$I^B I^B$	B
$2qr$	$I^B i$	B
$2pq$	$I^A I^B$	AB
r^2	ii	O

(b) Let $\overline{A}$, $\overline{B}$, and $\overline{O}$ represent the *phenotypic* frequencies of blood groups A, B, and O, respectively. Solving for the frequency of the recessive allele i, $r = \sqrt{r^2} = \sqrt{\overline{O}}$.

Solving for the frequency of the I^A allele,

$$p^2 + 2pr + r^2 = \overline{A} + \overline{O} \quad (p + r)^2 = \overline{A} + \overline{O} \quad p = \sqrt{\overline{A} + \overline{O}} - r = \sqrt{\overline{A} + \overline{O}} - \sqrt{\overline{O}}$$

Solving for the frequency of the I^B allele, $q = 1 - p - r$. Or, following the method for obtaining the frequency of the I^A allele, $q = \sqrt{\overline{B} + \overline{O}} - \sqrt{\overline{O}}$

Presenting the solutions in a slightly different form,

$$\underbrace{\sqrt{\overline{A}+\overline{O}} - \sqrt{\overline{O}}}_{p} + \underbrace{\sqrt{\overline{B}+\overline{O}} - \sqrt{\overline{O}}}_{q} + \underbrace{\sqrt{\overline{O}}}_{r} = 1.0$$

$$p = 1 - \sqrt{\overline{B}+\overline{O}} \qquad q = 1 - \sqrt{\overline{A}+\overline{O}} \qquad r = \sqrt{\overline{O}}$$

(c) Frequency of allele i = $\sqrt{\overline{O}}$ = $\sqrt{0.49}$ = $0.70 = r$

Frequency of I^B allele = $1 - \sqrt{\overline{A}+\overline{O}}$ = $1 - \sqrt{0.36+0.49}$ = $0.08 = q$

Frequency of allele I^A = $1 - \sqrt{\overline{B}+\overline{O}}$ = $1 - \sqrt{0.12+0.49}$ = $0.22 = p$

Check: $p + q + r = 0.22 + 0.08 + 0.70 = 1.00$

(d) $p^2 = I^A I^A = (0.22)^2 = 0.048$

$2pr = I^A i = 2(0.22)(0.7) = \underline{0.308}$

0.356 = total group A individuals

Thus $48/356 = 0.135$ or $13\tfrac{1}{2}\%$ of all group A individuals in this population is expected to be homozygous.

Sex-Linked Loci.
Codominant Sex-Linked Alleles.

10.11. The genetics of coat colors in cats was presented in Example 10.5: $C^B C^B$ ♀♀ or $C^B Y$ ♂♂ are black, $C^Y C^Y$ ♀♀ or $C^Y Y$ ♂♂ are yellow, $C^B C^Y$ ♀♀ are tortoise-shell (blotches of yellow and black). A population of cats in London was found to consist of the following phenotypes:

	Black	Yellow	Tortoise-Shell	Totals
Males	311	42	0	353
Females	277	7	54	338

Determine the allelic frequencies using all of the available information.

Solution:

The total number of C^B alleles in this sample is $311 + 2(277) + 54 = 919$. The total number of alleles (X chromosomes) in this sample is $353 + 2(388) = 1029$. Therefore the frequency of the C^B allele is $919/1029 = 0.893$. The frequency of the C^Y allele would then be $1 - 0.893 = 0.107$.

Dominant and Recessive Sex-Linked Alleles.

10.12. White eye color in *Drosophila* is due to a sex-linked recessive gene w and wild-type (red) eye color, to its dominant allele w^+. A laboratory population of *Drosophila* was found to contain 170 red-eyed males and 30 white-eyed males. (*a*) Estimate the frequency of the w^+ allele and the w allele in the gene pool. (*b*) What percentage of the females in this population would be expected to be white-eyed?

Solution:
(*a*)

Observed No. of Males	Genotypes of Males	Phenotypes of Males
170	$w^+ Y$	Wild type (red eye)
30	$w Y$	White eye
200		

Thus 30 of the 200 X chromosomes in this sample carry the recessive allele w.

$q = 30/200 = 0.15$ or 15% w alleles.
$p = 1 - q = 1 - 0.15 = 0.85$ or 85% w^+ alleles.

(*b*) Since females possess 2 X chromosomes (hence 2 alleles), their expectations may be calculated in the same manner as that used for autosomal genes.

$$p^2(w^+ w^+) + 2pq(w^+ w) + q^2(ww) = 1.0 \text{ or } 100\% \text{ of the females}$$

$q^2 = (0.15)^2 = 0.0225$ or 2.25% of all females in the population is expected to be white-eyed.

TESTING A LOCUS FOR EQUILIBRIUM

10.13. A human serum protein called haptoglobin has two major electrophoretic variants produced by a pair of codominant alleles Hp^1 and Hp^2. A sample of 100 individuals has 10 Hp^1/Hp^1, 35 Hp^1/Hp^2, and 55 Hp^2/Hp^2. Are the genotypes in this sample conforming to the frequencies expected for a Hardy-Weinberg population within statistically acceptable limits?

Solution:

First we must calculate the allelic frequencies.

$$\text{Let } p = \text{frequency of } Hp^1 \text{ allele} = \frac{2(10) + 35}{2(100)} = \frac{55}{200} = 0.275$$

$$q = \text{frequency of } Hp^2 \text{ allele} = 1 - 0.275 = 0.725$$

From these gene (allelic) frequencies we can determine the genotypic frequencies expected according to the Hardy-Weinberg equation.

$$
\begin{aligned}
Hp^1/Hp^1 &= p^2 \\
&= (0.275)^2 \\
&= 0.075625 \\
Hp^1/Hp^2 &= 2pq \\
&= 2(0.275)(0.725) \\
&= 0.39875 \\
Hp^2/Hp^2 &= q^2 \\
&= (0.725)^2 \\
&= 0.525625
\end{aligned}
$$

Converting these genotypic frequencies to numbers based on a total sample size of 100, we can do a chi-square test.

Genotypes	Observed	Expected	Deviation $(o - e)$	$(o - e)^2$	$(o - e)^2/e$
Hp^1/Hp^1	10	7.56	2.44	5.95	0.79
Hp^1/Hp^2	35	39.88	-4.88	23.81	0.60
Hp^2/Hp^2	55	52.56	2.44	5.95	0.11
Totals	100	100.00	0		$\chi^2 = 1.50$

$$\text{df} = k \text{ phenotypes} - r \text{ alleles} = 3 - 2 = 1 \quad P = 0.2\text{--}0.3 \text{ (Table 7.2)}$$

This is not a significant χ^2 value, and we may accept the hypothesis that this sample (and hence presumably the population from which it was drawn) is conforming to the equilibrium distribution of genotypes.

10.14. One of the "breeds" of poultry has been largely built on a single-gene locus, that for "frizzled" feathers. The frizzled phenotype is produced by the heterozygous genotype $M^N M^F$. One homozygote $M^F M^F$ produces extremely frizzled birds called "woolies." The other homozygous genotype $M^N M^N$ has normal plumage. A sample of 1000 individuals of this "breed" in the United States contained 800 frizzled, 150 normal, and 50 wooly birds. Is this population in equilibrium?

Solution:

$$\text{Let} \quad p = \text{frequency of the } M^F \text{ allele} = \frac{2(50) + 800}{2(1000)} = 0.45$$

$$q = \text{frequency of } M^N \text{ allele} = 1 - 0.45 = 0.55$$

Genotypes	Equilibrium Frequencies	Calculations		Expected Numbers
$M^F M^F$	p^2	$(0.45)^2$	$= 0.2025(1000) =$	202.5
$M^F M^N$	$2pq$	$2(0.45)(0.55)$	$= 0.4950(1000) =$	495.0
$M^N M^N$	q^2	$(0.55)^2$	$= 0.3025(1000) =$	302.5

Chi-square test for conformity to equilibrium expectations.

Phenotypes	o	e	$(o - e)$	$(o - e)^2$	$(o - e)^2/e$
Wooly	50	202.5	-152.5	23,256	114.8
Frizzle	800	495.0	$+305.0$	93,025	187.9
Normal	150	302.5	-152.5	23,256	76.9
					$\chi^2 = 379.6$

$$\text{df} = 1, \quad p < 0.01 \quad \text{(Table 7.2)}$$

This highly significant chi-square value will not allow us to accept the hypothesis of conformity with equilibrium expectations. The explanation for the large deviation from the equilibrium expectations is twofold. Much *artificial selection* (by people) is being practiced. The frizzled heterozygotes represent the "breed" type and are kept for show purposes as well as for breeding by bird fanciers. They dispose of (cull) many normal and wooly types. *Natural selection* is also operative on the wooly types because they tend to lose their feathers (loss of insulation) and eat more feed just to maintain themselves, are slower to reach sexual maturity, and lay fewer eggs than do the normal birds.

Supplementary Problems

HARDY-WEINBERG EQUILIBRIUM

10.15. At what allelic frequency is the heterozygous genotype (*Aa*) twice as frequent as the homozygous genotype (*aa*) in a Hardy-Weinberg population?

10.16. There is a singular exception to the rule that genetic equilibrium at two independently assorting autosomal loci is attained in a nonequilibrium population only after a number of generations of random mating. Specify the conditions of a population that should reach genotypic equilibrium after a single generation of random mating.

10.17. Let the frequencies of a pair of autosomal alleles (*A* and *a*) be represented by p_m and q_m in males and by p_f and q_f in females, respectively. Given $q_f = 0.6$ and $q_m = 0.2$, (*a*) determine the equilibrium gene frequencies in both sexes after one generation of random mating, and (*b*) give the genotypic frequencies expected in the second generation of random mating.

10.18. The autosomal gametic disequilibrium in a population is expressed as $d = 0.12$. The two loci under consideration recombine with a frequency of 16%. Calculate the disequilibrium (*d* value) that existed in the gamete pool of (*a*) the previous generation, and (*b*) the next generation.

10.19. The frequency of a sex-linked allele is 0.4 in males and 0.8 in females of a population (XY sex determination) not in genetic equilibrium. Find the equilibrium frequency of this allele in the entire population.

10.20. A laboratory population of flies contains all females homozygous for a sex-linked dominant allele and all males hemizygous for the recessive allele. Calculate the frequencies expected in each sex for the dominant allele in the first three generations of random mating.

10.21. For two independently assorting loci under Hardy-Weinberg conditions, (*a*) what is the maximum value of the disequilibrium coefficient (*d*)? (*b*) Specify the two conditions in which a population must be in order to maximize *d*.

10.22. Given gene *A* at frequency 0.2 and gene *B* at frequency 0.6, find the equilibrium frequencies of the gametes *AB*, *Ab*, *aB*, and *ab*.

CALCULATING GENE FREQUENCIES

Autosomal Loci with Two Alleles

Codominant Autosomal Alleles

10.23. A population of soybeans is segregating for the colors golden, light green, and dark green produced by the codominant genotypes $C^G C^G$, $C^G C^D$, $C^D C^D$, respectively. A sample from this population contained 2 golden, 36 light green, and 162 dark green. Determine the frequencies of the alleles C^G and C^D.

10.24. The MN blood group system in humans is governed by a pair of codominant alleles (L^M and L^N). A sample of 208 Bedouins in the Syrian Desert was tested for the presence of the M and N antigens and found to contain 119 group M ($L^M L^M$), 76 group MN ($L^M L^N$), and 13 group N ($L^N L^N$). (*a*) Calculate the gene frequencies of L^M and L^N. (*b*) If the frequency of $L^M = 0.3$, how many individuals in a sample of size 500 would be expected to belong to group MN?

Dominant and Recessive Autosomal Alleles

10.25. The ability of certain people to taste a chemical called PTC is governed by a dominant allele *T*, and the inability to taste PTC by its recessive allele *t*. If 24% of a population is homozygous taster and 40% is heterozygous taster, what is the frequency of *t*? *Hint:* Use the same method as that employed for codominant alleles for greatest accuracy.

10.26. Gene *A* governs purple stem and its recessive allele *a* produces green stem in tomatoes; *C* governs cut-leaf and *c* produces potato-leaf. If the observations of phenotypes in a sample from a tomato population were 204 purple, cut : 194 purple, potato : 102 green, cut : 100 green, potato, determine the frequency of (*a*) the cut allele, (*b*) the allele for green stem.

10.27. An isolated field of corn was found to be segregating for yellow and white endosperm. Yellow is governed by a dominant allele and white by its recessive allele. A random sample of 1000 kernels revealed that 910 were yellow. Find the allelic frequency estimates for this population.

10.28. The R locus controls the production of one system of antigens on the red blood cells of humans. The dominant allele results in Rh-positive individuals, whereas the homozygous recessive condition results in Rh-negative individuals. Consider a population in which 85% of the people are Rh-positive. Assuming the population to be at equilibrium, what is the gene frequency of alleles at this locus?

10.29. What is the highest frequency possible for a recessive lethal which kills 100% of its bearers when homozygous? What is the genetic constitution of the population when the lethal allele reaches its maximum?

10.30. Dwarf corn is homozygous recessive for gene *d*, which constitutes 20% of the gene pool of a population. If two tall corn plants are crossed in this population, what is the probability of a dwarf offspring being produced?

10.31. A dominant gene in rabbits allows the breakdown of the yellowish xanthophyll pigments found in plants so that white fat is produced. The recessive genotype *yy* is unable to make this conversion, thus producing yellow fat. If a heterozygous buck (male) is mated to a group of white fat does (females) from a population in which the frequency of *Y* is $\frac{2}{3}$, how many offspring with yellow fat would be expected among 32 progeny?

10.32. A metabolic disease of humans called phenylketonuria is the result of a recessive gene. If the frequency of phenylketonurics is 1/10,000, what is the probability that marriages between normal individuals will produce a diseased child?

10.33. Two recessive genes in *Drosophila*, *h* and *b*, producing hairy and black phenotypes, respectively, assort independently of one another. Data from a large population mating at random are as follows: 9.69% wild type, 9.31% hairy, 41.31% black, 39.69% hairy and black. Calculate the frequencies for the hairy and the black alleles.

Sex-Influenced Traits

10.34. Baldness is governed by a sex-influenced trait that is dominant in men and recessive in women. In a sample of 10,000 men, 7225 were found to be nonbald. In a sample of women of equivalent size, how many nonbald women are expected?

10.35. The presence of horns in some breeds of sheep is governed by a sex-influenced gene that is dominant in males and recessive in females. If a sample of 300 female sheep is found to contain 75 horned individuals, (*a*) what percentage of the females is expected to be heterozygous, (*b*) what percentage of the males is expected to be horned?

Autosomal Loci with Multiple Alleles

10.36. The genetics of the ABO human blood groups is presented in Problem 10.10. (*a*) A sample of a human population was blood grouped and found to contain 23 group AB, 441 group O, 371 group B, and 65 group A. Calculate the allelic frequencies of I^A, I^B, and i. (*b*) Given the gene frequencies $I^A = 0.36$, $I^B = 0.20$, and $i = 0.44$, calculate the percentage of the population expected to be of groups A, B, AB, and O.

10.37. The color of screech owls is under the control of a multiple allelic series: G^r (red) $> g^i$ (intermediate) $> g$ (gray). A sample from a population was analyzed and found to contain 38 red, 144 intermediate, and 18 gray owls. Calculate the allelic frequencies.

10.38. Several genes of the horse are known to control coat colors. The A locus apparently governs the distribution of pigment in the coat. If the dominant alleles of the other color genes are present, the multiple alleles of the A locus produce the following results: A^+ = wild-type (Prejvalski) horse (bay with zebra markings), A = dark or mealy bay (black mane and tail), a^t = seal brown (almost black with lighter areas), a = recessive black (solid color). The order of dominance is $A^+ > A > a^t > a$. If the frequency of $A^+ = 0.4$, $A = 0.2$, $a^t = 0.1$ and $a = 0.3$, calculate the equilibrium phenotypic expectations.

Sex-Linked Loci

10.39. A genetic disease of humans called hemophilia (excessive bleeding) is governed by a sex-linked recessive gene that constitutes 1% of the gametes in the gene pool of a certain population. (*a*) What is the expected frequency of hemophilia among men of this population? (*b*) What is the expected frequency of hemophilia among women?

10.40. Color blindness in humans is due to a sex-linked recessive gene. A survey of 500 men from a local population revealed that 20 were color blind. (*a*) What is the gene frequency of the normal allele in the population? (*b*) What percentage of the females in this population would be expected to be normal?

10.41. The white eyes of *Drosophila* are due to a sex-linked recessive gene and wild type (red eyes) to its dominant allele. In a *Drosophila* population the following data were collected: 15 white-eyed females, 52 white-eyed males, 208 wild-type males, 365 wild-type females (112 of which carried the white allele). Using all the data, calculate the frequency of the white allele.

TESTING A LOCUS FOR EQUILIBRIUM

10.42. A pair of codominant alleles governs coat colors in Shorthorn cattle: $C^R C^R$ is red, $C^R C^W$ is roan, and $C^W C^W$ is white. A sample of a cattle population revealed the following phenotypes: 180 red, 240 roan, and 80 white. (*a*) What is the frequency of the C^R allele? (*b*) What is the frequency of the C^W allele? (*c*) Does the sample indicate that the population is in equilibrium? (*d*) What is the chi-square value? (*e*) How many degrees of freedom exist? (*f*) What is the probability that the deviation of the observed from the expected values is due to chance?

10.43. A blood group system in sheep, known as the XZ system, is governed by a pair of codominant alleles (X and X^z). A large flock of Rambouillet sheep was blood grouped and found to contain 113 X/X, 68 X/X^z, and 14 X^z/X^z. (*a*) What are the allelic frequencies? (*b*) Is this population conforming to the equilibrium expectations? (*c*) What is the chi-square value? (*d*) How many degrees of freedom exist? (*e*) What is the probability of the observed deviation being due to chance?

10.44. The frequency of the T allele in a human population $= 0.8$, and a sample of 200 yields 90% tasters (T-) and 10% nontasters (tt). (*a*) Does the sample conform to the equilibrium expectations? (*b*) What is the chi-square value? (*c*) How many degrees of freedom exist? (*d*) What is the probability that the observed deviation is due to chance?

10.45. In poultry, the autosomal gene F^B produces black feather color and its codominant allele F^W produces splashed-white. The heterozygous condition produces Blue Andalusian. A splashed-white hen is mated to a black rooster and the F_2 was found to contain 95 black, 220 blue, and 85 splashed-white. (*a*) What F_2 ratio is expected? (*b*) What is the chi-square value? (*c*) How many degrees of freedom exist? (*d*) What is the probability that the observed deviation is due to chance? (*e*) May the observations be considered to conform to the equilibrium expectations?

Review Questions

Vocabulary   For each of the following definitions, give the appropriate term and spell it correctly. Terms are single words unless indicated otherwise.

1. The breeding structure of a population when each gamete has an equal opportunity of uniting with any other gamete from the opposite sex. (One or two words.)

2. The total genetic information possessed by the reproductive members of a population of sexually reproducing organisms. (Two words.)

3. The fundamental model of population genetics. (Three words.)

4. The condition of a locus that does not experience a change in allelic frequencies from one generation to the next.

5. An interbreeding group of organisms sharing a common gene pool. (Two words.)

6. Nonrandom assortment of chromosomes into gametes. (Two words.)

7. A deviation from Hardy-Weinberg expectations at any specific time in a population.

8. A phenotypically and/or geographically distinctive subspecific group, composed of individuals inhabiting a defined geographic and/or ecological region, and possessing characteristic phenotypic and gene frequencies that distinguish it from other such groups.

9. The hallmark criterion that demarcates one biological species from another. (Two words.)

10. Any change in the genetic composition of a population, such as a change in gene frequency.

True-False Questions   Answer each of the following statements either true (T) or false (F).

1. If a genetic locus in a population is not in Hardy-Weinberg equilibrium, it may be concluded that selection favors at least one of the genotypes.

2. Two populations with identical allelic frequencies need not have identical genotype frequencies.

3. Equilibrium at an autosomal locus can become fully established in a nonequilibrium population after one generation of random mating.

4. Evolutionary processes are at work whenever deviations from equilibrium exist.

5. The incidence of a dominant trait in a population is always greater than that of a recessive trait.

6. The frequencies of recessive autosomal alleles cannot be obtained easily unless the population is in genetic equilibrium.

7. When autosomal allelic frequencies are dissimilar in the sexes, the genotypic frequencies become equilibrated in one generation of random mating.

8. The frequency of a sex-linked gene in XY males is equivalent to the frequency of that gene in the females (XX) of the previous generation.

9. The frequency of a sex-linked gene in females (XX) is equal to the average of gene frequencies in males and females of the previous generation.

10. The frequencies of linked genes approach equilibrium more rapidly if they are far apart than if they are tightly linked.

Multiple-Choice Questions   Choose the one best answer.

For problems 1–4, use the following information. Snapdragon flowers may be red ($C'C'$), pink ($C'C^w$), or white (C^wC^w). A sample from a population of these plants contained 80 white, 100 pink, and 20 red-flowered plants.

1. The frequency of the red allele (C') in this sample is   (*a*) 0.10   (*b*) 0.20   (*c*) 0.30   (*d*) 0.45   (*e*) none of the above

2. The percentage of pink-flowered plants expected on the basis of the Hardy-Weinberg equation is approximately   (*a*) 35   (*b*) 45   (*c*) 50   (*d*) 55   (*e*) none of the above

3. A chi-square test of the sample data against the Hardy-Weinberg expectations produces a chi-square value of   (*a*) 1.96   (*b*) 2.43   (*c*) 2.87   (*d*) 3.02   (*e*) 3.11

4. Refer to Table 7.2 to answer this question. Assuming the sample is representative of its population in the above problem (3), it may be said that   (*a*) the chi-square test is significant and the sampled population is not in genetic equilibrium   (*b*) the chi-square test is nonsignificant and the sampled population is not in genetic equilibrium   (*c*) the chi-square test is significant and the sampled population is in genetic equilibrium   (*d*) the chi-square test is nonsignificant and the sampled population is in genetic equilibrium   (*e*) the chi-square value is significant, thereby invalidating the test.

For problems 5–7, use the following information. Black pelage is an autosomal dominant trait in guinea pigs; white is the alternative recessive trait. A Hardy-Weinberg population was sampled and found to contain 336 black and 64 white individuals.

5. The frequency of the dominant black gene is estimated to be   (*a*) 0.60   (*b*) 0.81   (*c*) 0.50   (*d*) 0.89   (*e*) none of the above

6. The percentage of black individuals that is expected to be heterozygous is approximately   (*a*) 46   (*b*) 57   (*c*) 49   (*d*) 53   (*e*) none of the above

7. The probability that a black male crossed to a white female would produce a white offspring is approximately   (*a*) 0.12   (*b*) 0.14   (*c*) 0.16   (*d*) 0.18   (*e*) none of the above

For problems 8–10, use the following information. Yellow body color in *Drosophila* is governed by a sex-linked recessive gene; wild-type color is produced by its dominant allele.

8. A sample from a Hardy-Weinberg population contained 1021 wild-type males, 997 wild-type females, and 3 yellow males. The percentage of the gene pool represented by the yellow allele is estimated to be (*a*) 0.04   (*b*) 0.16   (*c*) 0.21   (*d*) 0.42   (*e*) none of the above

9. If the frequency of the yellow allele is 0.01, the percentage of wild-type females expected to carry the yellow allele is   (*a*) 1.98   (*b*) 1.67   (*c*) 2.04   (*d*) 2.76   (*e*) none of the above

10. If the frequency of the yellow allele is 1.0 in females and 0 in males, the frequency of that allele in males of the next generation is expected to be   (*a*) 1.0   (*b*) 0.5   (*c*) 0.33   (*d*) 0.67   (*e*) none of the above

Answers to Supplementary Problems

10.15. 0.5

10.16. All individuals are *AaBb*.

10.17. (*a*) $p_m = p_f = 0.6$, $q_m = q_f = 0.4$ (*b*) $AA = 0.36$, $Aa = 0.48$, $aa = 0.16$

10.18. (*a*) $\frac{1}{7} = 0.143$ (*b*) 0.1008

10.19. $\frac{2}{3} = 0.67$

10.20. Males: (1) = 1.0, (2) = 0.5, (3) = 0.75; females: (1) = 0.5, (2) = 0.75, (3) = 0.625

10.21. (*a*) 0.25   (*b*) $\frac{1}{2}AABB : \frac{1}{2}aabb$ or $\frac{1}{2}aaBB : \frac{1}{2}AAbb$

10.22. $AB = 0.12$, $Ab = 0.08$, $aB = 0.48$, $ab = 0.32$

10.23. $C^D = 0.9$, $C^G = 0.1$

10.24. (*a*) $L^M = 75.5\%$, $L^N = 24.5\%$ (*b*) 210

10.25. $t = 0.56$

10.26. (*a*) $C = 0.30$ (*b*) $a = 0.58$

10.27. $Y = 0.7$, $y = 0.3$

10.28. $R = 0.613$, $r = 0.387$

10.29. 0.5; all individuals are heterozygous carriers of the lethal allele.

10.30. $\left(\dfrac{2pq}{1 - q^2}\right)^2 \left(\dfrac{1}{4}\right) = \dfrac{p^2 q^2}{(1 - q^2)^2} = \dfrac{1}{36} = 0.0277778$

10.31. 4

10.32. $\left[\dfrac{2(0.99)(0.01)}{(0.99)^2 + 2(0.99)(0.01)}\right]^2 (0.25) = 0.01\%$

10.33. $h = 0.7$, $b = 0.9$

10.34. 9775

10.35. (*a*) 50%   (*b*) 75%

10.36. (*a*) $I^A = 0.05$, $I^B = 0.25$, $i = 0.70$ (*b*) A = 44.6%, B = 21.6%, AB = 14.4%, O = 19.4%

10.37. $G^r = 0.1$, $g^i = 0.6$, $g = 0.3$

10.38. 64% wild type, 20% dark bay, 7% seal brown, 9% black

10.39. (*a*) 1/100   (*b*) 1/10,000

10.40. (*a*) 0.96   (*b*) 99.84%

10.41. $w = 0.19$

10.42. (*a*) 0.6 (*b*) 0.4 (*c*) Yes (*d*) 0 (*e*) 1 (*f*) 1

10.43. (*a*) $X = 0.75$, $X^z = 0.25$ (*b*) Yes (*c*) 0.7 (*d*) 1 (*e*) 0.3–0.5

10.44. (*a*) No (*b*) 18.75 (*c*) 1 (*d*) < 0.001

10.45. (*a*) $\frac{1}{4}$ black : $\frac{1}{2}$ blue : $\frac{1}{4}$ splashed-white (*b*) 4.50 (*c*) 1 (*d*) 0.01–0.05 (*e*) No

Answers to Review Questions

Vocabulary

1. random mating or panmixis
2. gene pool
3. Hardy-Weinberg law
4. equilibrium
5. Mendelian population
6. meiotic drive
7. disequilibrium
8. race or subspecies
9. reproductive isolation
10. evolution

True-False Questions

1. F (other violations of Hardy-Weinberg model conditions; e.g., migration) 2. T 3. T 4. T 5. F (frequencies of genes and heritable phenotypes are functions of evolutionary forces, not allelic interactions) 6. T 7. F (see Problem 10.20) 8. T 9. T 10. T

Multiple-Choice Questions

1. *e* (0.35) 2. *b* (45.5%) 3. *a* 4. *d* 5. *a* 6. *b* 7. *e* (0.286) 8. *e* (0.29) 9. *a* 10. *a*

Chapter 11

The Biochemical Basis of Heredity

NUCLEIC ACIDS

1. Deoxyribonucleic Acid (DNA).

The nucleic acid that serves as the carrier of genetic information in all organisms other than some viruses is **deoxyribonucleic acid** (DNA). The double-helical structure of this long molecule is shown in Fig. 11-1. The backbone of the helix is composed of two chains with alternating sugar (S)-phosphate (P) units. The sugar is a pentose (5-carbon) called **deoxyribose,** differing from its close relative **ribose** by one oxygen atom in the 2′ position (Fig. 11-2). The phosphate group (PO_4) connects adjacent sugars by a 3′→5′ phosphodiester linkage. In one chain the linkages are polarized 3′→5′; in the other chain, read in the same direction, they are in the reverse order 5′→3′. All nucleic acid chains pair in this **antiparallel** fashion, whether DNA with DNA chains, DNA with RNA chains, or RNA with RNA chains. The steps in the spiral staircase (i.e., the units connecting one strand of DNA to its polarized

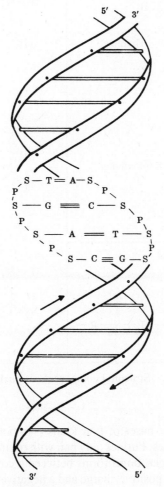

Fig. 11-1.
Diagram of Watson-Crick
model of DNA.

269

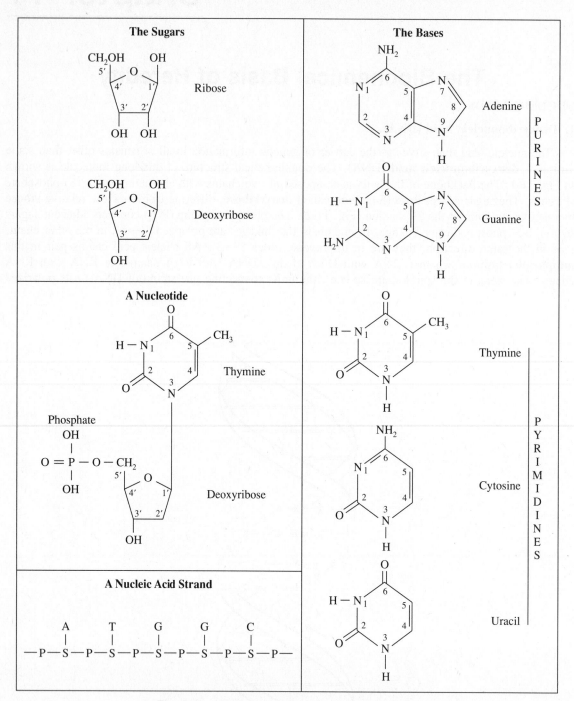

Fig. 11-2.   Structural components of nucleic acids.

complement) consist of paired organic bases of four kinds (symbolized A, T, G, C) classified into two groups, the **purines** and the **pyrimidines.** Purines only pair with pyrimidines and vice versa, thus producing a symmetrical double helix. A **hydrogen bond** forms between a covalently bound donor hydrogen atom (e.g., an imino group, NH) with some positive charge and a negatively charged covalently bound acceptor atom (e.g., a keto group, CO) by sharing of a hydrogen atom. Adenine (A) pairs with thymine (T) by two hydrogen bonds; guanine (G) and cytosine (C) pair by three hydrogen bonds (Fig. 11-3). A base-sugar complex is called a **nucleoside;** a nucleoside plus a phosphate is called a **nucleotide.** DNA is thus

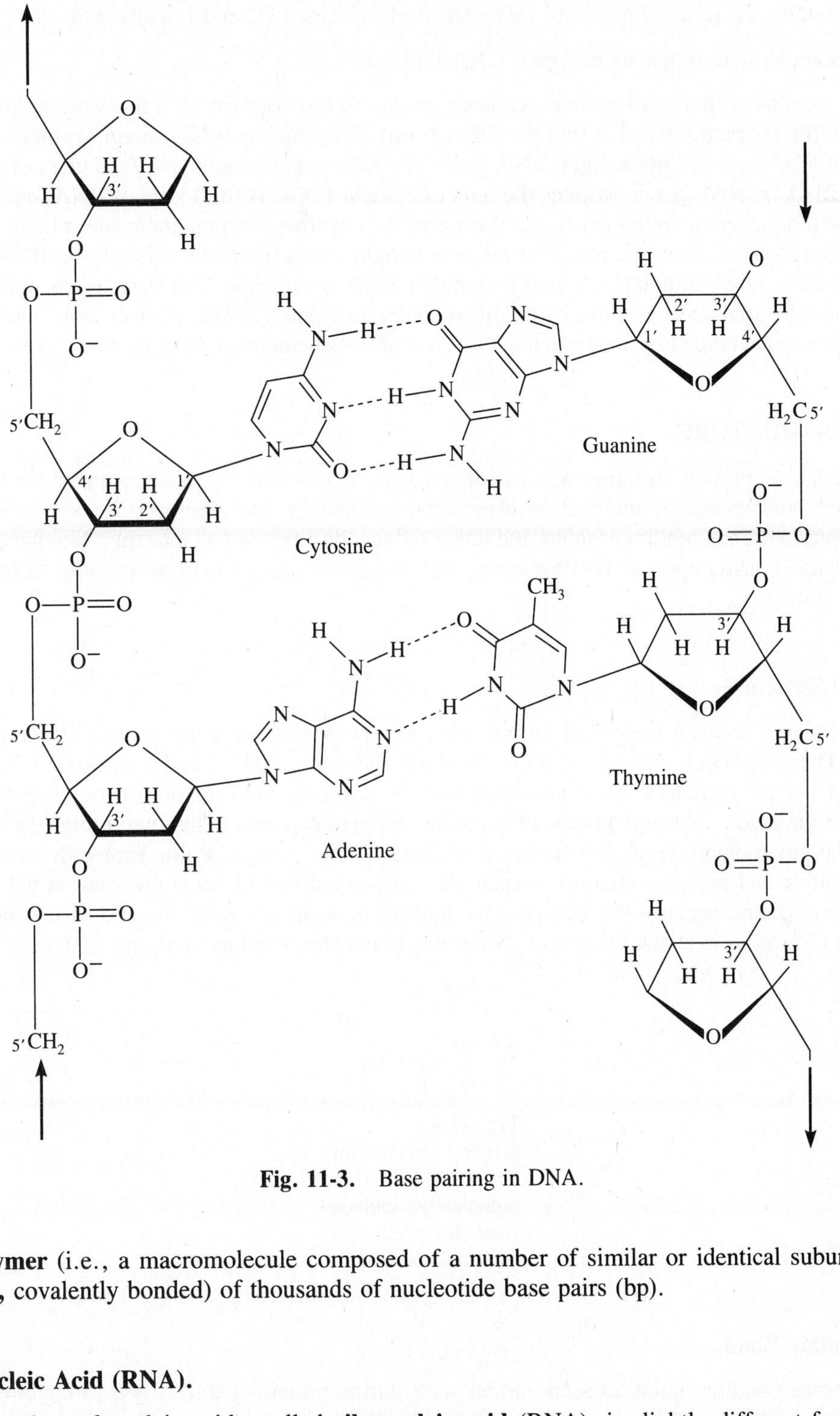

Fig. 11-3. Base pairing in DNA.

a long **polymer** (i.e., a macromolecule composed of a number of similar or identical subunits, called **monomers,** covalently bonded) of thousands of nucleotide base pairs (bp).

2. Ribonucleic Acid (RNA).

Another class of nucleic acids, called **ribonucleic acid** (RNA), is slightly different from DNA in the following respects:

(1) Cellular RNA is single-stranded; DNA is double-stranded. A few viruses have a single-stranded RNA genome; very few have a double-stranded RNA genome.

(2) RNA contains ribose sugars instead of the deoxyribose sugars that are found in DNA.

(3) RNA contains the pyrimidine uracil (U) instead of thymine (T), and U pairs with A.

(4) RNA molecules are much shorter than DNA molecules.

RNA functions primarily in protein synthesis, acting in one capacity as a messenger carrying information from the instructions coded into the DNA to the ribosomal sites of protein synthesis in the cell. This form of RNA is called **messenger RNA** (mRNA). Ribosomes contain a special class of RNA called **ribosomal RNA** (rRNA) that constitutes the bulk of cellular RNA. A third kind of RNA, called **transfer RNA** (tRNA), attaches to amino acids and during protein synthesis brings them into proper positioning with other amino acids using the mRNA-ribosome complex as a template. All cellular RNA molecules are made from a DNA template. A single-stranded RNA chain may fold back upon itself and form localized "double-stranded" sections by complementary base pairing. The "clover-leaf" model of tRNA in Fig. 11-8 was developed by maximizing this type of complementary base pairing.

PROTEIN STRUCTURE

Knowledge of protein structure and bonding forces is essential for a keen understanding of how various genetic factors (mutations) and environmental factors (e.g., pH, temperature, salt concentrations, chemical treatments) can modify proteins and either reduce, destroy, or enhance their biological activities. Such knowledge is also important for developing techniques to extract functional proteins from genetically engineered cells.

1. General Structure.

All completely ionized biological amino acids except proline have the general structure shown in Fig. 11-4. The α-carbon is the central atom to which an amino (NH^{3+}) and a carboxyl (COO^-) group are attached. As pH increases above neutrality (pH 7), the more basic nature of the environment tends to neutralize the acidic carboxyl groups of proteins. As pH decreases below neutrality, the more acidic nature of the environment tends to neutralize the basic amino groups. **Polar molecules** are those with separate positive and negative charges at each end, as exemplified by an amino acid at pH 7. Water is also a polar molecule because the two positive hydrogen atoms are near one end of the molecule and the oxygen (2^-) atom is at the other end. **Nonpolar molecules** (such as methane, CH_4) are uncharged.

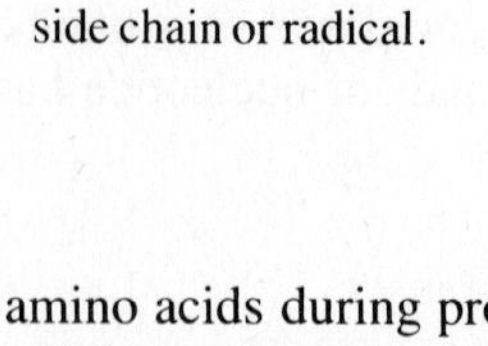

Fig. 11-4.
General structure of an amino acid in completely ionized form. R represents a side chain or radical.

2. The Peptide Bond.

The peptide bond that joins adjacent amino acids during protein synthesis is a strong covalent bond, in which atoms are coupled by sharing an electron. By the removal of water, the carboxyl group of one amino acid becomes joined to the amino group of an adjacent amino acid as shown in Fig. 11-5. This union, which is accompanied by the removal of water, is an example of dehydration synthesis. One of the ribosomal proteins, the enzyme **peptidyl transferase,** is responsible for making the peptide bond. Each complete polypeptide chain thus has an uncomplexed ("free") amino group at one end and a free carboxyl group at its other end. The amino end of the polypeptide corresponds to the 5' end of its

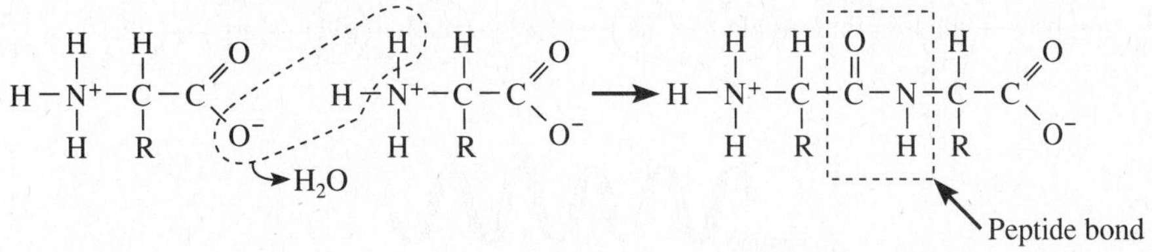

Fig. 11-5.   Dehydration synthesis of a dipeptide and formation of a peptide bond.

respective mRNA. The carboxyl end of the polypeptide corresponds to the 3′ terminus of the same mRNA.

3. Side Chains.

Each kind of amino acid differs according to the nature of the side chain or radical attached to the α-carbon. Glycine has the simplest side chain, consisting of a hydrogen atom. Other amino acids have hydrocarbon side chains of various lengths; some of these chains are ionized positively (basic proteins such as lysine and arginine), others are negatively charged (acidic amino acids such as aspartic and glutamic acids), and still others are nonionized (e.g., valine, leucine). Different proteins can be separated on the basis of their net electrical charges by a technique known as **electrophoresis.** Closely related proteins differing by a single amino acid can sometimes be resolved in this way. Some amino acids, such as phenylalanine and tyrosine, have aromatics (ring structures) in their side chains. The amino acid proline does not contain a free imino group (NH) because its nitrogen atom is involved in a ring structure with its side chain. Only two amino acids (cysteine and methionine) contain sulfur in their side chains. The sulfurs of different cysteines can be covalently linked into a disulfide bond (S—S) that is responsible for helping to stabilize the tertiary and quaternary shapes of proteins containing them.

4. Structural Levels.

The linear sequence of amino acids forms the **primary structure** of proteins (Fig. 11-6). Some portions of many proteins have a **secondary structure** in the form of an **alpha helix** in which the carbonyl group (C═O) next to one peptide bond forms a hydrogen bond with an imino group (NH) flanking a peptide bond a few amino acids further along the polypeptide chain. The protein chain may fold back upon itself, forming weak internal bonds (e.g., hydrogen bonds, ionic bonds) as well as strong covalent disulfide bonds that stabilize its **tertiary structure** into a precisely and often intricately folded pattern. Two or more tertiary structures may unite into a functional **quaternary structure.** For example, hemoglobin consists of 4 polypeptide chains (2 identical α-chains and 2 identical β-chains). A protein cannot function until it has assumed its full tertiary or quaternary configuration. Any disturbance of its normal configuration may inactivate the function of the protein. For example, if the protein is an enzyme, heating may destroy its catalytic activity because weak bonds that hold the protein in its secondary or higher structural forms are ruptured. The shape of an active enzyme molecule fits its **substrate** (the substance that is catalyzed by the enzyme) in a manner analogous to the way a key fits a lock (Fig. 11-7). An enzyme that is altered, either genetically (by mutation of the respective gene), physically (e.g., heat), or chemically (e.g., pH change) may not fit the substrate and therefore would be incapable of catalyzing the conversion of substrate to normal product.

5. Factors Governing Structural Levels.

Relatively weak bonds such as hydrogen bonds and **ionic bonds** (attraction of positively and negatively charged ionic groups) are mainly responsible for the secondary and higher structural levels of protein organization. Enzymes are not involved in the formation of weak bonds. The extent to which a protein

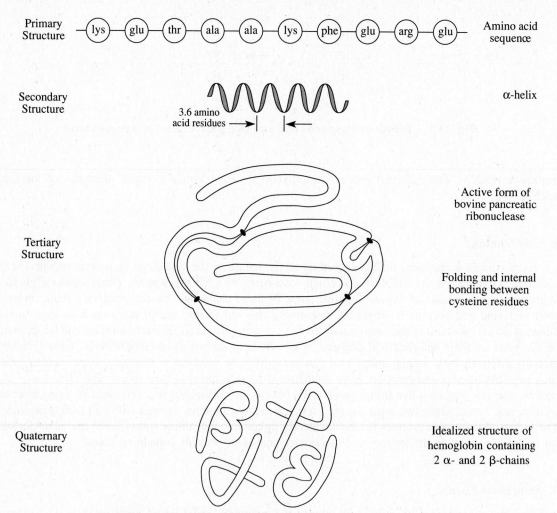

Primary Structure — lys — glu — thr — ala — ala — lys — phe — glu — arg — glu — Amino acid sequence

Secondary Structure — 3.6 amino acid residues → α-helix

Tertiary Structure — Active form of bovine pancreatic ribonuclease — Folding and internal bonding between cysteine residues

Quaternary Structure — Idealized structure of hemoglobin containing 2 α- and 2 β-chains

Fig. 11-6. Stages in the development of a functional protein.

contains alpha-helical regions is dependent upon at least three factors. The most important factor governing tertiary protein structure involves formation of the most favorable energetic interactions between atomic groupings in the side chains of the amino acids. A second factor is the presence of proline, which cannot participate in alpha-helical formation because it has no imino group. Proline is therefore often found at the "corners," or "hairpin turns," of polypeptide chains. Finally, the formation of intrastrand (on the same chain) disulfide bridges tends to distort the alpha helix.

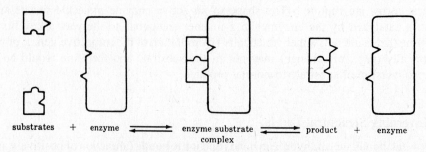

substrates + enzyme ⇌ enzyme substrate complex ⇌ product + enzyme

Fig. 11-7. Diagram of enzymatic action.

6. Formation of Quaternary Structure.

The ionized side chains of some amino acids readily interact with water and therefore are called **hydrophilic** (''water-loving'') amino acids. **Hydrophobic** (''water-fearing'') amino acids contain non-ionized side chains that tend to avoid contact with water. When a polypeptide chain folds into its tertiary shape, these forces cause amino acids with hydrophilic groups to predominate on the outside and hydrophobic segments of the chain to predominate in the interior of globular proteins. The multiple polypeptide chains of quaternary proteins are usually joined by hydrophobic forces. Nonpolar groups of the individual polypeptide chains come together as a way of excluding water. Hydrogen bonds, ionic bonds, and possibly interstrand (between chains) disulfide bonds may also participate in forming quaternary protein structures. Some quaternary proteins consist of 2 or more identical polypeptide chains (e.g., the bacterial enzyme β-galactosidase consists of 4 identical polypeptide chains). Such proteins are called **homopolymers.** Other quaternary proteins (such as hemoglobin) consist of nonidentical chains and are called **heteropolymers.** In order to become functional proteins, some polypeptide chains must be subject to modifications after they have been synthesized. For example, the protein chymotrypsinogen must be cleaved at one specific position by an enzyme to produce the active split-product chymotrypsin.

CENTRAL DOGMA OF MOLECULAR BIOLOGY

Each strand of the DNA double helix serves as a template for its own replication. All RNA molecules are synthesized from DNA templates in a process called **transcription.** Within a transcriptional unit, only one of the strands of DNA serves as a template for the synthesis of RNA molecules. Different transcriptional units may reside on the same or on different DNA strands. Genes are said to be **active** when they are transcribing RNA. Proteins are synthesized from mRNA templates by a process called **translation.** The central dogma of molecular biology is the concept that DNA is the genetic material of all cells, that all cellular DNA is synthesized from DNA templates, that DNA segments are transcribed into RNAs (of all classes), and that mRNAs (with the aid of tRNAs and rRNAs) are translated into polypeptide chains (proteins). This dogma was partly broken in 1990 by the discovery that DNA in telomeric regions of at least some chromosomes can be synthesized from an RNA template (see Example 14.4). Furthermore, certain viruses (viruses are not cells) use RNA as genetic material, and they contain or code for an enzyme that synthesizes a DNA strand from the viral RNA strand. Such viruses are called ''retroviruses'' (see Chapter 14) because they reverse the cellular dogma that all RNA strands are made from DNA templates.

GENETIC CODE

Biochemical reactions are mediated by enzymes. Virtually all enzymes are proteins. A few RNA molecules are known to have enzymatic activity; they are referred to as **ribozymes.** Some protein antibodies have also been found to exhibit enzymatic properties; they are called **abzymes.** Proteins are polymers of subunits (monomers) called **amino acids,** often spoken of as ''residues'' (especially during degradation of proteins to ascertain their amino acid sequences). Twenty different kinds of amino acids occur naturally in proteins. Each protein enzyme consists of a certain number of amino acids in a precisely ordered sequence. The blueprint that specifies this amino acid sequence is encoded in a nucleotide sequence of DNA. A **codon** is an adjacent group of 3 nucleotides in either the DNA or in its mRNA transcript that specifies an amino acid. The first experimental evidence supporting the ''triplet code'' concept was provided by a study of single base pair additions in a gene of a bacterial virus (phage T4). If the transcription of a functional genetic unit of DNA into mRNA is always read from a fixed position, then the first six codons in one chain of the corresponding DNA might be as follows.

	1	2	3	4	5	6
	TCA	GGC	TAA	AGT	CGG	TCG

The addition of a single base (e.g., G) at the end of the second codon would shift all other codons one nucleotide out of register and prevent the correct reading of all codons to the right of the base addition.

```
      1      2      3      4      5      6
     TCA    GGC    GTA    AAG    TCG    GTC    G
```

By successively adding bases in a nearby region, it should be possible to place the reading frame of the codons back into register. It was found that one or two base additions failed to produce a functionally normal protein. But three base additions apparently can place the reading frame of the codons back into register for all codons to the right of the third base addition.

```
      1      2      3      4      5      6      7
     TCA    AGG    CGT    ACA    AGT    CGG    TCG
            Missense codons            Codons in
            (out of register)       correct register
```

The same has also been found to be true for single nucleotide deletions. Three deletions or multiples thereof can correct the reading frame in the synthesis of an active protein. Several other lines of evidence indicate that the codon is a sequence of three nucleotides and the genetic code is generally referred to as a "triplet code."

High concentrations of ribonucleotides in the presence of the enzyme polynucleotide phosphorylase can generate synthetic mRNA molecules without a template *in vitro* by forming an internucleotide 3′-5′ phosphodiester bond. In this way a number of uracil molecules can become linked together to form a synthetic poly-U with mRNA activity. The addition of poly-U to bacterial cell extracts results in the limited synthesis of polypeptides containing only the amino acid phenylalanine. Thus 3 uracils probably code for phenylalanine. Mixtures of different ribonucleotides can also form synthetic mRNA molecules with the nucleotides in random order.

> **Example 11.1.** Poly-AU made from a mixture of adenine and uracil in concentrations of 2 : 1, respectively, is expected to form AAA triplets most frequently, AAU (or AUA or UAA) triplets would be next in frequency, AUU (or UAU or UUA) triplets next, and UUU triplets would be least frequent. The frequencies with which various amino acids are incorporated into polypeptides under direction of the synthetic poly-AU can then be correlated with the expected frequencies of various triplets, allowing tentative assignment of specific triplets to specific amino acids.

A combination of organic chemical and enzymatic techniques can be used to prepare synthetic polyribonucleotides with known repeating sequences as, for example, AUAUAUAU . . . , which alternately codes for the amino acids isoleucine and tyrosine, CUCUCUCU . . . , which codes for leucine and serine alternately, etc.

Even in the absence of mRNA and protein synthesis, an RNA trinucleotide will bind to a ribosome. Chemically synthesized trinucleotides of known sequence can thus be made to bind to ribosomes, and this complex will specifically bind one out of a mixture of 20 different tRNA–amino acid complexes *in vitro*. By radioactively labeling only one kind of amino acid in such a mixture, the specificity of the codon can be established. For example, UUG binds only leucine-tRNA complexes to ribosomes, and UGU binds only cysteine-tRNA complexes.

The genetic code is **degenerate** because more than one **samesense** codon exists for most amino acids. The nuclear code appears to be the same in all organisms, and thus is said to be a **universal code.** However, a few codons in some organelle DNAs have different meanings than those in nuclear DNAs (see Chapter 12). Apparently only 3 of the 64 possible three-letter codons fail to specify an amino acid. Such triplets are called **nonsense codons** or **stop codons,** and they serve as part of the translation termination signal. The mRNA codons for the 20 amino acids are listed in Table 11.1. These codons are conventionally written from the 5′ end (at the left) toward the 3′ end (at the right) because that is the direction in which translation (protein synthesis) occurs on mRNA.

Table 11.1. mRNA Codons

First Letter		Second Letter				Third Letter
		U	C	A	G	
U	U	UUU UUC } Phe UUA UUG } Leu	UCU UCC UCA UCG } Ser	UAU UAC } Tyr UAA UAG } Nonsense	UGU UGC } Cys UGA Nonsense UGG Trp	U C A G
	C	CUU CUC CUA CUG } Leu	CCU CCC CCA CCG } Pro	CAU CAC } His CAA CAG } Gln	CGU CGC CGA CGG } Arg	U C A G
	A	AUU AUC } Ile AUA AUG Met	ACU ACC ACA ACG } Thr	AAU AAC } Asn AAA AAG } Lys	AGU AGC } Ser AGA AGG } Arg	U C A G
	G	GUU GUC GUA GUG } Val	GCU GCC GCA GCG } Ala	GAU GAC } Asp GAA GAG } Glu	GGU GGC GGA GGG } Gly	U C A G

The three-letter symbols, names, and one-letter symbols (in parentheses) of the amino acids are as follows: ala = alanine (A), arg = arginine (R), asn = asparagine (N), asp = aspartic acid (D), cys = cysteine (C), glu = glutamic acid (E), gln = glutamine (Q), gly = glycine (G), his = histidine (H), ile = isoleucine (I), leu = leucine (L), lys = lysine (K), met = methionine (M), phe = phenylalanine (F), pro = proline (P), ser = serine (S), thr = threonine (T), trp = tryptophan (W), tyr = tyrosine (Y), val = valine (V).

PROTEIN SYNTHESIS

1. Transcription.

There are two major steps in protein synthesis: transcription and translation. The first step in the production of proteins is the transcription of DNA to an mRNA molecule. This process is carried out by the enzyme **RNA polymerase.** This enzyme attaches to the DNA at a specific nucleotide sequence called a **promoter** ahead of (upstream from) the gene to be translated. A number of enzymes stimulate the local unwinding of DNA, and this allows RNA polymerase to begin transcription of one of the DNA strands. Within a gene, only one of the DNA strands is transcribed into mRNA. This DNA strand is called the **anticoding strand** or **antisense strand;** the DNA strand that is not transcribed is called the **coding strand** or **sense strand.** In some other gene on that same DNA molecule, the other strand may serve as a template for RNA synthesis. Within a gene, however, RNA polymerase does not jump from one DNA strand to another to transcribe the RNA molecule. Termination of transcription occurs when RNA polymerase encounters a ''terminator nucleotide sequence'' at the end of a structural gene. In some bacterial genes, an accessory protein binds to the terminator sequence and thereby aids in dislodging RNA polymerase from the DNA. The mechanism of transcription termination in eucaryotes is still unknown.

In eucaryotic cells, primary mRNA transcripts are ''processed'' before they are released from the nucleus as mature mRNA molecules. Initially, most eucaryotic primary transcripts (pre-mRNAs) are mosaics of coding regions (**exons**) and noncoding regions (**introns**). Before the mRNA leaves the nucleus to become mature cytoplasmic mRNA, the noncoding regions must be precisely removed and the exons must be spliced together. In addition, an unusual guanine nucleotide (called a **cap**) is attached to the 5' end, and a string of adenine nucleotides (called a **poly-A tail**) is attached to the 3' end of the mRNA. In procaryotic cells, however, there is no nuclear membrane, and mRNA processing does not occur.

Except for the primitive archaebacteria (see Chapter 14), bacterial genes do not contain introns. Thus, translation of mRNA into protein can commence in bacteria even before the mRNA has been completely transcribed from the DNA.

2. Translation.

In the second major step of protein synthesis, ribosomes and tRNA-methionine complexes (called "charged" methionyl tRNAs) attach near the 5' end of the mRNA molecule at the first **start codon** or **initiation codon** (5'AUG3') and begin to translate its ribonucleotide sequence into the amino acid sequence of a protein. Ribosomes consist of 3 rRNA molecules and about 50 different proteins. Each amino acid is coded for by at least 1 tRNA molecule. Because the genetic code is so degenerate, many more than 20 tRNAs are actually involved in protein synthesis. Each amino acid becomes attached or loaded (at its carboxyl terminus) to the 3' end of its own species of tRNA (Fig. 11-8) by a specific enzyme **(amino-acyl synthetase).** Thus, there are at least twenty different synthetases. The "loaded" tRNA is said to be **activated** or **charged.** A loop of unpaired bases near the middle of the tRNA carries a triplet of adjacent bases called the **anticodon.** Other parts of the tRNA are thought to form complementary base pairs with rRNA of the ribosome during protein synthesis or to act as recognition sites for a specific amino-acyl synthetase.

Translation of all proteins begins with the start codon 5'AUG3', which specifies the amino acid methionine (refer to Fig. 11-9 throughout the following discussion). Two sites exist on a ribosome for activated tRNAs: the peptidyl site (P site) and the amino-acyl site (A site). The initiating methionine-loaded tRNA enters the P site (perhaps by passing through the A site). The 3'UAC5' anticodon of the

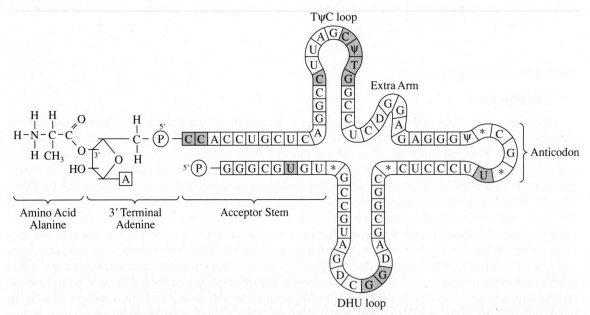

Fig. 11-8. A "cloverleaf model" of the yeast alanine transfer RNA molecule. All species of tRNA are about 75 ribonucleotides in length, with three major loops of unpaired bases. The middle loop contains the anticodon that can base pair with a codon in mRNA. The loop nearest the 3' end (called the TψC loop) is thought to interact with rRNA in the ribosome. There are several unusual bases (*) in tRNAs; pseudouridine (ψ) is one of them. The loop nearest the 5' end is called the DHU loop because it contains another unusual base, dihydrouridine (D). Enzymes in the nucleus modify the normal bases (A, U, C, G) in the preformed tRNA to create these unusual (rare) bases. All tRNAs end with CCA3'; the proper species of amino acid is attached to the terminal A by its cognate aminoacyl-tRNA synthetase enzyme. Some of the positions bearing identical bases in almost all tRNA species are indicated by shading.

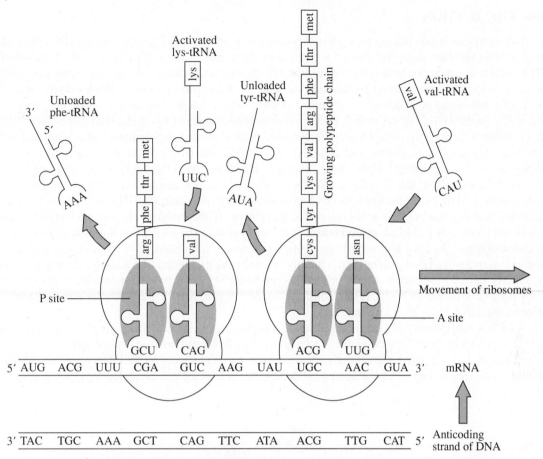

Fig. 11-9. Diagram of protein synthesis. (Reprinted, by permission, from William D. Stansfield, *The Science of Evolution,* © 1977 by Macmillan Publishing Co., Inc.)

tRNA pairs with the complementary 5′AUG3′ codon in the mRNA. The ribosome acts like a jig to hold all of the reactants in the proper alignment during translation. A second activated tRNA (e.g., one loaded with threonine) enters the A site (again by specific codon-anticodon base pairing). A peptide bond is formed between the two adjacent amino acids by the action of an enzymatic protein of the ribosome called peptidyl transferase. The amino-acyl bond that held the methionine to its tRNA is broken when the peptide bond forms. The now ''unloaded'' methionyl-tRNA in the P site leaves (usually to become activated again). The ribosome shifts (translocates) 3 nucleotides along the mRNA to position a new open codon in the vacant A site while at the same time moving the thr-loaded tRNA (now attached to a dipeptide) from the A to the P site. The third tRNA (e.g., one loaded with phenylalanine) enters the A site; a peptide bond forms between the second and the third amino acids; the second tRNA exits the P site; translocation of the ribosome along the mRNA displays the next codon for arginine in the A site while shifting the phe-loaded tRNA (now carrying a tripeptide) from the A to the P site; and so on. Eventually the system reaches one or more nonsense or stop codons (UAA, UAG, or UGA) causing the polypeptide chain to be released from the last tRNA, the last tRNA to be released from the ribosome, and the ribosome to be released from the mRNA. Thus, the 5′ end of mRNA corresponds to the amino terminus of the polypeptide chain; the 3′ end of the mRNA corresponds to the carboxyl terminus of the polypeptide chain.

The preceding story of protein synthesis presents only a broad outline of the process. Some important aspects of this process are performed differently in bacteria and in eucaryotes, details of which are presented in separate chapters dealing with these two major life forms.

DNA REPLICATION

The hydrogen bonds linking base pairs together are relatively weak bonds. During DNA replication, the 2 strands separate along this line of weakness in zipperlike fashion (Fig. 11-10). Each strand of the DNA molecule can serve as a template against which a complementary strand can form (according to the rules of specific base pairing) by the catalytic activity of enzymes known as **DNA polymerases.** This mode of replication, in which each replicated double helix contains one original (parental strand) and one newly synthesized daughter strand, is referred to as **semiconservative replication** (see Solved Problem 13.1). At least three forms of DNA polymerase have been identified in procaryotes (bacteria) and at least four in eucaryotes (fungi, plants, and animals). The three bacterial forms are denoted I, II, and III; the eucaryotic forms are denoted alpha, beta, gamma, and delta. All DNA polymerase enzymes can add free nucleotides only to the 3′ ends of existing chains, so that the chains will grow from their 5′ ends toward their 3′ ends. All three kinds of DNA polymerases can also degrade DNA in the 3′→5′ direction. Enzymes that degrade nucleic acids are called **nucleases.** If the enzyme cleaves nucleotides from the end of the chain it is called an **exonuclease;** if it makes cuts in the interior of the molecule it is termed an **endonuclease.** As long as deoxyribonucleotide precursors are present in even moderate amounts, the synthetic activity of a DNA polymerase is greatly favored over its degradation activity. During replication, incorrectly paired bases have a high probability of being removed by the exonuclease activity of the DNA polymerases before the next nucleotide is added. This is part of the ''proofreading system'' that protects the DNA from errors (mutations).

All DNA polymerases can extend existing polynucleotide chains only from their 3′ ends; they cannot initiate new chains from their 5′ ends. A special kind of RNA polymerase, called **primase,** constructs a short (about 10 base pairs) segment of ribonucleotides complementary to the DNA template. This **RNA primer** has a free 3′ end to which additional deoxyribonucleotides can be added by DNA polymerases.

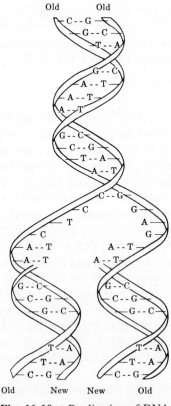

Fig. 11-10.   Replication of DNA.

In bacteria, DNA polymerase III is the enzyme primarily responsible for extending these chains in the replication process. Both DNA polymerases I and III have $5'{\rightarrow}3'$ as well as $3'{\rightarrow}5'$ exonuclease activity. However, it is primarily DNA polymerase I that removes the RNA primers $5'{\rightarrow}3'$ and simultaneously replaces them with deoxyribonucleotides. DNA polymerase II has only $3'{\rightarrow}5'$ exonuclease activity and therefore can perform a proofreading function, but it cannot replace primer ribonucleotides with deoxyribonucleotides simultaneously. A **nick** is the absence of a phosphodiester bond between adjacent nucleotides in one strand of duplex DNA. DNA polymerases cannot form a covalent phosphodiester bond between adjacent deoxyribonucleotides on either side of a nick; another enzyme, called **DNA ligase,** performs this task.

At least two other classes of enzymes are also required for DNA synthesis. The **helicases (unwinding proteins)** proceed ahead of the DNA polymerases, opening the double helix and producing single-stranded templates for replication. These single-stranded regions are stabilized when complexed with **single-stranded DNA binding proteins (SSB),** forming a **replication fork.**

Replication begins at the $3'$ end of a template (parental) strand (Fig. 11-11). A primer RNA is synthesized $5'{\rightarrow}3'$ toward the replication fork, and the primer is extended by DNA polymerase III, forming the **leading strand.** The opposite template strand has a $5'$ end, so no complementary primer can be formed $3'{\rightarrow}5'$. Instead, a **lagging strand** is replicated ($5'{\rightarrow}3'$) in short segments (a few hundred nucleotides each) in a direction opposite to the movement of the replication fork. These segments are called **Okazaki fragments** (named after their discoverer, Reji Okazaki). A **gap** is said to exist where one or more adjacent nucleotides are missing from one strand of a duplex DNA molecule. DNA polymerase I temporarily creates gaps by removing RNA primers, but quickly fills the gaps with replacement deoxyribonucleotides. Nicks between adjacent Okazaki fragments are rapidly joined by DNA ligase so that at any given time there is only a single incomplete fragment in the lagging strand. The **discontinuous replication** of the lagging strand results in its seemingly paradoxical overall growth from $3'$ to $5'$.

In eucaryotes, at least four DNA polymerases have been identified, all having the ability to extend primers in the $5'{\rightarrow}3'$ direction. The alpha DNA polymerase carries out DNA replication in the nucleus. Beta and delta DNA polymerases may play a role in gap filling and repair. Gamma DNA polymerase is only found in mitochondria and is required for replication of mitochrondrial DNA.

There is usually a single position (**ori site**) where initiation of DNA replication occurs on the circular DNA molecules of bacteria, viruses, plasmids, and organelles. The much longer linear nuclear-DNAs of eucaryotes have many sites at which replication can be simultaneously initiated. Each unit of replication is called a **replicon.** Other replication differences between bacteria and eucaryotes are presented in separate chapters devoted to these different forms of life.

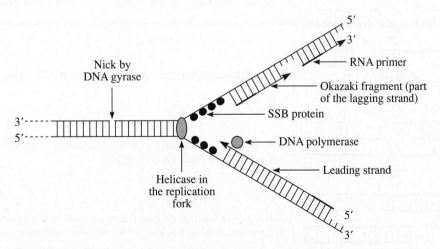

Fig. 11-11.   Production of Okazaki fragments on the lagging strand during DNA replication.

GENETIC RECOMBINATION

There is no effective pairing force between homologous DNA duplex molecules. Therefore, recombination is thought to involve the production of complementary single-stranded regions. This could be accomplished by an endonuclease nicking one strand of the double helix in each of two homologous DNA molecules. According to one theory (Fig. 11-12), DNA polymerase extends the broken ends, displacing one of the strands in the process. Complementary base pairing between the displaced segments creates a short double-stranded bridge. The other intact stands are then nicked by an endonuclease, producing one recombinant molecule and two fragments with overlapping terminal sequences. DNA polymerase fills the gaps and ligase seals the nicks to create reciprocal recombinant DNA molecules.

According to a second theory (Fig. 11-13), the broken strands of parallel-aligned double helices are reciprocally joined by ligase, creating a cross-bridge. Equivalent bases on the two original molecules can exchange places, causing the cross connection to move along the complex in a zipperlike fashion called **branch migration.** This action commonly produces long regions of hybrid DNA containing some base sequences that may not be completely complementary, referred to as a **heteroduplex.** Twisting the complex leads to steric rearrangement that converts the bridging strands to outside strands and vice versa ("isomerization"). Cross-bridges are removed by nuclease cuts, the gaps are filled by DNA polymerase, and the nicks are sealed by DNA ligase. This type of crossing over can produce either a single switch in all 4 strands or a double switch in 2 of the strands.

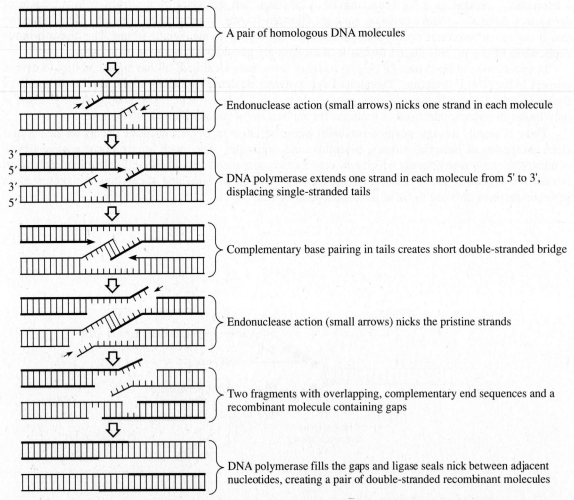

Fig. 11-12. Model of crossing over involving disruption of the individual DNA molecules. (After J. D. Watson, *Molecular Biology of the Gene,* 3rd ed., 1976, Benjamin-Cummings.)

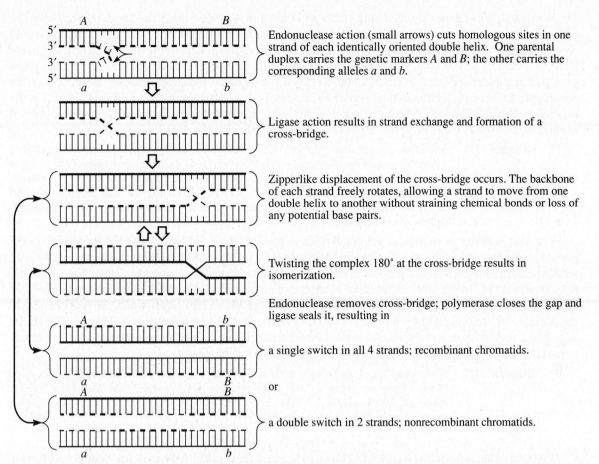

Endonuclease action (small arrows) cuts homologous sites in one strand of each identically oriented double helix. One parental duplex carries the genetic markers A and B; the other carries the corresponding alleles a and b.

Ligase action results in strand exchange and formation of a cross-bridge.

Zipperlike displacement of the cross-bridge occurs. The backbone of each strand freely rotates, allowing a strand to move from one double helix to another without straining chemical bonds or loss of any potential base pairs.

Twisting the complex 180° at the cross-bridge results in isomerization.

Endonuclease removes cross-bridge; polymerase closes the gap and ligase seals it, resulting in

a single switch in all 4 strands; recombinant chromatids.

or

a double switch in 2 strands; nonrecombinant chromatids.

Fig. 11-13. Model of crossing over without disruption of the individual DNA molecules. (After J. D. Watson, *Molecular Biology of the Gene*, 3rd ed., 1976, Benjamin-Cummings.)

MUTATIONS

Nonenzymatic or structural proteins constitute the bulk of organic matter in living systems. Most proteins are complex, high-molecular-weight molecules. The exact sequence of amino acids in proteins is known for only a few, including hemoglobin, insulin, bovine pancreatic ribonuclease, tobacco mosaic virus protein, lysozyme, and tryptophan synthetase. The normal human hemoglobin (Hb A) has about 140 amino acid residues in each of its α- and β- chains. The sequence in the β^A chain has been determined to be

$$\text{val - his - leu - thr - pro - glu - glu - lys - etc.}$$
$$\text{1} \quad \text{2} \quad \text{3} \quad \text{4} \quad \text{5} \quad \text{6} \quad \text{7} \quad \text{8}$$

An abnormal hemoglobin (Hb S) is produced by individuals with a mutant allele, resulting in a deformity of the red blood cell called "sickling." In a heterozygous condition this allele produces a mild anemia; in a homozygous condition the severity of the anemia may be lethal. The difference between Hb A and Hb S is that the latter has valine substituted for glutamic acid in the sixth position of the β^S-chain. Another potentially lethal abnormal hemoglobin (Hb C) is known in which the glutamic acid of the sixth position is replaced by lysine. One of the codons for glutamic acid is GAA. If a mutation occurred that changed the first A to a U, then the codon GUA (a **missense** triplet) would be translated as valine. The substitution of A for G would produce the missense codon AAA which codes for lysine. Thus a change in a single nucleotide in the hemoglobin gene can produce a substitution of one amino acid in a chain of about 140 residues with profound phenotypic consequences!

Fortunately most genes are relatively stable and mutation is a rare event. The great majority of genes have mutation rates of 1×10^{-5} to 1×10^{-6}, i.e., 1 gamete in 100,000 to 1 gamete in a million would contain a mutation at a given locus. However in a higher organism containing 10,000 genes, 1 gamete in 10 to 1 gamete in 100 would be expected to contain at least one mutation. The rate at which a given gene mutates under specified environmental conditions is as much a characteristic of the gene as is its phenotypic expression. The mutation rate of each gene is probably dependent to some extent upon the residual genotype. The only effect that some genes seem to exhibit is to increase the mutation rate of another locus. These kinds of genes are called "mutator genes."

> **Example 11.2.** A dominant gene called "dotted" (*Dt*) on chromosome 9 in corn causes a recessive gene *a* governing colorless aleurone, on chromosome 3, to mutate quite frequently to its allele *A* for colored aleurone. Plants that are *aaDt-* often have kernels with dots of color in the aleurone produced by mutation of *a* to *A*. The size of the dot will be large or small depending upon how early or late respectively during development of the seed the mutational event occurred.

The vast majority of mutations are deleterious to the organism and are kept at low frequency in the population by the action of natural selection. Mutant types are generally unable to compete equally with wild-type individuals. Even under optimal environmental conditions many mutants appear less frequently than expected. Mendel's laws of heredity assume equality in survival and/or reproductive capacity of different genotypes. Observed deviations from the expected Mendelian ratios would be proportional to the decrease in survival and/or reproductive capacity of the mutant type relative to wild type. The ability of a given mutant type to survive and reproduce in competition with other genotypes is an extremely important phenotypic characteristic from an evolutionary point of view.

> **Example 11.3.** White-eyed flies may be only 60% as viable as flies with pigmented eyes. Among 100 zygotes from the cross $w^+w\,♀$ (wild type) $\times$ $wY\,♂$ (white), the Mendelian zygotic expectation is 50 wild type : 50 white. If only 60% of white-eyed flies survive, then we would observe in the adult progeny

$$50 \times 0.6 = 30 \text{ white} : 50 \text{ wild type}$$

Ionizing radiations such as X-rays are known to increase the mutability of all genes in direct proportion to the radiation dosage. A linear relationship between dosage (in roentgen units) and the induction of sex-linked recessive lethal mutations in *Drosophila* is shown graphically in Fig. 11-14. This indicates that there is no level of dosage that is safe from the genetic standpoint. If a given amount of radiation is received gradually in small amounts over a long period of time (chronic dose) the genetic damage is sometimes less than if the entire amount is received in a short time interval (acute dose). In most cases,

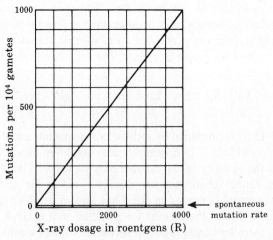

Fig. 11-14. X chromosome lethal mutations in *Drosophila* induced by X-rays.

dose rate effects are not demonstrable. Ionizing radiations produce their mutagenic effects most frequently by inducing small deletions in the chromosome.

The student's first encounter with the terminology involved in the study of mutations is sometimes a source of confusion. Mutations can be classified on the basis of several criteria. The outline in Table 11.2 may be useful in showing the interrelationships of concepts and terms.

Table 11.2   A Classification of Mutations

I. Size
  A. Point mutation—a change in a very small segment of DNA; usually considered to involve a single nucleotide or nucleotide pair
     1. Samesense (silent) mutation—change in a codon (usually at the third position) that fails to change the amino acid specificity from the unmutated state
     2. Nonsense mutation—a shortening of the protein product due to a chain-termination signal
     3. Missense mutation—a change in amino acid sequence with the wrong amino acid occupying a given position in the polypeptide chain
     4. Frameshift mutation—a shift of the reading frame, creating numerous missense or nonsense codons through the remainder of the cistron
  B. Gross mutations—changes involving more than one nucleotide pair; may involve the entire gene, the entire chromosome, or sets of chromosomes (polyploidy)

II. Quality
  A. Structural mutations—changes in the nucleotide content of the gene
     1. Substitution mutations—substitution of one nucleotide for another
        (*a*) *Transition* mutations substitute one purine for another or one pyrimidine for another
        (*b*) *Transversion* mutations substitute a purine for a pyrimidine or vice versa
     2. Deletion mutants—loss of some portion of a gene
     3. Insertion mutants—addition of one or more extra nucleotides to a gene
  B. Rearrangement mutations—changing the location of a gene within the genome often leads to "position effects"
     1. Within a gene—two mutations within the same functional gene can produce different effects, depending on whether they occur in the cis or trans position
     2. Number of genes per chromosome—different phenotypic effects can be produced if the numbers of gene replicas are nonequivalent on the homologous chromosomes
     3. Moving the gene locus may create new phenotypes, especially when the gene is relocated near heterochromatin
        (*a*) Translocations—movement to a nonhomologous chromosome
        (*b*) Inversions—movement within the same chromosome

III. Origin
  A. Spontaneous mutation—origin is unknown; often called "background mutation"
  B. Genetic control—the mutability of some genes is known to be influenced by other "mutator genes"
     1. Specific mutators—effects limited to one locus
     2. Nonspecific mutators—simultaneously affects many loci
  C. Induced mutations—through exposure to abnormal environments such as:
     1. Ionizing radiations—changes in chemical valence through the ejection of electrons are produced by protons, neutrons, or by α-, β-, γ-, or X-rays
     2. Nonionizing radiations—raise the energy levels of atoms (excitation), rendering them less stable (e.g., ultraviolet radiation, heat); UV often produces thymine dimers, i.e., bonding between thymines on the same strand
     3. Chemical mutagens—chemical substances that increase the mutability of genes
        (*a*) Copy errors—mutants arising during DNA replication (e.g., base analogue mutagens that are chemically similar to the nucleic acid bases may be incorporated by mistake; acridine causes single base additions or deletions possibly by intercalation between two sequential bases)
        (*b*) Direct gene change—produced in nonreplicating DNA (e.g., nitrous acid by deamination directly converts adenine to hypoxanthine and cytosine to uracil)

IV. Magnitude of Phenotypic Effect
  A. Change in mutation rate—some alleles can be distinguished only by the frequency with which they mutate

Table 11.2   Cont.

   B. Isoalleles—produce identical phenotypes in homozygous or heterozygous combinations with each other, but prove to be distinguishable when in combination with other alleles

   C. Mutants affecting viability:
1. Subvitals—relative viability is greater than 10% but less than 100% compared to wild type
2. Semilethals—cause more than 90% but less than 100% mortality
3. Lethals—kill all individuals before adult stage

V. Direction

   A. Forward mutation—creates a change from wild type to abnormal phenotype

   B. Reverse or back mutation—produces a change from abnormal phenotype to wild type
1. Single-site mutation—changes only one nucleotide in the gene
(e.g., adenine $\xrightarrow{\text{forward}}$ guanine $\xrightarrow{\text{reverse}}$ adenine)
2. Mutation suppressor—a gene change which occurs at a different site from the primary mutation, yet reverses its effect
   (*a*) Extragenic (intergenic) suppressor—occurs in a different gene from that of the mutant
   (*b*) Intragenic suppressor—occurs at a different nucleotide within the same gene; shifts the reading frame back into register

VI. Cell Type

   A. Somatic mutation—occurs in nonreproductive cells of the body, often producing a mutant phenotype in only a sector of the organism (mosaic or chimera)

   B. Gametic mutation—occurs in the sex cells, producing a heritable change

---

DNA REPAIR

One of the best understood repair mechanisms involves removal of pyrimidine dimers (usually covalently linked adjacent thymines in the same strand). Thymine dimers are easily induced in bacteria by ultraviolet (UV) light. These dimers are lethal if left unrepaired because they interfere with the normal replication of progeny DNA strands. There are at least three mechanisms known for repairing pyrimidine dimers.

(1) *Photoreactivation.* Some pyrimidine dimers can be removed by the action of an enzyme that becomes activated by absorption of blue light. This type of repair is more efficient if the bacteria are prevented from growing for a period of time after exposure to UV irradiation. Not much is known concerning the chemistry of this repair process.

(2) *Dark Repair.* This mechanism involves four steps. (*a*) A single-strand break is made on the 5′ side near the dimer by a specific endonuclease called UV endonuclease. (*b*) The 5′⊖3′ exonuclease activity of DNA polymerase I removes nucleotides near the cut, including the dimer. (*c*) One of the DNA polymerases (possibly pol I) synthesizes a correct replacement strand 5′ to 3′ using information from the intact complementary strand. (*d*) Polynucleotide ligase seals the break. Dark repair (excision repair) can begin as soon as a pyrimidine dimer is formed even if growth is not experimentally delayed.

(3) *SOS Repair.* This is a form of error-prone replication that repairs lesions in DNA without regard for restoring the original base sequence. This type of repair may be triggered by chemical mutagens that alter the hydrogen-bonding properties of bases or by radiation-induced mutations. Little is known concerning the nature of this emergency repair mechanism.

DEFINING THE GENE

Mendel's work suggested that each gene controls a given phenotype (e.g., a gene for tall vs. short pea vine growth). Later work showed that many genes may contribute to a single such character and, moreover, that each gene may have multiple phenotypic effects (pleiotropy). One of the earliest concepts of gene action to explain human metabolic disorders proposed that each such gene was responsible for a specific enzymatic reaction; hence the "one gene–one enzyme" hypothesis was born. Then it was discovered that some enzymes consist of more than one kind of polypeptide chain. For example, the bacterial enzyme tryptophan synthetase is a tetramer of 2 α-chains and 2 β-chains; each of the two types of chains is specified by a different genetic locus. The paradigm then became "one gene–one polypeptide chain."

It has become common to equate the term **cistron** with a region of DNA that specifies a complete polypeptide chain. However, the term "cistron" was originally given to a functional genetic unit as defined by the phenomenon of **complementation** as observed in the **cis-trans test.** Two mutations may be either in the same DNA molecule (**cis position**) or on different DNA molecules (**trans position**). A heterozygote containing two cis mutations in the same functional unit of one DNA molecule can be complemented to produce a normal phenotype by the other homologous DNA molecule that contains normal genetic information. A heterozygote containing two trans mutations (one on each homologous DNA molecule) in the same functional unit cannot complement to produce a normal phenotype because each DNA molecule contains defective information. Therefore, two point mutations are considered to be **functionally allelic** (in the same cistron) if they complement in cis position, but fail to complement in trans position.

Example 11.4.   Two point mutants (m_1 and m_2) in the same cistron are functionally allelic.

(a) Cis position (both mutant nucleotides on one homologue)

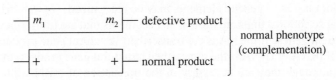

(b) Trans position (each homologue has a mutant and a nonmutant nucleotide)

However, if a heterozygote contains two point mutations in either cis or trans position in different functional units, complementation can produce a normal phenotype because for each mutant functional unit on one DNA molecule there is a corresponding normal functional unit on the other DNA molecule. Thus, two mutants are **functionally nonallelic** (in different cistrons) if they complement in either cis or trans position.

Example 11.5.   Two point mutants in different cistrons are functionally nonallelic.

(a) Coupling linkage

(b) Repulsion linkage

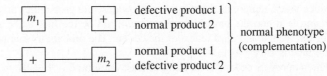

The structure of DNA reveals that multiple positions or sites potentially exist within a cistron where mutation or recombination can occur. The mutations may or may not lead to variance in expression of the corresponding trait. However, the name **muton** is given to the smallest amount of genetic material that when changed (mutated) produces a phenotypic effect. Experiments have shown that a single nucleotide may constitute a muton (as exemplified earlier in the case of sickle-cell anemia). Alternative forms of a cistron that differ at the same nucleotide site are referred to as **homoalleles.** Intragenic recombination between homoalleles is not possible. A **recon** is the smallest amount of genetic material within which recombination can occur. Two adjacent nucleotides are thought to constitute a recon. Intragenic (intracistronic) recombination is possible even between adjacent mutons. Such recombinationally defined forms of a gene are called **heteroalleles.**

Example 11.6.   An individual with a mutant phenotype has two mutant sites, m_1 and m_2, within homologous cistrons (diagrammed as boxes). These heteroalleles can recombine and be transmitted to the progeny as a functionally normal cistron.

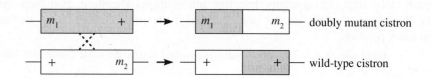

Two major classes of genetic elements may be recognized: (1) transcriptional units and (2) extragenic elements. Transcriptional units are those DNA segments that are transcribed into RNA; they are commonly called **structural genes.** If mRNA is the transcribed structural gene product, it will normally be translated into protein. If tRNA or rRNA is the transcribed structural gene product, these molecules are not translated into protein (although they are necessary in the translation of mRNA into protein). Some regions of the DNA that are not transcribed (e.g., promoters and transcription termination signals) control the transcription of structural genes. Although these kinds of regions have been called "control genes," the current trend is to refer to them as **extragenic elements.** It would be convenient if we could always equate a single gene with a single functional product (either an RNA molecule or a polypeptide chain), but this is seldom possible because the transcriptional product of a structural gene may be converted into more than one kind of functional RNA or polypeptide chain. For example, bacteria can produce polycistronic mRNAs; that is, a single mRNA can be translated into two or more different polypeptide chains. Although every eucaryotic mRNA is thought to be monocystronic, the single polypeptide chain synthesized from that mRNA might be enzymatically cleaved into more than one functional polypeptide chain. Should only "transcriptional units" be recognized as genes, or should a gene be equated with the smaller segments of a transcriptional unit that code for individual mature tRNAs, rRNAs, or polypeptide chains? This problem remains to be resolved.

Solved Problems

11.1. How many triplet codons can be made from the four ribonucleotides A, U, G, and C containing (*a*) no uracils, (*b*) one or more uracils?

Solution:

(*a*)   Since uracil represents 1 among 4 nucleotides, the probability that uracil will be the first letter of the codon is $\frac{1}{4}$; and the probability that U will not be the first letter is $\frac{3}{4}$. The same reasoning holds true for the second and third letters of the codon. The probability that none of the three letters of the codon are uracils is $(\frac{3}{4})^3 = \frac{27}{64}$.

(*b*)   The number of codons containing at least one uracil is $1 - \frac{27}{64} = \frac{37}{64}$.

11.2. A synthetic polyribonucleotide is produced from a mixture containing U and C in the relative frequencies of $5:1$, respectively. Assuming that the ribotides form in a random linear array, predict the relative frequencies in which the various triplets are expected to be formed.

Solution:

The frequencies with which the different triplets are expected to be formed by chance associations can be predicted by combining independent probabilities through multiplication as follows:

UUU should occur with a frequency of $(\frac{5}{6})(\frac{5}{6})(\frac{5}{6}) = \frac{125}{216}$.

Codons with 2U and 1C $= (\frac{5}{6})^2(\frac{1}{6}) = \frac{25}{216}$ each (UUC, UCU, CUU).

Codons with 1U and 2C $= (\frac{5}{6})(\frac{1}{6})^2 = \frac{5}{216}$ each (UCC, CUC, CCU).

CCC $= (\frac{1}{6})^3 = \frac{1}{216}$.

11.3. Suppose that synthetic RNAs were made from a solution that contained 80% adenine and 20% uracil. The proteins produced in a bacterial cell-free system under direction of these mRNAs were found to contain amino acids in the following relative proportions: 4 times as many isoleucine as tyrosine residues, 16 times as many isoleucine as phenylalanine residues, 16 times as many lysine as tyrosine residues. What triplet codons were probably specifying each of the above amino acids?

Solution:			**Codon**		**Ratio**	**Amino Acid**
AAA	=	$(0.8)^3$	=	0.512	64	Lysine
Some permutation of 2A and 1U	=	$(0.8)^2(0.2)$	=	0.128	16	Isoleucine
Some permutation of 1A and 2U	=	$(0.8)(0.2)^2$	=	0.032	4	Tyrosine
UUU	=	$(0.2)^3$	=	0.008	1	Phenylalanine

$$\text{phe} \xrightarrow{4x} \text{tyr} \xrightarrow{4x} \text{ileu} \xrightarrow{4x} \text{lys}$$

with $16x$ connecting phe to ileu, and $16x$ connecting tyr to lys.

11.4. H. J. Muller developed a system (*ClB* technique) for detecting recessive sex-linked lethal mutations induced by X-ray treatment in *Drosophila*. He used a heterozygous stock that had the dominant sex-linked gene "bar eye" (*B*) linked to a known recessive lethal gene (*l*). The segment of chromosome containing *B* and *l* was within an inversion (represented by the symbol *C*) that effectively prevented crossing over between the *B* and *l* loci. He began by mating these dihybrid bar-eye females to wild-type males that had been exposed to X-rays. He selected the F_1 bar-eye females and crossed them to unirradiated wild-type males in small vials, one female per vial. The incidence of sex-linked recessive lethals induced by the X-ray treatment was determined from inspection of the F_2. What criterion did he use for this determination?

Solution:

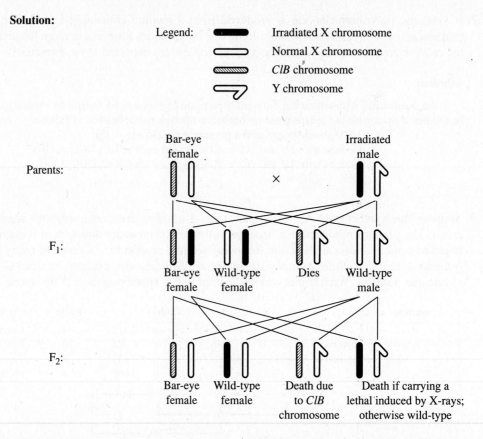

Any vials of the F_2 generation that are devoid of males can be scored as an X–ray-induced sex-linked lethal as long as spontaneous mutations are considered negligible. The same procedure could be followed without irradiation treatment of the parental males to obtain an estimate of the rate of spontaneous sex-linked lethals. The reason that the F_1 bar-eye females can survive even though carrying two recessive lethals is that the X–ray-induced lethal is, in all probability, at some locus other than the one in the ClB chromosome.

11.5. If 54 mutations are detected among 723 progeny of males that received 2500 roentgens and 78 mutations among 649 progeny of males that received 4000 roentgens, how many mutants would be expected to appear among 1000 progeny of males that received 6000 roentgens?

Solution:

The number of mutations induced by ionizing radiation is directly proportional to the dosage.

$$\frac{78}{649} = 12.02\% \text{ mutations at 4000 roentgens}$$
$$\frac{54}{723} = 7.47\% \text{ mutations at 2500 roentgens}$$
$$\text{Difference} = 4.55\% \text{ mutations for 1500 roentgens}$$

Among 1000 progeny at 6000 roentgens we expect $1000(6000/1500)(0.0455) = 182$ mutants.

11.6. Four single mutant strains of *Neurospora* are unable to grow on minimal medium unless supplemented by one or more of the substances A–F. In the following table, growth is indicated by + and no growth by 0. Both strains 2 and 4 grow if E and F or C and F are added to minimal medium. Diagram a biochemical pathway consistent with the data involving all 6 metabolites, indicating where the mutant block occurs in each of the 4 strains.

Strain	A	B	C	D	E	F
1	+	0	0	0	0	0
2	+	0	0	+	0	0
3	+	0	+	0	0	0
4	+	0	0	0	0	0

Solution:

Strain 1 will grow only if given substance A. Therefore the defective enzyme produced by the mutant gene in this strain must act sometime prior to the formation of substance A and after the formation of substances B, C, D, E, and F. In other words, this mutation is probably causing a metabolic block in the last step of the biochemical sequence in the synthesis of substance A.

$$\left(\begin{array}{c} B, C, D, E, F \\ \text{order unknown} \end{array} \right) \xrightarrow{\ 1\ } A$$

Strain 2 grows if supplemented by either A or D, but not by B. Therefore the metabolic block in strain 2 must occur after B but before A. Furthermore, since the dual addition of substances E and F or C and F allows strain 2 to grow, we can infer that the intervenient pathway is split, with E and C in one line and F in the other. Substance D could be at one of two positions as shown below.

Strain 3 grows if supplemented by A or C, but not by D. Therefore D cannot immediately precede A (as shown above), and the metabolic block in strain 3 must precede the formation of C but not E.

Strain 4 can grow if given dual supplementation of E and F or C and F but not if given D alone. The mutation in strain 4 apparently cannot split D into E and F.

Supplementary Problems

DNA AND PROTEIN SYNTHESIS

11.7. Given a single strand of DNA . . .$^{3'}$ TACCGAGTAC $^{5'}$ . . . , construct (*a*) the complementary DNA chain, (*b*) the mRNA chain which would be made from this strand.

11.8. If the ratio (A + G)/(T + C) in one strand of DNA is 0.7, what is the same ratio in the complementary strand?

11.9. How many different mRNAs could specify the amino acid sequence met-phe-ser-pro?

11.10. If the DNA of a species has the mole fraction of G + C = 0.36, calculate the mole fraction of A.

11.11. The size of a hemoglobin gene in humans is estimated to consist of approximately 450 nucleotide pairs. The protein product of the gene is estimated to consist of about 150 amino acid residues. Estimate the size of the codon.

11.12. Using the information in Table 11.1, convert the following mRNA segments into their polypeptide equivalents: (a) . . .⁵′ GAAAUGGCAGUUUAC ³′ . . . , (b) . . .³′ UUUUCGAGAUGUCAA ⁵′ . . . , (c) . . .⁵′ AAAACCUAGAACCCA ³′. . . .

11.13. Given the hypothetical enzyme below with regions A, B, C, and D (· = disulfide bond; shaded area = active site), explain the effect of each of the following mutations in terms of the biological activity of the mutant enzyme: (a) nonsense in DNA coding for region A, (b) samesense in region D, (c) deletion of one complete codon in region C, (d) missense in region B, (e) nucleotide addition in region C.

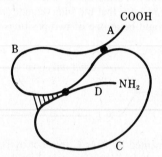

11.14. A large dose of ultraviolet irradiation can kill a wild-type cell even if the DNA repair system is unsaturated. Under what circumstances would this lethality likely occur?

11.15. In a system containing 70% U and 30% C and an enzyme that links ribonucleotides at random into a synthetic mRNA, determine the relative frequencies with which all possible triplet codons would be expected to be formed.

11.16. Acridine dyes can apparently cause a mutation in the bacteriophage T4 by the addition or subtraction (deletion) of a base in the DNA chain. A number of such mutants have been found in the r_{II} region of T4 to be single base addition type (+) or deletion type (−) mutants. A normal or wild-type r_{II} region produces a normal lytic period (small plaque size) in the host bacterium *Escherichia coli* strain B. Phage T4 mutant in the r_{II} region rapidly lyses strain B, producing a larger plaque. Several multiple mutant strains of T4 have been developed. Suppose the mutant sites are close together and also in a region of the chromosome which is not essential to the normal functioning of the protein specified by this gene. Determine the lytic phenotypes (large plaque or small plaque) produced by the following r_{II} single base mutations in *E. coli* B assuming a triplet codon: (a) (+), (b) (+)(−), (c) (+)(+), (d) (−)(−), (e) (+)(−)(+), (f) (+)(+)(+), (g) (−)(−)(+), (h) (−)(−)(−), (i) (+)(+)(+)(+), (j) (+)(−)(+)(+)(+).

11.17. A single base addition and a single base deletion approximately 15 bases apart in the mRNA specifying the protein lysozyme from the bacterial virus T4 caused a change in the protein from its normal composition . . . lys-ser-pro-ser-leu-asn-ala-ala-lys . . . to the abnormal form . . . lys-val-his-his-leu-met-ala-ala-lys. . . . (a) From the mRNA codons listed in Table 11.1, decipher the segment of mRNA for both the original protein and the double mutant. (b) Which base was added? Which was deleted?

11.18. In polynucleotides containing uracil and cytosine produced from a mixture of ribotides where uracil is in excess, more serine is incorporated into polypeptides than proline. However, when cytosine is in excess more proline is incorporated than serine. (*a*) Without reference to Table 11.1, list the codons containing uracil and cytosine that could possibly be coding for serine and for proline. (*b*) Using Table 11.1, determine the percentage of the various amino acids expected to be incorporated into polypeptides by a synthetic polynucleotide in which uracil constitutes 60% and cytosine 40% of the U-C mixture. (*c*) How much more phenylalanine is expected to be incorporated into protein than proline?

11.19. If the DNA of an *E. coli* has 4.2×10^6 nucleotide pairs in its DNA, and if an average cistron contains 1500 nucleotide pairs, how many cistrons does it possess?

11.20. The following experiment was performed: a short pulse of radioactive isotopes of the 20 amino acids is given to rabbit reticulocytes as they are synthesizing hemoglobin. The introduction of radioactive label occurs when some hemoglobin molecules are partly completed but unlabeled. Shortly after the pulse, completely finished hemoglobin molecules are isolated and analyzed for the location of the radioactive label. Where would you expect to find the label, and why?

11.21. The DNA of phage *lambda* has 1.2×10^5 nucleotides. How many proteins of molecular weight 40,000 could be coded by this DNA? Assume a molecular weight of 100 for the average amino acid.

11.22. In phage T4, deletion 1589 lacks part of the A and B cistrons of the r_{II} region and shows no A but partial B activity in *E. coli* strain B. When a single defect (deletion or addition) is induced in the A cistron by acridine, the B cistron activity is suppressed. What hypothesis is supported by these observations?

MUTATIONS

11.23. The "dotted" gene in maize (*Dt*) is a "mutator" gene influencing the rate at which the gene for colorless aleurone (*a*) mutates to its dominant allele (*A*) for colored aleurone. An average of 7.2 colored dots (mutations) per kernel was observed when the seed parent was *dt/dt, a/a* and the pollen parent was *Dt/Dt, a/a*. An average of 22.2 dots per kernel was observed in the reciprocal cross. How can these results be explained?

11.24. Assuming no intensity effect is operative, which individual would carry fewer mutations; an individual who receives 25 roentgens in 5 hours or an individual who receives only 0.5 roentgen per year for his or her normal lifetime (60 years)? In terms of percentage, how many more mutations would be expected in the individual with the higher total dosage?

11.25. If the mutation rate of a certain gene is directly proportional to the radiation dosage and the mutation rate of *Drosophila* is observed to increase from 3% at 1000 roentgens to 6% at 2000 roentgens, what percentage of mutations would be expected at 3500 roentgens?

11.26. The frequency of spontaneous mutation at the *R* (plant color) locus in maize is very high (492 per 10^6 gametes). The gene for red aleurone (*Pr*) is estimated to mutate in 11 out of 10^6 gametes. How many plants must be investigated on the basis of probability to find one with mutations at both loci?

11.27. A strain of *Drosophila* called Muller-5 contains the dominant sex-linked mutation for bar eye (*B*) and the apricot allele of the sex-linked white-eye locus (w^{ap}) together with an inversion (In) to prevent crossing over between them when a female is structurally heterozygous for the inversion. Homozygous In-bar-apricot females are crossed to x-irradiated wild-type males. Each F_1 female is placed in a separate vial together with one or more unirradiated wild-type males. Upon inspection of the F_2, what criterion can be used for scoring induced sex-linked recessive lethals?

11.28. Single wild-type female *Drosophila* possessing attached-X chromosomes ($X\hat{X}Y$) is mated to an irradiated wild-type male. (*a*) In which generation can a sex-linked mutation be detected? (*b*) What criterion is used to detect a sex-linked viable mutation? (*c*) What criterion is used to detect a sex-linked lethal mutation? (*d*) What percentage death loss is anticipated among the F_1 zygotes due to causes other than lethal mutations?

11.29. A method is known for rendering chromosome 2 of *Drosophila* homozygous so that all recessive mutants induced in that chromosome by irradiation can be detected. This method uses a balanced lethal system involving 3 genes on the second chromosome: curly wings (*Cy*), plum eye color (*Pm*), and lobe eye shape

(L). A ($Cy + L/+ Pm +$) female fly is mated to an X-irradiated wild-type male. A curly, lobed F_1 male is then backcrossed to a curly, plum, lobed female. From the backcross progeny, select and intercross curly-lobe flies. Predict the phenotypic ratios among the offspring when (a) no mutant was induced, (b) a viable recessive mutant was induced, (c) a semilethal or subvital was induced, (d) a lethal was induced.

11.30. The number of sex-linked lethals in *Drosophila* as detected by the *ClB* and Muller-5 techniques (Problems 11.4 and 11.27) increases in direct proportion to the amount of radiation at low dosage levels. However, at high dosage levels the amount of detectable lethal mutations falls below the linear expectations. How can this phenomenon be explained?

11.31. For single genes or single chromosome breaks, the number of mutations produced is directly related to the dose of x-rays received. For inversions and translocations, however, there is a "threshold effect"; i.e., a dosage below which no chromosomal rearrangements are detected. (a) Offer an explanation for the "threshold effect". (b) How is the dose-response curve for chromosomal rearrangements expected to appear? (c) Suppose that the exponential formula is $y = ax^2$, where y is the percentage of chromosome aberrations, a is a constant, and x is the dosage in Roentgens. If $y = 2.5$ when $x = 80$, find y when $x = 160$.

11.32. Assume that the rate of induced mutations is directly proportional to the radiation dosage. Further suppose that 372 individuals out of 6000 incur a mutation at 2000 roentgens, and that 610 out of 5000 individuals incur a mutation at 4000 roentgens. Estimate the spontaneous mutation rate.

11.33. Concerning a single nucleotide pair, list all possible (a) transitions, (b) transversions. (c) If purines and pyrimidines become replaced at random during evolution, what ratio of transversions to transitions is expected? (d) A comparison of homologous residues in the polypeptide chains of hemoglobins and myoglobins from various species indicates that 293 transitions and 548 transversions have probably occurred during evolution. Are these figures consistent with the hypothesis that transitions and transversions occur in a 1:2 ratio, respectively? Test the hypothesis by chi-square.

11.34. A number of nutritional mutant strains was isolated from wild-type *Neurospora* that responded to the addition of certain supplements in the culture medium by growth (+) or no growth (0). Given the following responses for single-gene mutants, diagram a metabolic pathway that could exist in the wild-type strain consistent with the data, indicating where the chain is blocked in each mutant strain.

(a)

Mutant Strain	Supplements Added to Minimal Culture Medium				
	Citrulline	Glutamic Semialdehyde	Arginine	Ornithine	Glutamic Acid
1	+	0	+	0	0
2	+	+	+	+	0
3	+	0	+	+	0
4	0	0	+	0	0

(b)

Strain	Growth Factors			
	A	B	C	D
1	0	0	+	+
2	0	0	0	+
3	+	0	+	+
4	0	+	+	+

(c)

Strain	Nutrients			
	E	F	G	H
1	+	0	0	+
2	0	0	+	+
3	0	0	0	+
4	0	+	0	+

11.35. Point mutations correlated with amino acids in the active site in widely separated regions of a cistron can render its enzymatic or antibody product inactive. What inference can be made concerning the structure of the active sites in such proteins?

11.36. A nonsense point mutation in one cistron can sometimes be at least partially suppressed in its phenotypic manifestation by a point mutation in a different gene. Offer an explanation for this phenomenon of intergenic suppression.

11.37. In addition to the kind of mechanism accounting for intergenic suppression of nonsense mutations (see previous problem), give two other possible mechanisms for intergenic suppression of missense mutations.

11.38. Intracistronic (interallelic) *in vitro* complementation has been observed in alkaline phosphatase enzymes and other proteins. How can a diploid heterozygote or a heterocaryon bearing two point mutations within homologous cistrons result in normal or nearly normal phenotypes (complementation)?

11.39. Why are most mutations in structural genes recessive to their wild-type alleles?

11.40. Forward mutation rates are usually at least an order of magnitude higher than back mutation rates for a given cistron. How can this be explained?

11.41. Bacterial cells that are sensitive to the antibiotic streptomycin (str^s) can mutate to a resistant state (str^r). Such "gain of function" mutations, however, occur much less frequently than "loss of function" mutations such as mutation from the ability to make the amino acid histidine (his^+) to the inability to do so (his^-), or mutation from the ability to metabolize the sugar lactose (lac^+) to the inability to do so (lac^-). Formulate a hypothesis that explains these observations.

Review Questions

Vocabulary   For each of the following definitions, give the appropriate term and spell it correctly. Terms are single words unless indicated otherwise.

1. The method of DNA replication in which each strand of the double-helical molecule serves as a template against which a complementary new strand is synthesized.

2. A genetic locus that serves as a recognition site for RNA polymerase attachment.

3. A group of 3 nucleotides in mRNA that specifies an amino acid.

4. A short RNA sequence onto which DNA polymerase III adds deoxyribonucleotides during bacterial DNA replication.

5. Development of a wild-type (normal) trait in an organism or cell containing two different mutations combined in a hybrid diploid or a heterocaryon.

6. A spiral secondary structure in parts of many peptide chains, constituting the secondary level of organization. (One or two words.)

7. The process whereby RNA is synthesized from a DNA template.

8. The single-stranded pieces of DNA produced by discontinuous replication of double-stranded DNA. (Two words.)

9. Regions within an eucaryotic primary transcript that are removed during processing of mRNA.

10. A DNA segment generated during recombination by base pairing between complementary single strands from different parental duplex molecules.

True-False Questions   Answer each of the following statements either true (T) or false (F).

1. There are 64 codons, 3 of which terminate transcription.

2. DNA ligase repairs gaps in DNA.

3. The coding strand of DNA is transcribed into mRNA.

4. All structural genes specify the amino acid sequences of proteins.

5. When two different mutations in trans position fail to restore normal function to the cell, they are considered to be in different cistrons.

6. Pyrimidines are smaller than purines.

7. The 5′ end of the coding segment in mRNA corresponds to the amino terminus of its nascent polypeptide chain.

8. All DNA polymerases can only extend polynucleotide chains; they cannot initiate new chains.

9. During DNA replication, the leading strand is synthesized from the 5′ end toward the 3′ end, whereas the lagging strand is synthesized from 3′ toward 5′.

10. A transition point mutation involves substitution of a purine for a pyrimidine or vice versa.

Multiple-Choice Questions   Choose the one best answer.

1. A genetic unit that codes for the amino acid sequence of a complete polypeptide chain is most closely related to a   (a) recon (b) promoter (c) muton (d) cistron (e) replicon

2. Without referring to a table of mRNA codons, solve the following problem. Given a hypothetical segment of antisense strand DNA 3′GGCAACCTTGGC5′, the corresponding polypeptide segment could be (a) H_2N-gly-asn-leu-pro-COOH (b) HOOC-his-arg-ser-tyr-NH_2 (c) HOOC-asp-val-ile-gln-NH_2 (d) H_2N-met-thr-phe-cys-COOH (e) H_2N-pro-leu-glu-pro-COOH

3. Given the antisense strand DNA codon 3′TAC5′, the anticodon that pairs with the corresponding mRNA codon could be (a) 3′CAT5′ (b) 5′AUG3′ (c) 3′UAC5′ (d) 5′GUA (e) none of the above

4. Which of the following is not a characteristic of cellular RNA? (a) contains uracil (b) is single-stranded (c) is much shorter than DNA (d) serves as template for its own synthesis (e) contains ribose

5. The lesion most commonly induced by ultraviolet radiation is (a) chromosome breaks (b) transitions (c) transversions (d) thymine dimers (e) frame shifts

6. An amino acid that cannot participate in alpha-helical formation is (a) proline (b) histidine (c) phenylalanine (d) threonine (e) more than one of the above

7. A coding system in which each word may be coded by a variety of symbols or groups of letters (e.g., the genetic code) is said to be (a) archaic (b) redundant (c) degenerate (d) polysyllabic (e) amplified

8. An amino-acyl synthetase is responsible for (a) formation of a peptide bond (b) attaching an amino group to an organic acid (c) causing a peptide chain to form secondary and higher structural organizations (d) movement of tRNA molecules from A to P sites on a ribosome (e) joining an amino acid to a tRNA

9. A class of mutations induced by addition or deletion of a nucleotide is called (a) missense (b) nonsense (c) substitution (d) frame shift (e) reversion

10. Which of the following E. coli DNA polymerases is correctly matched with its major function? (a) III, chain extension (b) II, replace RNA primer with DNA (c) I, primer formation (d) III, joining Okazaki fragments (e) none of the above

Answers to Supplementary Problems

11.7. (a) $^{5'}$ATGGCTCATG$^{3'}$ (b) $^{5'}$AUGGCUCAUG$^{3'}$

11.8. 1.43

11.9. $1 \times 2 \times 6 \times 4 = 48$

11.10. 0.32

11.11. Approximately 3 nucleotides code for each amino acid

11.12. (a) - glu - met - ala - val - tyr - (b) - phe - ala - arg - cys - asn - (c) - lys - thr - (nonsense), chain terminates prematurely

11.13. (a) The protein would be slightly shorter than normal. Since region A does not seem to interact with other portions of the polypeptide chain, the mutant enzyme should still function normally (barring unpredicted interaction of the side chain of the mutant amino acid with other parts of the molecule). If a nonsense mutation had occurred in region D, however, a very small chain would have been produced that would be devoid of a catalytic site, because proteins are synthesized beginning at the NH$_2$ end. (b) Samesense mutants produce no change in their polypeptide products from normal. (c) The polypeptide would be one amino acid shorter than normal. Since region C does not seem to be critical to the tertiary shape of the molecule, the mutant enzyme would probably function normally. (d) An incorrect amino acid would be present in region B. As long as its side chain did not alter the tertiary shape of the molecule, the mutant enzyme would be expected to function normally. (e) A frameshift mutant in region C is bound to create many missense codons (or perhaps a nonsense codon) from that point on through the carboxyl terminus, including the enzymatic site. Such a protein would be catalytically inactive.

11.14. Nonfunctional DNA fragments might be produced if DNA replication occurs before all of the critical repairs have been made.

11.15. 3U = 0.343, 2U + 1C = 0.441, 1U + 2C = 0.189, 3C = 0.027

11.16. (a), (c), (d), (e), (g), (i) = large; (b), (f), (h), (j) = small

11.17. (a)

	lys	-	ser	-	pro	-	ser	-	leu	-	asn	-	ala
normal mRNA	AA?		A GU		CCA		UCA		CUU		AAU		GC?
mutant mRNA	AA?		GUC		CAU		CAC		UUA		AUG		G C?
	lys	-	val	-	his	-	his	-	leu	-	met	-	ala

(b) G was added, A was deleted (at shaded positions)

11.18. (a) Serine: UUC, UCU, CUU; proline: CCU, CUC, UCC. (b) Phenylalanine = 0.36, leucine = 0.24, proline = 0.16, serine = 0.24. (c) $2\frac{1}{4}$

11.19. 2800 cistrons

11.20. Most molecules would be labeled more in the COOH end because synthesis is unidirectional starting at the NH$_2$ end.

11.21. 50 proteins, assuming only one chain of the DNA is transcribed into mRNA.

11.22. Codons of the r_{II} region are read unidirectionally beginning at the A end.

11.23. Seed parent contributes two sets of chromosomes to triploid endosperm; one *Dt* gene gives 7.2 mutations per kernel, two *Dt* genes increase mutations to 22.2 per kernel.

11.24. 20% more mutations in the individual receiving 0.5 roentgen per year.

11.25. $10\frac{1}{2}$%.

11.26. 1.848×10^8 (approx.)

11.27. Any vial which does not contain wild-type male progeny is probably the result of a sex-linked recessive lethal induced by X-ray treatment.

11.28. (*a*) F_1 (*b*) The appearance of the mutant trait in all F_1 males in a vial. (*c*) The absence of F_1 males in any vial. (*d*) 50%; superfemales (XXX) are usually inviable; all zygotes without an X chromosome die.

11.29. (*a*) 2/3 curly, lobe:1/3 wild type (*b*) 2/3 curly, lobe:1/3 recessive mutant (*c*) greater than 2/3 curly, lobe:less than 1/3 wild type (*d*) all curly, lobe

11.30. A single ionization ("hit") of a genetic element may destroy the functioning of a vital gene and result in death. Multiple hits at high dosage levels score as a single lethal event.

11.31. (*a*) Chromosomal rearrangements require at least two breaks. Thus at very low dosages of radiation a disproportionately low percentage of rearrangements would be expected. (*b*) Exponential; i.e., the rearrangements increase faster as radiation dosage increases only at higher dosage levels. (*c*) a = 1/2560, y = 10.

11.32. 0.2%

11.33. (*a*)

Original DNA	A:T	T:A	G:C	C:G
Transition DNA	G:C	C:G	A:T	T:A

(*b*)

Original DNA	A:T	A:T	T:A	T:A	G:C	G:C	C:G	C:G
Transversion DNA	T:A	C:G	A:T	G:C	T:A	C:G	A:T	G:C

(*c*) 2 transversions : 1 transition
(*d*) Yes. $\chi^2 = 0.86$, $p = 0.3$–0.5

11.34. (*a*)

(*b*)

(*c*)

11.35. The polypeptide chain folds into a configuration such that noncontiguous regions form portions of the catalytic or antibody-combining sites.

11.36. The suppressing mutation could be in that portion of a gene specifying the anticodon region of a tRNA molecule. For example, a tyrosine suppressor gene changes the anticodon of $tRNA_{tyr}$ from $^{3'}AUG^{5'}$ to $^{3'}AUC^{5'}$, thereby allowing it to recognize UAG mRNA nonsense codons. If the genes for $tRNA_{tyr}$ exists in multiple copies and only one of the $tRNA_{tyr}$ genes was mutated to a suppressor form, there would still be other normal (nonsuppressor) $tRNA_{tyr}$ genes to make some normal proteins. The efficiency of suppression must be low to be compatible with survival of the organism.

11.37. (1) A change in one of the ribosomal proteins in the 30S subunit could cause misreading of the codon-anticodon alignment, resulting in substitution of an "acceptable" (although perhaps not the normal) amino acid in a manner analogous to the misreading induced by the antibiotic streptomycin. In a cell-free system with synthetic poly-U mRNA, streptomycin causes isoleucine tRNA to be substituted for that of phenylalanine tRNA. (2) A mutation in a gene coding for an amino-acid-activating enzyme (amino-acyl synthetase) causes a different amino acid to occasionally be attached to a given species of tRNA. For example, if AUU (isoleucine mRNA codon) is mutated to UUU (phenylalanine mRNA codon), its effect may be suppressed by the occasional misattachment of isoleucine to $tRNA_{phe}$ by a mutant amino-acyl synthetase that is less than 100% specific in its normal action of attaching phenylalanine to $tRNA_{phe}$.

11.38. Such proteins are normally homopolymers (quaternary complexes consisting of two or more identical polypeptide chains). If two mutant polypeptide chains contain compensating amino acid substitutions, they may aggregate into a heterodimer that exhibits at least partial enzymatic activity.

11.39. Wild-type alleles usually code for complete, functional enzymes or other proteins. One active wild-type allele can often cause enough enzyme to be produced so that normal or nearly normal phenotypes result (dominance). Mutations of normally functioning genes are more likely to destroy the biological activities of proteins. Only in the complete absence of the wild-type gene product would the mutant phenotype be expressed (recessiveness).

11.40. A cistron contains numerous mutons, many of which if altered would destroy the biological activity of the gene product. Once a point mutation has occurred it usually requires a very specific back mutation of that same nucleotide to restore normal or wild-type gene activity.

11.41. Loss of function can potentially occur by point mutations at a number of sites within a cistron coding for a given fermentation enzyme or in any gene coding for one of the multiple enzymes in a common biosynthetic pathway such as those in histidine synthesis. The loss of such an indispensable function is lethal. Streptomycin distorts ribosomes, causing misreading of the genetic code. Only a limited number of changes in the ribosomal proteins or rRNA could render the ribosome immune from interference by streptomycin and still preserve the way these components normally interact with mRNA, tRNA, initiation factors, etc. during protein synthesis.

Answers to Review Questions

Vocabulary

1. semiconservative
2. promoter
3. codon
4. primer
5. complementation
6. alpha helix
7. transcription
8. Okazaki fragments
9. introns
10. heteroduplex

True-False Questions

1. F (terminate translation)   2. F (repairs nicks)   3. F (antisense or anticoding strand)   4. F (all structural genes are transcribed into RNA, but only mRNA is translated into protein)   5. F (same cistron)   6. T   7. T   8. T   9. F (both leading and lagging strands are synthesized $5' \rightarrow 3'$)   10. F (transversion mutation)

Multiple-Choice Questions

1. *d*   2. *e*   3. *c*   4. *d*   5. *d*   6. *a*   7. *c*   8. *e*   9. *d*   10. *a*

Chapter 12

Genetics of Bacteria and Bacteriophages

BACTERIA

1. Characteristics of Bacteria.

Each cellular organism is classified as either procaryote or eucaryote (acceptable alternative spellings are procaryote and eucaryote). A **procaryote** is a cell whose DNA is not confined within a nucleus. A **eucaryote** has its genetic material isolated from the rest of the cell by a nuclear membrane. All bacteria (including the Cyanobacteria, or "blue-green algae") are procaryotes. All other forms of life (fungi, plants, animals) are eucaryotes.

Most of the genetic information of a bacterial cell resides in a single, circular, double-stranded DNA molecule correctly called the **genophore,** but more commonly referred to as the bacterial "chromosome" or "chromatin." It has recently been discovered that at least some bacterial DNA is complexed with basic proteins to form a kind of bacterial chromatin analogous to the association of histone proteins with DNA in eucaryotic chromatin. Some bacteria may also contain small, self-replicating circles called plasmids, and they will be discussed later in this chapter. There seldom are any membrane-bound organelles in bacterial cells. The region (or regions, since there may be more than one genophore) of a procaryotic cell, mitochondrion, or chloroplast where a genophore(s) is located, is technically referred to as a **nucleoid,** but is more commonly called a "nucleus."

Bacteria do not reproduce sexually (i.e., by formation of haploid gametes produced by meiosis and fusion of gametes to form diploid zygotes). Bacteria do not reproduce asexually by mitosis, either. The "chromosome" does not condense; it has no centromere; no spindle develops. Instead, the circular bacterial "chromosome" is attached to the plasma membrane. Replication of the DNA produces copies that become adjacently attached to the plasma membrane. As the cell elongates, the chromosome copies move apart by growth of the membrane between them. This mode of asexual reproduction has long been called "binary fission." Bacteria can divide much more rapidly than eucaryotes (once every 20 minutes under ideal conditions, in contrast to 24–48 hours or longer for eucaryotic cells). Bacteria neither form interdependent clusters of cells nor differentiate into various morphological and physiological types of cells that characterize the tissues of multicellular plants and animals. Bacteria, which are about the size of a mitochondrion (0.5–1.0 micrometer in diameter; 5–10 micrometers long), are much smaller than most eucaryotic cells and near the limit (0.25 micrometer) of the light microscope.

2. Bacterial Culture Techniques.

Bacteria grown in the laboratory in an aqueous solution of nutrients and energy sources are referred to as a bacterial **culture.** If the culture medium is a complex mixture of organic nutrients, it is called a **broth.** Bacteria can also be grown on a medium that has been gelled by the addition of agar (a substance that most bacteria cannot digest). Solid media of this type are sometimes poured into flat, circular containers called **Petri dishes.** The depositing of bacteria on the agar surface in such a container is called **plating.** When a dilute sample from a culture is plated, each bacterial cell reproduces itself into a cluster of thousands of cells called a bacterial **colony** or **clone** that is visible to the naked eye. Barring mutation, all members of a clone are expected to be genetically identical. The number of cells in a culture can be estimated by plating.

> **Example 12.1.** Suppose that 0.1 milliliter of a 10^6-fold dilution of a bacterial culture is plated on nutrient agar and 200 colonies develop. If 0.1 milliliter produces 200 colonies, 1 milliliter should produce 10 times as many colonies. Furthermore, since the original culture was diluted 10^6, it must contain 10^6 more bacteria than the diluted sample. Thus, the cell density of the original culture is estimated to be $200 \times 10 \times 10^6 = 2 \times 10^9$ cells/milliliter.

When an undiluted sample of a dense culture is plated, the colonies are so numerous that they form a **lawn** of solid bacterial growth over the entire surface of the agar. Rare mutants can be easily isolated from such a lawn by several techniques to be explained later in this chapter.

3. Bacterial Phenotypes and Genotypes.

Bacteria exist in a number of morphological forms: bacilli (rod-shaped), cocci (spherical), spirilla (spiral), spirochetes (helical), and branched. Because they are so small, individual bacterial cells are rarely studied in genetics. However, bacterial colonies are large enough to examine macroscopically and often exhibit variations in size, shape or growth habit, texture, color, and response to nutrients, dyes, drugs, antibodies, and viral pathogens (bacterial viruses, called bacteriophage or phage). Some bacteria can grow on **minimal media** containing a carbon and energy source (e.g., glucose), a few inorganic salts, and water. Bacteria that can grow on such an ''unsupplemented'' medium are said to be **prototrophic.** If any other organic substance must be added to minimal medium to obtain growth, the bacteria are said ·to be **auxotrophic.** A medium that contains all the organic nutrients (amino acids, nucleotides, etc.) that could be required by any auxotrophic cell is called **complete medium.**

Five major types of phenotypic changes are commonly produced by bacterial mutations:

(1) A change from prototrophy to auxotrophy or vice versa, i.e., the loss or recovery of the ability to produce products of biosynthetic pathways. For example, a mutation that produces a defect in the gene that specifies the enzyme that converts glutamic acid to glutamine would cause the cell to be dependent on the environment for glutamine.

(2) The loss or recovery of the ability to use alternative nutrients. For example, a mutation in the gene for the enzyme that converts the sugar lactose into glucose and galactose renders the cell incapable of growing in a medium where lactose is the only carbon source. These kinds of mutations that are involved in catabolic (degradative) reactions are independent of prototrophy or auxotrophy.

(3) A change from drug sensitivity to drug resistance or vice versa. For example, most bacteria are sensitive to the antibiotic streptomycin, but resistant strains can be produced by mutation.

(4) A change from phage sensitivity to phage resistance or vice versa. For example, a mutation in the bacterial receptor for the phage would render the cell resistant to infection.

(5) The loss or recovery of structural components of the cell surface. For example, one pneumococcus strain may possess a polysaccharide capsule, whereas another strain may not have a capsule.

The symbols used to represent bacterial phenotypes and genotypes conform to the following rules:

(1) Phenotypic symbols consist of three roman letters (the first letter is capitalized) with a superscript ''+'' or ''−'' to denote presence or absence of the designated character, and ''s'' or ''r'' for sensitivity and resistance, respectively.

(2) Genotypic symbols are lowercase with all components of the symbol italicized.

> **Example 12.2.**   If the cell can synthesize its own leucine, its phenotype is symbolized Leu$^+$. The substance that characterizes the phenotype in this case (leucine) is symbolized Leu. The genotype that is auxotrophic for leucine is *leu* or *leu*$^-$, and the phenotype in this case is Leu$^-$ (unable to grow without leucine supplementation). If more than one gene is required to produce the substance, the three-letter symbol would be followed by an italicized letter, as *leuA*, *leuB*, etc. The genotype for resistance to the antibiotic drug penicillin is *pen*^{r} or *pen-r*; Pen^r or Pen-r is the corresponding phenotype. In partial diploids, the 2 haploid sets are separated by a diagonal line; thus, *leu*$^+$/*leuA*$^-$.

Genetically different members of the same bacterial species are sometimes recognized as different **strains** if the differences are small, or as different **varieties** if the differences are substantial.

> **Example 12.3.**   The most thoroughly studied bacterial species is *Escherichia coli*, or *E. coli*. Strains are designated by adding an unitalicized capital letter or number after the species name, thus

E. coli B, *E. coli* S, etc. The three most commonly used strains of *E. coli* are *E. coli* B (host for phages of the T series), *E. coli* C (host for the single-stranded DNA phage φX174, and *E. coli* K12 (harboring the lambda prophage). Note that variants within a strain are indicated by adding a number after the strain letter.

4. Isolation of Bacterial Mutations.

It is relatively easy to isolate phage- or drug-resistant mutant clones by plating the bacteria on a medium that contains a **selective agent** (phage or drug). Only resistant cells form colonies on such plates. Prototrophic mutants can be isolated from an auxotrophic culture by plating on minimal medium; only prototrophic colonies would grow on such a plate. Isolation of auxotropic mutants is more difficult. There are at least four methods for isolating auxotrophic mutants from prototrophic cultures. Each method is enhanced by first treating the culture with a mutagenic agent to increase the mutation rate.

(1) In the **delayed enrichment method,** a diluted culture is plated on minimal medium and then covered with an agar layer of the same medium. The plate is incubated and the locations of prototrophic colonies are marked on the plate. A layer of nutrient medium is then added, and the nutrient is allowed to diffuse through the minimal agar. After another incubation period, the appearance of any new colonies may represent auxotrophs that could only grow after supplementation.

(2) The **limited enrichment method** is a simplification of the delayed enrichment method. Bacteria are plated on minimal medium containing a small amount of nutrient supplementation. Under such conditions, auxotrophic bacteria will undergo limited growth until the supply of nutrients is exhausted, and hence will form small colonies. Prototrophic bacteria will continue to grow and produce large colonies.

(3) Penicillin interferes with the development of the bacterial cell wall only in growing cells, causing them to rupture. In the **penicillin enrichment technique,** the bacterial culture is exposed to penicillin in minimal medium. Growing prototrophic cells die, whereas auxotrophic cells cannot grow and therefore are not killed. The culture is then plated on nutrient medium without penicillin. Only auxotrophic colonies should form on the plate.

(4) In the **replica plating technique** (Fig. 12-1) the bacteria are first plated on nutrient agar and allowed to form colonies. A sterile velvet pad is then pressed onto the surface of this "master plate." The nap of the velvet picks up representatives from each colony on the plate. The pad is then pressed onto the sterile surface of one or more "replica plates" containing minimal medium. Only prototrophic colonies grow on the replica plate. Colonies on the master plate that are not represented on the replica plate may be auxotrophs. These colonies can be picked from the master plate to form a "pure" auxotrophic culture. The purity of cultures must be constantly monitored to remove newly formed mutants.

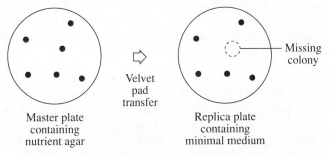

Fig. 12-1. The replica plating technique. The colony missing on the replica plate is likely to be an auxotrophic mutant. In reality, there would be about 100 colonies on each plate so that screening hundreds or thousands of such plates might be necessary to find a particular auxotrophic mutant.

5. Bacterial Replication.

The circular chromosomes of bacteria, mitochrondria, and phage present special problems for replication. The DNA of some species of bacteriophage (especially the tailed phages like lambda) is linear during infection of the cell, but quickly becomes enzymatically converted to a circular form after entry into the cell. Circular chromosomes usually have a single site at which replication originates, called the ori site. By contrast, many ori sites exist on each chromosome of eucaryotes. Once the replication process starts, it usually proceeds bidirectionally from the ori site.

As the 2 strands of a right-handed, double-helical, circular DNA unwind during replication, the molecule tends to become **positively supercoiled** or **overwound,** i.e., twisted in the same direction as the strands of the double helix. These supercoils would interfere with further replication if they were not removed. **Topoisomerases** are a group of enzymes that can change the topological or configurational shape of DNA. **DNA gyrase** is a bacterial topoisomerase that makes double-stranded cuts in the DNA, holds onto the broken ends so they cannot rotate, passes an intact segment of DNA through the break, and then reseals the break on the other side (Fig. 12-2). This action of DNA gyrase quickly removes positive supercoils and momentarily relaxes the DNA molecule into a more energetically stable state. However, with the expenditure of energy, DNA gyrase normally pumps **negative supercoiling** or **underwinding** (twisting in a direction opposite to the turns of the double helix) into relaxed DNA circles so that virtually all DNAs in both procaryotes and eucaryotes naturally exist in the negative supercoiled state. Relaxed circles and positively supercoiled DNA exist only in the laboratory. Localized regions of DNA transiently and spontaneously unwind to single-stranded "bubbles" and then return to their former topology as hydrogen bonds between complementary base pairs are broken and reformed by thermal agitation. This process is known as **breathing.** The strain of underwinding is thus momentarily relieved in a superhelix by an increase in the number, size, and duration of these bubbles. An equilibrium normally exists between these supercoiled and "bubbled" states. More bubbles form as the temperature increases.

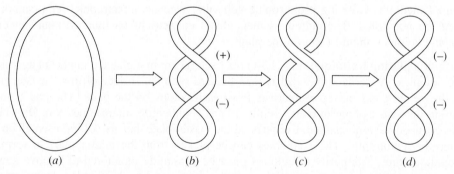

(a)   (b)   (c)   (d)

Fig. 12-2.   A proposed mechanism whereby DNA gyrase "pumps" negative supercoiling into DNA. A relaxed, covalently closed, circular DNA molecule (a) is bent into a configuration for strand passage (b). DNA gyrase makes double-stranded cuts (c), holds onto the ends, passes an intact segment through the break, and reseals the break on the other side (d).

At each replication fork, an enzyme called "helicase" unwinds the two DNA strands. Single-stranded, DNA-binding (SSB) proteins protect the single-stranded regions in the replication forks from forming intrastrand base pairings that could cause a tangle of partially double-stranded segments that would interfere with replication. The enzyme primase (plus a second enzyme coded by the gene *dnaB*) synthesize the RNA primers that are required by DNA polymerases. Three DNA polymerase enzymes have been found in *E. coli*, referred to as pol I, pol II, and pol III. Pol III is thought to be the principal replicating enzyme. Gaps left by pol III are filled by pol I, and DNA ligase seals the nicks. The function of pol II is unknown. In addition to their $5' \rightarrow 3'$ synthetic activity, both pol I and pol III have $3' \rightarrow 5'$ exonuclease activity, which plays an "editing" or "proofreading" role by removing mismatched bases inserted by error during chain polymerization. Pol I also has $5' \rightarrow 3'$ exonuclease activity by which it normally

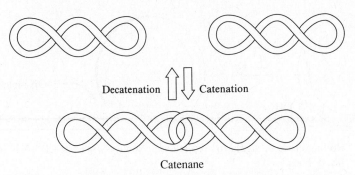

Decatenation ⇅ Catenation

Catenane

Fig. 12-3. Formation (catenation) and dissolution (decatenation) of
a catenane, mediated by DNA gyrase.

removes primers after polymerization has begun. Termination of replication is thought to occur primarily by collision of the replicating forks rather than at some specific base sequence. Termination by collision produces a pair of interlocked circles called a **catenane** (Fig. 12-3). In *E. coli*, the catenanes are separated by DNA gyrase. About half way through the above replication process, the replicative intermediate molecule looks like the Greek letter *theta* (θ). This type of replication is therefore referred to as **theta replication** (Fig. 12-4).

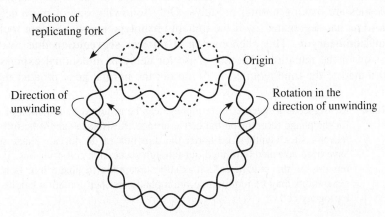

Motion of replicating fork

Origin

Direction of unwinding

Rotation in the direction of unwinding

Fig. 12-4. Theta (θ) replication. Newly synthesized DNA is indicated by broken lines. Overwinding of the unreplicated segment (caused by unwinding of the daughter branches) is removed by the nicking action of DNA gyrase.

Another type of bacterial replication is used to transfer a linear DNA molecule during bacterial conjugation or for the production of linear phage genomes. A nick occurs in one strand of a DNA double helix, creating free 3'-OH and 5'-P termini. Helicase and SSB proteins establish a replication fork. No primer is necessary because a strand with a free 3'-OH is available for elongation by pol I as the leading strand. Simultaneously with replication of the leading strand, the template for the lagging strand is displaced. The displaced strand is discontinuously replicated to produce Okazaki fragments in the usual way. The result of this replication model is a circle with a linear tail, resembling the Greek letter *sigma* (σ). Hence this model is called **sigma replication** or **rolling-circle replication** (Fig. 12-5). The circle may revolve several times, creating **concatemers** or covalently connected, linear repetitions of bacterial genomes. An endonuclease enzyme makes cuts at slightly different positions on each DNA strand of the concatemer to create genome-sized segments containing ''sticky ends'' (single-stranded complementary ends). The linear genomes circularize by base pairing of the sticky ends. DNA ligase seals each gap to create covalently closed (circular), double-stranded DNA molecules.

A replicating bacterial chromosome is thought to be attached to invaginations of the cell membrane, called **mesosomes,** at the 2 adjacent Y-forks. Mesosomes, however, have been seen only in certain

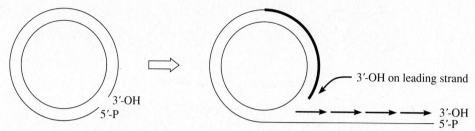

3'-OH on leading strand

3'-OH
5'-P

3'-OH
5'-P

Fig. 12-5.   Rolling circle or sigma (σ) replication. Newly synthesized DNA is indicated by heavy lines.

bacteria. After DNA replication, the cell elongates by growth of the sector between the 2 attachment points, causing the 2 chromosomal replicas to move apart. A septum of new cell membrane is then synthesized between the 2 chromosomes, creating 2 progeny cells (Fig. 12-6).

When bacteria are growing exponentially, most cells contain 2–4 identical chromosomes in various stages of replication. After a mutation occurs in a multinucleate cell, the number of mutant chromosomes present in the cell depends upon the time the mutation occurred and how it is repaired. If the cell contains genetically different chromosomes (nuclei), it is called a heterocaryon. If the mutation is one causing loss of a functional product, there will be no detectable change in the cell's phenotype because the unaltered chromosomes are making normal products. Only following one or more cell divisions, after the mutant chromosome has segregated, will the mutant phenotype appear. Such a multinucleate cell is said to be a mutant **homocaryon.** This phenomenon of **nuclear segregation** thus results in a delay of phenotypic expression of the mutation. Another cause for delay in mutational expression, called **phenotypic lag,** is attributed to the time required to dilute out the normal gene product that still resides in a mutant homocaryon.

Example 12.4.   Resistance to a specific bacteriophage can be acquired by mutation of a gene responsible for the phage receptor on the cell's surface. Resistance cannot be fully realized until the receptor sites (synthesized under the direction of the former phage-sensitive genotype) have been completely diluted out through successive cell divisions. If even one receptor remains on the mutant cell, it is still susceptible to phage infection. Thus, many cell generations may be required before a phage-resistant mutation can be fully expressed in a progeny cell.

6. Bacterial Transcription.

In bacteria, all RNA molecules (mRNAs, rRNAs, and tRNAs) are synthesized by the same enzyme, **RNA polymerase.** The complete, functional enzyme (**holoenzyme**) consists of 5 different polypeptide chains: β, β′, α, ω, and σ. The sigma (σ) subunit recognizes variants of a binding site (called a **Pribnow box**) in double-stranded DNA, and aligns the remainder of the enzyme (called the **core enzyme**) in the promoter region to begin transcription. In *E. coli* and its phages, the right end of the Pribnow box is 5–10 bases in front of (upstream from) the first base copied into mRNA. The most common sequence found in Pribnow boxes of various genes, called the **consensus sequence,** is TATAAT. RNA chains usually initiate with 5′ adenosine triphosphate (pppA) or guanosine triphosphate (pppG). After transcription has begun, sigma factor dissociates from the core enzyme and may then associate with the same or another core enzyme to get it started on a promoter. "Strong" promoters have high affinity for sigma factor and thereby favor many copies of RNA to be made from genes adjacent to the promoter. "Weak" promoters have low affinity for sigma factor, and foster only a few copies of RNA to be made from the nearby genes. Thus, one possible mechanism for controlling the amount of RNA synthesized from a gene is the relative strength of its promoter. The transcriptional activity of RNA polymerase may be blocked or its affinity for a promoter may be increased by the attachment of specific DNA-binding proteins near the transcription initiation site. Some DNA sequences that precede or follow the gene may control transcription as they are being transcribed. These regions of DNA are called **leader** and **trailer** regions, respectively.

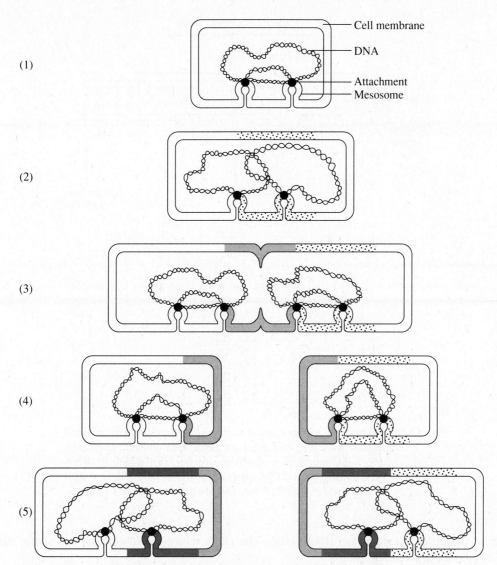

Fig. 12-6. A model for segregation of bacterial DNA ("chromosome") replicas. (1) A circular DNA molecule is attached to invaginations of the cell membrane (mesosomes) at two points. The DNA is a theta structure (about half replicated). (2) Replication is complete. The membrane region in strippled has just been formed. (3) Cell division is beginning via growth of the membrane region shown in medium gray. Both daughter chromosomes are already partially replicated. (4) Cell division is complete. (5) Daughter cells are midway through the next generation. Chromosome replication is completed. The mesosomes have moved to the center of the cell as a result of growth of new membrane (black) after cell division. (After G. S. Stent and R. Calendar, *Molecular Genetics*, 2nd ed., 1978, W. H. Freeman and Company.)

During elongation of the RNA molecule, ribonucleoside triphosphates of the bases A, U, G, and C pair with complementary bases in the sense strand of DNA and are then connected with 3'—5' phosphodiester bonds by RNA polymerase. The energy for driving the reaction is obtained by splitting phosphate groups from the triphosphate precursors. Thus, the RNA molecule grows from its 5' end toward its 3' end (5' → 3'). The DNA double helix unwinds ahead of the advancing RNA polymerase to expose more

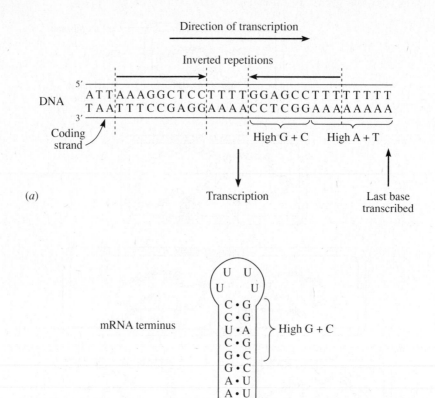

Fig. 12-7. Example of a transcription termination sequence. (*a*) Inverted repeats at the end of a gene are transcribed into (*b*), an mRNA that folds into a stem-and-loop structure that dislodges RNA polymerase from its DNA template. (After David Freifelder, *Molecular Biology,* 1987, Jones and Bartlett Publishing Company, Inc.)

of the sense strand for extending the RNA chain. The DNA reforms its double-helical shape after the enzyme has passed a given region.

RNA polymerase in bacteria stops transcription of an RNA chain at DNA sequences known as **terminators** [Fig. 12-7(*a*)], and dissociates from the DNA. To function properly, some terminators require an accessory protein called rho (ρ) factor, whereas the response to other terminators can be carried out by the core enzyme of RNA polymerase alone. The ρ-independent terminators have a diad symmetry in the double-stranded DNA, centered about 15–20 nucleotides before the end of the RNA, and have about 6 adenines in the sense strand that are transcribed into uracils at the end of the RNA. The RNA transcript of the diad symmetry folds back on itself to form a hairpin structure, ending with approximately 6 uracils [Fig. 12-7(*b*)]. Because an RNA-DNA hybrid consisting of polyribo-U and polydeoxyribo-A is very unstable, the RNA chain is quickly released from the DNA duplex. The ρ-dependent terminators lack this poly-A region. It is thought that even a weak hairpin structure causes RNA polymerase to pause, allowing ρ factor to attach to the terminator and cause dissociation of the RNA and RNA polymerase.

In bacteria, functional tRNAs and rRNAs are derived by enzymatic digestion of larger, short-lived precursor molecules. The 70S* bacterial ribosome consists of two major subunits: a larger 50S subunit and a smaller 30S subunit. The 50S subunit contains two rRNA molecules (23S and 5S); the 30S subunit contains a single 16S rRNA molecule. All three rRNAs are transcribed into a single 30S pre-rRNA

---

* S = Svedberg unit; a sedimentation coefficient for molecules in an ultracentrifuge. The S value tends to increase with the molecular weight of the molecule, but the geometry of the molecule also may be influential. Note that S units are not additive; i.e., 50S subunit + 30S subunit = 70S for the complete bacterial ribosome, not 80S.

transcript containing a leader sequence at the 5′ end, a trailer sequence at the 3′ end, and nonfunctional spacer regions between the three rRNA sequences. Likewise, all tRNAs are derived from longer pre-tRNA primary transcripts containing from one to as many as seven different tRNAs. Although rRNAs and tRNAs together constitute more than 98% of all the RNA in a bacterial cell, less than 1% of the DNA serves as their templates. The reason for this is that rRNAs and tRNAs are relatively stable molecules, whereas mRNAs are more easily degraded by RNase enzymes.

Enzymes that digest nucleic acids are called **nucleases.** If the nuclease digests the ends of the nucleic acid, it is called an **exonuclease.** If it cleaves within the nucleic acid, it is called an **endonuclease.** Ribonuclease P (RNase P) is an endonuclease that removes the extra 5′ nucleotides from every pre-tRNA in *E. coli.* This enzyme consists of a single polypeptide chain and an RNA molecule. Both components contribute to its enzymatic activity under physiological conditions. However, in nonphysiological buffers containing high concentrations of magnesium ions or spermidine, the RNA component alone can catalyze the same specific scission as the holoenzyme. Thus proteins are not the only macromolecules that can catalyze specific biochemical reactions, as was formerly believed. The name **ribozyme** is given to any ribonucleic acid that has enzymatic properties. An exonuclease called RNase D removes extra 3′ nucleotides from *E. coli* pre-tRNA molecules. Then still other enzymes modify certain bases (e.g., by addition of methyl groups) to produce the relatively high content of unusual bases (those other than A, G, C, or U) found in functional tRNA molecules.

Messenger RNA (mRNA) molecules of procaryotes and eucaryotes exist in a wide range of sizes, varying according to the number of amino acids in the polypeptide chains they specify. However, in bacteria, an mRNA may code for one or more polypeptide chains. Polycistronic mRNAs (coding for more than one polypeptide chain; Fig. 12-8) are common in bacteria.

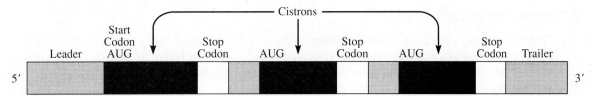

Fig. 12-8.   Example of a polycistronic mRNA molecule. Untranslated regions are stippled or white; coding regions are dark.

7. Bacterial Translation.

No membrane separates the DNA from the ribosomes in a bacterial cell. Hence, as soon as the 5′ end of an mRNA is transcribed, ribosomes can begin translation. In other words, transcription and translation are coupled processes in bacteria.

Translation occurs in three major steps: (1) initiation, (2) elongation, and (3) termination. A nucleotide sequence called the **Shine-Dalgarno sequence** (AGGAGG is the consensus sequence) in the leader of an mRNA molecule is complementary to a sequence at the 3′ end of 16S rRNA and thereby serves as a binding site for ribosomes. The initiation codon near the 5′ end of an mRNA molecule is 5′AUG, coding for the amino acid methionine. In bacteria, a formyl group (CHO) becomes attached to the amino group of the methionine after it has become attached to its tRNA molecule. A **deformylase** enzyme removes the formyl groups from some polypeptide chains soon after their synthesis commences. In other cases, an **aminopeptidase** enzyme removes the terminal methionine (or part of the amino terminal end), so that not all functional bacterial proteins have formyl-methionione or methionine at their N termini.

Initiation of protein synthesis begins with the formation of a complex involving the 30S ribosomal subunit, guanosine triphosphate (GTP), and three protein initiation factors (IF1, IF2, IF3). In the next step, formylated methionyl-tRNA and the mRNA attach to the IF-30S-GTP complex, forming a 30S initiation complex. Then IF3 is released, the 50S subunit is added, GTP is hydrolyzed, and IF1 and IF2 are released. The final complex is called a 70S initiation complex. Only the initiator region of the mRNA can simultaneously form two sets of base-pairing interactions (16S rRNA-mRNA and mRNA-fMet tRNA).

In this way, the AUG start codon is distinguished from other AUG codons downstream in the mRNA. Base pairing between the leader of the mRNA and the 16S rRNA somehow dissociates after formation of the 70S initiation complex, so that elongation can begin.

The elongation phase requires GTP, three protein elongation factors (EF-Tu, EF-Ts, and EF-G), and the enzyme **peptidyl transferase.** Two molecules of GTP are hydrolyzed for each amino acid added to the growing polypeptide chain. EF-Tu and EF-Ts cyclically interact to align each amino-acyl–tRNA complex (AA ~ tRNA) for effective codon-anticodon base pairing. EF-G (also called **translocase**) and GTP form a complex that mediates the movement of peptidyl-tRNA from the A site to the P site. Hydrolysis of GTP to GDP is required for entry of the ribosome into the next elongation cycle. Several ribosomes may simultaneously translate the same mRNA. A collection of ribosomes of this kind is called a **polysome** or **polyribosome.**

Termination of translation in *E. coli* requires at least two protein release factors. RF1 recognizes the mRNA stop codons UAG and UAA; RF2 recognizes UGA and UAA. These RFs cause peptidyl transferase to transfer the completed polypeptide chain to water instead of to an AA ~ tRNA. After chain termination, the 30S and 50S ribosomal subunits dissociate from the mRNA and are then free to recycle into new initiation complexes on the same or different mRNA templates.

If a translational product is to be transported across the plasma membrane to the cell's exterior, the protein usually contains 15–30 additional amino acids (called a **signal sequence**) at its N terminus. The signal sequence is rich in uncharged, usually hydrophobic amino acids that become anchored in the membrane, whereas the remainder of the polypeptide chain is extruded through the membrane as it is synthesized. A **signal peptidase** then cleaves the signal sequence to release the protein from the cell.

8. Genetic Recombination.

(*a*) *Transformation.*   Bacterial **transformation** is the transfer of naked DNA from one bacterial cell to another. When a bacterial cell ruptures (in a process called cellular **lysis**), its circular DNA becomes released into the environment as linear fragments of various lengths. The efficiency of transformation depends upon three factors: (1) size of the DNA fragment, (2) DNA concentration, and (3) cell competence. The DNA fragment must have a minimum molecular weight greater than 400,000 daltons, but apparently there is no upper limit. The number of cells transformed (transformants) increases directly with DNA concentrations up to the point at which all of the available receptor sites on the bacterial cells have become saturated with attached DNA molecules (approximately 10 fragments per cell). **Competence** is the ability of a cell to incorporate naked DNA. Most bacterial cells are only competent during a restricted part of their life cycle. During the competent state, the cell produces one or more proteins called "competence factors" that modify the cell wall so it can bind exogenous (foreign) DNA fragments. Thus, receptor sites are present only during the competent state. Adsorbed DNA fragments are then reduced in size to molecular weights of about 4 or 5 million by enzymatic cleavage. As the double-stranded DNA fragments penetrate the cell wall, one of the strands is degraded. Any fragment of DNA that has been transferred (by transformation or some other method) from a donor cell to a recipient cell is referred to as an **exogenote;** the **endogenote** is the native DNA of the recipient cell. A bacterial cell that has received an exogenote is initially diploid for part of its genome, and is said to be a **merozygote.** However, single-stranded exogenotes are unstable and will usually be degraded unless they are integrated into the endogenote. Any process of genetic exchange that transfers only part of the genetic material from one cell to another is called **meromixis.** It is thought that the single-stranded exogenote of transformation becomes coated with a protein (such as the RecA-protein of *E. coli*) that aids the exogenote to find a complementary region on the endogenote, to invade the double helix, to displace one of its strands, and to base-pair with the other strand. The displaced strand is enzymatically removed as the endogenote replaces it by homologous base pairing (a phenomenon known as **branch migration**). Trimming enzymes remove the free ends (either donor or recipient) and ligase seals the nicks. Once the exogenote is integrated into the endogenote and the displaced strand is degraded, the cell is no longer a merozygote.

If the exogenote contains an allele of the endogenote, the resulting recombinant double helix would contain one or more mismatched base pairs, and is referred to as a **heteroduplex.** If progeny cells are to receive the new allele, mismatch repair must occur by excising a segment of the endogenote strand and using the exogenote strand as a template for its replacement. Since incorporation of the exogenote into the endogenote requires homologous recombination, the donor cell would normally belong to either the same species as the recipient cell or to a closely related one. Two or more closely linked genes may reside on the same transforming piece of DNA. If 2 or more genes are incorporated together into the endogenote, the recipient cell would be **cotransformed.** The frequency of cotransformation is a function of the linkage distance between the respective genes.

Example 12.5. In 1928 Fred Griffith discovered the first example of bacterial transformation. *Streptococcus pneumoniae*, or *Pneumococcus*, is a bacterium that causes human pneumonia and can also kill mice. The virulent strain of this bacterium contains a polysaccharide capsule that tends to resist destruction by immune cells of the host species. A nonvirulent strain of the pneumococcus does not have a capsule. The virulent strain forms colonies with smooth borders on nutrient agar plates and is thus designated the S (smooth) strain; the nonvirulent strain forms colonies with rough borders and is designated the R (rough) strain. When mice were injected with both heat-killed S strain and live R strain, they died, and live S strain bacteria were recovered from their bodies. Griffith did not know how to explain these results, but he called the process "transformation" and named the responsible substance "transforming principle." Later studies by Avery and others demonstrated that the transforming principle was naked DNA. In the Griffith experiment, the exogenote from the S strain contained the gene responsible for capsule formation. When this exogenote was incorporated into the endogenote of the R strain the transformant cells had the ability to make the capsule and thus became virulent S-type cells.

(*b*) *Conjugation.*   Bacterial **conjugation** involves the temporary union of 2 cells of opposite mating type, followed by unidirectional transfer of some genetic material through a cytoplasmic bridge from the donor cell to the recipient cell, and then disunion of the cells **(exconjugants).** An **episome** is an extrachromosomal genetic element that may exist either as an autonomously replicating circular DNA molecule or as an integrated DNA sequence within the host chromosome (e.g., phage lambda). A **plasmid** was originally defined as a small, circular DNA molecule that replicates autonomously of the bacterial chromosome and is incapable of integration into the bacterial chromosome. Plasmids often carry genes for antibiotic resistance that confer a selective advantage upon their host cells when antibiotics are in their environment. Currently, however, the word "plasmids" is often used for both episomes and plasmids. Most plasmids are between $\frac{1}{10}$ and $\frac{1}{100}$ the size of the bacterial chromosome.

In some strains of *E. coli*, there is an episomal **fertility factor** (also known as a **sex plasmid** or **F plasmid**). Strains that carry an F plasmid are called **males,** designated F^+, and can manufacture a protein called **pilin** from which a conjugation tube, or **pilus,** can be constructed. Contraction of the pilus connecting 2 cells brings the conjugating cells into close contact. Cells that do not have an F plasmid are called **females** and are designated F^-. When an F^+ cell conjugates with an F^- cell, replication of the F plasmid is initiated. One strand of the F plasmid is broken, and replication by the rolling-circle mechanism (Fig. 12-5) causes the 5' end of the broken strand to enter the recipient cell through the pilus (Fig. 12-9), where it is copied into a double-stranded DNA molecule. The other strand of the F plasmid in the donor cell also replicates simultaneously so the donor cell does not lose its F plasmid (it remains F^+). The recipient cell thus becomes F^+.

An F plasmid has little homology with the bacterial chromosome, so homologus recombination between these two DNA circles rarely occurs. In approximately 1 in 10^5 cells, however, a nonhomologous recombination event causes F to become integrated into a site on the bacterial chromosome. Thus, F is an episome that can exist chromosomally or extrachromosomally. A cell with F integrated into its chromosome is called an **Hfr** (*h*igh *f*requency of *r*ecombination) cell. It is so designated because many chromosomal genes can now be transferred from donor to recipient with high frequency. In *E. coli*, integration of the F factor is known to occur (in either of two orientations) at about 10 specific sites on the chromosome. The integration site and the orientation of the integrated F determines the order with which chromosomal genes will be transferred during conjugation (Fig. 12-10). DNA replication begins in the Hfr cell at the F locus in such a way that a small part of F is at the beginning

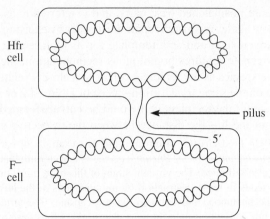

Fig. 12-9.   Transfer of a single strand of DNA from an Hfr (donor, male) cell to a recipient F⁻ (female) cell via the rolling-circle mechanism of replication. The same mechanism is used to transfer the circular DNAs of plasmids.

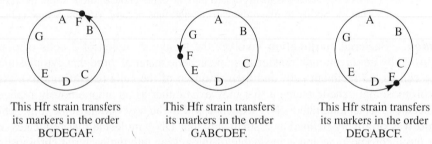

This Hfr strain transfers its markers in the order BCDEGAF.

This Hfr strain transfers its markers in the order GABCDEF.

This Hfr strain transfers its markers in the order DEGABCF.

Fig. 12-10.   Three examples of Hfr strains. Each strain transfers its genes in a unique sequence. Arrows indicate the directions of transfer.

of the donated segment; normal bacterial genes then follow in sequence, and finally the remaining portion of F is replicated last. About 90 minutes is required for *E. coli* to transfer its entire genome at 37°C under laboratory conditions. Thermal agitation of molecules (Brownian movement) usually causes the pilus to rupture before DNA transfer is complete, so a complete F particle is rarely recovered in the recipient cell. For this reason, the F⁻ recipient cell usually remains F⁻ after conjugation with an Hfr cell. The presence of the exogenote in the recipient cell activates a recombination system that causes genetic exchange to occur. In order to recover these recombinant bacteria, it is convenient to use an Hfr cell that is sensitive to some antibiotic and a recipient cell that is resistant to that same antibiotic. The locus of the antibiotic-resistance gene in the recipient cell ideally should be so far from the origin of the exogenote that the pilus will almost always rupture (stopping conjugation) before that locus can be transferred.

Example 12.6.   Suppose that an Hfr strain is able to synthesize leucine and is sensitive to the antibiotic streptomycin (*leu⁺*, *str-s*) and that a recipient F⁻ strain is unable to synthesize leucine, but is resistant to streptomycin (*leu⁻*, *str-r*). Mixing of these two strains allows conjugation to occur. Recombinants are selected by plating the mixture on minimal medium (without leucine) containing streptomycin. The Hfr strain cannot grow in the presence of streptomycin. The recipient strain cannot grow unless it has received the *leu⁺* gene by conjugation. Only the recombinants of genotype *leu⁺*, *str-r* will form colonies on the plate. In this case, *leu⁺* is the **selected marker**; *str-r* is the **counterselective marker** that prevents growth of any cell other than a recombinant on this type of medium.

The integration of F factor with the host chromosome is a reversible process. Normally the excision event that releases the F factor from the host chromosome involves a crossover at the same position at which it was integrated. Occasionally, however, the excision event is aberrant, and the released F factor contains one or a few bacterial genes that were close to the integrated F (Fig. 12-11). Such a plasmid is called an **F genote** and is symbolized F′. The cell that results from this aberrant release of the F′ factor is designated a **primary F′ cell.** This cell thus has a deletion in part of its chromosome; the missing material is present in the F′ plasmid. If the chromosomal genes in the plasmid are essential genes, the primary F′ cell becomes dependent upon both the host chromosome and the F genote for its survival. Normal binary fission of a primary F′ cell produces progeny that are also primary F′ cells. However, when a primary F′ cell conjugates with an F⁻ recipient cell, the recipient cell becomes a **secondary F′ cell** that is partially diploid for the small piece of chromosomal material carried in the F′ particle. Thus, a secondary F′ cell contains an F genote that was derived from a different cell. Because the F genote in a secondary F′ cell contains genetic material that is homologous with a segment of the host chromosome, it possesses "chromosomal memory" and therefore has a higher probability of becoming integrated at the homologous region. Furthermore, a secondary F′ cell can conjugate with F⁻ recipients and transfer the F genote to all its exconjugants with high frequency. The process whereby a fragment of genetic material from one bacterium is transported by an F′ plasmid to a second bacterium is called **sex-duction** or **F-duction.**

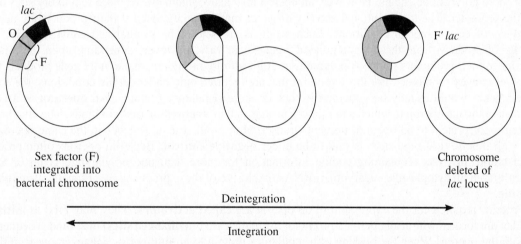

Fig. 12-11.   Formation of an F genote (F′). O is the origin of chromosome transfer when the sex or fertility factor F is integrated into the bacterial chromosome. If the lactose locus (dark segment) is adjacent to the F locus (gray region) an F′ *lac* genote can be formed by deintegration (breakage and reunion). Not drawn to scale; the F plasmid is approximately $\frac{1}{40}$ the length of the bacterial chromosome.

Plasmids carry genetic information for their own replication, but usually none that is essential for the life of the cell in normal environments. However, plasmids may carry one or more genes that confer selective advantage to the cell in certain environments, such as the presence of antibiotics. Plasmids that carry genes for resistance to one or more substances normally toxic to the host are designated **R plasmids** or **R factors.** One region of an R factor, called an **R determinant,** carries the genes for drug resistance. A second region of an R plasmid, termed the **resistance transfer factor (RTF),** conveys the ability to initiate conjugation. Some strains of *E. coli* carry a **colicinogenic plasmid (Col)** that can synthesize **colicin,** a protein that kills closely related bacterial strains that lack the Col plasmid. F, R, and Col are the best known of the bacterial plasmids.

(*c*) *Transduction.*   The transfer of genetic material from one bacterium to another, using a bacterial virus (bacteriophage, phage) as a vector, is called **transduction.** This aspect of bacterial genetic recombination is discussed later in this chapter under the heading of Bacteriophages.

9. Regulation of Bacterial Gene Activity.

Within any cell, all its genes are not active at the same time. Some gene products need to be continuously synthesized, whereas others are necessary only during certain phases of the life cycle or perhaps only when unusual environments are encountered. Even when genes are "turned on," the quantity of proteins they specify may need to be controlled. Some proteins need to be synthesized in large amounts and others, only in small amounts. Therefore, the activity of virtually all genes needs to be regulated in one or more ways to make the most efficient use of the energy available to the cell. These regulatory mechanisms over gene expression may act at one or more levels. Regulation may occur at the level of the gene itself by controlling the timing and/or rate of transcription. Other control mechanisms may operate during translation. After translation, some proteins must be modified to become functional.

Genes that are transcribed into RNA molecules are called structural genes. The proteins that are translated from mRNAs may be enzymatic or nonenzymatic. Among the nonenzymatic proteins are the **regulatory proteins** that interact with specific DNA nucleotide sequences to control the transcriptional activity of specific genes. The genes that synthesize these regulatory proteins are called **regulatory genes.** Each structural gene (or coordinately controlled group of structural genes) is preceded by a sequence (called a promoter) that can be recognized by RNA polymerase. Once the polymerase binds to the promoter it may then transcribe the adjacent anti-sense strand of DNA into an RNA molecule. An **operon** is a transcriptional unit consisting minimally of a promoter and adjacent mRNA coding sequences for one or more polypeptide chains. However, an operon may also contain one or more regulatory sites other than the promoter. The transcriptional activity of genes may be unregulated if their products are needed regardless of environmental conditions. Such products are said to be synthesized **constitutively.** The quantity of products from these "unregulated" genes can vary, however, depending upon the relative affinities of their promoters for RNA polymerase. High-affinity promoters make more gene products than do low-efficiency promoters. For those proteins that are required only under certain conditions, the action of their genes would usually be governed by one or more regulatory proteins. An **operator** is a DNA sequence within an operon to which a regulatory protein called a **repressor protein** binds. The attachment of a repressor protein to an operator prevents transcription of all structural genes in the same operon. A gene with this form of regulation is said to be under **negative control.** Bacterial operons often produce **polycistronic mRNAs** (containing coding information for more than one polypeptide chain or RNA molecule); but all cytoplasmic eucaryotic mRNAs (exclusive of those produced by organelles) are **monocistronic.**

Proteins required for the expression of an operon are called **activators.** They may bind to **initiator sites** that are located within an operon's promoter or (in the case of **enhancer sites**) may bind at sequences far from the operon. When the binding of a regulatory protein to an initiator or enhancer site stimulates transcription of structural genes in the operon, a **positive control** mechanism is said to be at work. The stimuli to which regulated genes respond may vary from relatively small molecules (e.g., sugars, amino acids) to relatively large substances (e.g., in eucaryotes, a complex of a steroid hormone and its protein receptor). A substance that turns on gene transcription is referred to as an **inducer,** whereas a substance that turns transcription off is said to be a repressor. **Inducible genes** are usually involved in **catabolic** (degradative) reactions, as in the breakdown of a polysaccharide into simple sugars. **Repressible genes** are usually involved in **anabolic** (synthetic) reactions, as in the construction of amino acids from simpler precursors. Thus, there are four possible combinations of the aforementioned transcriptional controls: (1) negative, inducible; (2) negative, repressible; (3) positive, inducible; and (4) positive, repressible (no example is presently known).

(*a*) *Negative, Inducible Control.* The prototype of negative control by way of an inducible operon is the "lactose system" of *E. coli*. **β-galactosidase** is an enzyme with dual functions. Its primary function is to catabolize lactose to glucose and galactose. Its secondary function is to convert the 1–4 linkage of glucose and galactose (in lactose) to a 1–5 linkage in allolactose. This enzyme is not normally present in high concentrations when lactose is absent from the cell's environment. Shortly after adding lactose to a medium in which glucose is absent, the enzyme begins to be produced. A transport protein called **galactoside permease** is required for the efficient transport of lactose across the cell membrane. This protein also appears in high concentration after lactose becomes available in the medium. The wild-type "lactose system" (Fig. 12-12) consists of a regulatory gene (i^+) and

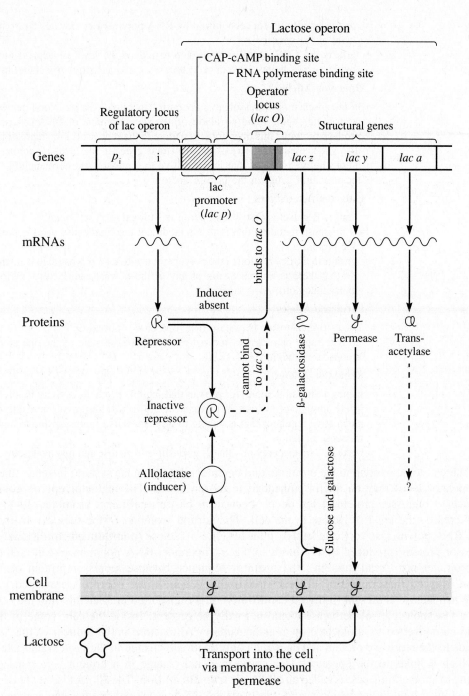

Fig. 12-12. Diagram of major elements controlling the lactose operon.

an operon containing a promoter sequence (p^+), an operator locus (o^+), and three structural genes for β-galactosidase (z^+), permease (y^+), and transacetylase (an enzyme whose function in lactose metabolism remains unresolved). Mutations at each of these loci have been found.

Example 12.7.   Some of the alleles of the lactose system are listed below.

Promoter Alleles

p^+ = wild-type promoter; normal affinity for RNA polymerase
p^- = mutant promoter cannot bind RNA polymerase; none of the structural genes in the lactose operon are transcribed

p^s = increased affinity for recognition by RNA polymerase; elevates the transcriptional level of the operon

$p^{i\ cr}$ = affects the CRP-cAMP binding site to reduce the level of expression of lactose operon genes below 10% of wild type; $i\ cr$ = insensitive to catabolite repression

Operator Alleles

o^+ = in the absence of repressor, this operator "turns on" the structural genes in its own operon; i.e., the z^+ and y^+ alleles in the same segment of DNA (cis position) can produce proteins; this operator is sensitive to the repressor; i.e., repressor will "turn off" the synthetic activity of the structural genes in the lactose operon

o^c = a constitutive operator that is insensitive to repressor and permanently "turns on" the structural genes in the lactose operon

Galactosidase Alleles

z^+ = makes β-galactosidase if its operon is "turned on" or "open"

z^- = a missense mutation that makes a modified, enzymatically inactive product called Cz protein

z^{-ns} = results in the destruction of the polycistronic message downstream from the mutation so that there is no expression of any of the downstream lactose operon genes (a polar mutation); ns = nonsense

Permease Alleles

y^+ = makes β-galactoside permease if its operon is "turned on"

y^- = no detectable permease is formed regardless of the state of the operator; probably a nonsense mutation

Regulator Alleles

i^+ = makes a diffusible repressor protein that inhibits synthetic activity in any o^+ operon in the absence of lactose; in the presence of lactose, repressor is inactivated

i^- = a defective regulator that is unable to produce active repressor due to a nonsense or missense mutation

i^s = makes a "superrepressor" that is insensitive to lactose and inactivates any o^+ operon

There is some overlap in the promoter and operator sites of the lac system; in some other operons the operator locus may be totally embedded in the promoter. The regulator operon constitutively produces a repressor protein at low levels because it has an inefficient promoter. Its synthesis is unaffected by the level of lactose in the cell. The normal promoter of the *lac* operon, by contrast, binds RNA polymerase very efficiently. In the absence of lactose (**noninduced conditions**), an active repressor protein (produced by i^+) binds to the o^+ operator. RNA polymerase can neither bind to the promoter nor "read through" the operator sequence because repressor protein occupies that region. Hence, transcription of all three structural genes in the *lac* operon is prevented.

When lactose is present (**induced conditions**), it is transported inefficiently into the cell because only a few molecules of permease would normally be present. Inside the cell, some of the lactose would be converted to allolactose by β-galactosidase. Allolactose is the inducer of the *lac* operon. It binds to the repressor protein and causes a conformational change in the protein that alters the site by which it binds to the operator. This conformational change in a protein as a consequence of binding to another molecule is called an **allosteric transformation.** The allolactose-repressor complex can no longer bind to the operator, and it falls off the DNA. RNA polymerase can now read through the operator to transcribe the structural genes in the operon. The increased amount of permease now transports lactose across the membrane in large quantities, and the sugar is then digested by β-galactosidase. When lactose becomes depleted from the medium, newly synthesized repressor proteins will not be coupled with allolactose, so they can bind to the operator and shut off transcription of the structural genes in the operon. Furthermore, allolactose can reversibly bind to repressor protein, so that under low levels of lactose in the cell allolactose would tend to dissociate from repressor-allolactose complexes. Even when the "lac system" is repressed, occasionally the repressor protein will diffuse from the operator momentarily. RNA polymerase may then be able to "sneak" past the open operator and synthesize a molecule of polycistronic mRNA, thus accounting for the very low levels of permease and β-galactosidase that are normally present in the cell. Bacterial mRNA molecules have a very short half-life (only a few minutes), so synthesis of proteins stops very soon after a cell is repressed. Proteins, on the other hand, are much more stable, but they would be diluted out with each subsequent cell division.

Example 12.8. Bacteria of genotype $i^+o^+z^+y^+$ grown on media devoid of lactose will produce neither galactosidase nor permease because i^+ makes repressor substance that inactivates the o^+ operator and "turns off" the synthetic activity of structural genes y^+ and z^+ in its own operon.

Example 12.9. Partial diploids can be produced in bacteria for this region of the chromosome. Cells of the genotype $\dfrac{i^-o^+z^+y^-}{i^+o^cz^-y^+}$ will produce Cz protein and permease constitutively (i.e., either with or without the presence of lactose inducer) because the allele o^c permanently "turns on" the genes in its operon (i.e., those in cis position with o^c). Galactosidase will be produced only inductively because in the presence of lactose (inducer) the diffusible repressor substance from i^+ will be inactivated and allow the structural gene z^+ in cis position with the o^+ operator to produce enzyme.

The operon of the regulatory gene (i) in the lactose system consists of just a promoter and the structural gene for the repressor protein. Its normal promoter is very inefficient, and only a few molecules of lac-repressor protein exist in the cell. In the operons of most regulatory genes in other systems, however, an operator locus is adjacent to its promoter, and **autoregulation** is possible. The repressor proteins made by these operons bind to their own operators to terminate transcription when the concentrations of their respective repressor molecules are elevated.

(b) **Negative, Repressible Control.**   An example of a repressible operon under negative control is found in the tryptophan system of *E. coli* (Fig. 12-13). The amino acid tryptophan is synthesized in five steps, each step mediated by a specific enzyme. The genes responsible for these five enzymes are arranged in a common operon in the same order as their enzymatic protein products function in the biosynthetic pathway. The regulatory gene for this system constitutively synthesizes a nonfunctional protein called **aporepressor.** When tryptophan is in oversupply, the excess tryptophan acts as a **corepressor.** The binding of corepressor to aporepressor forms a functional repressor complex. The functional repressor binds to the *trp* operator and coordinately represses transcription of all five structural genes in the operon. The promoter and operator regions overlap significantly, and binding of active repressor and RNA polymerase are thus competitive. When tryptophan is in low concentration, tryptophan dissociated from aporepressor, and the aporepressor protein falls off the operator. RNA polymerase could then synthesize the polycistronic mRNA for all five enzymes of the tryptophan pathway.

A secondary regulatory mechanism also exists in the tryptophan system. At the 5' end of the

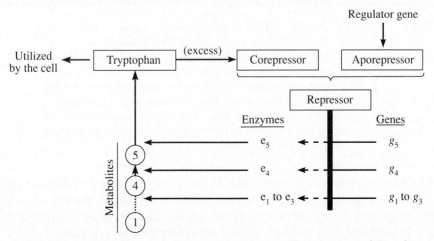

Fig. 12-13.   Negative repressible control in the tryptophan system of *E. coli*.

polycistronic mRNA of this operon, 162 bases precede the coding segments for the five enzymes. This region is called a leader sequence. Part of this sequence is transcribed into a **leader peptide** of 14 amino acids, the function of which is unknown. There are two adjacent tryptophan codons in the leader peptide. When tryptophan is present in excess, transcription of the rest of the *trp* operon is prevented because RNA polymerase generates a transcription termination sequence; this phenomenon is known as **attenuation.**

A model (Fig. 12-14) that explains attenuation assumes that (when tryptophan is abundant) movement of the bacterial ribosome follows closely behind the movement of RNA polymerase as it synthesizes mRNA, and all intramolecular base pairing is prevented in the mRNA segment in contact with the ribosome. In the experimental absence of ribosomes, only the leader mRNA is transcribed and no translation occurs [Fig. 12-14(*a*)]. Leader segments 1 and 2 become folded into stem and loop A by complementary base pairing, whereas segments 3 and 4 fold into stem and loop C that acts as a transcription termination signal. As RNA polymerase synthesizes the 7 uracils that follow segment 4, these uracils and the adjacent paired 3–4 region of mRNA (having just folded into stem and loop C) form a terminator signal that causes RNA polymerase to prematurely dissociate from the DNA before it can transcribe any of the DNA coding segments for the five enzymes of the *trp* operon.

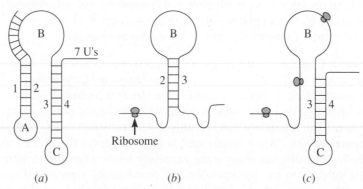

Fig. 12-14.   Three kinds of loops may form in the leader of an mRNA transcribed from the tryptophan operon. No translation occurs (*a*) if the cell is starved for tryptophan (or any other amino acid) or under experimental conditions when using purified tryptophan mRNA (no ribosomes). Loops A, B, and C form. Partial translation of the leader occurs (*b*) when the concentration of tryptophan (or other amino acids) in the cell is low. Ribosomes stall in region 1, allowing RNA polymerase to translate regions 2 and 3, forming loop B (the antiterminator). Loop C (a transcription termination signal) cannot form if loop B forms first. The tryptophan operon will be translated as tryptophan or the other amino acids become available. When all amino acids are abundant (*c*), ribosomes follow so closely behind RNA polymerase that loop B cannot form; hence loop C does form, causing RNA polymerase to dissociate from the mRNA. None of the structural genes of the tryptophan operon are transcribed.

When the concentration of activated trp-tRNAs is low [Fig. 12-14(*b*)] ribosomes begin to translate region 1, thereby preventing pairing of regions 1 and 2. However, the ribosome tends to stall momentarily (especially at the pair of tryptophan codons), and this allows pairing of regions 2 and 3 to form a B stem-and-loop structure (called an **antiterminator**); regions 3 and 4 are thereby prevented from forming the C termination signal, and RNA polymerase is allowed to continue transcription on into the *trp* operon.

If activated trp-tRNAs are abundant [Fig. 12-14(*c*)], the ribosome follows so closely behind RNA polymerase that the antiterminator B structure cannot form, and therefore the terminator C structure does form. Thus, all the leader peptide (but none of the five enzymes of the operon) can be translated from the prematurely terminated mRNA.

The repressor mechanism coarsely regulates the tryptophan system, whereas the attenuation mechanism fine-tunes the control over tryptophan concentrations. Attenuation of the *trp* operon is also sensitive to the concentrations of several amino acids other than tryptophan. Operons for the amino acids histidine and leucine, however, are thought to be regulated only by attenuation.

(*c*) **Positive, Inducible Control.** An example of a positive, inducible regulatory mechanism is found in the arabinose operon of *E. coli.* Arabinose is a sugar that requires three enzymes (coded by genes *araB, araA, araD*) for its metabolism. Two additional genes are needed to transport arabinose across the cell membrane, but they are located at a distance from the BAD cluster coding for the catabolic enzymes. The regulatory gene *araC* is close to the promoter for the BAD cluster. The protein product of *araC* (AraC) is a repressor of the BAD cluster when the substrate arabinose is absent. However, when arabinose is present, it binds to the repressor (AraC), forming an **activator** complex that facilitates the binding of RNA polymerase to the promoter, thus inducing transcription of the operon. The preceding story is a gross oversimplification of the complexity that is already known about the regulation of the arabinose system. For example, **cyclic adenosine monophosphate (cAMP)** and **catabolite gene activator protein (CAP;** also known as **cyclic AMP receptor protein, CRP)** are also involved in the regulation of the arabinose system. The action of these last 2 molecules in the phenomenon of catabolite repression is discussed in the next section.

(*d*) **Multiple Controls.** A genetic locus may be regulated by more than one mechanism. When glucose is available, there is no need to catabolize other sugars, and the genes coding for these other sugar-catabolizing enzymes can be turned off. For example, if glucose is absent and lactose is present in the medium, the *lac* operon would be induced. But if glucose is present, induction of the *lac* operon does not occur. This phenomenon was originally termed the **glucose effect;** it is now known as **catabolite repression.** A complex of 2 molecules acts as the activator in catabolite repression, namely, cAMP and CAP. Within the *lac* promoter (Fig. 12-12), there is a site for binding of a cAMP-CAP complex. RNA polymerase only binds effectively to the promoter if cAMP-CAP complex is also bound to this site. As the level of glucose increases within the cell, the amount of cAMP decreases and less cAMP-CAP complex is available to activate the *lac* operon. CAP is produced at low levels by its own genetic locus. The enzyme **adenylate cyclase** (adenylcyclase) converts adenosine triphosphate (ATP) to cyclic adenosine monophosphate (cAMP). Adenylate cyclase can become activated to **first messenger** status by the interaction of specific cell receptors with their target molecules; the cAMP thus produced (**second messenger**) can then regulate a battery of genes coordinately.

(*e*) **Post-translation Control.** The expression of genes can be regulated after proteins have been synthesized (post–translation control). **Feedback inhibition** (or end-product inhibition) is a regulatory mechanism involving inhibition of enzymatic activity. The end product of a synthetic pathway (usually a small molecule such as an amino acid) may combine loosely (if in high concentration) with the first enzyme in the pathway. This union does not occur at the catalytic site of the enzyme, but it does modify the tertiary or quaternary structures of the enzyme and hence inactivates the catalytic site. This allosteric transformation of the enzyme blocks its catalytic activity and prevents overproduction of the end product of the pathway and its intermediate metabolites.

> **Example 12.10.** The end product isoleucine in *E. coli,* when present in high concentration, unites with the first enzyme in its synthetic pathway and thus inhibits the entire pathway until isoleucine returns to normal levels through cellular consumption. Intermediates in the biosynthetic pathway are in numbered boxes; e = enzyme; g = gene.

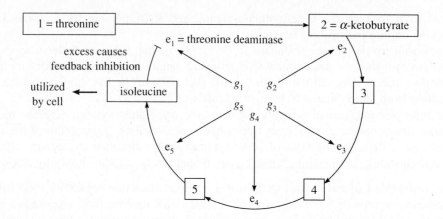

10. Transposable Elements.

Most genes reside at a specific locus or position on the chromosome. Some genes or closely linked sets of genes can mediate their own movement from one location to another and may exist in multiple copies dispersed throughout the genome. These elements have been variously called "jumping genes," "mobile elements," "cassettes," "insertion sequences," and "transposons." The formal name for this family of mobile genes is **transposable elements,** and their movement is called **transposition.** Transposable elements were first discovered in corn and later in phages, bacteria, fungi, insects, and viruses. The transposable elements of bacteria fall into two major classes. **Simple transposons** (also called **insertion sequences,** or **IS**) carry only the genetic information necessary for their transposition (e.g., the gene for the enzyme **transposase**). **Complex transposons** contain additional genetic material unrelated to transposition.

A transposable element is not a replicon (a sequence that contains a site for the origin of replication); thus, it cannot replicate apart from the host chromosome the way that plasmids and phage can. If an IS becomes inserted into an operon, it interrupts the coding sequence and inactivates the expression of the gene into which it inserts as well as any genes downstream in that same operon. This is because an IS contains transcription and/or translation termination signals that block the expression of other genes downstream in an operon. This "one-way" mutational effect (or polarity) is referred to as a **polar mutation.** Simple insertion sequences have no known effects beyond transposition and inactivation of the gene (or operon) into which they insert.

The hallmark of a **transposon (Tn),** whether it is known to transpose or not, is the presence of identical, **inverted terminal repeat (IR) sequences** of 8–38 base pairs (bp). Each type of transposon has its own unique inverted repeat. On either side of a transposon is a short (less than 10 bp) direct repeat (Fig. 12-15). If a transposon exists in multiple copies, these direct repeats are of different base composition at each site where the transposon exists in the chromosome; the inverted terminal repeats, however, remain the same for a given transposon. The sequence into which a transposable element inserts is called the **target sequence.** During insertion of a transposon, the singular target sequence becomes duplicated and thus appears as direct repeats flanking the inserted transposable element. The direct repeats are not considered part of the transposon. No homology exists between the transposon and the target site for its insertion. Many transposons can insert at virtually any position in the host chromosome or into a plasmid. Some transposons seem to be more likely to insert at certain positions (hot spots), but rarely at base-specific target sites. The enzyme(s) required for transposition is encoded in the central region of the transposon. Transposons usually generate a high incidence of deletions in their vicinity because of imprecise excision that removes some adjacent sequences along with the transposon.

Two copies of a transposable element can transpose a DNA sequence between them. For example, in bacteria, Hfr cells are formed by the integration of the sex factor F into the host chromosome. An integrated F sequence is always flanked by two copies (in direct repeat) of one of the insertion sequences located in an F plasmid. This kind of complex transposon obviously may have effects in addition to those of the simple insertion sequences at their ends. Some complex transposons carry one or more bacterial genes for antibiotic resistance in their central regions. Because transposons can shuttle in and

$$1\ 2\ 3\ 4\ 5\ a\ b\ c\ d\ e\ \ldots\ldots e'd'c'b'a'\ 1\ 2\ 3\ 4\ 5$$
$$1'2'3'4'5'\ a'b'c'd'e'\ \ldots\ldots e\ d\ c\ b\ a\ \ 1'2'3'4'5'$$

Target sequence ⟵ Transposon ⟶ Target sequence

Fig. 12.15. Diagram of a simple transposon. Letters and numbers are used instead of nucleotides to make the repeats easier to read. Primed and unprimed symbols of the same kind (e.g., 3 and 3′, d and d′) represent complementary base pairs. The ends of a transposon consist of inverted repeats (represented by letters). Direct repeats of the target sequence (represented by numbers) flank the transposon. The dotted central region of simple transposons contains only genes necessary for translocation, but in complex transposons it may contain one or more additional genes.

out of plasmids as well as chromosomes, it is thought that multiple drug resistance, characteristic of **R plasmids** ("R" for resistance) developed in this way. Such plasmids are easily transferred by conjugation to antibiotic-sensitive bacteria and, with the aid of natural selection, very quickly spread resistance throughout a bacterial species within a patient. Transposons do not carry genes that are essential for survival under normal conditions, but in hostile environments (e.g., the presence of antibiotics or an immune system) the genes carried by a transposon may make the difference between life and death of the bacterial cell.

Two models of transposition in procaryotes have been proposed, on the basis of the fate of the donor site. The transposon might be excised from the donor site, leaving no copy of itself at the donor site (**conservative mode**). Alternatively, the transposon might be replicated, allowing one copy to transpose to another site and leaving an identical copy at the donor site (**replicative mode**). Only the replicative mode could produce multiple copies at various sites in the genome. In bacteria, the number of copies of a transposon appears to be regulated, seldom exceeding 20 copies per genophore. In eucaryotes, however, the copy number can be very high.

11. Mapping the Bacterial Chromosome.

(a) *Interrupted Conjugation.* When Hfr and F^- cultures are mixed, conjugation can be stopped at any desired time by subjecting the mixture to the shearing forces of a Waring blender, which artificially disrupts the conjugation bridge. The sample is diluted immediately and plated on selective media, incubated, and then scored for recombinants. In addition to the selected marker, an Hfr strain must also carry a distal auxotrophic or sensitivity marker that prevents the growth of Hfr cells on the selective medium and thereby allows only recombinant cells to appear. This technique is called **counterselection** or **contraselection.** Because of the polarity with which the Hfr chromosome is transferred, the time at which various genetic markers appear in the recipient indicates their linear organization in the donor chromosome. At a given temperature, the transfer of the first half of the Hfr chromosome proceeds at a relatively uniform rate. Therefore the time of entry of different markers into a recipient (F^-) cell is a function of the physical distance between them. Because of errors introduced by experimental manipulations, this method is best suited for markers that are more than 2 minutes apart.

Example 12.11. An Hfr strain carrying the prototrophic markers a^+, b^+, c^+ is mixed with an F^- strain carrying the auxotrophic alleles a, b, c. Conjugation was interrupted at 5-minute intervals and plated on media that revealed the presence of recombinants.

Time (minutes)	Recombinants
5	ab^+c
10	ab^+c^+
15	$a^+b^+c^+$

The order of the genes in the Hfr donor strain is b^+-c^+-a^+; b is less than 5 time units from the origin; c is less than 10 time units from b; a is less than 10 time units from c.

(b) **Uninterrupted Conjugation.** When conjugation is allowed to proceed without artificial interruption, the time of rupture of the cytoplasmic bridge is apparently randomized among the mating pairs. The nearer a marker is to the origin (leading end of donor chromosome), the greater its chances of appearing as a recombinant in a recipient cell. Donor and recipient cells are mixed for about an hour in broth and then placed on selective media that allows growth of F^- recombinants only for a specific marker. Contraselection against Hfr must also be part of the experimental design. The contraselective marker should be located as distally as possible from the selected marker so that unselected recombinants will not be lost by its inclusion. The frequencies with which unselected markers appear in selected recombinants are inversely related to their distances from the selected marker, provided they lie distal to it. Obviously, any unselected marker between the selected marker and the origin of the chromosome will always be transferred ahead of the selected marker. Proximal markers more than three time units apart exhibit approximately 50% recombination, indicating that the average number of exchanges between them is greater than 1. Just at the point where gross mapping by conjugation becomes ineffective, i.e., for markers less than two time units apart, recombination mapping becomes very effective, permitting estimation of distances between closely linked genes or between mutant sites within the same gene. Distances between genes can be expressed in three types of units: (1) time units, (2) recombination units, or (3) chemical units.

   Example 12.12.   If 1 minute of conjugation is equivalent to 20 recombination units in *E. coli*, and the entire chromosome is transferred in 100 minutes, then the total map length is 2000 recombination units. If 10^7 nucleotide pairs exist in the chromosome, then 1 recombination unit represents $10^7/2000 = 5000$ nucleotide pairs.

(c) **Recombination Mapping.** Virtually all of the opportunities for recombination in bacteria involve only a partial transfer of genetic material (meromyxis) and not the entire chromosome. One or more genes have an opportunity to become integrated into the host chromosome by conjugation, depending upon the length of the donor piece received. Exogenotes usually must become integrated if they are to be replicated and distributed to all of the cells in a clone. Only a small segment of DNA is usually integrated during transformation or transduction. Thus if a cell becomes transformed for two genetic markers by the same transforming piece of DNA (double transformation), the two loci must be closely linked. Similarly, if a cell is simultaneously transduced for two genes by a single transducing phage DNA (cotransduction) the two markers must be closely linked. The degree of linkage between different functional genes (intercistronic) or between mutations within the same functional gene (intracistronic) may then be estimated from the results of specific crosses.

   In merozygotic systems where the genetic contribution of the donor parent is incomplete, an even number of crossovers is required to integrate the exogenote into the host chromosome (endogenote).

   Example 12.13.

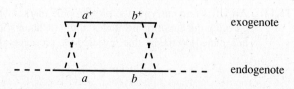

Prototrophic recombinants must integrate the exogenote from somewhere left of the a locus to right of the b locus. Two crossovers (an even number) are required for this integration.

Example 12.14.

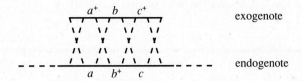

A prototrophic recombinant in this example requires a quadruple (even number) crossover for integration of all wild-type genes.

The total number of progeny is unknown in merozygotic systems so that recombination frequency cannot be expressed relative to this base. Therefore recombination frequencies must be made relative to some standard that is common to all crosses. For example, the number of prototrophic recombinants produced by crossing two mutant strains can be compared to the number emerging from crossing wild type by mutant type. However, many sources of error are unavoidable when comparing the results of different crosses. This problem can be circumvented by comparing the number of prototrophic recombinants to some other class of recombinants arising from the same cross.

Example 12.15. Ratio test for different functional genes. Suppose we have two mutant strains, a and b, where the donor strain ($a^+ b$) can grow on minimal medium supplemented with substance B, but the recipient strain (ab^+) cannot do so.

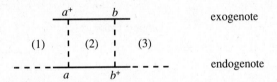

Crossing over in regions (1) and (2) produces prototrophic recombinants ($a^+ b^+$) able to grow on unsupplemented medium. If the medium is supplemented with substance B, then $a^+ b$ recombinants arising by crossing over in regions (1) and (3) can grow in addition to the prototrophs.

$$\text{Standardized recombination ratio} = \frac{\text{number of prototrophs}}{\text{number of recombinants}}$$

Example 12.16. Intracistronic ratio test. Consider two intracistronic mutations, b_1 and b_2, unable to grow in medium without substance B. The recipient strain contains a mutation in another functionally different gene (a), either linked or unlinked to b, which cannot grow unless supplemented by substances A and B.

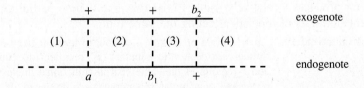

On unsupplemented medium, only prototrophs arising through crossovers in regions (1) and (3) appear. On medium supplemented only by substance B, recombinants involving region (1) and any of the other three regions can survive.

$$\text{Standardized recombination ration} = \frac{\text{number of colonies on unsupplemented medium}}{\text{number of colonies on B-supplemented medium}}$$

(d) *Establishing Gene Order.*   Mapping small regions in microorganisms has revealed that multiple crossovers often occur with much greater than random frequency, a phenomenon called "localized negative interference." The only unambiguous method for determining the order of very closely linked sites is by means of three-factor reciprocal crosses. Suppose that the location of gene a is known to be to the left of gene b but that the order of two mutants within the adjacent b cistron is unknown. Reciprocal crosses will yield different results, depending upon the order of the mutant sites.

Example 12.17.   Assume the order of sites is a-b_1-b_2.

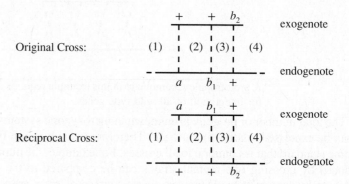

In the original cross, prototrophs ($+ + +$) can be produced by crossovers in regions (1) and (3). In the reciprocal cross, prototrophs arise by crossovers in regions (3) and (4). The numbers of prototrophs should be approximately equivalent in the two crosses.

Example 12.18.   Assume the order of sites is a-b_2-b_1.

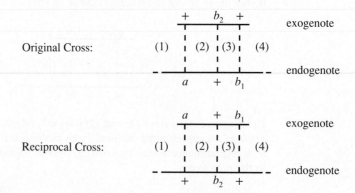

In the original cross, the production of prototrophs requires four crossovers, one in each of the regions (1), (2), (3), and (4). Only two crossovers [in regions (2) and (3)] in the reciprocal cross are needed to produce prototrophs. Therefore many more prototrophic recombinants are expected from the reciprocal cross than from the original cross.

(*e*) *Complementation Mapping.*   An F particle that carries another bacterial gene other than the sex factor produces a relatively stable F^+ merozygote. These partial diploids can be used for complementation tests of mutants affecting the same trait.

Example 12.19.   An Hfr strain of *E. coli* is unable to ferment lactose (z_1^-) and can transfer the z_1^- gene through sex-duction to a mutant (z_2^-) recipient, forming the heterogenote $z_2^-/(F$-$z_1^-)$. If z_1 and z_2 belong to the same cistron (functional alleles), then complementation does not occur and only mutant phenotypes are produced. If z_1 and z_2 are mutants in different cistrons, complementation could produce wild types able to ferment lactose.

Intracistronic complementation may sometimes be possible when the enzyme product is composed of two or more identical polypeptide chains. Experimental evidence has shown that an *in vitro* mixture of inactive enzymes from some complementing mutants can "hybridize" to produce an enzyme with up to 25% normal activity. Mutants that fail to complement with some but not all other mutants are assumed to overlap in function. A complementation map can be constructed from the experimental results of testing all possible pairs of mutants for complementary action in bacterial merozygotes or in fungal heterocaryons. A complementation map cannot be equated in any way with a crossover map, since the gene is defined by different criteria. A complementation map tells us nothing of the structure or location of the mutations involved. Complementation maps are deduced from merozygotes or heterocaryons; crossover maps from recombination experiments.

Example 12.20. Three mutants map by complementation as follows:

> This indicates that mutants 1 and 2 are complementary and do not overlap in function. Hence 1 and 2 are nonallelic mutations by this criterion. Mutant 3 fails to complement with either 1 or 2 and hence must overlap (to some degree) with both 1 and 2. Hence 3 is functionally allelic with both 1 and 2.

(*f*) *Mapping by Deletion Mutants.*   A deletion in some segment of a functional gene cannot recombine with point mutations in that same region even though two point mutations at different sites within this region may recombine to produce wild type. Another distinctive property of deletion mutants is their stability, being unable to mutate back to wild type. The use of overlapping deletions can considerably reduce the work in fine structure analysis of a gene.

Example 12.21. Determining the limits of a deletion. Suppose that a series of single mutants (1, 2, 3, 4) has already been mapped as shown below:

> A deletion that fails to recombine with point mutants 1 and 2 but does produce wild type with 3 and 4 extends over region X. A deletion that yields no recombinants with 3 and 4 has the boundaries diagrammed as Y. A deletion mutant that produces wild type only with point mutants 1 or 4 has the limits of Z.

Example 12.22. Assigning point mutations to deletion regions.

> Given the deletions R, S, and T as shown above, the point mutation that recombines to give wild type with deletions S and T, but not with R, is 1. Number 3 is the only one of the four mutants that fails to recombine with one of the three deletions.

BACTERIOPHAGES

1. Characteristics of All Viruses.

All viruses differ from cellular organisms in the following respects:

(1) Viruses are noncellular, obligate, intracellular parasites.

(2) Viruses have only one kind of nucleic acid (either DNA or RNA), whereas cells have both kinds.

(3) Viruses have no protein-synthesizing system of their own (e.g., they have no ribosomes); they have no energy-conversion system of their own (i.e., they do not metabolize food to generate ATP).

(4) Viruses are not contained by a lipid membrane of their own making (although some viruses become

invested by an **envelope** of modified host membrane as they leave the cell). They have no internal membranes.

(5) Viruses are not affected by levels of antibiotics that cells can tolerate.

(6) Viruses have no cytoskeleton or means of motility other than diffusion.

(7) Viruses do not "grow" in the classical sense of increasing in mass; i.e., once the virus is formed, it does not increase in size.

A fully formed virus is called a **virion,** and it has its genetic material protected within a protein coat known as a **capsid.** The individual protein subunits that make up the capsid are called **capsomeres.** Cells that are susceptible to viral infection have specific **receptors** on their surfaces to which each virus can attach. Cells without these receptors would be refractory to infection by virus.

2. Characteristics of Bacteriophages.

Viruses that infect bacteria are called **bacteriophages** or simply **phages.** The plural form "phages" is used when referring to different species (e.g., lambda and T4 are both phages). When referring to one or more virions of the same species, the word **phage** is used; thus a bacterial cell may be infected by one or more lambda phage. The most commonly studied phages have a roughly spherical icosahedral capsid, or head (consisting of 20 equilateral triangular faces), to which a tail is attached. The tail may be long or short, contractile or noncontractile. Other kinds of phage have tailless heads or filamentous structures. The genetic material of most phages is double-stranded DNA (dsDNA), although some single-stranded DNA (ssDNA), single-stranded RNA (ssRNA), and double-stranded RNA (dsRNA) phages are known. Enveloped forms are rare. Other characteristics that are useful for classification include molecular weight, genomic base composition (G + C content), antigenic specificities of the capsid, and species (or strains) of susceptible host cells **(host range). Host restriction** is the ability of a bacteriophage to replicate in only certain strains of bacteria.

> **Example 12.23.** Several bacterial species synthesize a site-specific endonuclease enzyme that can digest any foreign DNA containing the specific nucleotide sequence that constitutes the recognition site of the enzyme. According to the **restriction and modification model** proposed by W. Arber, such a bacterium would also contain a methylase enzyme to modify (by methylation) these same sequences in its own DNA, and thus protect it from digestion by endogenous endonuclease. Foreign DNA from a different strain would not have these recognition sites methylated and hence would be destroyed (and thus restricted from surviving in that strain) by the host's endonuclease.

The nucleic acid from a single phage particle (virion) typically infects a bacterial cell, replicates itself many times, produces viral proteins to make numerous viruses, and ruptures the cell to release several hundred progeny phage. Repetitions of this vegetative reproductive process can cause a turbid bacterial culture to rapidly become clear owing to lysis of the host cells. The various types of viral reproductive processes are sometimes referred to as "life cycles"; this is a misnomer because viruses are not considered to have all of the properties attributed to living cells. If a dilute solution of phage is plated on a confluent growth of bacterial cells ("lawn") on nutrient agar in a Petri dish, a cleared area, or "hole," will develop around each position where a phage particle was deposited. These holes, referred to as **plaques,** contain millions of progeny phage that have been released from lysed cells. By counting the number of plaques on a plate, and knowing the amount and dilution of the phage suspension added to the plate, one can estimate the total number of phage particles in the original phage culture.

3. Bacteriophage Life Cycles.

Most phages (such as phage T4 that infects *E. coli*) have only a vegetative or lytic life cycle in which they kill the host cell in the production of progeny phage. Such phages are said to be **virulent.**

A few phages (such as phage lambda that also infects *E. coli*) have a lysogenic life cycle in which they may either act as a **temperate** (nonvirulent) phage or enter a lytic cycle.

(a) *Lytic Cycles.*   The first step in the life cycle of phage T4 (Fig. 12-16) involves the adsorption of a virion to a specific receptor site on the surface of the host cell. Any cell lacking this receptor would be immune to infection by T4. Each type of phage can usually infect only one species of bacteria, and in some cases only a particular strain or strains of that species; the number of such cell types in which a phage can carry out its lytic cycle constitutes its host range. Following adsorption, T4 injects its DNA through its tail into the host cell. The empty phage capsid remains outside the bacterium as a **ghost** (so named because of the empty appearance of the head in electron micrographs). The DNA of a tailless phage is released onto the cell surface, and the phage "genome" is taken into the cell by an unknown mechanism. A filamentous phage (e.g., M13) is able to penetrate the cell wall and then has its nucleic acid released by host-cell enzymes that digest the coat proteins. Once the naked phage DNA is inside the cell, different phages may use different strategies to produce progeny particles. Generally, however, the phage DNA initially is transcribed by the host's DNA polymerase into "early mRNAs." Later mRNAs may be synthesized by a phage RNA polymerase that was made from an early mRNA; or perhaps the bacterial RNA polymerase becomes modified to transcribe phage genes preferentially or exclusively. These later mRNAs become translated into catalytic (enzymatic), regulatory, and structural proteins. The regulatory proteins of the phage control the timing at which various phage genes become active. The structural proteins form heads, tails, and other protein parts of the complete phage particle (virion) as needed. The phage enzymes mediate replication of many copies of the phage genome, further transcription, and sometimes even the destruction of the host's DNA.

> **Example 12.24.**   Phage T4 specifies the enzyme hydroxymethylase that modifies the cytosine bases in its own DNA to 5-hydroxymethyl cytosine. Such modified bases are resistant to degradation by nucleases of either the host cell or the phage. A T4 encoded nuclease can thus digest the host DNA at unprotected cytosines without harming the DNA of the phage.

Several different mechanisms are known for packaging phage DNAs into their protein coats. In *E. coli* phage T4, rolling-circle replication of its double-stranded DNA produces long, tandemly

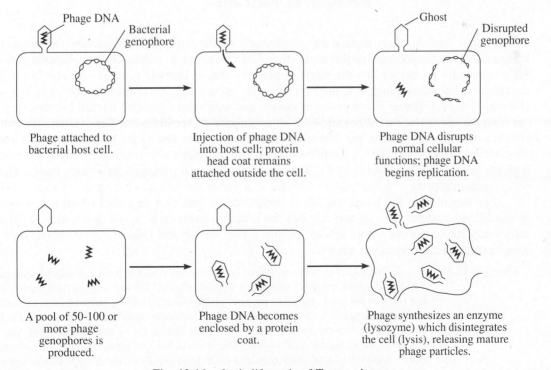

Fig. 12-16.   Lytic life cycle of T-even phages.

linked series (concatemers) of phage genomes. It is thought that the end of the concatemer enters the head, followed by enough DNA to fill the head. The concatemer is then cleaved at a nonspecific site by what is known as the **headful mechanism.** Since the DNA capacity of the head is greater than the length of one phage genome (monomer), the gene order will be different in each linear fragment cut from the concatemer. Terminal regions will be present twice within each monomer **(terminally redundant).** Since each phage monomer cut from a concatemer begins at a different gene sequence, they collectively form a **cyclically permuted** set (Fig. 12-17).

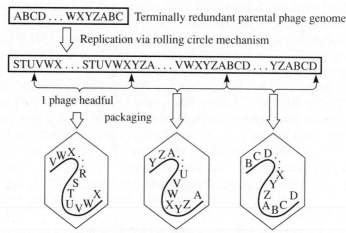

Fig. 12-17. Production of a terminally redundant and cyclically permuted set of progeny phage by cutting (vertical arrows) the linear tail produced by sigma replication according to the "headful rule." Terminal redundancy can be present without cyclic permutation in some phages that do not use a headful mechanism, but the converse has not been observed.

In phage lambda, theta replication occurs early in the lytic cycle to increase the number of templates for transcription and further replication. Later in the cycle, rolling-circle replication provides the genomes for packaging into the heads of progeny phage. Lambda genomes are also cut from a concatemer, but unlike phage T4, the cuts are made at base-specific sequences known as **cos sites** (for *co*hesive *s*ite). Linear phage genomes always end with single-stranded termini because they are cut from the concatemer at the *cos* site by a sequence-specific **terminase** or **Ter system.** Ter-cutting requires that two *cos* sites or one *cos* site and a free cohesive end ($\frac{1}{2}$ *cos*) be present on a single concatemeric DNA molecule. A modified lambda genome that is 79–106% the length of a normal λ phage genome will still be cut by the Ter system and become packaged into phage heads. This is an important property of λ that makes it useful as a vector for genetic cloning (see Chapter 14).

After assembly of the phage capsids is completed, a lytic protein called **lysozyme** is usually produced that ruptures the cell and releases the progeny phage in a typical **burst size** of 50–300 infective particles per cell. Most virulent phages follow the general lytic life cycle outlined above. Some exceptions, however, are known.

Example 12.25. *E. coli* phage M13 is filamentous and contains a circular, single-stranded DNA molecule. Among all known phages reproducing vegetatively, M13 is the only one that neither kills nor lyses its host cell. Infective progeny phage leave the cell by budding from its surface without causing cell damage. Upon infection, the entire phage particle penetrates the cell wall by being absorbed at the end of an F-pilus. The entry of coat proteins into the cell is another feature unique to this phage. One strain of M13 (M13mp7) contains the promoter (*lacP*), operator (*lacO*), and β-galacosidase gene (*lacZ*) of the *E. coli* lactose operon. Insertion of a foreign DNA segment into *lacZ* would inactivate the gene and no enzyme would be produced. Lac⁻ bacterial cells infected with normal M13mp7 would be able to ferment lactose. On EMB agar, lactose-fermenting colonies would appear dark purple. Cells exposed to an M13mp7 carrying a foreign DNA insert in *lacZ* would be unable to ferment lactose; therefore, they grow into colorless colonies. Like lambda, phage M13 has been widely used as a cloning vehicle in genetic engineering (Chapter 13).

Example 12.26. The temperate phage Mu inserts its DNA obligatorily into its *E. coli* host chromosome during its lytic cycle. These insertions are at random, and they often inactivate host genes or regulatory sequences. Insertion always results in duplication of a terminal target sequence. Thus Mu is a giant transposon that has acquired phage functions enabling it to be packaged into phage coats and to escape its host by lysis. Transposition is obligatory during Mu DNA replication. Insertion of progeny Mu DNA occurs at various sites throughout the lytic cycle. Various host DNA sequences are always found at the termini of Mu DNA. However, only Mu DNA inserts; the duplicated terminal bacterial sequences are not inserted.

(b) *Lysogenic Cycles.* There are two types of lysogenic cycles. In the most common type, typified by *E. coli* phage lambda (λ), the phage DNA becomes integrated into the host chromosome. In the other type, represented by *E. coli* phage P1, the phage DNA does not integrate into the host chromosome, but somehow replicates in synchrony with it as a plasmid. Both the integrated and plasmid forms of phage DNA are called **prophage.**

The establishment of an integrated lambda prophage occurs in four major steps:

(1) Linear phage DNA is injected into the host bacterial cell; the phage DNA is circularized by base pairing of its terminally redundant tails.

(2) Some early phage genes are transcribed to produce a few molecules of a repressor protein and an **integrase** enzyme. The repressor then turns off transcription of phage genes.

(3) The phage DNA is usually **integrated** or inserted at a specific site into the host chromosome as a prophage with the aid of integrase.

(4) The bacterium survives and multiplies; the prophage is replicated along with the host chromosome.

The mechanism whereby an infected cell is switched to either the lytic or the lysogenic cycle is incompletely known. Many details of the lysogenic cycle are known for phage lambda, but they are too complex to be presented here. However, two conditions seem to favor the establishment of the lysogenic cycle of a temperate phage: (1) depletion of nutrients in the growth medium and (2) high **multiplicity of infection** (MOI)—i.e., many adsorbed phages per bacterium. Phage can carry out the lytic cycle only in cells that are actively metabolizing. When nutrients are depleted, bacteria degrade their own mRNAs and proteins before they become dormant. When nutrients become available to an uninfected dormant bacterium, it can again resume growth. A phage-infected cell that becomes dormant interrupts the lytic cycle, and usually loses the ability to produce phage. The cell dies. On the other hand, if the cell can become **lysogenized** (containing a prophage), both the phage and the bacterium can survive a dormant period, and the potential for production of phage by induction persists (Fig. 12-18).

If a lysogenic bacterium sustains damage to its DNA, it would be advantageous for the prophage to **deintegrate** from the bacterial chromosome, enter the lytic cycle, produce progeny phage, and leave that cell. When bacterial DNA is damaged, a protease (**RecA protein**) of the SOS repair mechanism is activated. This protease cleaves the lambda repressor that has kept the prophage in its inactive state. The prophage DNA becomes **derepressed,** an **excisionase** enzyme is synthesized, and the prophage deintegrates from the host chromosome to enter the lytic cycle. This is the process known as **prophage induction.** If ultraviolet radiation has damaged the host DNA, the ensuing prophage induction is termed **UV induction.** When a nonlysogenic F⁻ bacterial cell receives, by conjugation, a prophage from a lysogenic Hfr donor, the recipient cell dies by induction of the lytic phage cycle. This form of prophage induction is termed **zygotic induction.**

In the lysogenic cycle of phage P1, the prophage is not integrated into the bacterial chromosome.

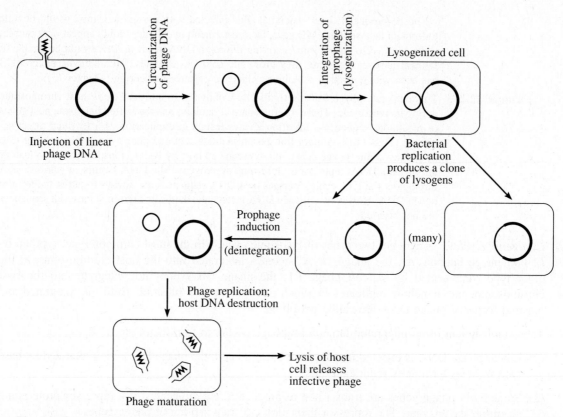

Fig. 12-18. Lambda-type lysogenic cycle. Thin lines represent phage DNA; thick lines represent bacterial chromosome.

Upon entry into the cell, P1 DNA circularizes and is repressed. It remains as a free, supercoiled, plasmidlike molecule, and replicates once with each cell division so that each daughter cell receives one copy of the prophage. The mechanism for this orderly assortment is unknown.

4. Transduction.

Transduction is the virus-mediated transfer of DNA from a donor cell to a recipient cell. There are two types of transduction: specialized and generalized.

(a) *Specialized (Restricted) Transduction.*   There are four distinguishing characteristics of specialized transduction: (1) the only bacterial genes that can be transduced are those very near the site at which the prophage is integrated, (2) only λ-type prophage are involved, (3) it results from defective excision of the prophage from the host chromosome, and (4) recombinant progeny bacteria may be partial diploids. The only site at which lambda phage integrates into the host chromosome (Fig. 12-19) is between the genes for galactose fermentation (*gal*) and biotin synthesis (*bio*). The head of the phage can only contain a limited amount of DNA, so if the prophage deintegrates abnormally from the host chromosome (taking some bacterial DNA in place of its own DNA), only the *gal* or *bio* genes could be transduced. Thus, all transducing lambda phages are defective in part of their own genome and cannot replicate on their own. A lambda phage that transduces the galactose genes is therefore called λ*gal* or λdg (d = defective; g = galactose). If a *gal*⁻ cell is infected by λdg (bearing the gene *gal*⁺), integration of the defective prophage into the host chromosome produces a partial diploid (for the *gal* locus) recombinant chromosome. Aberrant excision of the prophage is usually a rare event, so restricted transduction is an event of low frequency. However, high-frequency transduction can be attained under laboratory conditions. If a bacterial cell is doubly infected with a wild-type lambda phage and a λdg phage, the wild-type phage can supply the functions missing in the defective phage, and the progeny will contain about equal numbers of both types. When the lysate is used for

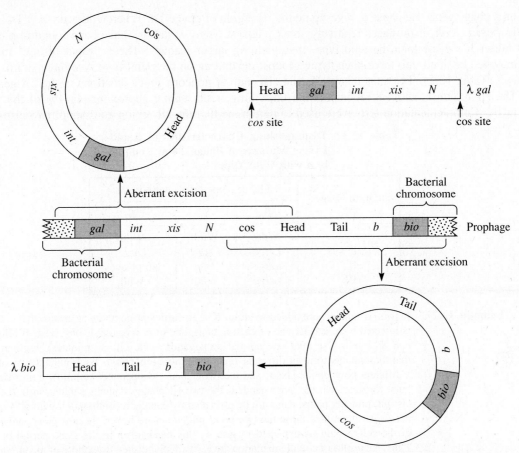

Fig. 12-19. Formation of λ *bio* (or λ *gal*) by aberrant excision of the prophage from the bacterial chromosome (stippled).

transduction, the process is referred to as **high-frequency transduction.** In many cases, because of its defective genome, λdg fails to be integrated into the host chromosome (and therefore is not replicated). At each division, only one of the two progeny cells contains the defective phage genome; this process is called **abortive transduction.**

(b) *Generalized Transduction.* The hallmarks of this type of transduction are as follows: (1) the transduction usually involves P1-type phage, (2) any bacterial gene can be transduced, (3) the transduction results from a packaging error during phage maturation, and (4) haploid recombinants are produced. Since there is no homology between DNA sequences in these phage and the sequences of their host, there is no preferential site at which the prophage integrates. Any gene can be transduced because the head of the phage can package an entire headful of bacterial DNA. **Cotransduction** is the process of transducing 2 or more genes via the same defective phage. Reciprocal crossing over is required to integrate the transduced genes, so recombinant bacteria tend to be haploid rather than diploid. The endogenote segment replaced by the exogenote fails to replicate for lack of an *ori* (*ori*gin of replication) site and becomes lost in the culture through dilution or digestion.

5. Fine-Structure Mapping of Phage Genes.

(a) *Complementation Mapping.* Because so little of the phage or bacterial genome consists of non-functional sequences, virtually all crossing over occurs within, rather than between, genes. Before the discovery that DNA is genetic material, the gene was thought to be the smallest genetic unit by three criteria: mutation, recombination, and function. Semour Benzer set out to determine the limits of these operational units by performing the most definitive fine-structure mapping ever performed on a phage gene. He chose to investigate the rII region of phage T4. When wild-type (r^+) T4 infects its host *E. coli,* it produces relatively small plaques. Many mutations have been found that have a shorter life cycle than the wild type, thus yielding larger plaques. These "rapid lysing" mutants may be classified into three phenotypic groups, depending on their ability to lyse three strains of *E. coli* (Table 12.1). The sites of *r*I, *r*II, and *r*III map at noncontiguous locations in the T4 genome. The *r*II region is about 8 recombination units long, representing approximately 1% of the phage DNA. Complementation tests were used to determine that the *r*II region consists of two cistrons.

Table 12.1. Distinguishing Characteristics of Rapid-Lysing Mutants of Phage T4 in Comparison with Wild Type

Strain of Phage T$_4$	Plaque Type on *E. coli* Strains		
	B	S	K
r^+	Wild	Wild	Wild
*r*I	Large	Large	Large
*r*II	Large	Wild	No plaques
*r*III	Large	Wild	Wild

Example 12.27.   If two *r*II mutants are added to strain K12 in sufficient numbers to ensure that each cell is infected with at least one of each mutant, one of two results is observed. If all the *E. coli* K12 cells lyse after one normal propagation cycle (20–30 minutes), we may infer that the mutants were in different functional units (**cistrons**). Each mutant was making a different polypeptide chain, and the two chains "cooperated" to allow a normal-sized burst to occur. On the other hand, if the two *r*II phages contain a mutation in the same cistron, progeny phage can only be produced by genetic recombination with a frequency dependent upon how close the two point mutations are linked. In any event, only a few of the cells would be expected to lyse by this mechanism in the same period of time. Thus, the results of complementation are easily distinguished from those of recombination. Benzer found that all of the point mutations in the *r*II region mapped into 2 cistrons (A and B).

*(b) **Deletion Mapping.***   Benzer also found that about 10% of his more than 2000 *r*II mutants did not backmutate to wild type because they were deletions of various lengths. By infecting cells with two different deletions, wild-type recombinants could be produced if the deletions did not overlap. Of course, wild-type recombinants cannot be produced if the two deletions overlap to any extent. Thus, by a series of crosses he was able to draw a topological map in which deletions were shown to overlap or not overlap. The lengths of the deletions or the degree of overlap or nonoverlap is arbitrary at this point, although they can be determined by crosses with point mutations.

Having obtained a topological map, it is then possible to assign one or more point mutations to a relatively small segment of a cistron by crossing them with deletion mutants. A point mutation cannot recombine with a deletion over the same site. This principle allowed Benzer to group mutants within relatively small regions of each cistron. He did not attempt to order the point mutations within each of these small segments, but he did subject them to recombination tests to ascertain identity or nonidentity. This was accomplished by doubly infecting strain B with a pair of *r*II point mutants (e.g., *r*IIa and *r*IIb) in broth, and then allowing them to lyse the culture. The total number of progeny phage can be estimated by plating dilutions of this lysate on *E. coli* B and counting the resulting plaques. Wild-type recombinants are scored by plating the lysate on strain K. For every wild-type (r^+IIa, r^+IIb) plaque counted on strain K, we assume that an undetected double mutant (*r*IIa, *r*IIb) reciprocal recombinant was formed.

$$\text{Recombination percentage} = \frac{2(\text{number of plaques on K})100}{\text{number of plaques on B}}$$

The smallest reproducible recombination frequency Benzer observed between two sites in the *r*II region was about 0.02%, corresponding to approximately $\frac{1}{400}$ of a genetic region whose total length is only 8 recombination units. Thus it was concluded that the cistrons of the *r*II region each contained hundreds of possible mutation sites, and that recombination could occur between the closest of these mutant sites. He reasoned that the smallest distance within which recombination occurs (**recon**) might be as small as adjacent nucleotide pairs. The smallest bit of DNA that when mutated could cause a phenotypic effect (**muton**) was found to be as small as five nucleotide pairs or smaller. Since Benzer's observations, the muton has been shown to be a single nucleotide base pair.

A surprising finding of this work was that the point mutants were not randomly located in the *r*II region; a few locations in both cistrons had many more mutations than elsewhere (over a hundred in a couple of positions vs. about 1 to 10 elsewhere). The reason for these so-called **hot spots** is presently unknown.

Solved Problems

BACTERIA

12.1. The discipline of bacterial genetics began in 1943 when S. E. Luria and M. Delbrück published a paper entitled "Mutations of bacteria from virus sensitivity to virus resistance." Before this time, it was not known if the heredity of bacteria adaptively changed in specific ways as a consequence of exposure to specific environments, or whether specific mutants existed in the population prior to an environmental challenge, the latter acting as a selective agent to increase the numbers of the adaptive mutants. The former idea was Lamarckian, the latter was neo-Darwinian. Luria and Delbrück found that there was great variation from one trial to another in the number of *E. coli* that were resistant to lysis by phage T1. In order to determine which of the two hypotheses was correct, they devised the following "fluctuation test." Twenty 0.2-milliliter "individual cultures" and one 10-milliliter "bulk culture" of nutrient medium were incubated with about 10^3 *E. coli* cells per milliliter. The cultures were incubated until they contained about 10^8 cells/milliliter. The entire 0.2 milliliter of each individual culture was spread on a nutrient agar plate heavily seeded with T1 phages. Ten 0.2-milliliter samples from the bulk culture were also treated in similar fashion. After overnight incubation, the total number of T1-resistant (Ton^r) bacterial cells was counted; the results are presented in the following table. What inferences can be drawn from this "fluctuation test"?

Individual Cultures		Samples from Bulk Culture	
Culture Number	Number of Resistant Colonies	Sample Number	Number of Resistant Colonies
1	1	1	14
2	0	2	15
3	3	3	13
4	0	4	21
5	0	5	15
6	5	6	14
7	0	7	26
8	5	8	16
9	0	9	20
10	6	10	13
11	107		
12	0		
13	0		
14	0		
15	1		
16	0		
17	0		
18	64		
19	0		
20	35		

Solution:

Variances for each experiment can be calculated from the square of formula (9.2); the individual cultures have a variance of 714.5, whereas the variance of samples from the bulk culture is 16.4. In a Poisson distribution, the mean and the variance are essentially identical; hence, the variance/mean ratio should be unity (1.0). The variance/mean ratio for the bulk culture samples is $16.4/16.7 = 0.98$ or nearly 1.0, as expected from a random distribution of rare events. The samples from the bulk culture collectively serve as a control for the individual cultures. The same ratio for the individual cultures, however, is $714.5/11.3 = 63.23$, indicating that there are extremely wide fluctuations of the numbers of Ton^r cells in each culture around the mean. If resistance to the T1 phages occurs with a given probability only after contact with the phages, then each culture from both the individual and batch experiments should contain approximately the same average number of resistant cells. On the other hand, if Ton^r mutants occurred prior to contact with the phages, great variation around the mean is expected from one individual culture to another because some will incur a mutation early and others late (or not at all) during the incubation period. This experiment argues in favor of the mutation hypothesis and against the induced resistance hypothesis.

Certain mutations, such as that to phage resistance, are *preadaptive* in that their selective advantage only becomes manifest when phages are in the environment as a selective agent; in this case, T1-sensitive bacteria (Ton^s) are killed by T1 phages, allowing only the few Ton^r cells to survive and multiply. Phage resistance depends upon altering the structure of the bacterial receptor sites to which T1 phages normally attach. Immunity to superinfection by a specific phage is based upon production of a repressor of phage replication by a lysogenic cell.

12.2. Two triple auxotrophic strains of *E. coli* are mixed in liquid medium and plated on complete medium, which then serves as a master for replica plating onto 6 kinds of media. From the position of the clones on the plates and the ingredients in the media, determine the genotype for each of the 6 clones. The gene order is as shown.

$$thr^- \; leu^- \; thi^- \; bio^+ \; phe^+ \; cys^+ \quad \times \quad thr^+ \; leu^+ \; thi^+ \; bio^- \; phe^- \; cys^-$$

Gene symbols are abbreviated as follows:

thr = threonine	*bio* = biotin
leu = leucine	*phe* = phenylalanine
thi = thiamin	*cys* = cystine

Master Plate
(complete medium)

Replica plates: Each dish contains minimal medium plus the supplements listed below each dish.

Thr, Leu   Leu, Thi   Bio, Phe

Phe, Cys   Thr, Thi   Bio, Cys

Solution:

Clone 1 grows when supplemented with Thr and Leu or Thr and Thi, but not with Leu and Thi. Therefore this colony is auxotrophic for Thr alone ($thr^- leu^+ thi^+ bio^+ phe^+ cys^+$).

Clone 2 appears only on the plate supplemented with Phe and Cys. This is a double auxotrophic colony of genotype $thr^+ leu^+ thi^+ bio^+ phe^- cys^-$.

Clone 3 appears on all replica plates and therefore must be prototrophic ($thr^+ leu^+ thi^+ bio^+ phe^+ cys^+$).

Clone 4 grows only when supplemented with Thr and Leu and therefore must be a double auxotroph of genotype $thr^- leu^- thi^+ bio^+ phe^+ cys^+$.

Clone 5 and clone 1 always appear together on the replica plates and therefore have the same genotype.

Clone 6 can grow in the presence of Phe and Cys or Bio and Cys. The common factor is Cys, for which this strain is singly auxotrophic ($thr^+ leu^+ thi^+ bio^+ phe^+ cys^-$).

12.3. Under optimal conditions, some bacteria can divide every 20 minutes. Suppose each cell has a mass of 2×10^{-9} milligrams. The mass of the earth is approximately 5.97×10^{27} grams. Determine the time (in hours) required for the progeny of a single cell dividing without restriction at the above rate to equal the weight of the earth.

Solution:

At time zero we have 1 cell; 20 minutes later we have 2 cells; at 40 minutes there are 4 cells; at 60 minutes there are 8 cells; etc. The number of cells at any hour, t, is obviously 2^{3t}. The number of cells equivalent to the weight of the earth is

$$(5.97 \times 10^{27})/(2 \times 10^{-12}) = 2.98 \times 10^{39} = 2^{3t}$$

from which $3t \log 2 = \log 2.98 + \log 10^{39}$, $\quad t = \dfrac{\log 2.98 + 39}{3 \log 2} = \dfrac{39.475}{3(0.301)} = 43.7$ hours.

12.4. A strain of *E. coli* unable to ferment the carbohydrate arabinose (ara^-) and unable to synthesize the amino acids leucine (leu^-) and threonine (thr^-) is transduced by a wild-type strain (ara^+ $leu^+ thr^+$). Recombinants for leucine are detected by plating on minimal medium supplemented with threonine. Colonies from the transduction plates were replicated or streaked onto plates containing arabinose. Out of 270 colonies that grew on the threonine-supplemented plates, 148 could also ferment arabinose. Calculate the amount of recombination between *leu* and *ara*.

Solution:

In order for a transductant to be $leu^+ ara^+$, crossing over in regions (1) and (3) must occur; for leu^+ ara^- to arise, crossing over in regions (1) and (2) must occur.

$$\text{Standardized recombination ratio} = \frac{\text{no. of } leu^+ ara^-}{\text{no. of } leu^+} = \frac{270 - 148}{270} = 0.45 \text{ or } 45\%$$

12.5. Several z^- mutants, all lacking the ability to synthesize β-galactosidase, have been isolated. A cross is made between Hfr ($z_1^- ade^+ str^s$) $\times$ F$^-$ ($z_2^- ade^- str^r$) where ade^- = adenine requirement, str^s and str^r = streptomycin sensitivity and resistance, respectively. Many of the ade^+ exconjugant clones were able to ferment lactose, indicating β-galactosidase activity. Only a few ade^+ clones from the reciprocal cross Hfr ($z_2^- ade^+ str^s$) $\times$ F$^-$ ($z_1^- ade^- str^r$) were able to ferment lactose. What is the order of the z_1 and z_2 mutants relative to the *ade* locus?

Solution:

Assume that the order is z_2-z_1-*ade*. In the first mating, four crossovers are required to produce a streptomycin-resistant prototroph able to ferment lactose ($z_2^+ z_1^+ ade^+ str^r$).

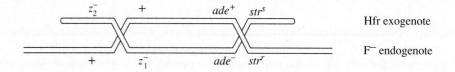

The reciprocal mating requires only two crossovers to produce a prototroph able to ferment lactose.

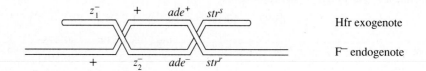

Double crossovers are expected to be much more frequent than quadruple crossovers. The above scheme does not fit the data because the first mating was more frequent than the reciprocal mating. Our assumption must be wrong.

Let us assume that the order is z_1-z_2-ade. The first cross now requires a double crossover.

The reciprocal cross requires four crossover events.

The reciprocal cross is expected to be much less frequent under this assumption and is in agreement with the observations.

12.6. Six mutations are known to belong to three cistrons. From the results of the complementation tests, determine which mutants are in the same cistron.

	1	2	3	4	5	6	
1	0	+	+				1
2		0		+	+		2
3			0	+	0		3
4				0		+	4
5					0	+	5
6						0	6

+ = complementation
0 = noncomplementation
blank = not tested

Solution:

Obviously mutations 3 and 5 are in the same cistron, since they fail to complement each other. Mutations 1 and 3 are in different cistrons, since they do complement each other. We will arbitrarily assign these to cistrons A and B.

(3, 5)	1	
Cistron A	Cistron B	Cistron C

1 and 2 are in different cistrons, but we do not know whether 2 is in A or C. However, 5 and 2 complement and therefore 2 cannot be either in cistron A or B and thus must be in C.

(3, 5)	1	2
Cistron A	Cistron B	Cistron C

3 and 4 complement; thus 4 must be in either B or C. But 2 and 4 also complement; thus 4 cannot be in C and must reside in B.

(3, 5)	(1, 4)	2
Cistron A	Cistron B	Cistron C

6 cannot be in A since it complements with 5. Thus 6 is either in B or C. Since 6 and 4 complement, they are in different cistrons. If 6 cannot be in A or B, it must be in C. The mutants are grouped into cistrons as shown below.

(3, 5)	(1, 4)	(2, 6)
Cistron A	Cistron B	Cistron C

BACTERIOPHAGES

12.7. In an attempt to determine the amount of recombination between two mutations in the rII region of phage T4, strain B of *E. coli* is doubly infected with both kinds of mutants. A dilution of $1:10^9$ is made of the lysate and plated on strain B. A dilution of $1:10^7$ is also plated on strain K. Two plaques are found on K, 20 plaques on B. Calculate the amount of recombination.

Solution:

In order to compare the numbers of plaques on B and K, the data must be corrected for the dilution factor. If 20 plaques are produced by a 10^9 dilution, the lesser dilution (10^7) would be expected to produce 100 times as many plaques.

$$\text{Recombination percentage} = \frac{200(\text{no. of plaques on K})}{\text{no. of plaques on B}} = \frac{200(2)}{20(100)} = 0.2\%$$

12.8. Seven deletion mutants within the A cistron of the rII region of phage T4 were tested in all pairwise combinations for wild-type recombinants. In the table below of results, + = recombination, 0 = no recombination. Construct a topological map for these deletions.

	1	2	3	4	5	6	7
1	0	+	0	0	+	0	0
2		0	0	0	+	+	0
3			0	0	+	+	0
4				0	+	0	0
5					0	0	0
6						0	0
7							0

Solution:

If two deletions overlap to any extent, no wild-type recombinants can be formed.

(1) Deletion 1 overlaps with 3, 4, 6, and 7 but not with 2 or 5.

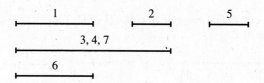

(2) Deletion 2 overlaps with 3, 4, and 7 but not with 1, 5, or 6.

(3) Deletion 3 overlaps with 1, 2, 4, and 7 but not with 5 or 6.

(4) Deletion 4 overlaps with 1, 2, 3, 6, and 7 but not with 5.

(5) Deletion 5 overlaps with 6 and 7 but not with 1, 2, 3, or 4. To satisfy these conditions we will shift 5 to the left of 1 and extend 7 into part of region 5 so that the overlaps in step (4) have not changed. Now segment 5 can overlap 6 and 7 without overlapping 1, 2, 3, or 4.

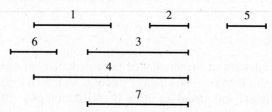

(6) Deletion 6 overlaps with 1, 4, 5, and 7 but not with 2 or 3. No change is required.

(7) Deletion 7 overlaps with all other regions, just as it was temporarily diagrammed in step 5. This completes the topological map. Altough the overlaps satisfy the conditions in the table, we have no information on the actual lengths of the individual deletions.

12.9. Five point mutations (*a–e*) were tested for wild-type recombinants with each of the seven deletion mutants in Problem 12.8. Determine the order of the point mutations and modify the topological map accordingly.

	1	2	3	4	5	6	7
a	0	+	0	0	+	+	0
b	+	+	+	0	+	0	0
c	+	+	+	+	0	0	0
d	0	+	+	0	+	0	0
e	+	0	0	0	+	+	0

Solution:

A deletion mutation cannot recombine to give wild type with a point mutant that lies within its boundaries. The topological map was developed in Problem 12.8.

(1) Mutant *a* does not recombine with 1, 3, 4, and 7 and therefore must be in a region common to all of these deletions.

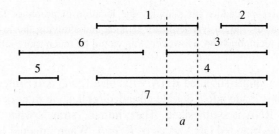

(2) Mutant *b* does not recombine with 4, 6, and 7 and thus lies in a region common to these three deletions. As the topological map stands in step (1), a point mutant could not be in regions 4, 6, and 7 without also being in region 1. Therefore this information allows us to modify the topological map by shortening deletion 1, but still overlapping deletion 6. This now gives us a region in which *b* can exist.

(3) Mutant *c* lies in a region common to deletions 5, 6, and 7. Mutant *d* lies in a region common to deletions 1, 4, 6, and 7. Mutant *e* lies in a region common to deletions 2, 3, 4, and 7.

Thus the order of these point mutations is *c-b-d-a-e* and the topological map is modified as shown in step (2).

12.10. Propose a procedure for establishing the location of a lambda prophage with respect to other bacterial genes.

Solution:

Cross a donor Hfr cell (lysogenic for lambda) with a nonlysogenic F⁻ recipient. Once the lambda genome has been transferred via conjugation to the F⁻ recipient cell, the cell often will die by lysis (a phenomenon known as zygotic induction). Using the interrupted mating technique (blender treatment), it should be possible to determine the point at which the frequencies of origin-proximal recombinants decrease with time. At this point, all of the lambda genome has been donated and can therefore be related on the temporal map to the location of other bacterial genes.

Since recipient cells contain no repressor (and no unbound repressor is likely to be transferred during conjugation), the exogenous prophage has a good chance of entering the lytic cycle because relatively high levels of repressor are required to establish the lysogenic state within the F⁻ recipient cell. A lysogenic cell usually contains sufficient unbound ("cytoplasmic") repressor to inhibit superinfection by one or a few lambda phages, but a nonlysogenic cell has no immunity to infection by exogenous lambda phages or lambda prophages. Hence, in the latter case, zygotic induction of exogenous lambda prophages has a good chance of occurring.

An alternative procedure for mapping the location of prophage lambda is by mating a nonlysogenic Hfr strain with an F⁻ strain lysogenic for lambda and studying the loss of immunity to superinfection by lambda through recombination. However, this would be much more laborious than the previous procedure.

12.11. Phage MS2 is a single-stranded RNA virus of *E. coli*. After infecting a cell, the phage RNA (the "plus" strand) is made into a double-stranded replicative intermediate form ("plus–minus") from which "plus" RNA is synthesized. The "minus" strands when isolated are not infective. Phage X174 is a single-stranded DNA virus of *E. coli*. When infected into a bacterium, the same events as described for MS2 occur, but the "minus" strands when isolated are infective. Devise a reasonable hypothesis to account for these observations.

Solution:

The DNA "minus" strand can serve as a template and can utilize the bacterial enzyme DNA polymerase for replication. The "minus" strand of RNA does not code for the enzyme that replicates RNA (RNA synthetase), and this enzyme is absent in uninfected bacteria. The "plus" strand of RNA carries the coded instructions for this enzyme and acts first as mRNA for enzyme synthesis. In the presence of the enzyme, single-stranded RNA can form a complementary strand and becomes a double-helical replicative form.

Supplementary Problems

BACTERIA

12.12. Approximately 10^8 *E. coli* cells of a mutant strain are plated on complete medium forming a bacterial lawn. Replica plates are prepared containing minimal medium supplemented by the amino acids arginine, lysine, and serine. (*a*) From the results, determine the genotype of the mutant strain. (*b*) Explain the colonies which appear on the replica plates.

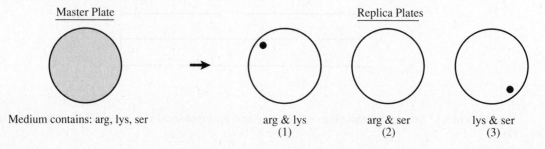

Master Plate

Replica Plates

Medium contains: arg, lys, ser

arg & lys
(1)

arg & ser
(2)

lys & ser
(3)

12.13. Two triple auxotrophic bacterial strains are conjugated in broth, diluted and plated onto complete agar (master plate). Replica plates containing various supplements are then made from the master. From the position of each clone and the type of media on which it is found, determine its genotype.

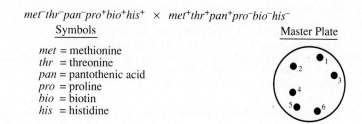

$$met^-thr^-pan^-pro^+bio^+his^+ \ \times \ met^+thr^+pan^+pro^-bio^-his^-$$

Symbols   Master Plate

met = methionine
thr = threonine
pan = pantothenic acid
pro = proline
bio = biotin
his = histidine

Replica plates: Each dish contains minimal medium plus the supplements shown at the bottom.

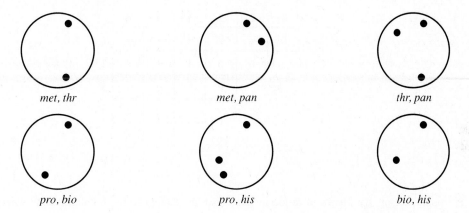

met, thr met, pan thr, pan

pro, bio pro, his bio, his

12.14. A bacterial strain unable to synthesize methionine (met^-) is transduced by a strain unable to synthesize isoleucine ($ileu^-$). The broth culture is diluted and plated on minimal medium supplemented with isoleucine. An equivalent amount of diluted broth culture is plated on minimal medium. Eighteen clones appeared on the minimal plates and 360 on the isoleucine plates. Calculate the standardized recombination ratio.

12.15. Calculate the standardized recombination ratio between two mutants of the arginine locus, using the following information. A bacterial strain that is doubly auxotrophic for thymine and arginine ($thy^-arg_{E1}^-$) is transformed by using a high concentration of DNA from a single auxotrophic strain ($thy^+arg_{E2}^-$). Identical dilutions are plated on minimal medium and on minimal plus arginine. For every colony which appears on the unsupplemented plates there are about 120 colonies on the serine-supplemented plates.

12.16. Two mutants at the tryptophan locus, trp_A^- and trp_B^-, are known to be close to a cysteine locus (cys). A bacterial strain of genotype $cys^+ \ trp_A^-$ is transduced by phage from a bacterial strain that is $cys^- \ trp_B^-$. The reciprocal cross is also made wherein the strain $cys^- \ trp_B^-$ is transduced by phage from a strain that is cys^+ trp_A^-. In both cases, the numbers of prototrophic recombinants are equivalent. Determine the order of the tryptophan mutants relative to the cysteine marker.

12.17. A cross is made between the streptomycin-resistant (str^r) F^- strain of genotype $gal^- thr^- azi^r lac^- Ton^r$ $mal^- xyl^- leu^-$ and the prototrophic Hfr strain having opposite characters. After 60 minutes of contact, samples are transferred to plates with minimal medium plus streptomycin. The original mixture is in the ratio 2×10^7 Hfr to 4×10^8 F^-. The percentages of each Hfr gene transferred are: 72% Ton^s, 0% mal^+, 27% gal^+, 91% azi^s, 0% xyl^+, 48% lac^+. (a) How many F^- cells exist in the original mixture for every Hfr cell? (b) What is the counterselective agent that prevents Hfr individuals from obscuring the detection of recombinants? (c) In what order are these genes probably being transferred by the Hfr strain?

12.18. Four Hfr strains of *E. coli* are known to transfer their genetic material during conjugation in different sequences. Given the time of entry of the markers into the F^- recipient, construct a genetic map that includes all of these markers and label the time distance between adjacent gene pairs.

Strain 1.	Markers:	*arg - thy - met - thr*
	Time in minutes:	15 21 32 48

Strain 2.	Markers:	*mal - met - thi - thr - try*
	Time in minutes:	10 17 22 33 57

Strain 3.	Markers:	*phe - his - bio - azi - thr - thi*
	Time in minutes:	6 11 33 48 49 60

Strain 4.	Markers:	*his - phe - arg - mal*
	Time in minutes:	18 23 35 45

12.19. Abortive transductants are relatively stable merozygotes which can be used for complementation tests. Six mutants were tested in all pairwise combinations, yielding the results shown in the table ($+$ = complementation, 0 = noncomplementation). Construct a complementation map consistent with the data.

	1	2	3	4	5	6	
	0	+	0	+	+	+	1
		0	0	+	+	+	2
			0	+	+	+	3
				0	0	+	4
					0	0	5
						0	6

12.20. Six point mutants are known to reside in three cistrons. Complete the following table where $+$ = complementation and 0 = noncomplementation.

	1	2	3	4	5	6
1	0	+		+	+	+
2		0	+			+
3			0	0		
4				0		
5					0	+
6						0

12.21. Given the topological map of 6 deletion mutants shown below, predict the results of recombination experiments involving the 5 point mutants (*a–e*) with each of the 6 deletions (1–6). Complete the accompanying table of results by using $+$ for recombination and 0 for no recombination.

	Deletions					
	1	2	3	4	5	6
a						
b						
c						
d						
e						

12.22. Five point mutations (*a–e*) were tested for wild-type recombinants with each of the five deletions shown in the topological map below. The results are listed in the table below (+ = recombination, 0 = no recombination). Determine the order of the point mutations.

Deletions

	1	2	3	4	5
a	0	0	+	+	+
b	+	+	+	0	+
c	0	0	+	+	0
d	0	+	0	0	0
e	0	+	0	0	+

12.23. Several lines of evidence suggest that the circular chromosome of *E. coli* has two replicating Y-forks. The length of one whole unreplicated chromosome is 1300 micrometers (about 500 times longer than the *E. coli* cell). There are ten base pairs per one complete turn of the DNA double helix, equivalent to 34 angstroms or 3.4×10^{-3} micrometers. (*a*) How many nucleotide base pairs are in the *E. coli* DNA complement or genome? (*b*) If the *E. coli* genome is replicated in 40 minutes at 37°C by two replicating forks, how many revolutions per minute (rpm) must the parental double helix make to allow separation of its complementary nucleotide strands during replication?

12.24. DNA damage (mutation) is an essential initiation event for a cell to transform into a cancerous state, but it is not the only event causing cancer. Therefore, DNA-damaging agents (mutagens) are only *potential* carcinogens (agents causing cancer). Most chemical carcinogens are not biologically active in their original form; they must first be metabolized to carcinogenic metabolites. Bruce Ames devised a test for screening chemicals for their potential carcinogenic properties. The **Ames test** is currently the standard test for a quantitative estimate of the mutagenic potency of a chemical. This test employs an auxotrophic strain of *Salmonella typhimurium* that cannot make the amino acid histidine (*his*⁻). To increase the sensitivity of the tester strain (1) it carries a mutation that makes the cell envelope more permeable to allow penetration of the test chemicals, (2) its capacity for excision repair is eliminated so that most of the primary lesions remain unhealed, and (3) a genetic element that makes DNA replication more error prone is introduced via a plasmid. Rat liver extract is added to a minimal medium culture plate coated with a thin layer of these bacteria. The chemical to be tested is impregnated in a disc of filter paper; the paper is placed in the center of the plate. After 2 days of incubation, the number of colonies are counted. (*a*) What events are being scored by the colony counts? (*b*) Why was mammalian liver extract added to the test? (*c*) Diagram the expected distribution of colonies on a plate containing a known carcinogen. Explain why this distribution develops. (*d*) Suppose that the test chemical (e.g., nitrosoguanidine) is mixed with the bacteria prior to plating at two dosages (low and high). A control is run simultaneously with these two doses. Diagram the expected distribution of colonies on these three plates.

12.25. When bacterial DNA is damaged by a mutagenic agent, excision repair normally operates to repair the lesion. This process is less than 100% efficient, however, so that some residual lesions remain unrepaired. If these lesions delay replication of DNA, an error-prone "SOS repair" system becomes operative involving activation and increased production of a multifunctional protein called RecA protein (for "recombination"). RecA protein interferes with cell partition, resulting in elongation of cells into filaments. RecA protein also cleaves lambda repressor; this repressor must remain intact for the virus to remain dormant as a prophage. *E. coli* strain B is lysogenic for lambda; strain A is not lysogenic for lambda. This knowledge led Moreau, Bailone, and Devoret to devise a "prophage induction test" or "inductest" for potential carcinogens. Lysogenic strain B of *E. coli* is made defective in its excision repair system and genetically modified to make the cell envelopes permeable to a wide variety of test chemicals. This special strain is mixed with indicator strain A and rat liver extract; the mixture is then plated; the medium is covered with a thin layer of indicator bacteria interspersed with a few lysogenic bacteria. The test chemical is applied to a filter paper disc and placed in the center of the plate for a "spot test." (*a*) After incubation, how is DNA damage assayed? (*b*) Why is strain A required as an indicator? (*c*) What advantage does an inductest have over an

Ames test? (*d*) Explain the selective advantage of lysogenic induction. (*e*) Genetic engineers have spliced the gene for galactokinase into a bacterial chromosome, thereby creating an organism for assaying mutagens by an enzymatic activity test. Where was this gene inserted into the chromosome and how does the system work?

12.26. A given transposable element becomes duplicated at a fairly constant (although usually low) rate. Therefore, over evolutionary time, the descendants of a bacterial cell might be expected to contain thousands of copies of such a transposon. However, the number of copies of bacterial transposons is very low (usually only one or two per cell). (*a*) Offer an explanation for this low copy number. (*b*) Why have most bacterial transposons been isolated from plasmids rather than from the bacterial chromosome?

REGULATION OF GENE ACTIVITY

12.27. In addition to the i^+ allele, producing repressor for the lactose system in *E. coli* and the constitutive i^- allele, a third allele i^s has been found, the product of which is unable to combine with the inducer (lactose). Hence the repressor ("superrepressor") made by i^s remains unbound and free to influence the operator locus. (*a*) Order the three alleles of the i locus in descending order of dominance according to their ability to influence the lactose operator. (*b*) Order the 4 alleles of the p locus in descending order of dominance according to their ability to bind RNA polymerase. (*c*) Using + for production and 0 for nonproduction of the enzymes permease (P) and β-galactosidase (β-gal), complete the following table. *Hint:* See Example 12.7.

Genotype	Inducer Absent		Inducer Present	
	P	β-gal	P	β-gal
(1) $i^+o^+y^+z^+$				
(2) $i^-o^+y^+z^+$				
(3) $i^so^+y^+z^+$				
(4) $i^+o^cy^+z^+$				
(5) $i^-o^cy^+z^+$				
(6) $i^so^cy^+z^+$				

12.28. For each of the following partial diploids, determine whether enzyme formation is constitutive or inductive: (*a*) i^+/i^+, o^+/o^+; (*b*) i^+/i^+, o^+/o^c; (*c*) i^+/i^+, o^c/o^c; (*d*) i^+/i^-, o^+/o^+; (*e*) i^-/i^-, o^+/o^+.

12.29. In the lactose system of *E. coli*, y^+ makes permease, an enzyme essential for the rapid transportation of galactosides from the medium to the interior of the cell. Its allele y^- makes no permease. The galactoside lactose must enter the cell in order to induce the z^+ gene to produce the enzyme β-galactosidase. The allele z^- makes a related but enzymatically inactive protein called *Cz*. Predict the production or nonproduction of each of these products with a normal operator o^+ by placing a + or 0, respectively, in the table below.

Genotype	Inducer Absent			Inducer Present		
	P	β-gal	Cz	P	β-gal	Cz
(*a*) $i^+y^+z^-$						
(*b*) $i^+y^+z^+$						
(*c*) $i^-y^+z^+$						
(*d*) $i^+y^-z^+$						
(*e*) $i^-y^-z^-$						
(*f*) $i^-y^-z^+$						

12.30. In genotype (1) of the table below, the i^- allele allows constitutive enzyme production by the y^+ and z^+ genes in an operon with a normal operator gene o^+. The action of i^- might be explained by one of two hypothesis: (1) i^- produces an internal *inducer,* thus eliminating the need for lactose in the medium to induce enzyme synthesis; i^+ produces no internal inducer, or (2) i^+ produces a *repressor* substance that, in the absence of lactose inducer, blocks enzyme formation, but in the presence of lactose inducer the repressor becomes inactivated to allow enzyme synthesis; i^- produces no repressor. (*a*) Assuming dominance of the i^- allele under the first hypothesis in an *E. coli* partial diploid of the constitution i^+/i^-, would internal inducer be produced? (*b*) Under the conditions of part (*a*), would enzymes be produced constitutively or inductively in a wild-type *lac* operon? (*c*) Assuming dominance of the i^+ allele under the second hypothesis in a partial diploid of the constitution i^+/i^-, would repressor be produced? (*d*) Under the conditions of part (*c*), would enzymes be produced constitutively or inductively in a wild-type *lac* operon? (*e*) From the pattern of reactions exhibited by genotypes (2) and (3) in the table below, determine which of the two hypotheses is consistent with the data. (*f*) Is the repressor substance diffusible, or can it only act on loci in cis position with the *i* locus? How can this be determined from the information in the table?

Partial Diploid Genotype	Lactose Absent		Lactose Present	
	P	β-gal	P	β-gal
(1) $o^+y^-z^-i^-/o^+y^+z^+i^-$	+	+	+	+
(2) $o^+y^-z^-i^-/o^+y^+z^+i^+$	0	0	+	+
(3) $o^+y^-z^-i^+/o^+y^+z^+i^-$	0	0	+	+

12.31. The repressor for an inducible operon has two binding sites. (*a*) What are the specificities of these two sites? (*b*) List four kinds of single mutations that change the functions of such a repressor.

12.32. List two kinds of single mutations that can change the function of an operator.

12.33. The entry of lactose into a bacterial cell is mediated by a permease enzyme. In cells that have not previously been exposed to lactose, how can lactose enter an uninduced $i^+z^+y^+$ cell to affect induction of β-galactosidase synthesis?

12.34. A bacterial mutation renders a cell incapable of fermenting many sugars (e.g., lactose, sorbitol, xylose) simultaneously. The operons of genes specifying the respective catabolic enzymes are wild type (unmutated). Offer an explanation for this phenomenon.

12.35. The enzymes necessary for glucose catabolism are made constitutively by bacterial cells. When both glucose and lactose are added to the growth medium, glucose enters the cell by its own permease molecules embedded in the cell membrane. The operons for catabolizing lactose and other sugars fail to be activated even though a few respective permease molecules for these other sugars are normally present in the cell membrane. Explain.

12.36. Shown below is a hypothetical biosynthetic pathway subject to feedback inhibition; letters represent metabolites; numbers represent enzymes. Identify the enzymes that are most likely to be subject to feedback inhibition and their inhibitor(s). *Note:* The inhibitor may consist of more than one metabolite.

12.37. An antibiotic is a microbial product of low molecular weight that specifically interferes with the growth of microorganisms when it is present in exceedingly small amounts. Specify some of the physiological activities that might be interrupted by an appropriate antibiotic and the reason why human cells are not harmed.

BACTERIOPHAGES

12.38. Six deletion mutants within the A cistron of the *r*II region of phage T4 were tested in all pairwise combinations for wild-type recombinants. In the following table, + = recombination, 0 = no recombination. Construct a topological map for these deletions.

	1	2	3	4	5	6
1	0	0	0	0	0	0
2		0	0	0	0	+
3			0	+	0	0
4				0	+	+
5					0	+
6						0

12.39. Five depletion mutants within the B cistron of the *r*II region of phage T4 were tested in all pairwise combinations for wild-type recombinants. In the following table of results, + = recombination, 0 = no recombination. Construct a topological map for these deletions.

	1	2	3	4	5
1	0	+	+	0	0
2		0	+	0	+
3			0	+	0
4				0	0
5					0

12.40. The DNA of bacteriophage T4 contains approximately 200,000 nucleotide pairs. The *r*II region of the T4 genome occupies about 1% of its total genetic length. Benzer has found about 300 sites are separable by recombination within the *r*II region. Determine the average number of nucleotides in each recon.

12.41. The molecular weight of DNA in phage T4 is estimated to be 160×10^6. The average molecular weight of each nucleotide is approximately 400. The total genetic map of T4 is calculated to be approximately 2500 recombination units long. With what frequency are r^+ recombinants expected to be formed when two different *r* mutants (with mutations at adjacent nucleotides) are crossed?

12.42 A number of mutations were found in the *r*II region of phage T4. From the recombination data shown in the table below, determine whether each mutant is a point defect or a deletion (+ = recombination, 0 = no recombination). Two of the four mutants have been known to undergo back mutation; the other two have never been observed to backmutate. Draw a topological map to represent your interpretation.

	1	2	3	4
1	0	0	0	+
2		0	+	0
3			0	+
4				0

12.43. *Escherichia coli* strain B is doubly infected with two *r*II mutants of phage T4. A 6×10^7 dilution of the lysate is plated on *E. coli* B. A 2×10^5 dilution is plated on *coli* K. Twelve plaques appeared on strain K, 16 on strain B. Calculate the amount of recombination between these two mutants.

12.44. A nonlytic response usually is observed in lysogenic (λ) *E. coli* cells when conjugated with nonlysogenic Hfr donors or in crosses between Hfr (λ) $\times$ F$^-$(λ). The donated prophage is almost never inherited by the recombinants. Lysis is very anomalous in crosses of Hfr (λ) $\times$ F$^-$. Explain these observations.

12.45. Temperate phages such as lambda sometimes produce turbid plaques on lambda-sensitive indicator cells; virulent phages that cannot lysogenize always produce clear plaques on cells of their host range. (*a*) Offer an explanation for the turbid plaques. (*b*) Some lambda mutants produce only clear plaques. What genetic locus is most likely mutant in these cases?

Review Questions

Matching Questions   For each item in the numbered column choose an item from the lettered column with which it is most closely associated. Each letter may be used only once.

1.	Rolling circle	A.	Topoisomerase
2.	DNA gyrase	B.	Restricted transduction
3.	Velvet	C.	Concatemers
4.	Competence	D.	Bacteriolysis
5.	Pilus	E.	"Male" cells
6.	Lambda phage	F.	Tryptophan operon
7.	Sex-duction	G.	Transformation
8.	Plaque	H.	Viral protein
9.	Capsid	I.	Replica plating
10.	Attenuation	J.	F′ plasmid

Vocabulary   For each of the following definitions, give the appropriate term and spell it correctly.

1. Descriptive of all mutant strains of bacteria requiring supplementation to minimal medium for their growth.

2. A colony of genetically identical bacterial cells.

3. The Greek letter representing an intermediate structure of the bacterial genophore when it is halfway through bidirectional replication from a single origin.

4. A region of the bacterial cell membrane to which the bacterial DNA is attached.

5. A solid mass of bacterial cells covering the surface of nutrient agar medium in a Petri dish.

6. A form of bacterial recombination requiring cell-to-cell contact.

7. A form of genetic recombination between bacterial cells that is mediated by a bacteriophage.

8. A partially diploid exconjugant.

9. A bacteriophage genophore that is integrated into the chromosome of a host cell.

10. A small, circular DNA molecule capable of replication independent of the genophore in its bacterial host.

True-False Questions   Answer each of the following statements either true (T) or false (F).

1. A single lambda phage particle cannot be cyclically permuted.

2. Phage M13 infects *E. coli* but neither kills nor lyses its host cell.

3. An "F minus" (F⁻) cell usually remains F⁻ after conjugation with an "F plus" (F⁺) cell.

4. When the F factor integrates into the host cell's genophore, the cell becomes Hfr.

5. Zygotic induction occurs by exposure of a nonlysogenic F⁻ cell to an antibiotic.

6. Restricted transduction occurs only with a phage that has a specific site at which it regularly integrates into the genophore of the host cell.

7. Abortive transduction occurs when a transducing phage fails to become integrated into the genophore of the host cell.

8. Viruses do not increase in mass once the virion is formed.

9. As in cells, DNA has been found to be the genetic material of all viruses investigated thus far.

10. Catabolite repression occurs when an active repressor protein binds to an operator.

Multiple-Choice Questions   Choose the one best answer.

1. Which of the following is classified as a procaryote?   (*a*) protozoa   (*b*) yeast   (*c*) bacteria   (*d*) algae   (*e*) more than one of the above

2. Which of the following is found in procaryotes?   (*a*) mitochondria   (*b*) histones   (*c*) actin and myosin   (*d*) formylated methionine   (*e*) more than one of the above

3. Which of the following is not characteristic of viruses?   (*a*) only one kind of nucleic acid per virion   (*b*) inhibited by antibiotics   (*c*) nonmotile   (*d*) pass through bacterial filters   (*e*) more than one of the above

4. Which of the following DNA modifications is normally used by bacteria to prevent digestion of the genophore by the cell's own endonucleases?   (*a*) methylation   (*b*) glycosylation   (*c*) phosphorylation   (*d*) deamination   (*e*) intercalation

5. Lambda phage can transduce bacterial genes only at or near the gene concerned with   (*a*) interferon synthesis   (*b*) immunity repressor   (*c*) CAP   (*d*) lactose fermentation   (*e*) galactose fermentation

6. The physiologically receptive state in which a bacterial cell is able to be transformed is called   (*a*) sensitized   (*b*) activated   (*c*) competent   (*d*) lysogenic   (*e*) inducible

7. Which of the following is not a method for genetic recombination in bacteria?   (*a*) translocation   (*b*) conjugation with Hfr transfer   (*c*) transformation   (*d*) sex-duction   (*e*) transduction

8. The most commonly used trait for counterselection when mapping genes by interrupted conjugation is   (*a*) lactose fermentation   (*b*) antibiotic resistance   (*c*) phage resistance   (*d*) vitamin synthesis   (*e*) pilus formation

9. Which of the following modes of replication is not used by bacteria?   (*a*) binary fission   (*b*) rolling circle   (*c*) theta replication   (*d*) mitosis   (*e*) bidirectional replication

10. The distances between bacterial genes, as determined from interrupted conjugation experiments, are measured in units of   (*a*) recombination   (*b*) nucleotide pairs   (*c*) minutes   (*d*) micrometers   (*e*) percentage of genophore

Answers to Supplementary Problems

12.12. (*a*) *arg⁻ lys⁻ ser⁻* (triple auxotroph)   (*b*) Plate (1) contains a mutation to *ser⁺*, plate (3) contains a mutation to *arg⁺*.

12.13.

Clone	Genotype of Clone					
	met	*thr*	*pan*	*pro*	*bio*	*his*
1	+	+	+	+	+	+
2	+	−	−	+	+	+
3	−	+	−	+	+	+
4	+	+	+	+	+	−
5	+	+	+	−	+	+
6	+	−	+	+	+	+

12.14. 20% recombination

12.15. 0.83% recombination

12.16. cys - trp_B - trp_A

12.17. (*a*) 20   (*b*) Streptomycin; Hfr is streptomycin-sensitive (str^s).   (*c*) Origin - (thr^+ leu^+) - azi^s - Ton^s - lac^+ - gal^+ - str^s - (mal^+ xyl^+). The genes for synthesizing the amino acids threonine and leucine must have entered first, otherwise none of the other recombinants could survive on unsupplemented medium. *Note:* The order of markers within parentheses has not been determined.

12.18. arg - thy - mal - met - thi - thr - azi - bio - try - his - phe - arg
  6   4   7   5   11   1   15   8   14   5   12

12.19.

12.20.

Cistron A   Cistron B   Cistron C

	1	2	3	4	5	6
1	0	+	+	+	+	+
2		0	+	+	0	+
3			0	0	+	0
4				0	+	0
5					0	+
6						0

Note: Name of cistron is arbitrary.

12.21.

Point Mutations	Deletions					
	1	2	3	4	5	6
a	0	+	+	0	0	+
b	+	+	0	+	+	0
c	+	0	0	+	+	+
d	0	0	+	+	0	+
e	+	0	0	+	+	0

12.22. a - c - d - e - b

12.23. (a) $\dfrac{1300 \text{ micrometers} \times 10 \text{ base pairs/turn}}{3.4 \times 10^{-3} \text{ micrometers/turn}} = 3.9 \times 10^{6}$ or 3900 kilobase pairs

(b) Rate of chain growth $= \dfrac{3900 \text{ kilobases}}{2(2400 \text{ seconds})} = 0.8$ kilobase/second

$\dfrac{800 \text{ base pairs/second}}{10 \text{ bp/rev}} \times 60 \text{ seconds/minute} = 80 \text{ revolutions} \times 60 \text{ minutes}^{-1} = 4800$

revolutions/minute

or about as fast as a laboratory centrifuge.

12.24. (a) Back mutations (reverse mutations) from his^{-} to his^{+}.   (b) It supplies the mammalian metabolic functions that are usually required to convert a chemical into its carcinogenic metabolites.   (c) After 2 days, most of the his^{-} bacteria have died for lack of histidine. Back mutation rates are expected to be proportional to concentration of the chemical that forms a radially diminishing concentration gradient around the paper disc. Close to the disc there is a zone in which no cells grow because of toxic levels of the chemical. Beyond this zone there may be so many his^{+} revertants that the cells almost form a continuous lawn. At the periphery are a few larger clones (because they are isolated) representing spontaneous his^{+} mutants that have not been exposed to the chemical.

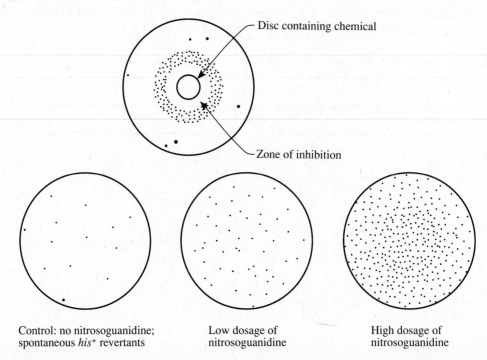

Disc containing chemical

Zone of inhibition

Control: no nitrosoguanidine;   Low dosage of   High dosage of
spontaneous his^{+} revertants   nitrosoguanidine   nitrosoguanidine

12.25. (a) DNA damage activates RecA protein that then cleaves lambda repressor and opens up the viral genome for replication (induction). The cell bursts and releases viruses that infect and lyse the indicator strain A, causing plaques (holes) to appear in the bacterial "lawn" surrounding the paper disc.   (b) If a cell of strain B is induced to lysis, the viruses cannot multiply in other cells of the same strain because active lambda repressor is present in these cells as a product of their prophages. Therefore, a nonlysogenic strain (A) is required to indicate how many viruses have been induced by the chemical treatment.   (c) The inductest can assay a potential carcinogen at doses that would kill the tester bacteria in an Ames test (giving a false-negative reaction). The Ames test only detects the rare backmutations of his^{-} to his^{+}, whereas DNA damage at any site can initiate lysogenic induction (a mass effect, independent of cell survival by toxic chemicals). (d) If DNA of the host cell cannot replicate, the cell is likely to die. Under these conditions it would be advantageous for a prophage to enter the lytic cycle and thereby possibly infect a "healthier" cell (like a "rat leaving a sinking ship").   (e) The gene for galactokinase was inserted adjacent to (and under the control of) the lambda repressor. When the mutagen damages DNA, RecA protein is activated and cleaves the repressor; this opens the operon to RNA polymerase and allows synthesis of the enzyme galactokinase, the activity of which can be quantitated spectrophotometrically when supplied with its substrate.

12.26. (*a*) Most of the DNA in bacteria, unlike the DNA in eucaryotic cells, is coding information. There is relatively little DNA that is not serving some function. Thus, the movement of most transposons to a new location would inactivate one or more vital genes, causing cell death or weakening it so that it cannot compete with normal cells.   (*b*) Plasmids rarely are essential to their host cells, and therefore could tolerate the integration of transposable elements without interfering with vital gene functions.

12.27. (*a*) i^s, i^+, i^- (*b*) p^s, p^+, p^{icr}, p^-

		Inducer Absent		Inducer Present	
		P	β-gal	P	β-gal
	(1)	0	0	+	+
(*c*)	(2, 4, 5, 6)	+	+	+	+
	(3)	0	0	0	0

12.28. (*a*), (*d*) = inductive;   (*b*), (*c*), (*e*) = constitutive

12.29.

	Inducer Absent			Inducer Present		
	P	β-gal	Cz	P	β-gal	Cz
(*a*)	0	0	0	+	0	+
(*b*)	0	0	0	+	+	0
(*c*)	+	+	0	+	+	0
(*d*)	0	0	0	0	+	0
(*e*)	0	0	+	0	0	+
(*f*)	0	+	0	0	+	0

All + answers for parts (d), (e), and (f) are due to new level of products by sneak synthesis.

12.30. (*a*) Yes   (*b*) Constitutively   (*c*) Yes   (*d*) Inductively   (*e*) Note that in genotypes (2) and (3) the i^- allele fails to produce enzymes in the absence of the external inducer (lactose); it fails to exhibit dominance. Therefore the first hypothesis is incorrect. Under the second hypothesis, i^+ is dominant and produces a repressor that (in the absence of lactose inducer) blocks enzyme synthesis as seen in genotypes (2) and (3). (*f*) Genotype (3) has y^+ and z^+ on one DNA molecule and i^+ on a different DNA molecule. Yet in the absence of lactose inducer, the repressor made by i^+ still prevents the production of enzymes by y^+ and z^+. Therefore, the repressor must be able to act at a distance (it behaves as a diffusible substance) on genes that are either on the same DNA molecule (cis position) or on a different DNA molecule (trans position).

12.31. (*a*) One site is for the operator locus; the other site is for the inducer.   (*b*) (1) Inactivation of the operator binding site causes the repressor to be incapable of binding to the operator. (2) Increasing the operator binding affinity results in permanent repressor binding even in the presence of inducer. (3) Inactivation of the inducer binding site makes derepression impossible. (4) Increasing the inducer binding affinity results in permanent allosteric change, and once the inducer is bound, the repressor can never bind to an operator.

12.32. (1) A change that prevents repressor binding. (2) Modifications that increase repressor binding so that operons cannot be derepressed even when inducer is bound.

12.33. Occasionally a repressor molecule will momentarily become dissociated from the operator and RNA polymerase will attach and begin transcription of the β-galactosidase and permease genes before the repressor reattaches. This so-called sneak synthesis endows the cell with enough enzymes to transport a few lactose molecules through the plasma membrane; these will be catabolized to the true inducer (allolactose) so that derepression can occur.

12.34. The mutation could be in the gene for adenyl cyclase or in the gene for catabolite activator protein (CAP).

12.35. Glucose enters the cell via its own permease and is metabolized. One or more glucose metabolites somehow decrease the intracellular level of cAMP. In the absence of cAMP, CAP cannot bind to the left end of the lactose (or other sugar) promoter(s) and hence the binding of RNA polymerase to the right end of the promoter(s) is not fostered. Some lactose gains entry into the cell via its permease and inactivates the lactose repressor so that the lactose operator locus is open. However, little or no mRNAs are made from such operons if RNA polymerase binding is inefficient at the respective promoter site(s).

12.36. I inhibits 7; J inhibits 9; G alone or (I, J) together inhibits 5; E inhibits 3; enzyme 1 could be inhibited by (I, J, E), (G, E), (I, J, C), or (C, G).

12.37. Cell wall formation is interfered with by penicillins and cephalosporins. DNA replication is prevented by the bleomycins and anthracyclines. Rifamycins interrupt the transcription of DNA into RNA. Translation is disrupted by erythromycin, the tetracyclines, chloramphenicol, and streptomycin. Antibiotics are toxic for microorganisms but safe for humans because all of these metabolic processes are subtly different in bacteria and humans.

12.38.

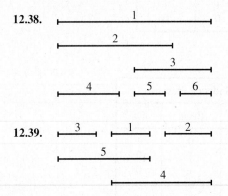

12.39.

12.40. Approximately 7 nucleotides per recon.

12.41. 0.00625% of all progeny are expected to be r^+ recombinants.

12.42. m_1 and m_2 are deletions; m_3 and m_4 are point mutations.

12.43. 0.5% recombination

12.44. Repressor is already present in the cytoplasm of the $F^-(\lambda)$ recipient cell. It binds to the operators that prevent prophage induction (vegetative reproduction of the phage) in either the $F^-(\lambda)$ or the Hfr (λ) donated chromosome segment. Early enzymes are therefore not produced, and recombination (leading to the inheritance of the donated lambda genes) cannot occur. Nonlysogenic F^- cells do not contain repressor. There are so few repressor molecules in a lysogenized cell that it is unlikely that free repressor would be bound to the newly synthesized donor fragment that moves almost immediately through the pilus into the F^- recipient. When the prophage from Hfr (λ) enters the F^- cell, a race occurs between the production of lambda repressor and an early protein of vegetative phage development. The outcome of this race is not predictable; hence lysis is unpredictable in such crosses.

12.45. (*a*) Turbid plaques are due to secondary growth of lysogenized bacteria derived from the lambda-sensitive indicator strain. (*b*) Mutations of the gene coding for the lambda repressor of lytic activity are likely to produce an inactive (nonfunctional) repressor; hence these mutants cannot lysogenize the indicator strain.

Answers to Review Questions

Matching Questions

1. C   2. A   3. I   4. G   5. E   6. B   7. J   8. D   9. H   10. F

Vocabulary

1. auxotrophic
2. clone
3. theta (θ)
4. mesosome
5. lawn
6. conjugation
7. transduction
8. merozygote
9. prophage
10. plasmid

True-False Questions

1. T   2. T   3. F (usually becomes F$^+$)   4. T   5. F (exposure to a lysogenic Hfr donor)   6. T   7. T   8. T   9. F (a few have RNA genophores)   10. F (cAMP-CAP complex binds to promoter)

Multiple-Choice Questions

1. *c*   2. *d*   3. *b*   4. *a*   5. *e*   6. *c*   7. *a*   8. *b*   9. *d*   10. *c*

Chapter 13

Molecular Genetics

HISTORY

Prior to discovery of the chemical structure of the genetic material, the "gene" was an abstract, indivisible unit of heredity (comparable to the old concept of the indivisible atom). This period in history is referred to as **classical** or **formal genetics.** The word "formal" pertains to the extrinsic aspect of something as distinguished from its substance or material. Classical genetics has been extremely successful in elucidating many basic biological principles without understanding the nature of the gene. The era of **molecular genetics** followed the discovery of DNA structure when the fundamental unit of heredity was determined to be the DNA nucleotide and the "gene" was found to consist of an aggregate of nucleotides.

The histories of most scientific disciplines are generally characterized by relatively long periods of stagnation punctuated by bursts of rapid progress. Most of these flurries of research are initiated by new technical developments. This is certainly true of biochemistry and molecular biology. At least three major areas of technology have been influential in this respect: (1) instrumentation and techniques, (2) radioactive tracers, and (3) nucleic acid enzymology.

1. Instrumentation and Techniques.

(a) *Instrumentation.* The analytical ultracentrifuge was developed in the 1920s by Theodor Svedberg. The sedimentation rate of a substance during ultracentrifugation is mainly a function of its density and secondarily of its shape. The unit of sedimentation (S, in honor of Svedberg) is an expression of these parameters. This instrument has been modified for isolating organelles such as nuclei, ribosomes, mitochondria, and chloroplasts. It can be used for determining the minimum number of kinds of macromolecules in a biological specimen and for estimating the molecular weights of macromolecules.

The electron microscope was invented in the 1930s, and eventually enabled the direct visualization not only of cellular substructures but also of viruses and macromolecules. Circular genetic maps of microorganisms have been shown by electron microscopy to have a corresponding circular physical structure. Multiple ribosomes attached to an mRNA molecule (polysomes) have also been visualized by this instrument.

Electrophoresis is a technique that separates molecules according to their shapes, net charges and molecular weights in an electric field, usually on solid or semisolid support media such as paper or agar. Linus Pauling used this technique to differentiate sickle-cell hemoglobin from normal hemoglobin and determined (by protein sequence analysis) that the difference in electrophoretic mobilities of these proteins was due to a single amino acid difference in the β-chains. Nucleotide sequencing is usually performed on (poly)acrylamide gels; agarose gels are usually employed to isolate DNA fragments and in estimation of their molecular weights. Electrophoresis has been extensively used to differentiate **isozymes,** i.e., proteins possessing the same enzymatic properties but differing in primary structure.

X-ray-diffraction data from crystalline materials have been analyzed by electronic computers to help elucidate the three-dimensional shapes of nucleic acids (e.g., DNA, tRNAs) and proteins (e.g., myoglobins, viral capsomeres, enzymes).

During the mid 1940s and early 1950s, various forms of chromatography were perfected, enabling molecules to be separated by differences in solubilities in organic solvents, electrical charge, molecular weight, and specific binding properties for the support medium, or combinations of these factors. Erwin Chargaff used paper chromatography to determine the base compositions of DNAs from various sources. He found that the molecular ratio of adenine was equivalent to that of thymine and the ratio of guanine equals that of cytosine. This was a vital clue in the search for DNA structure utilized by James Watson and Francis Crick.

Automated equipment is now available for doing many repetitive biochemical tasks. DNA synthesizers ("gene machines") can be programmed to make oligonucleotide sequences of any desired composition. Automated instrumentation is now available for sequencing DNA or protein fragments. Computer programs have been developed to interpret data from electropherograms, and to scan data bases for similar or identical sequences.

(b) *Techniques.*   Several techniques have been developed to separate, rejoin, or break nucleic acid molecules. Separation of the complementary chains of a DNA molecule is known as **denaturation.** DNA is denatured if placed in alkali (0.2N NaOH) or when boiled. The latter process is referred to as **melting.** Separation of DNA strands can be detected by spectrophotometric instruments; **optical density** (OD) or **absorbance** at 260 nanometers increases during the melting process. The temperature at which the increase in OD_{260} is 50% of that attained when strand separation is complete is known as the **melting temperature (T_m).** Because G and C base-pair by three hydrogen bonds, whereas A and T base-pair by two hydrogen bonds, the higher the G-C content in DNA the higher the melting temperature. Melting is enhanced where there are clusters of A's and T's, and also when the purines (A, G) are on one strand and all the pyrimidines (T, C) are on the other strand.

If DNA is boiled and then quickly cooled, the strands will remain single; if cooled slowly, complementary strands will base-pair and reform double-helical DNA molecules. This process is called **renaturation** or **annealing.** Hybrid DNA-RNA molecules can be produced by analogous processes from single strands. RNA can be totally hydrolyzed to nucleotides by exposure to high pH (alkali). This property can be used to purify DNA from a mixture of DNA and RNA. Single-stranded DNA will bind to membranous filters made of nitrocellulose; RNA will pass through such filters. However, if single-stranded RNA is complementary to nitrocellulose-bound single strands of DNA, it will form DNA-RNA hybrid molecules and be retained by such a filter.

There are three main methods for breaking long DNA molecules into fragments of suitable size for base sequencing or for recombinant engineering: (1) shear degradation, (2) ultrasound, and (3) restriction endonuclease treatment. If a solution of DNA is subjected to the stirring forces of a Waring blender or forced through a narrow tube or orifice, the ends of long DNA strands will usually move at different speeds; this stretches the DNA and tends to break it near the middle. This phenomenon is called **shear degradation.** The higher the stirring speed or velocity of flow through an orifice, the greater the shearing force. The effectiveness of any shearing force increases with molecular size of the DNA, but decreases with concentration (because entanglement of DNA molecules reduces the effective stretching).

2. Radioactive Tracers.

Radioactive elements can be used as highly sensitive labels for detecting minute amounts of specific macromolecules.

> **Example 13.1.**   A. D. Hershey and M. Chase differentially labeled the nucleic acid and the protein components of T2 phages. They used radioactive ^{32}P in place of normal ^{31}P to label DNA; radioactive ^{35}S was used in place of normal ^{32}S to label protein (cysteine and methionine are two amino acids that contain sulfur). Since there is no phosphorus in phage proteins and no sulfur in nucleic acids, the fate of both viral components could be followed during the viral life cycle. After allowing the phages to become attached to sensitive *Escherichia coli* host cells, the mixture was subjected to the shearing forces of a Waring blender. The mixture was centrifuged to sediment the cells and then activity characteristic of each radionuclide was assayed in the pellet and in the supernatant fluid. All of the ^{32}P activity was found in the bacterial pellet and virtually all of the ^{35}S was found in the supernate. ^{32}P was found in some progeny phages, but no ^{35}S was found. The inference is that phages inject their DNA into host cells. Blender treatment shears the phage tail fibers from receptor sites on host cells; the empty phage protein capsids (ghosts) are therefore left free in the supernate. Semiconservative replication from the infecting ^{32}P-labeled DNA caused some progeny phages to be released with one of the original radioactively labeled infecting strands. This experiment was the first to demonstrate that DNA and not protein is genetic material in phages.

DNA labeled with radioactive nuclides can reveal its own presence in a photographic technique called **autoradiography** or **radioautography.** A preparation of DNA on a slide or on filter paper can be covered with a photographic film or emulsion. As the radionuclides undergo **radioactive disintegration,** or **decay,** they release charged particles and/or photons that cause a chemical reaction on the film. After development of the film, the location of the labeled DNA is revealed by dark spots. It was by autoradiography that John Cairns discovered the theta intermediate of circular DNA replication in bacteria.

Radioactively labeled thymidine can be used to differentiate DNA from RNA molecules because uracil usually replaces thymine in RNA. Tritium (^{3}H) is a radioactive isotope of hydrogen commonly used to label thymidine; the labeled nucleoside is called **tritiated thymidine.** By allowing thymine-deficient (thy^-) *E. coli* to grow in the presence of tritiated thymidine, its DNA becomes radioactively labeled. The **half-life** of tritium is 12.46 years, meaning that its radioactivity decreases by one-half each 12.46 years. Tritium-labeled thymidine and uridine are often used to tag or label newly synthesized DNA and RNA molecules, respectively. Tritium is often the radioisotope of choice in radioautography because it emits an extremely weak beta particle when it undergoes radioactive disintegration or decay. In a medium of unit density, the average tritium beta particle will penetrate only 1 micrometer. Therefore, in autoradiographs of tritium-labeled cells, darkened grains of the photographic emulsion will be localized within 1 micrometer of the decaying atoms.

A radioactive isotope of phosphorus (^{32}P) is also widely used to label nucleic acids; it emits a strong beta particle and has a half-life of 14.3 days. It is thus more radioactive ("hotter") than tritium and can reveal itself in much lower amounts than can tritium during the same decay period. An instrument called a **scintillation counter** is used to detect radioactive disintegrations. High-energy γ-rays can be detected by a crystal scintillation counter. A liquid scintillation counter must be used to detect weaker beta particles, although it can also detect γ-rays.

Any organic substance can be labeled with radioactive carbon (^{14}C). This isotope emits a weak beta particle and has a relatively long half-life of 5730 years. All living organisms incorporate a predictable amount of ^{14}C while alive. After death, ^{14}C decays to ^{14}N at the predictable rate of its half-life. This knowledge allows the dating of organic remains from the time of death up to about 40,000 years before the present.

Radioactive iodine (^{125}I) has a half-life of about 60 days, emits γ-rays, and is extensively used to label proteins of all kinds. This isotope is easily coupled to the amino acid tyrosine. Radioactive sulfur (^{35}S) is similarly used to label the amino acids cysteine and methionine; ^{35}S can also be used to label nucleic acids. ^{35}S is actually more desirable than ^{32}P for most autoradiography because it has a half-life of 87.1 days and emits a much weaker beta particle that gives sharper bands. It is much less hazardous to handle than ^{32}P and poses less waste disposal problems. Quantitation of small amounts (nanograms or picograms per milliliter) of these proteins can be accomplished by sophisticated techniques such as competitive protein binding assays and radioimmunoassays.

Even nonradioactive isotopes (e.g., ^{15}N) have been useful in solving fundamental problems in molecular biology (see Solved Problem 13.1).

3. Nucleic Acid Enzymology.

Nucleases are enzymes that hydrolyze nucleic acids. Those that detach terminal nucleotides, one at a time, are called exonucleases; those that break the sugar-phosphate backbone at nonterminal sites are called endonucleases. A deoxyribonuclease (DNase) attacks DNA molecules; a ribonuclease (RNase) degrades RNA molecules, especially at their single-stranded regions, where they are not internally base paired. Some endonucleases act specifically, cleaving the phosphodiester bonds of many different nucleotide sequences. Others, such as the bacterial **restriction endonucleases (RE),** break the backbone only at specific DNA sequences (RE recognition sites). Most RE recognition sites consist of 4–8 bp that are symmetrical around a midpoint, or axis of symmetry, formed on opposite DNA strands by inverted base sequences called **palindromes.** RE sites consisting of an odd number of base pairs cannot be completely symmetrical.

Example 13.2. A restriction endonuclease called EcoRI (derived from the bacterium *E. coli*) cuts bonds within the palindromic sequence at the arrows shown below.

┌ axis of symmetry

$^{5'}$G A A T T C$^{3'}$

$^{3'}$C T T A A G$^{5'}$

Notice that the $5' \rightarrow 3'$ nucleotide sequence within the palindrome is the same on both strands of the DNA. Another restriction endonuclease (HaeIII), derived from the bacterium *Haemophilus aegypticus*, snips DNA in the axis symmetry as shown below.

$^{5'}$G G C C$^{3'}$

$^{3'}$C C G G$^{5'}$

Many other enzymes are known to be involved in the replication, recombination, repair, modification, transcription and translation of nucleic acids, but those already discussed are the main ones utilized by recombinant DNA technology.

It is usually possible to construct a **restriction enzyme map** for any given DNA segment (linear or circular). Such a map diagrams the location of sites on the DNA segment where one or more restriction enzymes cleave the molecule. The sizes of the various restriction fragments can be expressed by molecular weight, but more commonly they are given in terms of base pairs (bp).

Example 13.3. A linear 10,000-bp segment of DNA is cut at two places by restriction enzyme HindIII into three fragments of sizes ($\times 10^4$ bp) 5, 3, and 2. There are three possible orders for these two cut sites.

(1) ___5___↓_3_↓_2_

(2) ___5___↓2↓___3___

(3) _2↓___5___↓___3___

To determine the correct order, a radioactive label can be attached to each $3'$ end of the double-stranded DNA segment before digesting it with HindIII. If fragments 5 and 2 are labeled, then order (1) must be correct; i.e., fragment 3 is in the middle.

DNA MANIPULATIONS

During the late 1970s, the science of genetics entered a new era dominated by two developments: (1) the use of **recombinant DNA technology (genetic engineering)** to endow cells with new synthetic capabilities and (2) the ability to both synthesize and determine the linear order of nucleotides (**sequencing**) of DNA molecules. Through these manipulations, it has been possible to transfer genes between bacteria or from eucaryotes into bacteria (or vice versa), causing the engineered cells to become tiny factories for making (in relatively large quantities) proteins of great economic importance such as enzymes, hormones (e.g., insulin, growth hormone), and **interferons** (lymphocyte proteins that prevent replication of many viruses). These proteins are made in such small quantities in human cells that the cost of their extraction and purification from blood or cadaver tissues has been very expensive, thus restricting their medical use in **prophylaxis** (prevention) and **therapeutics** (treatment) of disease. By genetic engineering techniques it has been possible to produce various blood-clotting factors (e.g., **tissue plasminogen activator,** or **TPA,** used to activate the breakdown of blood clots and to prevent recurrence of blood clots in heart attack patients), **complement** components (part of the immune system), and other substances for the amelioration of genetic deficiency diseases **(euphenics).** In 1980, the United States Supreme Court decreed that new life forms created by genetic engineering could be patented. This decision has contributed to the investment of large sums of money by private corporations into the development of many useful genetic recombinants. It is hoped that recombinant DNA technology can someday infuse the genes from nitrogen-fixing bacteria into cereal crops. This would allow these plants to "fertilize themselves" from the boundless supply of nitrogen in the atmosphere. These few examples suffice to demonstrate the possibilities of this new technology and explain why there is such great excitement in the scientific, medical, agricultural, and pharmaceutical communities concerning its further exploitation.

There are four major steps in most genetic engineering work. (1) A nucleotide sequence (or gene) of interest is isolated. (2) The fragment is spliced into a **cloning vector,** or **vehicle,** such as a phage or a plasmid. (3) The vector is introduced into a host cell where it is replicated many times in an amplification process known as **cloning.** (4) The gene or its protein product is isolated from the clone.

There are two major purposes for cloning DNA segments: (1) to obtain large amounts of a segment for DNA sequencing (e.g., in order to discover how an abnormal gene differs structurally from its normal allele) and (2) to produce large amounts of a structural gene product (RNA or protein) (e.g., in order to produce quantities of a viral capsid protein for use as a vaccine). Such a genetically engineered vaccine would not be capable of causing disease the way some attenuated microbial vaccines have been known to do.

A good cloning vector should be able to autonomously form many replicas within the host cell to **amplify** its foreign DNA insert. The vector should have a single recognition site for one of the known restriction endonucleases so that it can be opened at only one position to receive a foreign piece of DNA. Ideally, a vector containing a foreign DNA insert should impart to its host cell some property that distinguishes it from cells that do not contain an insert so that the insert can be easily isolated.

1. Isolation of a Specific DNA Segment.

There are two general methods for isolating a specific nucleotide sequence (or gene) of interest: (*a*) by cloning all of the genes of an organism into a gene library and (*b*) by cloning individual genes or DNA sequences of interest.

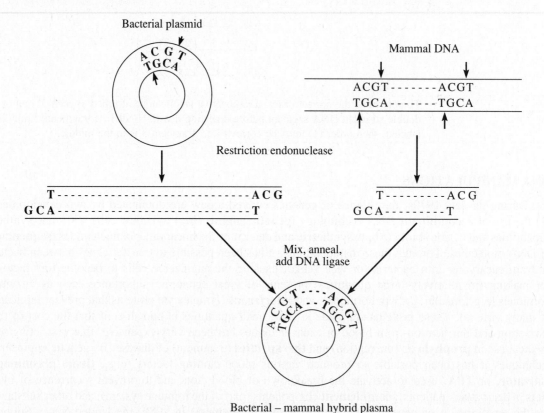

Fig. 13-1.   Formation of hybrid (chimeric) DNA molecules by cutting with the same restriction endonuclease.

(a) ***Construction of a Gene Library.***   In **shotgun** experiments, donor genomic DNA is cut into many pieces by the same restriction endonuclease (RE) used to cleave the plasmid vector at its single RE site. (Cloning in phages is discussed later in this chapter.) The two kinds of fragments are mixed *in vitro* and allowed to randomly rejoin by their complementary (**cohesive,** or ''sticky'') ends to form circles (Fig. 13-1). DNA ligase seals the nicks, creating stable, covalently closed, circular recombinant DNA molecules. If it is important that an insert be connected in the proper orientation into a vector for expression of the foreign DNA, vector and insert can be cleaved with two REs that generate different cohesive tails at the ends of each fragment. The insertion can then occur in only one orientation (Fig. 13-2).

Some of these circles are **chimeric** (partly vector and partly foreign insert). The concentrations of donor and plasmid DNAs are adjusted so that each chimeric vector is likely to contain a different segment of the donor's DNA. Recipient bacterial cells are made permeable for transformation by the naked DNA of the plasmids via treatment with a cold calcium chloride solution. When plated on nutrient agar medium, each transformed cell will multiply many times to form a colony or clone, all cells of which contain multiple copies (sometimes hundreds) of the same chimeric plasmid. The large set of clones that collectively contains all the donor's DNA is known as a **gene library.** Identification of the clone(s) containing the gene of interest will be discussed in section 3.

(b) ***Cloning Individual Genes.***   The other method for isolating genes is much more selective. Instead of cloning all of the donor's DNA, only the gene or segment of interest is cloned. If the desired protein is very small (15–20 amino acids) and its primary structure is known, it should be possible

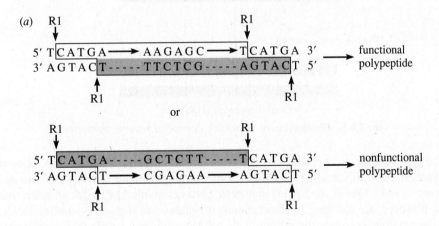

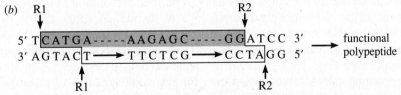

Fig. 13-2.   A method for ensuring that a foreign DNA insert (box) will be joined to a cloning vector in the proper orientation for production of the desired protein. (*a*) If insert and vector are cleaved (vertical arrows) by the same restriction enzyme (R1), the anticoding strand (serving as a transcriptional template for mRNA synthesis) may or may not be in the desired orientation with respect to the promoter, which is upstream (to the left) of the insert. Horizontal arrows indicate direction of transcription of the mRNA. Shaded strand indicates the desired antisense strand. (*b*) If the insert and the vector are cleaved by two different restriction enzymes (R1 and R2), only the desired orientation is possible.

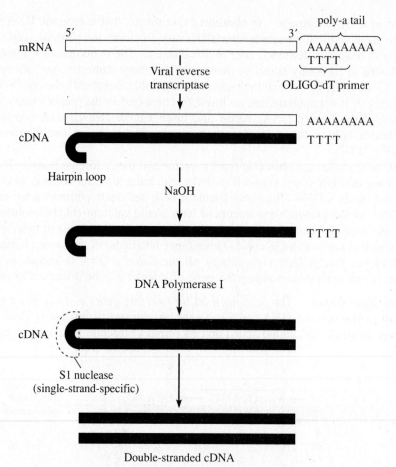

Fig. 13-3. Production of cDNA by the use of reverse transcriptase.

(using the genetic code) to chemically synthesize a corresponding DNA molecule. One of the earliest genes synthesized in this manner was that for the hormone somatostatin (14 amino acids; 42 bases in the sense strand). One of the largest **synthetic genes** contains 514 bp for an interferon gene. Most proteins, however, are too long to allow chemical synthesis of the corresponding DNA. In this case it might be possible to isolate the homologous mRNA from those cells that are specialized to make the protein. For example, human insulin is produced only by the pancreas, even though the insulin gene is present in all human nucleated body cells. A purified preparation of insulin mRNA is isolated from pancreatic cells. A synthetic oligonucleotide of thymidines (oligo-dT) is hybridized to the poly-A tail of the mRNA strand. The viral enzyme **reverse transcriptase (RNA-dependent DNA polymerase)** is added to make a single-stranded DNA copy (**cDNA** or **complementary DNA**) that ends in a hairpin loop (Fig. 13-3). The mRNA template is then destroyed with alkali. The hairpin end of the remaining cDNA serves as a primer for extension synthesis of a complementary strand by DNA polymerase I. The loop is then removed by an enzyme called **S1 nuclease** to produce a double-stranded cDNA molecule. This blunt-ended molecule can now be spliced into a suitable vector and cloned as before.

2. Joining Blunt-Ended Fragments.

There are several methods for joining nucleotide fragments with blunt ends.

(*a*) *Homopolymer Tails.*   An enzyme called **terminal nucleotidyl transferase** can add any available deoxyribonucleotides to the 3′ end of a single-stranded region of DNA without need of a template.

A single-stranded region can be produced by partial digestion of a blunt-ended fragment with a 5'-specific exonuclease. If a string of nucleotides bearing adenines (A) are added onto the vector DNA and thymines (T) are added onto the foreign DNA, **homopolymer tails** are produced that should base-pair in complementary fashion. The gap (absence of one or more nucleotides in a DNA molecule) can be filled by DNA polymerase I using the other complete strand as a template. The nick (absence of a phosphodiester bond between adjacent deoxyribose sugars) can be sealed by DNA ligase (Fig. 13-4).

(b) **Blunt-End Ligation.**   Another method for joining RE fragments with blunt ends is called **blunt-end ligation.** A DNA ligase from *E. coli* phage T4 can be used to join blunt ends of double-stranded DNA (dsDNA) fragments. The tendency of each fragment to form a circle with itself is largely avoided by using a high concentration of DNA that favors hybridization. An advantage of this method is that it can join two defined sequences without introducing any additional material between them. The inability to control which pairs of blunt ends become joined is an obvious disadvantage (Fig. 13-5).

(c) **Linkers.**   A third method employs short DNA segments containing an RE site, called **linkers** or **adapters,** that can be synthesized chemically. Linkers can be added covalently to the ends of a plasmid or to an insert by blunt-end ligation (Fig. 13-6). This method imposes no restriction on the choice of sites to generate the ends, yet allows retrieval of the insert by cleavage with the appropriate RE.

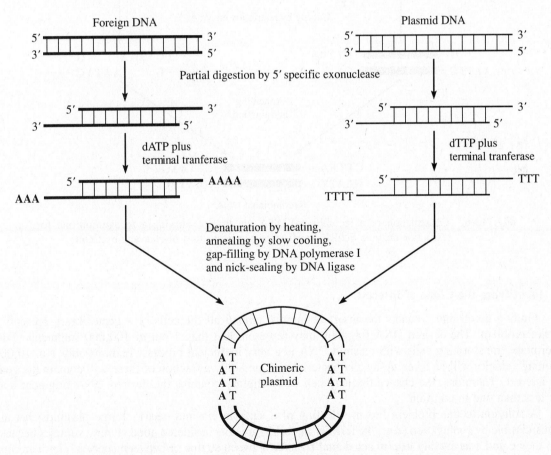

Fig. 13-4.   Production of a chimeric plasmid by the formation of homopolymer tails.

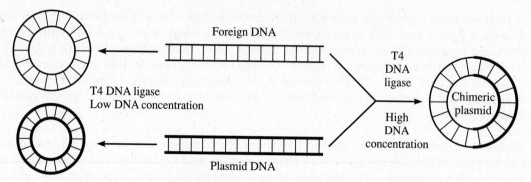

Fig. 13-5. Two possible results of blunt-end ligation via T4 DNA ligase.

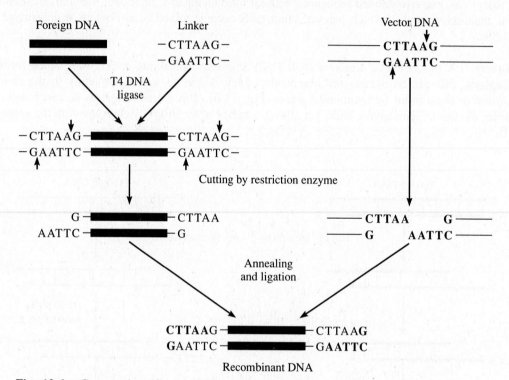

Fig. 13-6. Construction of a recombinant DNA via linkers carrying a recognition site for restriction enzyme EcoRI. Small arrows indicate sites of cleavage by EcoRI.

3. Identifying the Clone of Interest.

Finding a cell that contains the insert of interest among all the cells of a gene library presents a major problem. The desired DNA fragment may represent less than 1 out of 100,000 fragments. Furthermore, transforming cells with plasmid DNA is a very inefficient process. Perhaps only 1 in 10,000 cloning vehicles will be taken up by any bacterial cell, and only a fraction of these will contain the gene of interest. Therefore, the chance that any cell of the library contains the desired DNA fragment may be less than one in a billion.

A solution to this problem lies in selection of a suitable plasmid vector. Large plasmids that are transmissible by conjugation (e.g., the fertility factor, F) are not considered good cloning vehicles because (1) they could conceivably lead to accidental transfer between strains or between species, (2) their copy number per cell is usually very low, and (3) they contain multiple sites for almost any RE. Therefore, smaller [2–4 kilobase pairs (kbp)], nontransmissible plasmids that contain 2 different antibiotic-resistance genes are normally used as vectors. One of the most popular vehicles of this kind is the *E. coli* plasmid pBR322. It consists of 4363 bp and contains resistance genes for the antibiotics tetracycline and ampicillin. There is a single RE site for the restriction enzyme BamHI in the entire pBR322 plasmid, and that site is within the tetracycline-resistance gene (*tet-r*). If both the donor DNA and the plasmid DNA are cut with BamHI, the donor fragments can be spliced into the plasmid as described previously. The insertion of a foreign piece of DNA within the *tet-r* gene destroys the ability of this plasmid to confer resistance to tetracycline on the recipient bacterial cell, a process known as **insertional inactivation** (Fig. 13-7). Recipient cells that are sensitive to both antibiotics are exposed to the plasmids, some of which contain the foreign insert of interest. Three types of cells are produced. Those cells that were not transformed remain Amp-s, Tet-s; those that were transformed (took up the plasmid) are Amp-r. A few of the Amp-r cells are expected to be Tet-s because of insertional inactivation of the *tet-r* gene by the foreign DNA. Cycloserine, ampicillin, and tetracycline are then added to the broth culture. Cycloserine kills any growing cell; ampicillin kills growing cells that are Amp-s; tetracycline inhibits growth without killing cells. Hence, Amp-r, Tet-r cells start to grow and are killed in the presence of cycloserine. When surviving cells are plated on nutrient agar containing ampicillin, only Amp-r, Tet-s cells (containing a foreign DNA insert) grow into colonies.

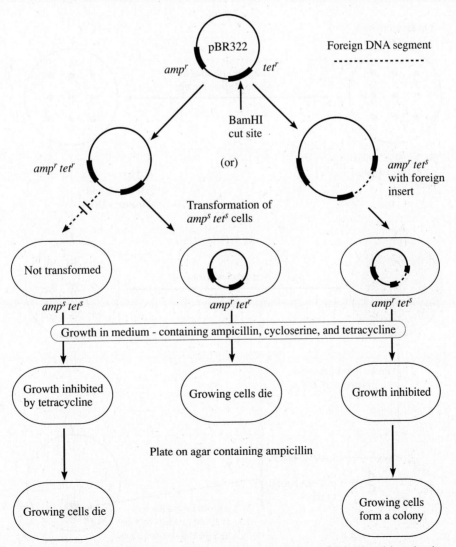

Fig. 13-7. Isolation of a chimeric plasmid by the technique of insertional inactivation.

Locating the few clones that contain the specific segment of interest can be accomplished by an *in situ* **hybridization technique** known as **colony hybridization** (Fig. 13-8). A sample from each tetra-cycline-sensitive colony is spotted onto nutrient agar plates in a gridlike fashion and allowed to grow into colonies there. A piece of nitrocellulose paper is pressed into the plate, thereby transferring some cells from each clone onto the paper in the same gridlike pattern they had on the plate. The paper is then treated with a dilute sodium hydroxide solution to lyse the cells and denature the DNA to single strands. The cell contents are released, and its DNA binds tightly to the paper. Next, the sodium hydroxide is neutralized with acid. The paper is then covered with a solution containing a radioactive or enzyme-labeled **probe,** a single-stranded synthetic oligonucleotide, cDNA or RNA specifically complementary to some portion of the gene of interest. The probe hybridizes wherever such complementary regions exist on the paper, and thereby becomes indirectly bound to the paper. The paper is washed to remove any probe that has not hybridized, and is then covered with X-ray film for autoradiography or the substrate for the enzyme is added. Dark spots on the developed film or colored enzyme products correspond to colonies that contain the gene of interest. Cells from the corresponding clones on the Petri plates can be grown in broth culture to any desired amount. The gene of interest can be liberated from the plasmid by digestion with the same RE used for its insertion. It can then be isolated from the larger plasmid DNA by electrophoresis.

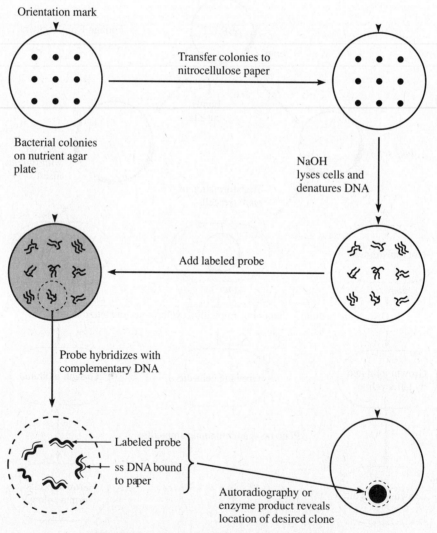

Fig. 13-8. The colony hybridization technique.

4. Expression Vectors.

Expression vectors contain very efficient regulatory sequences that allow genes to be highly expressed in host cells. For example, the gene for resistance to ampicillin in plasmid pBR322 has a very active promoter. Foreign genes inserted into the *amp-r* gene can produce large amounts of the corresponding protein.

The most common procedures for detecting protein-secreting clones usually involve antibodies (immunoassays). Antibodies against one protein antigen are usually highly specific and do not react with other proteins. A **label** or **tag** can be attached to antibodies to reveal whether they have bound to a corresponding antigen. The most sensitive labels are radioactive isotopes used for radioimmunoassay (RIA) or enzyme labels used in enzyme-linked immunosorbent assay (ELISA). The latter are often preferred over the handling and disposal problems associated with radioactive materials.

> **Example 13.4.** A bacterial clone that has been genetically engineered to secrete human insulin can be identified among all other colonies on a plate by exposure to anti–insulin antibodies that are bound to a plastic disc. The disc is stamped onto the plate, and the antibodies pick up any insulin secreted by a clone. The disc is placed in a solution containing radioactive anti–insulin antibodies, then washed to remove any unbound radioactivity. Autoradiography of the disc reveals the location of any insulin-secreting clones on the plate.

If the protein of interest is not secreted by the genetically engineered cells, other techniques may be used.

> **Example 13.5.** A temperature-sensitive (Ts) mutant lambda repressor (designated c1857) is inactivated at 42°C, allowing the phage to replicate vegetatively in its lytic cycle. Cells that are known to contain a gene of interest may or may not be producing the corresponding protein. Such cells can be exposed to the phage and incubated at 37°C. The phage enters the cell but is unable to replicate because of its active repressor. To locate any clones on a plate that synthesize a desired protein but do not secrete it, a replica plate is made and incubated at 42°C. The repressor is inactivated, allowing phage replication. Lysis of host cells releases their proteins. The bacterial colonies of interest can then be detected by an immunoassay as explained in the previous example.

> **Example 13.6.** Agar containing lysozyme and antibodies to a specific protein of interest is poured on bacterial colonies and allowed to harden. Colonies lysed by lysozyme release their proteins. If the protein of interest is present, the antibodies will react with it and form a ring of precipitate around the colony.

5. Phage Vectors.

The central region of phage lambda contains genes involved in establishing and maintaining the lysogenic state, and hence is not essential for its lytic cycle. This region can be replaced with a foreign DNA insert if it is of an appropriate size [approximately 15,000 bp or 15 kilobase pairs (kbp)] and still allow the phage DNA to be packaged into phage heads. Large foreign inserts tend to be unstable in plasmids, so the two vectors complement one another. Furthermore, transduction is a much more efficient process than transformation, and it avoids the problem of the vector closing up without an insert. Genetically manipulated phage DNA without such an insert will not be packaged properly to become functional (infective) virions. The restriction enzyme EcoRI cuts lambda DNA at both ends of the nonessential region. The two essential end regions can be isolated by electrophoresis and ligated *in vitro* with foreign DNA cut by that same enzyme (Fig. 13-9).

Lambda-sensitive bacteria are grown on agar plates in high density to form a lawn of confluent growth. The artificially synthesized transducing phage are added in a concentration resulting in about 100 phage particles per plate, hence producing about 100 plaques of lysed bacterial cells per plate. Each plaque is a phage clone containing millions of identical phage genomes. In a gene library of such phage clones, at least one of the phage clones contains the foreign insert of interest. The library can then be screened by an *in situ* hybridization technique (e.g., by using a radioactive probe) to locate the rare

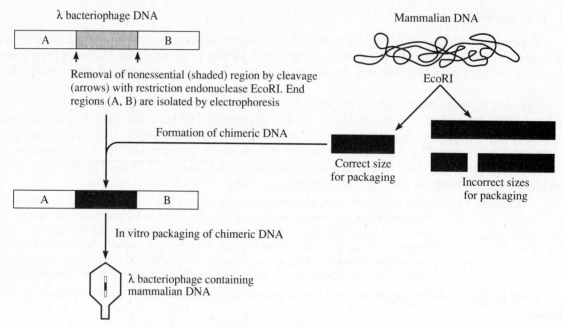

Fig. 13-9. Cloning of foreign DNA in λ bacteriophage.

clones containing the insert of interest. The insert can be extracted from such a clone by cutting lambda DNA with EcoRI and isolated by electrophoresis.

Cosmids are plasmids into which have been inserted the *cos* sites (*cohesive end sites*) required for packaging lambda DNA into its capsid. Cosmids can be perpetuated in bacterial cells or purified by packaging *in vitro* into phages. The main advantages of using cosmids are that inserts much longer than 15 kb can thereby be cloned and the ease of selecting a recombinant plasmid is greatly improved.

> **Example 13.7.** Plasmid ColE1 carries a gene for resistance to rifampicin (*rif-r*) and the *cos* sites of phage lambda, which can be recognized by the *cos*-site-cutting (Ter) system of *E. coli*. Cosmids such as this can function properly, provided that two *cos* sites are present and the *cos* sites are separated by no less than 38 kb and no more than 54 kb. Cleavage of ColE1 and foreign DNA by the restriction enzyme HindIII can be used to produce linear, chimeric, recombinant molecules (Fig. 13-10). Transducing phage particles can be formed if the insert between the two cos sites is 38–54 kb in length. No particles are produced if no insert is made or if the insert is larger or smaller than that range. *In vitro* **packaging** (adding heads and tails) forms transducing particles containing cosmids with cohesive termini. Upon infection of a rifampicin-sensitive (Rif-s) cell with a transducing phage particle, the linear chimera becomes circularized and replicates using the ColE1 replication system. Plating cells on medium containing rifampicin selects for those cells containing the *rif-r* gene, the ColE1 region, and a foreign insert.

6. Polymerase Chain Reaction.

Cloning DNA segments for the purpose of nucleotide sequencing used to be a relatively laborious process. However, in 1985, an *in vitro* technique, called the **polymerase chain reaction (PCR),** was developed for making large amounts of any DNA sequence without the need for cloning. The PCR (Fig. 13-11) requires a pair of "primers" that are usually short pieces of chemically synthesized DNA (**oligonucleotides**), having nucleotide sequences specifically complementary to those in opposite strands flanking the target region. These primers thus define the ends of the DNA segment that will be duplicated. The original template source of DNA does not have to be highly purified, and even a very small amount of template can serve as the initiator for the PCR. The DNA sample is heated, allowing the complementary DNA chains to separate. The primers are then added together with a DNA-polymerizing enzyme. The primers bind to the single-stranded chains during the cooling phase, and the polymerizing enzyme extends

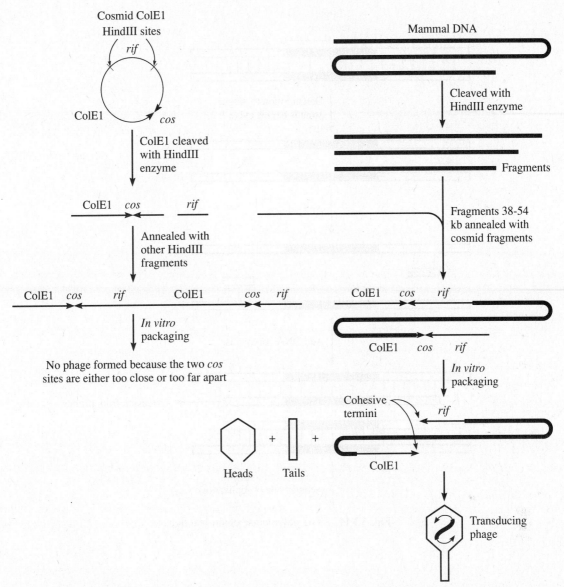

Fig. 13-10. Formation of transducing phage via a cosmid. Thick lines represent mammal DNA; thin lines, cosmid DNA.

the primer through the rest of the fragment, creating double-stranded DNA molecules. The process is then repeated; i.e., the mixture is reheated, and during the ensuing cooling phase the excess primers (or newly added primers) bind to template strands and become extended by the polymerizing enzyme to produce more double-stranded molecules. About 20–30 cycles of heating plus DNA synthesis are normally run during gene amplification by the PCR. After 20 cycles, a single DNA molecule can theoretically be amplified to about one million copies, and after 30 cycles to about one billion copies. With this quantity of DNA, nucleotide sequencing can be done easily.

Probes can also be used to locate genes or DNA segments of interest. Because of the large quantity of DNA generated by the PCR, highly radioactive probes are not required, and the target segments can be detected by using nonradioactive probes or stains.

Example 13.8. Human immunodeficiency virus type 1 (HIV-1) is the cause of **acquired immunodeficiency syndrome (AIDS).** Only about 1 in 10,000 susceptible cells actually harbors the virus in an infected person. It is estimated that 1–10 copies of viral DNA per million cells can be detected through the use of the PCR and suitable probes.

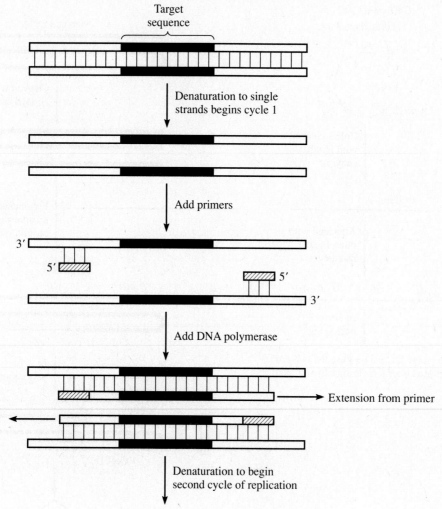

Fig. 13-11.   The polymerase chain reaction.

7. Site-Specific Mutagenesis.

It is possible, by several techniques, to introduce one or more nucleotide alterations of known composition and location into specific genes or regulatory sequences. For example (Fig. 13-12), a plasmid carrying a gene of interest can be nicked at one position with an endonuclease. The plasmid DNA is then denatured and intact single-stranded circles are isolated. Short (13–30 bases) oligonucleotides of known complementary structure (either synthesized *de novo* or from cleavage by a restriction enzyme) can be made to have a mutant base at a desired site in the gene. This oligonucleotide is then renatured with the intact single-stranded circles to serve as a primer for *in vitro* replication of a strand that is not completely complementary to that of the plasmid strand. The replicated circles are sealed with DNA ligase. The covalently closed circles are isolated and used to transform bacteria. During *in vivo* replication, each strand of the plasmid serves as a template for producing a progeny strand. Thus some plasmids are produced with wild-type gene sequences and some with a single base pair mutation at a known site. After isolation, these mutants can be evaluated for their effects on the functioning of the gene or regulatory sequence.

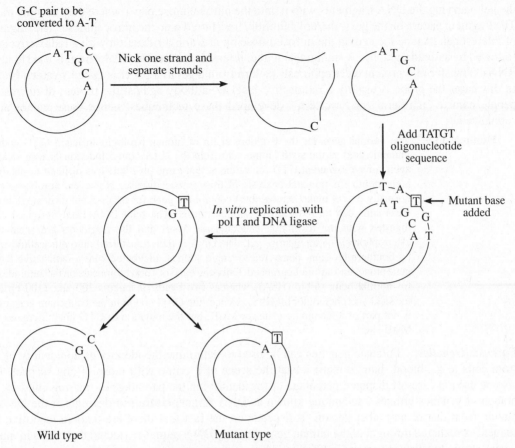

Fig. 13-12. Site-specific mutagenesis.

8. Polymorphisms.

A **polymorphism** is the existence of two or more contrasting genetic elements in a population at frequencies greater than can be accounted for by recurrent mutation. Conventionally, a polymorphic element or locus is one at which the frequency of the most common allele is less than 0.99. Polymorphisms may exist minimally at three levels: (1) chromosome, (2) gene, and (3) restriction fragment length. Chromosomal polymorphisms that are large enough to be detected in the light microscope may involve euploidy, aneuploidy, translocations, inversions, duplications, or deficiencies. A polymorphic gene locus has 2 or more alleles that produce different phenotypes (e.g., blood groups). A **restriction fragment length polymorphism (RFLP)** exists if the DNAs of different individuals in a population produce different fragment length profiles when their DNAs are cut by the same restriction endonuclease. Variation in the spacing of restriction enzyme recognition sites may be due to a base change that either creates or removes such a site near a probed region. Alternatively, the addition or deletion of one or more DNA segments can change the spacing of recognition sites without creation or abolition of such sites. There are two major uses for RFLPs: in medical genetics and in forensic genetics.

(*a*) **Medical Genetics.**   The technique used to analyze RFLPs is **Southern blotting,** named after E. M. Southern, who first developed it. A restriction enzyme digest of an individual's DNA is electrophoresed on an agarose gel and then denatured to single strands. The single-stranded fragments are then transferred from the gel to nitrocellulose paper in the following manner. The gel is placed on normal filter paper that has been soaked in concentrated salt solution. The nitrocellulose paper is placed on top of the gel, with dry blotting paper and a weight on top of that. The salt solution moves through the gel, carrying the DNA fragments with it onto the nitrocellulose paper where they become trapped. The fragment pattern on the gel is thereby faithfully transferred onto the nitrocellulose. The fragment(s) of interest can then be located on the nitrocellulose by *in situ* hybridization with a radioactive probe, followed by autoradiography. A similar technique, referred to as **northern blotting,** is used to identify RNAs. Transfer of a protein electrophoresis pattern from a gel to a paper is called **western blotting.** In this case, the probe is usually a radioactive-labeled antibody against the protein of interest. (No people named ''northern'' or ''western'' developed these techniques; hence these names are not capitalized.)

> **Example 13.9.** The normal gene for the β-globin chain of human hemoglobin has a GAG codon for glutamic acid as the sixth amino acid from the N terminus. Individuals with sickle-cell anemia have a mutant GTG for valine at that same position. It is difficult to obtain fetal hemoglobin for prenatal analysis of this genetic disease. However, fibroblasts (which normally do not make hemoglobin) contain the gene for the β-chain of hemoglobin, and these cells can be retrieved by amniocentesis. The total DNA from fibroblast cells is digested with the restriction endonuclease MstII and the fragments are separated by electrophoresis on an agarose gel. The DNA is then transferred onto nitrocellulose paper by Southern blotting, denatured to single strands, incubated with a radioactive β-globin gene probe, and autoradiographed. Only one band of 1300 bp appears on the autoradiograph for normal hemoglobin (HbA), whereas two bands of lengths 200 and 1100 bp appear for sickle-cell hemoglobin (HbS). Hence, the GAG codon in the beta-chain gene of HbA is not part of a recognition site for MstII, but the mutation to GTG in HbS creates a new MstII site.

(b) ***Forensic Genetics.*** Forensic genetics can be used to determine the identity or nonidentity of DNA from cells (e.g., blood, hair, semen) left at the scene of a crime with those of any suspect. It can also be used in cases of disputed parentage or for identifying the parentage of missing children. This branch of genetics utilizes a technique known as **DNA fingerprinting** to distinguish the DNA of a human from that of any other person. It depends on the fact that there are tandem repetitive DNA sequences scattered throughout the human genome. Any DNA sequence (locus) that exists in multiple copies strung together in various lengths one after another in tandem order is referred to as a **variable number of tandem repeats locus (VNTR locus).** The number, the pattern, and the length of these repeats are unique for each individual. Regardless of its length, each repeat contains a common (usually 10–15 bp) core sequence that can be recognized by an appropriate radioactive probe. The DNA of an individual is extracted from a convenient sample of that person's cells (e.g., from white blood cells) and subjected to cleavage by one or more restriction endonucleases. The fragments are separated on an agarose gel, denatured to single strands, transferred to a nitrocellulose filter by Southern blotting, exposed to the probe, and then autoradiographed. The bands that develop on the autoradiograph are unique for each individual.

DNA SEQUENCING

A relatively large quantity of identical single-stranded DNA fragments is required for any sequencing method. These fragments can be prepared by either an *in vivo* cloning procedure or by the *in vitro* polymerase chain reaction procedure. The DNA must then be purified of all proteins by phenol extraction before sequencing can commence.

1. Enzyme Method.

The first rapid method for determining the nucleotide sequences of DNA fragments was developed in 1975 by F. Sanger and A. R. Coulson (Fig. 13-13). This procedure, referred to as the enzyme method, is also known as a **primed synthesis method** or **the plus and minus methods.** The following preliminary steps are common to both the plus and minus systems. A primer must be annealed to the single-stranded DNA template. Such a primer can be obtained by digestion of the fragment with a different restriction

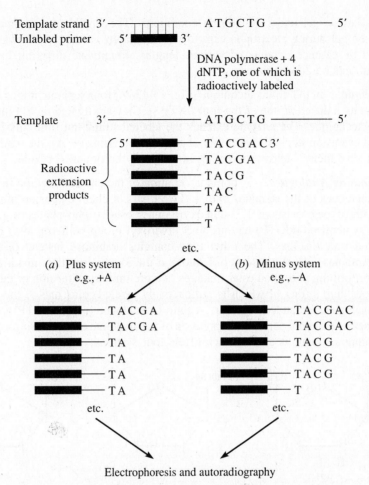

Fig. 13-13. Primed synthesis methods of DNA sequencing. An autoradiograph for the sequence illustrated here is Supplementary Problem 13.22.

endonuclease or by chemical synthesis of a short oligonucleotide sequence. The primers undergo limited extension by *E. coli* DNA polymerase I when given a restricted supply of all four deoxyribonucleoside triphosphates (dntp), one of which is radioactively labeled. Different primed complexes are extended in a random manner, so ideally, every chain length over the region to be sequenced should be present. The unincorporated labeled nucleotides and DNA polymerase I are then removed. The labeled strand, which remains attached to the template, is then treated by either the "plus method" or the "minus method."

(*a*) **Plus Technique.** In the plus technique [Fig. 13-13(*a*)] one aliquot of the reaction mixture is exposed to only one of the four dNTP's (unlabeled). A DNA polymerase is added that lacks the normal 5′ exonuclease activity of DNA polymerase I (e.g., a mutant DNA polymerase I, or a protease-treated DNA polymerase I known as "Klenow" fragment, or T4 DNA polymerase). The exonuclease activity of these enzymes removes one base at a time from the 3′ end. Four separate reaction systems are set up, one for each type of dntp (A, T, G, C). If an adenine dntp is the base added (+A), the enzyme will chew away the 3′ end until it encounters an A on the "extension strand." As long as the added dntp remains in excess, the synthetic activity of DNA polymerase predominates over its exonuclease activity. Thus, the A will be maintained at the end of that strand. Each length of primed chain will therefore terminate at its 3′ end with an A. The same process is repeated in the three other systems, adding a different dntp in each case. The extension products are separated from the template (e.g., by heating in formamide), followed by simultaneous electrophoresis of all four systems on the same acrylamide gel under denaturing conditions. The smaller the fragments, the faster they travel along the gel during electrophoresis. Autoradiography of the gel allows visualization of the bands formed by extended chains of various lengths. Fragments differing in length by a single nucleotide can thus be differentiated.

(b) *Minus Technique.*   In the minus technique [Fig. 13-13(b)] four separate minus reactions are carried out, each missing a different one of the four dNTP's. They are treated in all other respects the same as in the plus technique. The enzyme extends the labeled strand until the missing dntp is required, at which point extension stops. For example, if adenine is missing ($-$A), the random length extension products will have their 3′ ends terminating immediately before an A residue.

(c) *Chain-Terminating Analogues.*   A popular variation of the enzyme method involves use of chain-terminating analogues of the standard dntp's. Two kinds of chain extension inhibitors are available (Fig. 13-14). One type consists of 2′3′-dideoxyribonucleoside triphosphates (e.g., dideoxyguanosine triphosphate, symbolized ddGTP) having no 3′ hydroxyl group with which to form internucleotide 3′-5′ phosphodiester linkages. The other type contains arabinose instead of ribose as the sugar component. Arabinose is a sterioisomer of ribose at the 3′ position, thus making its hydroxyl group unavailable for forming phosphodiester linkages. No preliminary extension of the primer is required. Instead, all four dntp's (one of which is radioactively labeled) plus one of the four specific chain-terminating analogues are added together. A ratio of analogue (e.g., ddGTP) to normal dntp (e.g., dGTP) is chosen so that only partial incorporation of the analogue occurs during extension. A different chain-terminating analogue is used in each of the four systems.

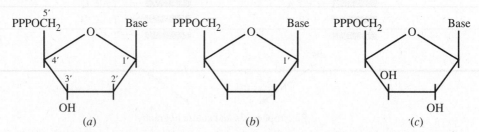

Fig. 13-14.   Structure of chain extension inhibitors. (*a*) Normal deoxyribonucleoside-5′-triphosphate. (*b*) Dideoxynucleoside-5′-triphosphate. (*c*) Arabinonucleoside-5′-triphosphate.

2. Chemical Method.

A second method for rapidly sequencing DNA fragments was developed in 1977 by A. M. Maxam and W. Gilbert (Fig. 13-15). The sequence may be determined separately in both strands of a fragment of interest for the purpose of checking the accuracy of the data (according to the rules of base pairing) or for extending the length of the sequence capable of being analyzed.

(1) In the first major step, the 5′-phosphate group is removed from both ends of a double-stranded DNA fragment by treatment with alkaline phosphatase and replaced with a radioactive phosphate from radioactive ATP using the enzyme polynucleotide kinase.

(2) The two 5′-labeled ends are then separated by one of two methods. The DNA fragment can be denatured in alkali and the two strands isolated by electrophoresis. Alternatively, the DNA fragment can be cleaved with a different restriction enzyme (RE) than that used to generate the fragment. This second RE must cut at one position, producing two fragments, each labeled at only one end; these double-stranded fragments are then separated by gel electrophoresis.

(3) The two sets of 5′-labeled products (either single-stranded or double-stranded) are then independently subjected to attack by chemical reagents that cause modification and removal of one or two specific bases from the DNA. One treatment cleaves G bases alone; another treatment cleaves both G and A bases; a third removes T and C bases; a fourth removes only C bases. Reaction conditions are chosen such that usually only one base-specific reaction occurs randomly per DNA strand in the region to be sequenced, thus generating a series of labeled fragments of all possible lengths. Similar breaks

1. Radioactive labeling at 5′ ends of each strand of a restriction fragment.

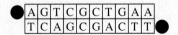

2. Separation and isolation of the two strands. Sequence analysis can be performed separately on each strand up to about 50 nucleotides.

3. Chemical treatments cleave the strand at specific bases. For example, a strand with three Gs would be cut randomly at one of three places (arrows), producing radioactive fragments of three lengths.

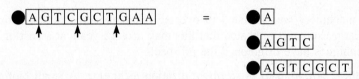

4. The shorter fragments move faster during electrophoresis. Only the fragments bearing the radioactive tag will be revealed by autoradiography.

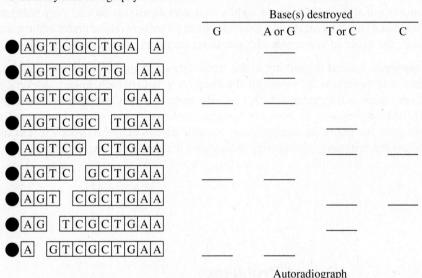

Autoradiograph

Fig. 13-15.   Major steps in DNA sequence analysis by the chemical method.

occur in both the labeled and unlabeled strands of double-stranded fragments (if this mode of separation was chosen), but the unlabeled strand can be ignored because it will not be detected by autoradiography. If the 5′-labeled double-stranded fragments were separated by cleavage with a second RE, the labeled strands are separated from the unlabeled strands by heating in formamide.

(4) Simultaneous electrophoresis of all four treatment groups is performed on the same 20% acrylamide gel containing 7M urea (denaturing conditions). Autoradiography is carried out at $-20°C$ to minimize diffusion of very small products.

3. Automated DNA Sequencing.

The currently most promising methods for automated DNA sequencing use fluorescent labels instead of radioactive labels. Computerized analysis of the autoradiographic sequence data is made difficult, in part, by the lane-to-lane variations of the electrophoretic mobilities of the DNA fragments. This problem can be overcome (and productivity can be increased fourfold) by electrophoresing all of the reactants in one lane. To do this, a different fluorophore is attached to each of the four dideoxyribonucleoside triphosphates used in the chain-termination technique. The distinctive emission spectrum of each fluorophore is identified as it migrates past a stationary fluorescence detector during electrophoresis. The data acquired by the detector are stored and analyzed by microcomputer to yield the DNA sequence. The theoretical throughput capability of such an instrument is about 10,000 bases of raw sequence data per day, but the realized capability is probably only 30–40% of that. Undoubtedly further technological developments of such instrumentation and new techniques will enhance the realized capability in the future.

4. The Human Genome Project.

During 1989, the administrative machinery was initiated to oversee the sequencing of the entire human genome—some 3 billion bp. Early estimates indicated that this may take 15 years at a cost of 3 billion dollars. Two new mapping techniques have brightened the prospects.

(*a*) **In Situ *Hybridization*.**   One of these is a kind of *in situ* hybridization technique. A small biotin-labeled probe of single-stranded DNA is hybridized to a denatured metaphase chromosome spread. Any unhybridized probe is washed away. The spread is then exposed to the protein avidin that has been tagged with a fluorescent dye. Avidin binds tightly and specifically to biotin. Any unbound, labeled avidin is then washed away. The location of the hybridized probe is revealed under a fluorescent microscope. In this way, the order of numerous chromosomal fragments can be established.

(*b*) ***Radiation Hybrid Mapping*.**   Instead of looking at the frequency of recombination between linked genes, or markers, this new technique is based on the frequency with which linked markers are separated after the chromosome is fragmented by X-rays. By these two new techniques, it is hoped that mapping of 5000–7000 probes will be possible, creating landmarks spaced an average of one million base pairs apart over the entire human genome. Specific clones of these probes would then be assigned to the various participating laboratories throughout the world for sequencing.

Solved Problems

13.1. In 1953, Watson and Crick proposed that DNA replicates *semiconservatively;* i.e., both strands of the double helix become templates against which new complementary strands are made so that a replicated molecule would contain one original strand and one newly synthesized strand. A different hypothesis proposes that DNA replicates *conservatively,* i.e., the original double helix remains intact so that a replicated molecule would contain two newly synthesized strands. Bacterial DNA can be ''labeled'' with a heavy isotope of nitrogen (^{15}N) by growing cells for several generations in a medium that has $^{15}NH_4Cl$ as its only nitrogen source. The common ''light'' form of nitrogen is ^{14}N. Light and heavy DNA molecules can be separated by high-speed centrifugation (50,000 rpm = $10^5 \times$ gravity) in a 6M (molar) CsCl (cesium chloride) solution, the density of which is 1.7 gram/centimeter^3 (very close to that of DNA). After several hours of spinning, the CsCl forms a density gradient, being heavier at the bottom and lighter at the top. In 1957, Matthew Meselson and Franklin W. Stahl performed a density-gradient experiment to clarify which of the two replication hypotheses was correct. How could this be done, and what results are expected after the first, second, and third generations of bacterial replication according to each of these hypotheses?

Solution:

Bacteria from ^{15}N-labeled culture are transferred into medium containing ^{14}N as the only source of nitrogen. A sample is immediately taken and its DNA is extracted and subjected to density-gradient equilibrium centrifugation. The DNA forms a single band relatively low in the tube where its density matches that of the CaCl in that region of the gradient. After each generation of growth and replication of all DNA molecules, DNA is again extracted and measured for its density. According to the semiconservative theory, the first generation of DNA progeny molecules should all be "hybrid" (one strand containing only ^{14}N and the other strand only ^{15}N). Hybrid molecules would form a band at a density intermediate between fully heavy and fully light molecules. The second generations of DNA molecules should be 50% hybrids and 50% totally light, the latter forming a band relatively high in the tube where the density is lighter. After three generations, the ratio of light:hybrid molecules should be 3:1, respectively. The amount of hybrid molecules should be decreased by 50% in each subsequent generation.

According to the conservative replication scheme, the first generation of DNA molecules should be 50% heavy : 50% light. The second generation should be 25% heavy : 75% light. The third generation should be $12\frac{1}{2}$% heavy : $87\frac{1}{2}$% light. No hybrid molecules should be detected. The results of the Meselson and Stahl experiment supported the semiconservative theory of DNA replication.

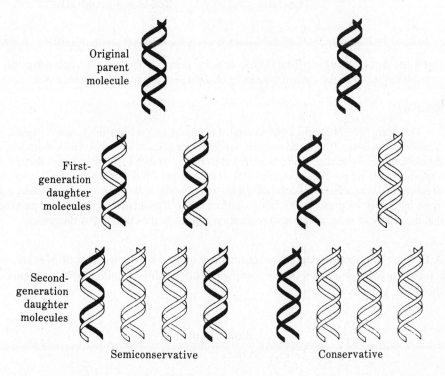

Original parent molecule

First-generation daughter molecules

Second-generation daughter molecules

Semiconservative   Conservative

13.2. The Meselson-Stahl density-gradient experiment (Problem 13.1) demonstrated that some elementary DNA unit replicates conservatively, but it could be argued that it failed to prove conclusively that this unit applied to the entire DNA molecule. For example, at least two other models of DNA replication could have produced the same first-generation results as those observed by Meselson-Stahl: (1) dispersive and (2) end-to-end conservative. In both of these models, about half of each strand is newly synthesized and half is old parental material.

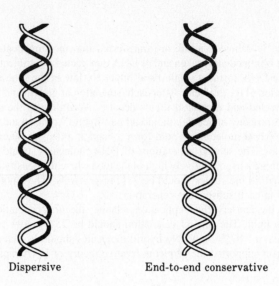

Dispersive   End-to-end conservative

Using the first-generation hybrid double helices, devise a method for confirming that semiconservative replication applies to the entire DNA molecule, not just to certain segments of the molecule.

Solution:

Denature ^{14}N-^{15}N hybrid DNA (strand separation) and subject the isolated strands to density-gradient equilibrium analysis. If semiconservative replication applies to the entire DNA molecule, half of the strands should find equilibrium at a density identical to that of isolated ^{15}N strands and the other half should form a band at the same position as isolated ^{14}N strands. If the DNA replicates according to either the dispersive or end-to-end conservative models, all single strands would seek an intermediate density equilibrium between those for totally light and totally heavy single strands. The actual results of such an experiment confirmed that the theory of semiconservative replication applies to the entire DNA molecule.

13.3. A DNA restriction endonuclease fragment is treated by the method of Maxam and Gilbert. From the autoradiograph shown below, determine the double-stranded DNA sequence of this fragment including polarity of the strands.

	Bases Destroyed		
G	A or G	T or C	C

Solution:

Since the distance of movement of fragments from the origin on the gel increases with decreasing fragment size, the fragment at the bottom of the gel is the smallest one containing the radioactive label at its 5′ end. Any band appearing only in the T or C column indicates that the corresponding fragment must have been derived by cleaving at T. Any fragment in the C column was cleaved at C. Similarly, a fragment that appears only in the A or G column must have been cut at A. Any fragment in the G column must have been cut at G. Therefore, the nucleotides in this strand of DNA can be read sequentially from the 5′ end starting at the bottom of the gel.

$$^{5'}\text{T G G A G G A C C C G G A A T}^{3'}$$

The complementary strand runs in an antiparallel direction and its base sequence is determined by the conventional base pairing rules (A with T; G with C).

$$^{5'}\text{T G G A G G A C C C G G A A T}^{3'}$$
$$^{3'}\text{A C C T C C T G G G C C T T A}^{5'}$$

13.4. The relative position of recognition sites for various restriction endonucleases can be determined by a procedure known as *restriction-enzyme mapping,* the 3′ ends of a DNA molecule are labeled with radioactive ^{32}P. The DNA is then completely digested in separate experiments with two restriction endonucleases (X and Y), the resulting fragments are separated by polyacrylamide gel electrophoresis (PAGE), and the labeled end fragments are identified by autoradiography. The mobilities of nucleic acid fragments in PAGE are inversely proportional to the logarithms of their lengths. Treatment with enzyme X produced fragments A*, B, and C* (* = radioactively labeled); treatment with enzyme Y produced fragments D*, E, and F*. Fragments A–C were then digested by enzyme Y into subfragments 1–5; fragments D–F were digested by enzyme X into subfragments, some of which overlap with those of Y. These subfragments can be homologized between the two enzyme digests because they occupy similar positions after PAGE. Fragment A contains a single subfragment 1; fragment F contains only subfragment 5. B was digested into subfragments 2 and 3; likewise C into 4 and 5, D into 1 and 2, and E into 3 and 4. Reconstruct the order of subfragments in this DNA molecule and show where the recognition sites for enzymes X and Y reside.

Solution:

Since three fragments were generated by each enzyme, there must be two recognition sites for each enzyme (cut a string twice and three pieces are produced). Fragment B was unlabeled, indicating it must be between labeled end fragments A and C; similarly E must be between end fragments D and F. Fragment B contains a site for enzyme Y because treatment with Y produced subfragments 2 and 3. Likewise C also contains a site for Y. But A does not contain a site for Y because Y could not digest A (contains only subfragment 1). Similarly D and E each have a site for enzyme X, but F does not. Because subfragment 4 is produced by digestion of C and E, they must overlap. By the same token, B and E must overlap (both contain subfragment 3), C and F must overlap (both contain 5), B and D must overlap (both contain 2), and A and D must overlap (both contain 1). These facts can now be used to reconstruct the original DNA molecule.

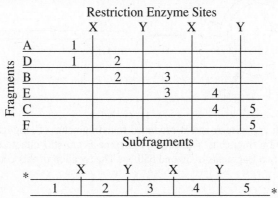

13.5. Suppose that a circular plasmid contains 1000 bp. It is cut by three different restriction endonucleases, both singly and in pairs, with the results as shown below.

Enzyme(s)	Fragment Length(s)
A	1000
B	100, 300, 600
C	200, 800
A + B	50, 100, 300, 550
A + C	200, 375, 425
B + C	75, 100, 125, 225, 475

Reconstruct the plasmid, indicating where each enzyme cuts and the distances between all cuts.

Solution:

Enzyme A cuts the circular plasmid at only one position, producing a linear molecule 1000 base pairs (bp) in length.

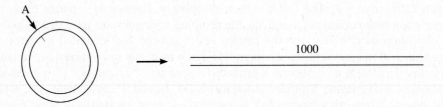

Enzyme B cuts the plasmid at three positions, producing fragments 100, 300, and 600 bp in length. Let us label these fragments B1, B2, and B3, respectively.

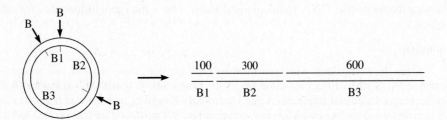

Enzyme C cuts the plasmid at two places, giving fragments 200 and 800 bp in length. Let us label them C1 and C2, respectively.

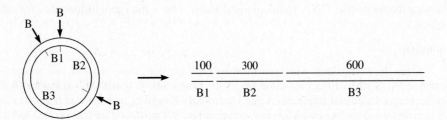

Digestion by both enzymes A and B produced four fragments of lengths 50, 100, 300, and 550 bp. Since the 100- and 300-bp fragments generated by enzyme B are still intact, enzyme A must have cut fragment B3 (600 bp) into two fragments of 50 and 550 bp. The location of this cut could be either closer to or farther from B2.

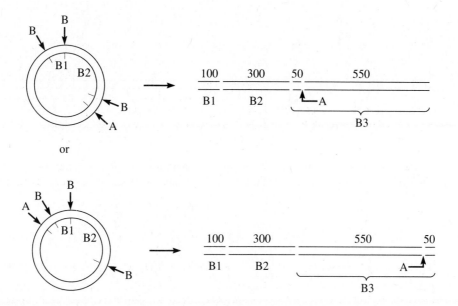

Digestion with both enzymes A and C produced three fragments of lengths 200, 375, and 425 bp. Obviously, the single cut by enzyme A must have been in fragment C2 (800 bp). The smaller 425 bp fragment could be either to the left or right of C1 in the circular map.

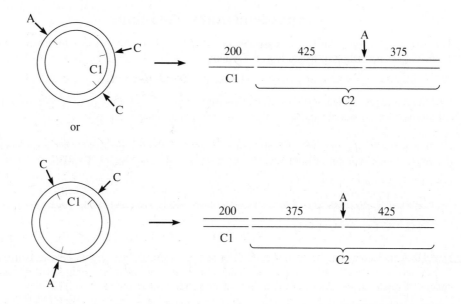

Double digestion with enzymes B and C yields five pieces: 75, 100, 125, 225, and 475 bp in length. Fragment B1 (100 bp) is still intact, but B2 (300 bp) and B3 (600 bp) have been degraded. Therefore, one cut by enzyme C occurs in B2 and the other cut occurs in B3. The sum of the 75- and 225-bp fragments is 300 bp, corresponding to the length of B2. Thus, one cut by enzyme C is 75 bp from one end of B2. Likewise, the other cut by enzyme C is 125 bp from one end of B3. Recall that the single digest with enzyme C produced fragments of 200 bp (C1) and 800 bp (C2). Therefore, the only way the double digest of B and C can make sense is to have the 75 bp and 125 bp fragments adjacent to one another so that they total 200 bp as in C1.

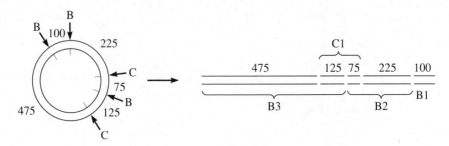

The results of all three double digests can only be combined in one meaningful way. Since the cut made by enzyme A is in fragment B3, 50 bp from a B cut, and far from either C cut, A must map as follows:

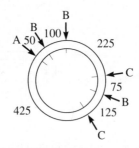

Supplementary Problems

13.6. The buoyant density (ρ) of DNA molecules in *6M* CsCl solution increases with the molar content of G + C nucleotides according to the following formula:

$$\rho = 1.660 + 0.00098 \,(G + C)$$

Find the molar percentage of (G + C) in DNA from the following sources: (*a*) *Escherichia coli:* ρ = 1.710, (*b*) *Streptococcus pneumoniae:* ρ = 1.700, (*c*) *Mycobacterium phlei:* ρ = 1.732.

13.7. Given two DNA molecules, the overall composition of which is represented by the segments shown below, determine which molecule would have the highest melting temperature. Explain.

(*a*) T T C A G A G A A C T T
     A A G T C T C T T G A A
(*b*) C C T G A G A G G T C C
     G G A C T C T C C A G G

13.8. Two DNA molecules having identical (G + C)/(A + T) ratios are shown below. If these molecules are melted and subsequently annealed, which one would require a lower temperature for renaturation of double helices? Explain. *Hint:* Consider the effects of intrastrand interactions.

(*a*) A A T A G C C C C A T G G G G C T A
     T T A T C G G G G T A C C C C G A T
(*b*) C T G C A T C T G A T G C A G C T C
     G A C G T A G A C T A C G T C G A G

13.9. The primary mRNA transcript for chicken ovalbumin contains seven introns (light, A–G) and eight exons (dark) as shown below.

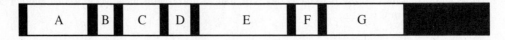

If the DNA for ovalbumin is isolated, denatured to single strands and hybridized with cytoplasmic mRNA for ovalbumin, how would the hybrid structure generally be expected to appear in an electron micrograph? *Note:* Double-stranded regions appear thicker than single-stranded regions.

13.10. RNA can be translated into protein only when it is single-stranded; if DNA hybridizes with RNA, no translation occurs. This fact suggests a way by which one can identify those recombinant bacterial clones that are synthesizing rat insulin. Bacterial DNA is first isolated from the clones being tested and then denatured to single strands. Unpurified RNA (the same source used to make insulin cDNA) is added to the single-stranded DNA under conditions that promote annealing between the RNAs and any homologous DNA. A "translation system" containing radioactive amino acids, ribosomes, tRNAs, enzymes, energy sources, etc., is added to the mixture. Small plastic beads (coated with antibodies specifically reactive with rat insulin) are later introduced into the system. The tube is centrifuged and the supernatant fluid is discarded leaving the antibody-coated beads in the tube. The tubes are then assayed for radioactivity. Rat insulin was detected in some of the tests; it was not detected in other tests. How does one know which clones contained the insulin gene?

13.11. The *E. coli* genome contains about 4000 kilobase pairs (kb; kilo = 1000); there are about 1.5 kb in 16S rRNA. If 0.14% of the genome forms hybrid double helices with RNA complementary to one strand of DNA, estimate the number of genetic loci encoding 16S rRNA.

13.12. About half the weight of RNA synthesized at any given time within a bacterial cell is rRNA. The 30S subunit of bacterial ribosomes contains one 16S rRNA molecule (1.5 kb); the 50S subunit contains one 23S rRNA (3 kb) and one small 5S rRNA (0.1 kb). Hybridization tests of 16S and 23S rRNAs with complementary single strands of DNA reveal that about 0.14% of DNA is coding for 16S rRNA and about 0.18% for 23S rRNA. Estimate the relative activity of rRNA genes as transcription templates compared to the average gene of the bacterial genome that gives rise to mRNA. *Note:* Assume that the amount of DNA allocated to 5S rRNA synthesis is negligible; likewise for all kinds of tRNAs.

13.13. Some bacterial proteins are normally secreted from the cell. If insulin could be attached by genetic engineering to such a bacterial protein, it too might be secreted from the cell. Suppose that you are given an agar plate containing several recombinant bacterial clones known to contain the gene for rat insulin. Propose an autoradiographic method for identifying those clones that are secreting rat insulin. *Hint:* Antibodies can be attached to certain kinds of plastic in a way that leaves their antigen-combining sites free to react.

13.14. Restriction endonuclease EcoRI makes staggered cuts in a 6-nucleotide DNA palindrome; restriction endonuclease HaeIII cleaves at one point in the middle of a 4-nucleotide palindrome. If different aliquots of a purified DNA preparation are treated with these enzymes, which one would be expected to contain more restriction fragments? Explain (give the rationale for) your choice.

13.15. Only about 200 molecules of lambda repressor are made by lysogenic bacteria when lambda is normally integrated at its specific attachment site between *E. coli* genes *gal* and *bio*. Some bacterial genes such as *lac* can be induced to produce more than 20,000 molecules of an enzyme per cell. If you could cut and splice structural and regulatory genes at your discretion, how would you design a bacterial cell for maximum synthesis of lambda repressor protein?

13.16. Suppose that we are trying to clone a specific human gene. After human DNA fragments have been spliced into plasmid vectors (shotgun method) and the plasmids have been exposed to recipient bacterial cells, how many kinds of cells exist? List their characteristics.

13.17. The polymerase chain reaction (PCR) was originally performed with a DNA polymerase from the bacterium *E. coli,* a common inhabitant of the human gut (37°C). Each cycle of heating denatured the enzyme added during the previous cycle. In order to reduce costs and automate the PCR, another source of the enzyme had to be found. Where is the most likely place to find this alternative source?

13.18. Protein P is synthesized in relatively high amounts in the human pancreas. This protein has been isolated and purified, but its amino acid sequence has not been determined. We wish to clone the gene for protein P.

(a) How can a probe be prepared to identify the gene for protein P?

(b) If we have prepared a radioactive messenger RNA as our probe in part (a), how could we verify that it is the mRNA for protein P?

(c) If we wish to make a gene library from the DNA of human pancreatic cells, we proceed by digesting the DNA with the restriction enzyme BamHI and then separating the fragments by agarose gel electrophoresis. The fragments are transferred (by Southern blotting) onto a nitrocellulose filter and flooded with the radioactive probe. Following incubation, the filter is washed to remove any probe that has not specifically bound to one or more DNA fragments. Autoradiography of the filter reveals two bands of sizes 300 and 700 bp. When the experiment is repeated using restriction enzyme PstI, only one band of 1000 bp appears. If it is already known that pancreatic cells contain a single copy of the gene for protein P, which of these enzymes should be used to construct our gene library?

(d) We can construct our gene library by cloning the PstI fragments into either plasmid pBR322 or phage lambda. Which one should we choose and why?

(e) Suppose that we want to insert the PstI fragments into the BamHI site within the gene for tetracycline resistance (tet^r) in the plasmid pBR322. If both of these restriction enzymes produce cohesive ends, how can this be done?

(f) After transforming E. coli with the plasmids, how can we identify the cells that contain a chimeric plasmid (containing a DNA insert)?

(g) If a million tetracycline-sensitive, ampicillin-resistant clones are grown on nutrient agar plates, how are we going to detect the rare clone or clones that carry the gene for protein P?

(h) After selecting a clone carrying the gene for protein P, its cells are propagated to high density in nutrient broth. The chimeric plasmid (with an insert of the gene for protein P) is then extracted and purified from the rest of the cellular DNA. How can we now isolate the gene from the plasmid?

(i) How can we demonstrate that the gene we have isolated is indeed the one for protein P?

(j) The ampicillin-resistance gene of plasmid pBR322 contains a single PstI restriction site. Genes that are inserted into an *amp-r* region are highly expressed. If an antibody specific for protein P is available, how would we now construct our gene library and detect the clones of interest?

(k) After we have cloned the gene for protein P into the amp^{-n} region of pBR322, suppose that we had to rely only on the drug-resistance properties of the plasmid to select from the gene library those cells carrying the plasmid plus the gene for protein P. What drug-resistance characteristics would the desired cells exhibit?

(l) How would we select for tet^r, amp^{-s} cells?

(m) Suppose that the base sequence of the gene for protein P is known. A defective protein P has been discovered, and its gene has also been cloned and sequenced. Both genes are 1000 bp in length and are flanked on either side by a site (—GAATTC—) for the restriction enzyme EcoRI. A base sequence —GCATTC— exists 300 bp from one end of the normal gene for protein P, but the sequence —GAATTC— exists at that same position in the abnormal gene. We want to find out if fetal cells contain the normal gene. So we cleave DNA from fetal cells with EcoRI and separate the fragments on an agarose gel. A probe for the normal gene will also hybridize with the abnormal gene if it differs by only a few bases from the normal gene. The size of the fetal DNA fragments can be estimated by running DNA fragments of known sizes on the same gel. What band pattern is expected if the fetal cells contain the abnormal gene?

13.19. A purified segment of DNA if labeled at its 5′ ends with ^{32}P and partially digested with the restriction enzyme Alu (from *Arthrobacter luteus*). The concentration is adjusted so that only about one of every fifty sites is recognized by the enzyme and cleaved. Therefore, each DNA molecule, if broken, is only broken once. This creates five fragments of various sizes. The fragments were electrophoresed, autoradiographed and the longest one (slowest migrating band) is selected for partial digestion (in separate experiments) with Alu and with another restriction endonuclease HaeIII (from *Haemophilus aegyptius*). These new fragments are separated by electrophoresis and located on the gel by autoradiography. The bands appear as shown below.

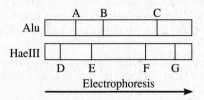

(a) Determine the sequence of restriction sites in this DNA segment. (b) How can the relative distances between cleavage sites be determined?

13.20. Diagram the electrophoretic pattern expected from a triple digest of the plasmid in Solved Problem 13.5 by restriction enzymes $A + B + C$.

13.21. Given the following information regarding digestion of a circular plasmid by three different restriction endonucleases, diagram the restriction map showing the distances between each cut.

Restriction Endonuclease	Fragment Length(s) (bp)
A	1000
B	50, 375, 575
C	400, 600
A + B	50, 175, 200, 575
A + C	225, 375, 400
B + C	25, 50, 150, 375, 400

13.22. (a) The following diagram represents six bands on an electrophoretic gel. The plus technique of the enzyme method was used for sequencing the DNA fragment. Determine the base sequence of the fragment and specify its polarity.

(b) If the minus technique had been performed on the same fragment as in part (a), diagram the expected location of the six bands in four columns adjacent to those in part (a).

(c) When more than one identical nucleotide is adjacent in a DNA sequence (e.g., AA or CCC), one or more bands will be missing from the plus and minus columns. Only the first (5′) nucleotide of the run is present in the minus system, and only the last (3′) nucleotide is represented in the plus system. The total number of residues in a sequence is revealed by running an aliquot of the initial extension reactions alongside the plus and minus reactions on the same gel as a control. Diagram the bands expected by sequencing the DNA segment $^{5′}$TAACGGGATCCCC$^{3′}$ with both the plus and minus techniques.

13.23. (a) From the following electrophoretic banding pattern, representing a fragment sequenced by the dideoxy (chain-termination) technique, determine the base sequence and orientation of the fragment.

(b) List all possible extension chains in each of the four reaction systems.

Review Questions

Vocabulary For each of the following definitions, give the appropriate term and spell it correctly. Terms are single words unless indicated otherwise.

1. A technique that separates molecules according to their net charge in an electric field, usually on solid or semisolid support media such as paper or agarose.

2. Separation of complementary chains of a DNA molecule, usually by heating.

3. Reassociation of complementary single-stranded regions of DNA with DNA or DNA with RNA.

4. Exposure of a photographic film to DNA labeled with a radioactive isotope.

5. Symmetrical sequences of nucleotide base pairs in double-stranded DNA that read the same on each strand from 5' to 3'.

6. Bacterial enzymes that break phosphodiester bonds in DNA at specific base sequences. (Two words.)

7. The random collection of a sufficiently large sample of cloned fragments of the DNA of an organism to ensure that all of that organism's DNA is represented in the collection. (Two words.)

8. An enzyme used to add deoxyribonucleotides to the 3' ends of DNA chains without a template. (Two or three words.)

9. An *in vitro* technique for copying the complementary strands of a target DNA sequence simultaneously for a series of cycles until the desired amount is obtained. (Three words.)

10. The name of the product produced by reverse transcriptase enzyme from an mRNA template. (One or two words.)

True-False Questions Answer each of the following statements either true (T) or false (F).

1. The unit of sedimentation (S) during ultracentrifugation was adopted in honor of its inventor, Sanger.

2. Double-stranded DNA molecules that are rich in G–C base pairs have a higher melting temperature than those that are rich in A–T base pairs.

3. The most common method for destroying RNA in the purification of DNA is exposure of the mixture to alkali.

4. Chargaff's rule states that in double-stranded DNA the molar amount of adenine is equivalent to that of thymine, and guanine is equivalent to that of cytosine.

5. The longer the half-life of a radioisotope, the higher its specific activity.

6. Single-stranded DNA binds to nitrocellulose; RNA does not.

7. Thymine is never found as a normal base in RNA molecules.

8. Euphenics is the science of improving the genetic constitution of the human gene pool.

9. DNA molecules that code for biologically active polypeptide chains are too large to be chemically synthesized (i.e., without biological synthesis).

10. During electrophoresis for nucleotide sequencing, the smaller the fragment the faster it moves.

Multiple-Choice Questions   Choose the one best answer.

1. A radioisotope used to label proteins differentially from nucleic acids is   (a) ^{32}P   (b) ^{14}C   (c) tritium   (d) ^{35}S   (e) ^{15}N

2. Which of the following single strands would be part of a palindrome in double-stranded DNA? (a) GAATTC   (b) ATGATG   (c) CTAATC   (d) CCCTTT   (e) none of the above

3. Which of the following is an enzyme used to form a phosphodiester bond in a nick between a 3′ end of one DNA chain and a 5′ end of another?   (a) DNA polymerase   (b) restriction endonuclease   (c) DNA ligase   (d) S1 nuclease   (e) phosphodiesterase

4. Bacterial cells are rendered more permeable to uptake of plasmids by treatment with   (a) heat   (b) calcium chloride   (c) alkali   (d) blender   (e) ultrasound

5. The melting temperature of a DNA molecule is determined by using   (a) electrophoresis   (b) change in electrical conductivity   (c) column chromatography   (d) density-gradient ultracentrifugation   (e) change in optical density

6. Which of the following is a desirable characteristic for a cloning plasmid?   (a) a site at which replication can be initiated   (b) a single restriction endonuclease site   (c) one or more antibiotic-resistance or drug-resistance genes   (d) one or more highly active promoters   (e) all of the above

7. Among the products of genetic engineering are the interferons. These substances are involved in   (a) viral replication   (b) blood clotting   (c) neuron function   (d) pain suppression   (e) tissue transplantation

8. Many of the genes in lambda phage are clustered according to similarity of function. Which of these gene clusters could most likely be deleted and replaced with foreign DNA, making the recombinant phage a useful cloning vector?   (a) nucleases to destroy host DNA   (b) head capsomeres   (c) phage-specific RNA polymerase   (d) establishment and maintenance of lysogeny   (e) tail proteins

9. Eucaryotic genes may not function properly when cloned into bacteria because of   (a) inability to excise introns   (b) destruction by native endonucleases   (c) failure of promoter to be recognized by bacterial RNA polymerase   (d) different ribosome binding sites   (e) all of the above

10. In the chemical method of DNA sequencing, four chemical treatments remove nucleotides as follows: (a) A, T, G, C   (b) G, G or C, A, A or T   (c) A or G, T or C, G, C   (d) A or C, G or T, C, G   (e) T, C, A, A or G

Answers to Supplementary Problems

13.6. (a) 51.02   (b) 40.82   (c) 73.47

13.7. (b), because it has a higher (G + C)/(A + T) ratio.

13.8. (b) would renature at a lower temperature because the long stretches of G–C pairs in (a) will tend to form *intrastrand* hydrogen bonds during cooling and therefore will require a higher temperature to disrupt these intrastrand interactions.

13.9.

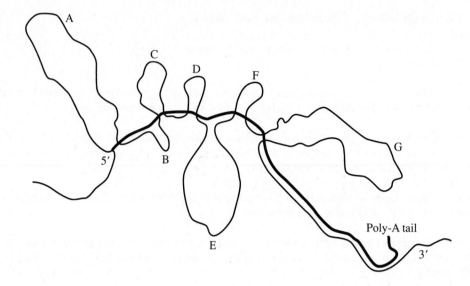

13.10. The fact that insulin was detected in some tests indicates that the RNA source contained the necessary information for *in vitro* insulin synthesis. Those clones that did not possess the insulin gene allowed single-stranded insulin mRNAs to make insulin; insulin was then specifically bound to the antibody-coated beads. Tubes that contain insulin are radioactive. However, if a clone contains rat insulin cDNA homologous with insulin mRNAs in the unpurified mixture, hybrid DNA-RNA molecules form, preventing such RNAs from making insulin. If no insulin is made, radioactive amino acids will not be bound by the antibody-coated beads. Little or no radioactivity should be detected in the tube after decantation of the supernate.

13.11. $(0.0014)(4000)/1.5 = 4$

13.12. Of all the RNAs that hybridize with DNA, the 16S and 23S rRNAs account for only $0.0014 + 0.0018 = 0.0032$ or 0.32%. Since these rRNAs and mRNAs are about equally represented in a cell, the ratio $1/0.0032 = 312.5$ expressed how much more active in transcription are the genes for the rRNAs.

13.13. Attach anti-rat insulin antibodies to a plastic disc about the size of an agar plate. Impress the disc onto the plate and allow any secreted insulin to be specifically bound by the antibodies. Remove the plastic disc and expose it to radioactive anti-insulin antibodies, forming an "immunological sandwich" with the antigen (insulin) between two antibody molecules. Wash away any unattached radioactive antibodies and then make an autoradiograph of the disc. Images on the film can be used to identify the locations of insulin-secreting clones on the agar plate.

13.14. More fragments are expected from HaeIII because the probability of a specific four-base sequence is greater than the probability of a specific six-base sequence if the nucleotides are distributed along a chain in essentially a random order.

13.15. Insert the gene for lambda repressor protein immediately adjacent to the *lac* promoter in a plasmid. With no operator locus between these two genes, thousands of repressor molecules should be made per cell constitutively.

13.16. Five kinds of cells:
   (1) Bacteria that do not contain any plasmid DNA.

   (2) Bacteria that took up the plasmid DNA, but do not contain any human DNA.

   (3) Bacteria that contain the plasmid DNA with human DNA spliced in, but not the desired human gene sequence.

   (4) Bacteria that contain plasmid DNA and a portion of the desired human gene, but not all of it.

   (5) Bacteria that contain plasmid DNA and all of the desired human gene.

13.17. Organisms that live in hot springs must have heat-stable enzymes. A DNA polymerase was isolated for use in automating the PCR from the bacterium *Thermus aquaticus* that normally lives in hot springs at a temperature of 70–80°C.

13.18. (*a*) It should be possible to purify a major species of messenger RNA from pancreatic cells that codes for protein P. It can then be tagged with a radioactive label for use as a probe. Alternatively, if a gene for protein P has already been isolated from some other mammal, it could also be made radioactive and used as a probe.

(*b*) Use the mRNA in an *in vitro* (cell-free) translational system that allows it to direct the synthesis of its protein. Isolate the protein and compare its amino acid sequence with that of protein P.

(*c*) PstI, because it does not cut the gene for protein P.

(*d*) Since the gene for protein P is 1000 bp or less in length, it is too small to clone into phage lambda, which requires fragments of approximately 15,000 bp. Thus we should choose plasmid pBR322.

(*e*) By attaching BamHI linkers to the PstI fragments, they can be inserted by hybridization between their complementary single-stranded tails into the BamHI site on the plasmid.

(*f*) By employing the replica plating technique, we can select cells that are tetracycline-sensitive and ampicillin-resistant. Only those cells that have incorporated the plasmid are ampicillin-resistant, and of these only the cells with an insert in the *tet-r* gene are tetracycline-sensitive.

(*g*) Blot each Petri plate with a nitrocellulose filter paper, thereby transferring some cells of each clone onto the filter for *in situ* hybridization. Lyse the cells and denature the DNA with a dilute sodium hydroxide solution. Single strands of the denatured DNA thus will stick to the filter. Flood the filter with the radioactive probe. After washing to remove any of the unhybridized probe, subject the filter to autoradiography. Select cells from the plate that correspond in position to the radioactive loci on the filter.

(*h*) By cutting the chimeric plasmid with BamHI, the gene can be released. It can then be isolated from the plasmid by electrophoresis on an agarose gel.

(*i*) The gene for protein P should hybridize specifically with the probe made from protein P mRNA. It might be possible in an *in vitro* system to synthesize both the mRNA and the protein it codes for from the gene. By sequencing both the gene and the protein, it would be possible to ascertain by the genetic code if the 2 molecules were compatible (allowing for removal of any introns). The biological activity of the protein thus produced might also be demonstrable in an *in vivo* system.

(*j*) Cleave human pancreatic cell DNA with PstI and insert the DNA fragments into the PstI site in the *amp-r* region of the plasmid. Clones that contain the plasmid bearing the gene for protein P might produce large amounts of protein P that could then be detected by an appropriate immunoassay.

(*k*) They would be ampicillin-sensitive and tetracycline-resistant because the *tet-r* gene is still functional, but the gene for protein P has been inserted into the *amp-r* gene and thereby has inactivated it.

(*l*) Expose the cells to a medium containing tetracycline. Cells that do not harbor plasmid pBR322 will not grow. Then, by replica plating, identify those tetracycline-resistant clones that do not grow in the presence of ampicillin.

(*m*) The normal gene for protein P should produce one band, 1000 bp long. The mutant gene for an abnormal protein P should produce a band of 300 bp and another band of 700 bp in length because a single base mutation has created a new EcoRI site.

13.19. (*a*)

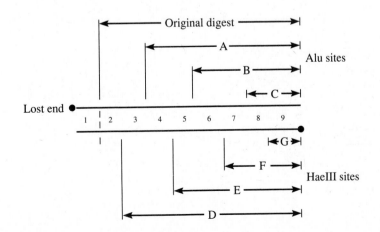

(b)   Since the distances the various fragments travel in the gel are related (by a log function) to their sizes, the relative distances between cleavage sites can be determined.

13.20. *Note:* The migration distance is not linear with increasing fragment length, but more like a log function.

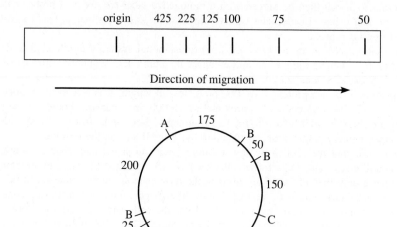

13.21.

13.22.   (a) ⁵′TACGAC³′

(b)

	+C	+T	+A	+G	−C	−T	−A	−G
7	—							
6				—		—		
5					—		—	
4	—							—
3				—		—		
2		—					—	
1				—				

Notice that the ''negative bands'' are shifted one step lower than the ''positive bands.'' For example, bands at positions 3 and 6 in the −C column indicate that these fragments were terminated just prior to C, hence bands should appear at positions 4 and 7 in the +C columns. DNA base sequencing can be done by either the plus or minus system, but they are usually analyzed together on the same gel to provide mutual confirmation of the sequence.

(c)

Control		−C	−T	−A	−G	+C	+T	+A	+G
14	___						—		
13	___								
12	___								
11	___								
10	___		—				—		
9	___			—				—	
8	___				—				—
7	___								
6	___								
5	___			—	—				
4	___	—					—		
3	___								
2	___			—			—		
1	___		—						

13.23. (a)   5′CGACGGT3′

(b)   ddGTP-terminated fragments (d)

> 5′CGACGGT
> CGACG*d*
> CGAC*d*
> C*d*

ddATP-terminated fragments (d)

> 5′CGACGGT
> CG*d*

ddTTP-terminated fragments (d)

> 5′CGACGGT
> CGACGG*d*

ddCTP-terminated fragments (d)

> 5′CGACGGT
> CGA*d*
> *d*

Answers to Review Questions

Vocabulary

1. electrophoresis
2. denaturation or melting
3. renaturation or annealing
4. autoradiography
5. palindrome
6. restriction endonucleases
7. gene (DNA) library or genomic library
8. terminal (deoxyribonucleotidal) transferase
9. polymerase chain reaction
10. complementary DNA (cDNA)

True-False Questions

1. F (Svedberg)   2. T   3. T   4. T   5. F (lower)   6. T   7. F (in some tRNAs)   8. F (eugenics)   9. F (e.g., somatostatin, interferon)   10. T

Multiple-Choice Questions

1. *d*   2. *a*   3. *c*   4. *b*   5. *e*   6. *e*   7. *a*   8. *d*   9. *e*   10. *c*

Chapter 14

The Molecular Biology of Eucaryotic Cells and Their Viruses

The cells of fungi, plants, and animals contain a double-membraned organelle called the nucleus. The term **eucaryote** (eukaroyte is a variant spelling) refers to cells that contain such an organelle. The protoplasm between the nucleus and the plasma membrane constitutes the cell's cytoplasm. Other double-membraned organelles exist in the cytoplasm, including mitochondria in both plants and animals, and chloroplasts in plants. Bacteria do not have double-membraned organelles, but some may contain single-membraned organelles such as the chlorobium vesicles involved in photosynthesis. The term **procaryote** refers to cells that do not have a nucleus. Bacterial cells are much smaller than most eucaryotic cells and have smaller DNA genomes. Most of what we know about molecular genetics has been discovered by studying these simpler bacterial systems and their viruses. It was hoped that much of what we learned about procaryotes would be directly applicable to eucaryotes. Unfortunately, that has not proved to be true. Greater fundamental differences exist between a simple single-celled eucaryote (such as a yeast or an algal cell) and a bacterium than between a yeast cell and a human cell. In this chapter, we shall investigate some of the most striking differences between these two major forms of life.

QUANTITY OF DNA

The amount of DNA present in a typical mammalian cell is approximately 800 times that found in a bacterium such as *E. coli*. While a eucaryotic cell might possibly be 50 or 100 times more genetically complex than a bacterium, it could hardly be 800 times more complex. So a paradox exists as to why eucaryotes have so much DNA. A roughly similar number of genes is probably required to carry out housekeeping functions (such as coding for the enzymes of metabolism) in both procaryotes and eucaryotes. Most eucaryotic genes coding for proteins are present in only one or a few copies in each genome; however, some genes (e.g., genes for rRNAs, tRNAs, and histones) exist in tens, hundreds or thousands of copies; and a few short DNA segments may be repeated over 10^5 times per genome (Table 14.1).

Table 14.1. Frequency Classes of Eucaryotic DNA Sequences

DNA Frequency Class	Number of Copies per Genome	Percentage of the Genome	Examples
Unique	1	10–80	Structural genes for ovalbumin, silk fibroin, hemoglobin
Middle repetitive	10^1–10^5	10–40	Genes for tRNA, rRNA, histones
Highly repetitive	$> 10^5$	0–50	Satellite sequences (5–300 nucleotides)

By contrast, procaryotes almost exclusively have unique DNA sequences. Undoubtedly many eucaryotic DNA sequences are needed to code for tissue-specific proteins, to regulate the activation and deactivation ("silencing") of large batteries of genes at appropriate times, and to control the quantity of proteins synthesized during cellular differentiation. Even so, the eucaryotic cell is estimated to contain at least an order of magnitude more DNA than it needs. Estimates of "unnecessary" DNA in humans run as high as 95% of the genome. The question of what all this DNA is doing has not been answered satisfactorily. Perhaps it is "junk" or "selfish" DNA with no function other than to make more copies of itself, as some have suggested. In any event, this massive amount of DNA (e.g., 3×10^9 bp in the haploid human genome) is packaged into the linear chromosomes found in the cell's nucleus.

CHROMOSOME STRUCTURE

Eucaryotic DNA is primarily associated with a basic class of proteins known as **histones.** Together, the DNA and histones form **nucleoprotein,** or **chromatin.** In the first level of packaging (Fig. 14-1), about 150 bp of the double-stranded DNA molecule are wrapped around an octomer of four pairs of different histone proteins to form a **nucleosome** core particle. A fifth kind of histone protein occupies the **linker DNA** that connects one core particle with another (analogous to beads on a string). This "string" first coils up into a solenoid of 30-nanometer diameter and then into a filament of 300-nanometer diameter. Even higher levels of compaction occur during cell division when the chromatin material appears in the light microscope to condense from an amorphous chromatin mass into distinctive chromosomes. Nonhistone proteins (including various DNA and RNA polymerases, regulatory proteins, etc.) can also be found associated with chromatin, but they are not responsible for the basic structure of chromatin.

The highly compacted chromatin that can be seen in the light microscope during interphase is called **heterochromatin;** the much more open form of chromatin that is difficult to see is called **euchromatin.** Eucaryotic genes cannot be expressed (i.e., cannot serve as templates for RNA sythesis) if they are tightly bound to histones. So the first step in gene activation requires a dissociation of the DNA from the histones. Thus, euchromatic regions are thought to contain active genes whereas heterochromatic regions are thought to contain silenced genes. Various mechanisms exist to regulate which regions become heterochromatic.

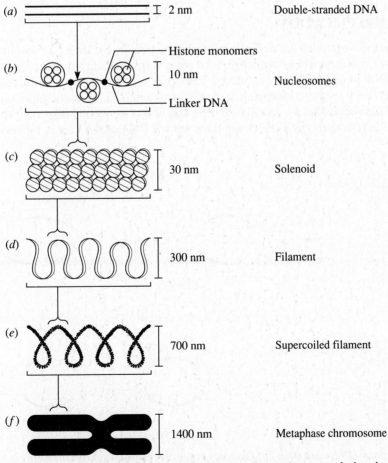

Fig. 14-1.   Structural levels of organization hypothesized to occur during the condensation of a chromosome. (After J. D. Watson et al., 1987, *Molecular Biology of the Gene,* 4th ed., Benjamin/Cummings Publishing Company, Inc.).

Example 14.1.   In female mammals, one of the two X chromosomes in each somatic cell appears highly condensed (heterochromatic), indicating that it is genetically inactive. In some cells one of the X chromosomes is inactive, and in other cells the other X chromosome is inactive. Thus the female is a mosaic consisting of a mixture of two cell types with regard to X gene activity.

Example 14.2.   The stained giant polytene chromosomes of *Drosophila* (Fig. 8-1) consist of alternating dark and light bands. The dark bands are heterochromatin; the light bands are euchromatin. At various stages during larval development, specific regions appear to decondense and form fluffy puffs of open chromatin material. At least some of the genes in these puffs are actively synthesizing RNA. Furthermore, the pattern of these puffed regions changes during larval development, indicating that different groups of genes are being activated and silenced as cellular differentiation proceeds.

Example 14.3.   The regions around the centromeres of chromosomes are normally heterochromatic. They contain highly repetitive DNA sequences that are so different from the rest of chromatin that they can be easily separated by differential centrifugation. Such sequences are referred to as **satellite** sequences. The exact function of these regions is presently unknown.

The DNA in a metaphase chromosome appears to be attached to a protein **scaffold** constructed from two high-molecular-weight proteins. This association persists in metaphase chromosomes that have had their histones and most of their nonhistones removed. How this elegent scaffold becomes assembled and its role in the induction of superhelicity of the DNA is not known.

CHROMOSOME REPLICATION

Three elements are essential for replication of eucaryotic chromosomes: (1) origins of replication, (2) telomeres, and (3) centromeres. Each chromatid (or unreplicated chromosome) is thought to contain a single, linear DNA molecule. DNA replication can occur simultaneously at numerous places in each such chromosome. Each of these independent "replication units" is called a **replicon.** The origins of replication in adjacent replicons are usually 50–250 kbp apart. Replicons may correspond to the independently supercoiled domains that lie between the points of DNA attachment to the metaphase scaffold.

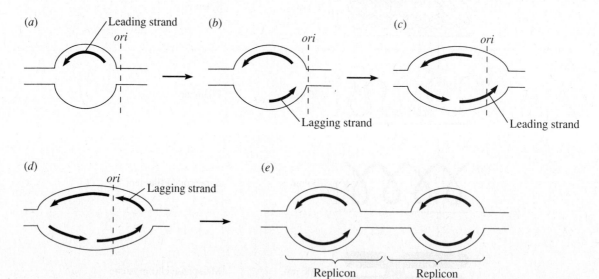

Fig. 14-2.   Bidirectional DNA replication. (*a*) From any origin of replication site (*ori*) a leading strand is synthesized. (*b*) Initiation of lagging strand synthesis. (*c*) The first precursor (Okazaki) fragment has passed the *ori* site and has become the rightward leading strand. (*d*) Initiation of leftward lagging strand begins with establishment of a second complete replication fork. (*e*) Two replication bubbles about to coalesce. Each independently replicating unit is a replicon.

Within each replicon, a special RNA polymerase (primase) synthesizes an RNA primer (called an **initiator**) that binds to the 3′ end of each template DNA strand to be replicated. DNA polymerase then extends the primer in the 5′ → 3′ direction. Replication is normally bidirectional. Numerous "replication bubbles" appear during DNA replication (Fig. 14-2); each bubble grows in length, and eventually fuses with flanking bubbles to complete the process.

Since RNA primers for DNA replication are normally excised, the ends of eucaryotic chromosomes (called **telomeres**) are maintained by special ribonucleoprotein enzymes (called **telomerases**) that add new terminal DNA sequences to replace those lost during each replication cycle.

Example 14.4.   The ends of the linear chromosomes in the macronucleus of the ciliated protozoan *Tetrahymena* have 30–70 tandemly repeated blocks of the sequence

$$3'\text{-AACCCC-}5'$$
$$5'\text{-TTGGGG-}3'$$

A special enzyme adds 5′-TTGGGG-3′ to the 3′ end of any such sequence in single-stranded DNA. After the enzyme has extended the 3′ end of the telomere, synthesis of the repeats in the complementary DNA strand could be primed by a primase. Similarly, the ends of all yeast chromosomes end with approximately 100 bp of the irregularly repeated sequence

$$5'\text{-}C_{1-3}\,A\,\ldots$$
$$3'\text{-}C_{1-3}\,T\,\ldots$$

The mechanism that determines the length of such telomeres is not known.

In the ciliate *Euplotes crassus,* the RNA component of the telomerase serves a template function for synthesis of telomeric T_4G_4 repeats. Thus, at least some portions of certain eucaryotic DNA molecules are known to be replicated from RNA templates. Enzymes that make DNA from RNA templates are called reverse transcriptases; this kind of telomerase represents a specialized kind of reverse transcriptase.

Little is presently known about the centromeric regions where sister chromatids are joined. The centromeric sequences in yeast are about 130 bp long and very rich in A-T. It is thought that the chromatin material is not organized into nucleosomes in the centromeric region either because the histones have become modified or because a complex of proteins other than the normal histones are specifically bound to the centromeric sequences. This proteinaceous region of the centromere (called the **kinetochore**) somehow attaches to microtubule bundles of the spindle. Each sister chromatid has its own kinetochore. The centromeric sequence is generally bordered (flanked) by heterochromatin containing repetitive DNA sequences (see Example 14.3). The centromeric sequences replicate during the contracted metaphase state, and thus are the last DNA segments to do so in eucaryotic cells prior to normal cell division.

ORGANIZATION OF THE NUCLEAR GENOME

Functionally related bacterial genes are often clustered together in operons that produce polycistronic mRNAs. Eucaryotes have only monocistronic cytoplasmic mRNAs and their genes are not organized into operons. Many eucaryotic **reiterated genes** that exist in multiple identical copies (e.g., genes for rRNAs, tRNAs, and histones) are clustered together on specific chromosomes, as components of **multigene families.** Other multiple-gene families may consist of a set of genes descended by duplication and mutation from one ancestral gene; they may be clustered together on the same chromosome or dispersed on different chromosomes. Such genes are usually coordinately controlled.

Example 14.5.   In humans, there are two families of hemoglobin genes. The alpha (α) family consists of a cluster of genes (including zeta [ζ], α_2, and α_1) on chromosome 16. The beta (β) family cluster on chromosome 11 includes epsilon (ε), gammas (γ^G, γ^A), delta (δ), and β. In addition, each family has one or more nonfunctional DNA sequences that are very similar to those of normal globin genes. These nonfunctional DNA gene–like sequences are referred to as **pseudogenes.** During the embryonic stage (less than 8 weeks) of development, the ζ- and ε-chains are synthesized. During the fetal period (8–41 weeks) the γ- and α-chains replace the embryonic chains. Beginning around birth and continuing for life, β-chains replace the gammas. A small fraction of adult hemoglobin has δ-chains in place of β-chains. The signals that control this switching on or off of the various hemoglobin genes is not known. The similarity in nucleotide structure of all these genes, however, suggests that early in evolution (perhaps 800 million years ago) a single ancestral globin gene began a series of duplications, followed by mutations and transpositions, to produce the two families and their multiple constituent genes and pseudogenes that exist today.

GENOMIC STABILITY

Each gene normally resides at a specific location on a particular chromosome, thus allowing the construction of gene maps. However, multiple chromosomal breaks can be repaired in abnormal ways to produce translocations and inversions that rearrange the genetic architecture. This type of genetic relocation is not self-generated by the segments moved. As in bacteria, however, there are some chromosomal segments that encode proteins responsible for their own movement; they are called **transposons** or **transposable elements.**

Example 14.6. Movable controlling elements ("jumping genes") were first discovered in maize by Barbara McClintock in the 1950s. Insertion of the controlling element *Ds* into or adjacent to a locus governing kernel color inhibits the production of color and results in a colorless phenotype. Excision of *Ds* reverses the effect and produces colored spots on a colorless background. The *Ds* elements occur in different sizes as deleted forms of a larger complete gene called *Ac*. The *Ds* elements are **nonautonomous** because they remain stationary unless an *Ac* element is also present, whereas *Ac* elements are **autonomous** because they can move independently. Both *Ac* and *Ds* elements have perfect inverted repeats of 11 bp at their termini, flanked by 6- to 8-bp direct repeats of the target site. Thus, *Ac* and *Ds* are transposons. *Ac* need not be adjacent to *Ds* or even on the same chromosome in order to activate *Ds*. When *Ds* is so activated, it can alter the level of expression of neighboring genes, the structure of the gene product, or the time of development when the gene expresses itself, as a consequence of nucleotide changes inside or outside a given cistron. An activated *Ds* element can also cause chromosomal breakage, which can yield deletions or generate a bridge-breakage-fusion-bridge cycle. Several other systems like the *Ac/Ds* system are now known in maize. Each has a **target gene** that is inactivated by insertion of a **receptor element** into it, and a distant **regulator element** that is responsible for the mutational instability of the locus. The receptor and regulator elements are both considered to be **controlling elements** of the target gene.

In bacteria, the number of copies of a transposon appears to be regulated, seldom exceeding 20 copies per genome. In eucaryotes, however, the copy number can be very high.

Example 14.7. In a human genome, there exist about 300,000 members of a sequence (approximately 300 bp) that is cut by a base-specific DNase called AluI. Members of this Alu family are related, but not identical in base sequence. Each member is flanked by direct repeats. Although transposition has not been observed for any member, the Alu family is thought to have evolved from a DNA copy of an RNA molecule that plays a role in protein synthesis. Since no function, essential or otherwise, has been attributed to this family, it may represent an example of "selfish DNA" whose only function is to make copies of itself.

As a generalization, however, the genetic architecture of eucaryotic cells usually remains quite stable even during the differentiation of various cell and tissue types during embryological development. Only a couple of exceptions to this rule have been found, and they are limited to the immune system (see Example 14.23).

GENE EXPRESSION

1. Transcription.

The synthesis and processing of ribosomal RNA (rRNA) occurs in one or more specialized regions of the genome called **nucleoli.** Multiple copies of rRNA genes in tandem array are found in each nucleolus.

In contrast to the single RNA polymerase of procaryotes, there are three such enzymes in eucaryotes, one for each major class of RNA. The enzyme that synthesizes rRNA is RNA polymerase I (pol I). The promoter regions for pol I lie upstream from the start site of transcription. A **Hogness box** (TATA box) lies within the promoter as the eucaryote analogue of the Pribnow box in procaryotes. The initiation of rRNA synthesis is highly species-specific; within a species, one or more proteins (essential for the transcription process) recognize promoters only in the rDNA of the same species.

RNA polymerase II (pol II) has its own specific initiation factors for sythesis of all eucaryotic mRNAs. Its promoters lie upstream from the start site of each gene, but the activity of the promoters may be increased by physically linked (i.e., in cis position) DNA sequences called **enhancers.** Enhancers may function in either orientation, and may reside either within or upstream or downstream from their target genes (sometimes at great distances). The enhancing effect is mediated through sequence-specific DNA-binding proteins. It is hypothesized that once the DNA-binding protein attaches to the enhancer sequence, it causes the intervening nucleotides between the enhancer and the promoter to loop out and bring the enhancer into physical contact with the promoter of the gene it enhances. This loop structure then facilitates the attachment of RNA polymerase II molecules to the promoter of the transcribing gene.

The transcription termination signals for eucaryotic mRNA molecules is not known. RNA polymerase II continues elongating mRNA chains beyond the sequences found in mature mRNAs before termination occurs by an unknown mechanism. The transcript is then somehow specifically cleaved to form the correct 3' end.

Complex mechanisms (too involved to be presented here) ensure that the introns are removed from the pre-mRNA (primary transcript) and that the exons are spliced together in the proper order. Thereafter, the pre-mRNAs of eucaryotes undergo a number of covalent modifications before they are released from the nucleus as mature messenger molecules. The enzyme **poly-A polymerase** adds (without a template) a long stretch of adenine nucleotides to the 3' end of each pre-mRNA, forming a poly-A tail. Since only mRNA molecules (not rRNAs or tRNAs) have these tails, it might be suggested that they have something to do with translation. In contrast to most mRNAs, however, those for histone proteins in most species do not acquire poly-A tails. So the function of these tails remains a mystery. The 5' ends become "capped" with an unusual guanine nucleotide (3'-G-5'ppp5'-N-3'p). A methyl group is subsequently added to this backward guanine cap. Thus, both the 5' and 3' ends of most eucaryotic mRNAs possess free 2'- and 3'-OH groups on their terminal ribose sugars. Bacterial mRNAs contain specific ribosome-binding sites in their leader sequences; eucaryotic mRNAs do not have these sites. Instead, a eucaryotic ribosome usually binds to the mRNA cap and then moves downstream along the mRNA until it encounters the first AUG initiation codon, and begins translation there.

Eucaryotic ribosomes, like their bacterial counterparts, consist of two major subunits, but they are more complex, existing as 40S and 60S subunits that together form an 80S complex. The rRNA components in more evolutionarily advanced ("higher") eucaryotes having sedimentation coefficients of 18S, 5.8S, and 28S are transcribed from 50 to 5000 identical genes tandemly arranged in that order into massive clusters located on one or more chromosomes as **nucleolar organizing regions (NORs).** When active, these rRNA repeat units extend out from the main chromosome fiber as elongated threads. When complexed with specific proteins involved in rRNA synthesis and processing, these clusters become visible in the light microscope as nucleoli where the assembly of ribosomes begins. The number of NORs per haploid genome varies with the species from one to several. In *E. coli*, there are only seven copies of the rRNA genes. Very few bacterial genes exist in multiple copies, and even then the copy number is very small. As much as half of the eucaryotic primary rRNA transcript may be lost during processing of the mature rRNA molecule. Some of this loss is due to the removal of introns. In the protozoan ciliate *Tetrahymena thermophila,* the rRNA transcripts appear to be self-splicing. RNA molecules with autocatalytic properties are called **ribozymes.**

The eucaryotic genes encoding tRNAs generally also exist in multiple copies, from 10 to several hundred for each tRNA species per haploid genome. The identical genes within each tRNA family tend to be widely dispersed in species with relatively low numbers of tRNA gene copies. In organisms with more highly reiterated tRNA genes, they may form heteroclusters containing several kinds of tRNA genes. RNA polymerase III (pol III) is responsible for synthesizing not only all of the tRNAs but also 5S ribosomal RNA and other small RNAs. These transcripts are usually short (less than 300 nucleotides), with complementary end sequences that may allow formation of a stable base-paired stem. Sequences within the tRNA genes are required for transcription by pol III. Internal control regions (located inside the genes themselves) also direct termination of transcription by pol III. Thus, the same region can function both biosynthetically (in the gene) and structurally (in the RNA product).

2. Translation.

The process of translating an mRNA into a polypeptide chain in eucaryotes is essentially the same as that in bacteria, but differs in several important ways. Whereas only three well-defined initiation factors are required for translation of *E. coli* mRNAs, many more are needed in eucaryotes. Eucaryotic initiation factors are designated **eIFs** to distinguish them from their bacterial counterparts. Other examples follow.

Example 14.8.   A tRNA^{Met} (symbolized Met-tRNA^{Met} when activated) brings an unformylated methionine into the first position on the ribosome. Hydrolysis of ATP to ADP is required for mRNA binding. The 40S ribosomal subunit is then thought to attach to the mRNA at its capped 5' terminus, and then it slides along (consuming ATP) until it reaches the first AUG codon. Normally only AUG is an efficient initiator codon in eucaryotes, whereas UUG, GUG, and AUU may also be used in *E. coli*.

Example 14.9.   Three different elongation factors (EFs) in eucaryotes replace those found in bacteria. However, a single termination factor (RF) replaces RF1 and RF2 of bacteria. RF recognizes all three stop codons (UAC, UAA, and UGA).

3. Post–translation Modifications.

A nascent polypeptide chain may not become biologically active until after it has been modified in one or more specific ways, such as being enzymatically phosphorylated, glucosylated, or partly digested.

Example 14.10.   Protein kinases are enzymes that transfer terminal phosphate groups from ATP to specific amino acids on target proteins. Phosphorylation of these proteins may either raise or lower their biological activities. For example, the skeletal muscle enzyme glycogen synthetase is inactivated after phosphorylation, whereas phosphorylation of the enzyme glycogen phosphorylase increases its activity.

Example 14.11.   The hormone insulin is synthesized as a single-chain precursor (proinsulin) with little or no hormonal activity. Two internal cuts remove 31 amino acids from proinsulin, producing the two polypeptide chains of the functional dimer. Likewise, human growth hormone that circulates in blood is a "clipped" version of the pituitary form of that hormone.

REGULATION OF GENE EXPRESSION

Much less is known about gene regulation in eucaryotes than in procaryotes. In contrast to bacteria, most eucaryotic cells (some algae, yeast, and protozoa are a few notable exceptions) are not free-living single cells. Multicellular eucaryotes usually show cellular differentiation. Differentiation allows cells to become specialized for certain tasks; e.g., liver cells are highly metabolic, muscle cells contract, nerve cells conduct impulses, red blood cells carry oxygen. The signals that cause eucaryotic cells to differentiate is largely endogenous (within the multicellular body). Eucaryotic cells cooperate with one another to maintain a fairly uniform internal environment despite variation in environmental conditions exterior to the organism; this regulatory phenomenon is known as **homeostasis.** Bacteria can turn their genes on or off repeatedly in response to various nutrients such as glucose or lactose in their environment. Switching genes on or off during development of eucaryotic cells, however, is usually a permanent change. Once a cell has started to differentiate, it can seldom be diverted to another developmental pathway. Because eucaryotic cytoplasmic mRNAs are monocistronic, operons that coordinately control multiple structural genes (as in bacteria) are not found in plants and animals. Furthermore, the somatic cells of eucaryotes are produced by mitosis and sexual cells, by meiosis; neither of these processes is found in bacteria. Thus, the regulatory systems of eucaryotes must be far more complex than those of prokaryotes.

1. Six Points of Control.

Gene expression in eucaryotes involves six major steps:

(1) Uncoiling of nucleosomes

(2) Transcription of DNA into RNA

(3) Processing of the nuclear RNA (nRNA) or pre-mRNA

(4) Transport of mRNA from nucleus to cytoplasm

(5) Translation of mRNA into a polypeptide chain

(6) Processing of the polypeptide chain into functional proteins

Each of these steps represents a potential point at which the expression of eucaryotic gene may be turned on or off.

2. Genetic Regulation by Altering the Structure or Genomic Content of DNA.

Evolution progresses by sequential modifications of preexisting developmental patterns. Whatever mechanism that works initially to solve a biological problem tends to become so integrated into the overall developmental program with the passage of many generations that it cannot be changed thereafter. Thus it is not surprising that different organisms may use quite different mechanisms to solve common biological problems. The abundance of a species of RNA molecules may be regulated at the gene level by several mechanisms. In order to understand some processes of selective **gene amplification,** a distinction must be made between **germ-line genes** (those that are passed on to offspring) and **somatic genes** (not hereditary).

> **Example 14.12.** In the ciliate protozoans, there are two kinds of nuclei: a polyploid somatic macronucleus (controlling all transcription during vegetative growth and asexual reproduction) and a haploid micronucleus containing the germ line. Fusion of haploid nuclei from conjugation of opposite mating types produces a diploid zygotic nucleus. The old macronucleus then degenerates and the zygotic nucleus divides to produce a new haploid micronucleus and an immature macronucleus. The macronuclear genome then becomes polyploid like the polytene chromosomes of *Drosophila*. The macronuclear chromosomes, however, become highly fragmented, and most of the fragments (up to 95% in some species) are degraded. The surviving fragments contain the genes required for vegetative growth and asexual reproduction. The mechanisms controlling this selective degradation and the distribution of surviving fragments into progeny cells during cell division are essentially unknown.

> **Example 14.13.** Amphibian oocytes contain a hundred to a thousand times more rRNA genes than are found in somatic cells, almost all of the increase being due to large numbers of extrachromosomal nucleoli. Each nucleolus contains one or more circular DNA molecules having 1–20 tandemly arranged rRNA genes coding for the 45S rRNA precursor. Most of these nucleolar circles are produced by the rolling-circle mechanism (as discussed in Chapter 12). These circles contain somatic genes and cannot replicate themselves. Extrachromosomal rRNA genes must be derived from the tandemly repeated rRNA germ-line genes.

Unlike the amphibian rRNA genes in Example 14.13, the chorion (eggshell) genes of *Drosophila* can be amplified without extrachromosomal replication. A large number of follicle cells surround the egg and produce the chorion. The genes encoding the chorionic proteins exist in two clusters (one on the X chromosome and one on an autosome). Only a single copy of each somatic gene is present. A developmentally controlled origin of replication, located within each gene cluster, is programmed to fire 3–6 times during interphase within the 5 hours of choriogenesis. The process shown in Fig. 14-3 usually produces a 32- to 64-fold amplification of the chorion genes.

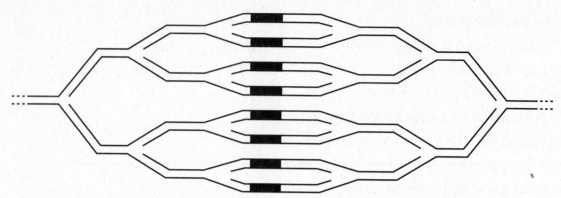

Fig. 14-3.   Gene amplification of chorion genes (dark segments) in *Drosophila*. Three rounds of replication from a single replication origin near the chorion genes has occurred.

3. Transcription Regulation.

In procaryotic operons, regulatory genes and the promoters that they control are adjacent, but in eucaryotes the regulatory genes are rarely adjacent to the promoters that they control. As previously noted, a class of regulatory sites called "enhancers" may be several hundred base pairs either upstream or downstream from the promoters they stimulate. Also difficult to understand is how sets of genes on different chromosomes are coordinately regulated. Some models of gene regulation in eucaryotes have proposed that each gene in a coordinated set is preceded by the same regulatory sequence so that they will all respond to the same signal, but perhaps not to the same extent. It is also possible that a set of genes might respond to more than one signal or combinations of signals. In a model, these possibilities could be accommodated by proposing that some genes are adjacent to multiple receptor sequences, only one of which needs to receive a signal for activation, or by having single receptors and multicomponent signal molecules.

(*a*) *Exogenous Signals.*   Gene regulation in procaryotes occurs mainly in response to exogenous signals such as the presence or absence of nutrients (e.g., glucose or lactose). Most gene regulation in eucaryotes occurs in response to endogenous signals, but not exclusively so.

> **Example 14.14.**   When plants are grown in darkness for several days they start to lose their green color (etiolation) because of loss of the enzymes that catalyze chlorophyll synthesis. Within a few hours after exposure of an etiolated plant to sunlight, more than 60 photosynthetic enzymes, chloroplast rRNA, and chlorophyll synthesis occurs. A protein called **phyto-chrome** is covalently bound to a light-absorbing pigment. In the dark, phytochrome is inactive; in sunlight, it becomes activated and is thought to become a transcription factor for production of an unknown number of photosynthetic enzymes.

(*b*) *Endogenous Signals.*   The best-known endogenous regulators of gene activity in eucaryotes are the **hormones.** These are substances produced by one cell type that have effects on other cell types. Hormones are usually transported throughout the organism (e.g., via the bloodstream in animals) but interact only with those cells that have the corresponding receptors. These receptors would have to be on the cell surface to react with large hormones such as proteins. For small hydrophobic molecules such as steroids that may pass freely through the cell membrane, the hormone receptor could be in the cytoplasm or in the nucleus. The interaction of hormone and receptor eventually would cause a signal to be transmitted to the DNA at one or more specific sites to activate the appropriate gene or set of genes.

> **Example 14.15.**   Only the oviduct cells of the chicken respond to an injection of the steroid hormone estrogen by synthesizing ovalbumin mRNA. Other cell types fail to respond to estrogen because they lack the corresponding receptor. It is proposed that estrogen enters the cell by diffusion and binds to a cytoplasmic protein receptor. The hormone-receptor complex then migrates into the nucleus and initiates transcription of the ovalbumin gene.

A family of membrane proteins called **G proteins** are interposed between some signal molecules (e.g., hormones or neurotransmitters) and an "amplifier enzyme." If the hormone binds to a cell surface receptor, it induces a conformational change in the receptor. This change is transmitted through the cell membrane to a G protein, making it able to bind guanosine triphosphate (GTP); hence the G in the name for these proteins. Binding of GTP causes a conformational change in the G protein that enables it to activate an amplifier enzyme. If the amplifier enzyme is adenyl cyclase, its activation results in the production of cyclic AMP (the second messenger). The cAMP can then regulate the activity of one or more genes coordinately.

Hormones might promote transcription by any of the following mechanisms:

(1) The hormone could cause DNA to become uncoupled from histones (dissolution from nucleosomes) and thereby allow RNA polymerase to begin transcription.

(2) The hormone might act as an inducer by inactivating a repressor molecule.

(3) The hormone may bind directly to specific DNA sequences to facilitate binding of RNA polymerase or of a protein transcription factor.

(4) The hormone may activate an effector protein (comparable to the CRP protein of the bacterial *lac* operon) so that the complex can bind to a site on the DNA and thereby stimulate binding of RNA polymerase.

(5) The hormone could become attached to a protein already bound to DNA and thereby form an active complex that stimulates binding of RNA polymerase.

Luxury genes are those whose products are usually synthesized only in particular cell types (e.g., hemoglobin in erythrocytes; immunoglobulins in plasma cells). These genes appear to be heavily methylated in cells that do not express the corresponding gene products and unmethylated in cells where those genes are expressed. The genes involved in general metabolism common to all cells (called **housekeeping genes**) are rarely methylated in or near their initiation regions. Methylation is rare in invertebrates and nonexistent in insects, and in mammals many examples are known in which methylation seems to have no effect on transcription. The regulatory role of methylation thus remains controversial.

4. Regulation of mRNA Processing.

Eucaryotic genes contain introns (noncoding regions) interspersed among the coding regions (exons). Part of the process that converts primary transcripts to complete mRNA molecules involves removal of the introns and splicing the exons together. Variations in the excision and splicing jobs can lead to different mRNAs and, following translation, to different protein products.

> **Example 14.16.** Immunoglobulins of class IgM have μ-type heavy chains that are produced in two varieties as a consequence of differences in intron/exon excision/splicing events. When processed in one way, the μ-chains are longer, ending with a group of hydrophobic amino acids at their carboxyl ends. This "water-fearing" tail tends to lodge in the lipid membrane and extends into the cytoplasm. The amino terminus extends outside the cell where it participates with an L chain to form an antigen-combining site (see Example 14.23). Thus it becomes a cell receptor for a specific antigen. An alternative processing step removes from the primary transcript the sequence responsible for the hydrophobic tail. This shorter version of the μ-chain readily passes out of the cell and becomes part of the secretory antibody population found in the blood and other body fluids.

5. Regulation of Translation.

There are three major methods by which eucaryotic cells are known to regulate translation: (1) by altering the life of the mRNA, (2) by controlling the initiation of translation, and (3) by changing the overall rate of translation. A typical eucaryotic mature mRNA consists of four major regions: (1) a 5′

noncoding region (leader), (2) a coding region, (3) a 3' noncoding region (trailer), and (4) a poly-A tail. Each of the four segments may affect the half-life of mRNA molecules.

Example 14.17. The mRNA transcribed from a normal human gene *c-myc* is relatively unstable, with a half-life of about 10 minutes. A mutant form of *c-myc* that is missing some of the 5' noncoding region of the normal *c-myc* produces an mRNA 3–5 times more stable than full-length mRNA.

Within the coding region of a histone gene, repositioning of the stop codon closer to the 5' end of its transcript not only produces abnormally short histone proteins but also at least doubles the half-life of such mutant mRNAs.

The mRNAs for human β-globin and δ-globin (Example 14.5) differ mainly in their 3' noncoding segments, yet δ-globin mRNA is degraded 4 times faster than β-globin mRNA.

Mature mRNA molecules do not normally exist as naked mRNAs but as ribonucleoprotein. One of the proteins normally bound to mRNAs is a poly(A)-binding protein (PABP). Experimental removal of PABP from normal mRNAs decreases their half-lives. Removal of poly-A tails from otherwise normal mRNAs greatly reduces their half-lives. Just how these changes in mRNA molecules influence their susceptibility to digestion by ribonuclease enzymes is not presently known.

Example 14.18. Unfertilized sea urchin eggs store large quantities of mRNA complexed with proteins as ribonucleoprotein particles. In this inactive form it is called **masked mRNA.** Within minutes after fertilization, the mRNA somehow becomes "unmasked" and translation begins.

6. Post-Translation Controls.

In procaryotes, the synthesis of several gene products can be coordinately controlled by the production of a polycistronic mRNA. Eucaryotes synthesize only monocistronic mRNAs, but the resulting single polypeptide chains may be cleaved into two or more functional protein components. A multicomponent protein such as this is termed a **polyprotein.**

Example 14.19. A polyprotein called pro-opiomelanocortin is synthesized by the anterior lobe of the pituitary gland. A cut near the C (carboxy) terminus first produces β-lipotropin. Then a cut near the N terminus produces adrenocorticotropic hormone (ACTH). In the intermediate lobe of the pituitary, β-lipotropin is further digested, releasing the C-terminal peptide β-endorphin; the ACTH is also cleaved to release α-melanotropin.

Polypeptides that are destined to be released (after being processed in the Golgi apparatus) from the cell possess a **signal peptide.** This peptide usually consists of about 20 amino acids at or near the N terminus of a polypeptide chain. It serves to anchor the nascent polypeptide (as it is being synthesized) and its ribosome to the endoplasmic reticulum.

DEVELOPMENT

The term **ontogeny** represents the development of an individual from zygote to maturity; **embryology** is the study of early ontogenic events. **Epigenesis** is the modern concept that development of differentiated cells, tissues, and organs proceeds by building upon the relatively small amount of organization in the fertilized egg, as opposed to the now discredited notion that an organism develops simply by growth of tiny entities that are essentially fully formed in the fertilized egg (**preformation theory**). **Epigenetics** is the study of the mechanisms by which genes bring about their phenotypic effects. The series of interrelated developmental pathways through which the adult is formed is referred to as the **epigenotype.**

Undifferentiated cells of the embryo develop epigenetically into morphologically and physiologically different types (e.g., muscle cells that contract, neurons that transmit impulses, fibroblast cells that manufacture extracellular collagen or elastic fibers). Cells become **committed,** or **determined,** to differentiate along certain lines before changes in their morphology can be detected. It is thought that relatively few master control switches exist, and that they are arranged in a hierarchy, with early-acting genes controlling the expression of other genes that act at later times in development. The products of these master control genes that determine specific developmental pathways are called **morphogens.** **Induction** is the determination of the developmental fate of one cell mass by another. This morphogenetic effect is brought about by a living part of an embryo (called an **inducer** or **organizer**) acting upon another part (competent tissue) via one or more morphogens. An undifferentiated cell may, under the influence of a mutant master control gene, follow a developmental pathway different from that which it normally would pursue **(transdetermination),** usually with bizarre (if not lethal) consequences.

Example 14.20. In the fruit fly *Drosophila*, the genes that control development of its body plan can be grouped into three classes. **Maternal effect genes** are those genes of the mother that establish the organization of the egg (e.g., gradients of chemicals from the anterior pole to the posterior pole). The embryo contains **segmentation genes** that establish the segmentation pattern of the fly. The embryo's **homeotic genes** (homoeotic is an alternative spelling) switch on after the segmentation genes and establish the kind of structure that will develop in each body segment. A common conserved DNA sequence of about 180 bp (called a **homeobox**) is shared by most of the known homeotic genes and with at least some of the segmentation genes. A homeobox constitutes only part of a gene and hence codes for only one domain of its protein product. That very basic domain, however, has a **helix-turn-helix** motif that characterizes several well-known procaryotic DNA-binding proteins (e.g., CAP and lambda phage repressor). Although the precise functions of homeoboxes are not yet known, they are thought to form a network of master control genes that switch on batteries of other genes whose activities specify the kind of body structure that will develop. Similar homeoboxes have been found in other invertebrates as well as in some vertebrates, including mammals. But at present it is not known if they function in the same way as in *Drosophila*.

Maternal effect genes may provide certain substances or organize the egg cytoplasm in such a way that development of certain progeny phenotypes is essentially totally controlled by the maternal genotype rather than by the genotype of the embryo. Such effects may be ephemeral or may persist throughout the life of an individual. The substances that produce maternal effects are not self-perpetuating, and therefore must be synthesized anew for each generation of progeny by the appropriate maternal genotype.

Example 14.21. A dominant gene *K* in the meal moth *Ephestia* produces a hormonelike substance called *kynurenine* that is involved in pigment synthesis. The recessive genotype *kk* is devoid of kynurenine and cannot synthesize pigment. Females of genotype *Kk* can produce *k*-bearing eggs containing a small amount of kynurenine. For a short time during early development, a larva may use this supply of kynurenine to develop pigment even though its own genotype might be *kk*. The color fades as the larva grows older because the maternally supplied kynurenine becomes depleted.

Example 14.22. The direction in which the shell coils in the snail *Limnaea* can be *dextral* like a right-hand screw or *sinistral* like a left-hand screw. The maternal genotype organizes the cytoplasm of the egg in such a way that cleavage of the zygote will follow either of these two patterns regardless of the genotype of the zygote. If the mother has the dominant gene s^+, all her progeny will coil dextrally; if she is of the genotype *ss*, all her progeny will coil sinistrally. This coiling pattern persists for the life of the individual.

Depending on the signals it receives, the cell type and the species, a differentiated cell may or may not be able to **dedifferentiate** (revert to an unspecialized state). Differentiation is usually reversible at the nuclear level, as evidenced from nuclear transplantation experiments. However, fully differentiated cells often are incapable of replication. For example, spinal nerve cells, mature red blood cells (erythrocytes) that carry oxygen, and plasma cells that make antibodies can no longer divide. The undifferentiated **stem cells** from which mature blood cells are derived retain the capacity to replicate and differentiate into various blood cell types. Differentiation is seldom due to gain or loss of chromosomes or of genetic material (lymphocytes are a notable exception).

Example 14.23. Antibodies are made by white blood cells (lymphocytes) known as **plasma cells.** Lymphoid stem cells in the bone marrow differentiate into B cells that can complete their maturation into antibody-secreting plasma cells after making specific contact with an antigen via their membrane receptor (an antibody molecule). An immunoglobulin (antibody) molecule is

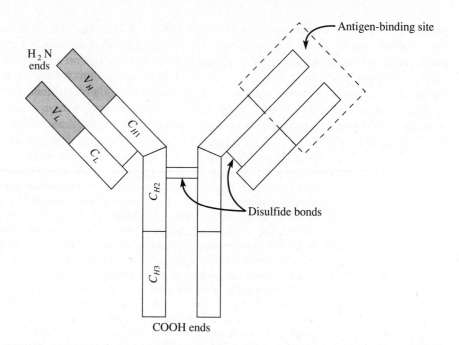

a tetramer composed of two identical heavy (H) polypeptide chains and two identical light (L) chains. There are five classes of immunoglobulin molecules (IgG, IgM, IgA, IgE, and IgD) based upon the structure of their heavy chains (γ, μ, α, ϵ, and δ, respectively). There are only two types of L chains (κ and λ). The carboxy ends of heavy and light chains possess amino acid sequences (called constant regions, designated ''C'') that are invariate within each H chain class and L chain type. The free amino ends of each chain differ in amino acid sequence and are referred to as variable (''V'') regions. The V regions of an L chain and an H chain together form an antigen-binding site. The C_H region consists of three or four similar segments, presumably evolved by duplication of an ancestral gene, followed by subsequent mutational modifications; these similar segments are called ''domains'' and are labeled C_{H1}, C_{H2}, C_{H3}, and so on.

A mature plasma cell produces antibodies bearing a single class of H chain and a single class of L chain, hence also a single antigen-binding specificity. Although an individual may inherit different genes for the H and L chains, an unknown mechanism allows expression of only one gene for each of these chains, a phenomenon known as **allelic exclusion.** The first antibodies produced by a plasma cell are usually of class IgM. Later in that same cell, the same antigen-binding specificity may be associated with H chains of a different class (e.g., IgG or IgA). At any given time, however, a plasma cell is thought to synthesize primary mRNA H-chain transcripts of a single kind.

There are three immunoglobulin gene families: two for the light chain types (κ and λ) and one for the heavy chains, each on a different human autosome. Within each gene family, there usually are multiple DNA sequences (sometimes hundreds) coding for the V region of an immunoglobulin chain. There are also one or more sequences coding for the C region of that same chain. In embryonic lymphoid cells, the V and C segments of a gene family that ultimately code for a given immunoglobulin chain are not adjacent to one another, but are only loosely linked. As the cell matures into an antibody-secreting plasma cell, the V and C sequences become more tightly linked. The V and C sequences are ''exons'' that code for portions of the immunoglobulin polypeptide chain. An apparently random choice is made to connect one of the V exons to one of the C exons, and all unnecessary intervening material (exons or introns) is deleted (sometimes at the *DNA level*).

Between the V and C regions there are a few J (for ''joining'') exons in both L- and H-chain families; the H-chain family also contains a few additional D (for ''diversity'') exons. These J and D segments contribute to hypervariable regions (also known as complementarity determining regions, CDRs) that form part of an antigen-binding cavity in an immunoglobulin molecule. A light-chain V exon is joined to a J exon by a single recombination event. The V-J complex is then connected to a C exon at the level of mRNA by the standard RNA-splicing mechanism. Two recombination events are required to assemble a heavy-chain gene. The first event joins the J and D exons; the second event joins the V exon with the D-J complex to form a V-D-J complex. Since the joining of V-J or V-D-J is imprecise, this produces the phenomenon termed **junctional diversity** in the possible kinds of immunoglobulin chains. As a heavy-chain gene is being assembled, extra nucleotides (called **N regions**) can be inserted in a template-free fashion between the V-D or D-J segments. The random association of any V exon with any J or J-D complex is called **combinatorial translocation.** A V-D-J complex can be coupled to a C exon by either of two mechanisms. RNA splicing can connect the V-D-J group with one of the nearest C exons (either μ or δ). Alternatively, the V-D-J group can be connected to more remote C exons (γ, α, or ϵ) by a third DNA recombination; this latter mechanism is known as **class switching.** A high level of point mutations in fully assembled antibody genes is another source of diversity called **somatic hypermutation.** In the formation of a tetrameric immunoglobulin molecule, any L chain can be associated with any H chain, an option known as **combinatorial association.**

Estimates of the number of immunoglobulin components in the mouse are as follows. L chains (κ type only) have 250 V and 4 J regions, and 3 sites for junctional diversity; total number of κ L chains $= 250 \times 4 \times 3 = 3000$. H chains have 250 V, 10 D and 4 J regions, and plus 3 sites for junctional diversity at both V-D and D-J joints; total number of H chains $= 250 \times 10 \times 4 \times 3 \times 3 = 90,000$. Combinatorial association of 3000 L chains with 90,000 H chains $= 2.7 \times 10^8$ possible antibody molecules. This is an underestimate because it does not consider lambda L chains, N regions, somatic hypermutation, or the five classes (C exons) of the heavy chains. Moreover, in humans there are four different C_H exons for the four subclasses (unrelated to the number of C_H domains) of IgG, two each for IgM and IgA, and one each for IgD and IgE; for L chains there are four C_L exons for the four subtypes of the lambda family and one in the kappa family. Different C_H classes endow the immunoglobulin molecules with special **effector functions** such as complement binding (IgG and IgM), placental passage (IgG), secretion into body fluids (IgA), and binding to mast cells (IgE). Thus the union of one kind of variable region with one kind of constant region in H chains contributes to an antibody-combining site that specifically binds antigen and also allows the immunoglobulin molecule to become biologically active.

ORGANELLES

Both mitochondria and chloroplasts share several characteristics with modern procaryotic cells. All three generally have a circular double-stranded DNA genome (exceptions include some protozoans such as *Paramecium* and *Tetrahymena* that have linear mitochondrial DNA molecules). Their genomes are neither enclosed within a nuclear membrane nor associated with histone proteins (hence no nucleosomal organization). They each code for part of their own protein-synthesizing systems (all rRNAs, tRNAs, and at least some of the ribosomal proteins). Many of the enzymes and other proteins that function in these organelles, however, are encoded by nuclear genes, synthesized on 80S ribosomes, and transported into these organelles. Their ribosomes are usually 70S or smaller and are sensitive to antibiotics and other substances that have no effect on the 80S eucaryotic cytoplasmic ribosomes. Protein synthesis is initiated by formyl-methionyl-tRNA. The nucleus, mitochondrion, and chloroplast are bounded by a double-membrane envelope, but only the nuclear membrane contains pores. Mitochondria and chloroplasts grow in size and then seem to split in two, in a process akin to binary fission in bacteria.

1. Mitochondria.

Mitochondria are organelles found in the cytoplasm of both plants and animals. They contain the enzymes of the electron-transport chain that carry out oxidative phosphorylation in the production of adenosine triphosphate (ATP, the main source for energy-requiring biochemical reactions). Unlike chloroplasts, the mitochondrial genome (**mtDNA**) varies markedly in length between species. For example, it is about 20 micrometers in *Neurospora,* 25 micrometers in yeast, 30 micrometers in higher plants, but only 5 micrometers in some metazoan (multicellular) animals. Most of the mtDNA of fungi and plants is thought to be noncoding (perhaps ''junk'' or ''selfish'' DNA). One or more mitochondrial DNA molecules reside within each of the several nucleoid regions within the mitochondrion. If a cell contained 250 mitochondria, each with 5 mtDNA molecules, there would be 1250 mtDNA copies in that cell. Mitochondrial ribosomes are also highly variable between species (e.g., 55S in animals, 73S in yeast). There is also some interspecific variation in mitochondrial tRNAs. Some codons are read differently by mitochondrial tRNAs than by nuclear-encoded tRNAs. For example, AUA codes for methionine (not isoleucine) and UGA codes for tryptophan (not translation termination) in mammalian mitochondria. Mitochondrial mRNAs of fungi and higher plants contain introns, but those of animals lack introns and are transcribed as polycistronic mRNAs that become cut into monocistronic mRNAs before translation. Mitochondria have no DNA repair systems. Hence the mutation rate of mictochondrial DNA is much higher than that of nuclear DNA.

2. Chloroplasts.

Chloroplasts contain the enzymes for photosynthesis and are thus characteristic only of plant cells. Most plant cells contain numerous chloroplasts. A few plants such as the unicellular alga *Chlamydomonas* (Fig. 5-1) contain a single chloroplast. In most plants, however, each chloroplast genome is usually present in multiple copies. For example, a typical leaf cell of *Euglena* may contain 40–50 chloroplasts. Every chloroplast usually contains several nucleoid regions, each containing 8–10 DNA molecules; thus the entire cell may contain over 500 copies of the chloroplast genome (**ctDNA**). The length of the *Euglena* ctDNA is estimated to be capable of coding well over 100 proteins. Evidence indicates that ctDNA from liverworts to the higher plants have essentially the same genome (highly conserved). Some of the ctDNA genes (both for tRNAs and mRNAs) are known to contain introns. The RNA polymerase of the liverwort *Marchantia polymorpha* contains α- and β-subunits that are homologous in amino acid sequences to those found in the bacterium *E. coli.*

3. Origin of Organelles.

According to one classification scheme, all organisms fall into one of two superkingdoms: Procaryotes and Eucaryotes. Cells of the former lack a nucleus or any other double-membraned organelles. Cells of the latter possess a nucleus and other double-membraned organelles. Within the Procaryotes there are two subkingdoms. Most bacteria belong to the subkingdom **Eubacteria.** The subkingdom **Archaebacteria** contains less familiar bacteria that lead unusual life-styles; e.g., salt-loving halophiles, anaerobic (without oxygen) ''marsh-gas''-producing bacteria called ''methanogens,'' sulfur-metabolizing forms, and some that require high temperatures (>80°C) and acidic environments (pH < 3) known as ''thermoacidophiles.'' However, the archaebacteria and the eubacteria seem to be as distinct from each other as they are from the eucaryotes. Hence, it is hypothesized that all three groups may have arisen from a common ancestor, or **progenote,** that is now extinct.

There are no clues in extant organisms as to the evolution of the nucleus. It is thought that the eucaryotic nuclear membrane probably evolved independently of the procaryotes, possibly by invaginations and coalescences of the cell membrane. The nucleus is a double-membraned organelle like mitochondria and chloroplasts, so any theory regarding the origins of these organelles would have to take this into consideration. On the other hand, several lines of evidence support the theory that mitochondria evolved from eubacteria. According to the **endosymbiosis theory,** a primitive anaerobic-phagocytic type of nucleated cell (called the **urcaryote**) engulfed aerobic bacteria that were able to generate energy by oxidative phosphorylation. The engulfed bacteria somehow escaped digestion by the feeder cell and replicated within the cytoplasm. These early symbiotic relationships gradually evolved into a mutualism whereby they could not survive apart from one another. During the evolution of this organelle, the bacteria gave up many of its genes to the nucleus, so that now many of the proteins needed for mitochondrial functions are specified by nuclear genes, made on cytoplasmic ribosomes, and transported into the mitochondria. This is how fully aerobic, nucleated cells (like modern eucaryotic cells) are proposed to have evolved.

At some later time, some of these fully aerobic, nucleated, feeder cells may have engulfed photosynthetic **cyanobacteria** (blue-green "algae"). A mutualism gradually developed between these two entities in the evolution of the chloroplasts that characterize the plant kingdom.

Although the shape of mitochondria is different from that of the purple, nonsulfur bacteria from which they presumably were derived, the mitochondria resemble bacteria in many ways. Both of their genomes are circular and histone-free. Their transcription and translation systems are also similar. On the other hand, some archaebacterial genes (like those in the eucaryote nucleus) have introns. But introns are unknown in modern eubacteria. Hence it has been suggested that the progenote may have had introns but they became lost during the evolution of the eubacteria. Interestingly, the mitochondrial DNA of mammalian cells does not contain introns, but many mitochondrial genomes of more primitive eucaryotes do. In addition, eubacteria and eucaryotes contain ester-linked, unbranched lipids containing L-glycerophosphate, whereas the branched lipids of archaebacteria are ether-linked, containing D-glycerophosphate.

4. Inheritance of Organelles.

In most plants and animals, mitochondria and chloroplasts are strictly inherited only from the female parent (**maternal transmission**) because the male gamete (or that part that enters into fertilization) is essentially devoid of these organelles. It is estimated that in about two-thirds of plant species the inheritance of chloroplasts is strictly maternal. The smallest heritable extranuclear (extrachromosomal, cytoplasmic) element is called a **plasmagene.** All of the plasmagenes of a cell constitute the **plasmon.** Traits with an extranuclear basis may be identified on the basis of several diagnostic criteria.

(1) Differences in reciprocal crosses that cannot be attributed to sex linkage or some other chromosomal basis tend to implicate cytoplasmic factors.

    (*a*) If progeny show only the characteristics of the female parent that can be attributed to unequal cytoplasmic contributions of male and female parents, then plasmagene inheritance is suspect (Example 14.24).

    (*b*) If the uniparental inheritance of a trait cannot be attributed to unequal cytoplasmic contributions from the parents, this does not necessarily rule out cytoplasmic factors (Example 14.25).

(2) Extranuclear factors may be detected by either the absence of segregation at meiosis (Example 14.26) or by segregation that fails to follow Mendelian laws (Example 14.27).

(3) Repeated backcrossing of progeny to one of the parental types for several generations causes their chromosomal endowment to rapidly approach 100% that of the recurrent parental line. The persistence of a trait in the progeny, when the backcross parent exhibits an alternative character, may be considered evidence for plasmagene inheritance (Example 14.28).

> **Example 14.24.**   In higher plants, pollen usually contributes very little, if any, cytoplasm to the zygote. Most of the cytoplasmic elements are transmitted through the maternal parent. In the plant called "four-o'clock" (*Mirabilis jalapa*), there may be normal green, pale green, and variegated branches due to two types of chloroplasts. Plants grown from seeds that developed on normal green branches (with all normal chloroplasts) will all be normal green; those that developed on pale-green branches (with abnormal chloroplasts) will all be pale green; those on variegated branches (with both normal and abnormal chloroplasts) will segregate green, pale green, and variegated in irregular ratios. The type of pollen used has no effect in this system. The irregularity of transmission from variegated branches is understandable if plasmagenes exist in the chloroplasts, because there is no mechanism to ensure the regular distribution of chloroplasts to daughter cells as there is for chromosomes.

Example 14.25. The uniting gametes of the single celled alga *Chlamydomonas reinhardi* (Fig. 5-1) are morphologically indistinguishable. One strain of the alga that is streptomycin-resistant (*sr*) and of the "plus" mating type (*mt*$^+$) is crossed to a cell of "negative" mating type (*mt*$^-$) that is streptomycin-sensitive (*ss*). All progeny are resistant, but the nuclear genes for mating type segregate as expected: $\frac{1}{2}mt^+$, $\frac{1}{2}mt^-$. The reciprocal cross *ss mt*$^+$ × *sr mt*$^-$, again shows the expected segregation for mating type, but all progeny are sensitive. Repeated backcrossings of *sr mt*$^+$ to *ss mt*$^-$ fail to show segregation for resistance. It appears as though the plasmagenes of the *mt*$^-$ strain become lost in a zygote of *mt*$^+$. The mechanism which inactivates the plasmagenes of *mt*$^-$ in the zygote is unknown.

Example 14.26. Slow-growing yeast cells called *petites* lack normal activity of the respiratory enzyme cytochrome oxidase associated with the mitochondria. Petites can be maintained indefinitely in vegetative cultures through budding, but can sporulate only if crossed to wild type. When a haploid neutral petite cell fuses with a haploid wild-type cell of opposite mating type, a fertile wild-type diploid cell is produced. Under appropriate conditions, the diploid cell reproduces sexually (sporulates). The four ascospores of the ascus (Fig. 6-2) germinate into cells with a 1:1 mating type ratio (as expected for nuclear genes), but they are all wild type. The petite trait never appears again, even after repeated backcrossings of both mating types to petite. The mitochondrial factors for petite are able to perpetuate themselves vegetatively, but are "swamped," lost or permanently altered in the presence of wild-type factors. Neutral petite behaves the same in reciprocal crosses regardless of mating type, and in this respect is different from the streptomycin resistance factors in *Chlamydomonas* (Example 14.25).

Example 14.27. Another type of petite in yeast called *suppressive* may segregate, but in a manner different from chromosomal genes. When haploid suppressive petites are crossed to wild types and each zygote is grown vegetatively as a diploid strain, both petites and wild types may appear, but in frequencies that are hardly Mendelian, varying from 1 to 99% petites. Diploid wild type cells may sporulate producing only wild-type ascospores. By special treatment, all diploid zygotes can be made to sporulate. The majority of the ascospores thus induced germinates into petite clones. Some asci have 4, 3, 2, 1, or 0 petite ascospores, suggesting that environmental factors may alter their segregation pattern. Nuclear genes, such as mating type, maintain a 1:1 ratio in all asci.

Example 14.28. The protoperithecial parent in *Neurospora* (Fig. 6-3) supplies the bulk of the extra-chromosomal material of the sexually produced ascospores. Very slow spore germination characterizes one strain of this fungus. The trait exhibits differences in reciprocal crosses, maternal inheritance, and fails to segregate at meiosis. When the slow strain acts as protoperithecial parent and the conidial strain has normal spore germination, all the progeny are slow, but possess 50% of the nuclear genes of the conidial parent. Each generation is then backcrossed to the conidial parent, so that the F_2 contains 75%, F_3 contains 87.5%, etc., of nuclear genes of the conidial parent. After the fifth or sixth backcross, the nuclear genes are almost wholly those of the conidial parent, but the slow germination trait persists in all of the progeny.

Exceptions are known to the generalization that cytoplasmic factors are maternally inherited.

Example 14.29. When a green strain of geranium (*Pelargonium*) is crossed to a strain with white-margined leaves, the progeny may have green, white, or white-margined leaves. Since the results of reciprocal crosses are the same it has been hypothesized that plastids can be transmitted to offspring by both the male and female gametes. Cells that contain a mixture of plastid genomes are said to be **heteroplasmic;** those that contain only one type of plastid genome are called **homoplasmic.**

EUCARYOTIC VIRUSES

Eucaryotic viruses differ in many respects from virulent bacteriophages; some of the more obvious differences are outlined in Table 14.2.

Table 14.2.   Some Differences between Virulent Bacteriophages and Eucaryotic Viruses

Bacteriophage	Eucaryotic Viruses
20–60-minute life cycle	Typically 6–48-hour life cycle
DNA virus = 50–1000 burst size	500–10^5 virions per cell per generation
Fraction of burst size capable of infection is very high (at or near 1.0)	Fraction of progeny virions capable of infection is very low (10^{-4} to 10^{-1})
Life cycle terminates in cell death (M13 is an exception); all phage simultaneously released	Some infected cells die; others continue to grow and release progeny viruses continuously
Cessation of synthesis of host DNA, mRNA, and protein is an early event after infection	Impairment of host functions usually occurs in late states of infection
Tailed forms inject DNA into host cells	No tailed forms; viral DNA is never injected into host cells
No segmented genomes	Some single-stranded RNA viruses have segmented genomes; double-stranded RNA viruses always have segmented genomes and are isocapsidic
No 5' capping	5' end of each ssRNA virion (+) strand or viral mRNA is capped
No poly-A tails	3' end of ssRNA animal viruses have poly-A tail
Phage proteins rarely penetrate the host cell (phage M13 is an exception)	Viral proteins commonly enter the cell; removal of the capsid (uncoating) is an early event in infection
No replicative intermediate	Replicative intermediate required for ssRNA virions
Many rounds of recombination common with multiple infections	Genetic recombination between viral genomes rare
No known highly mutable forms	Some highly mutable forms; e.g., HIV-1, influenza virus
Restriction sites specifically methylated	No RE sites specifically methylated

1. Animal Viruses.

Some animal viruses cause relatively mild diseases such as the common cold; others cause more severe problems or even life-threatening conditions such as rabies, acquired immune deficiency syndrome (AIDS), and cancer. Much of what is known about the molecular biology of eucaryotic cells has come from studying their viruses.

Viral capsids are usually constructed from only one or a few types of proteins and thus do not require much coding information. The viruses that infect animal cells have been classified into four morphological types: (1) naked **icosahedral** (20 faces), (2) naked helical, (3) enveloped icosahedral, and (4) enveloped helical. **Naked viruses** have a protein capsid but no lipid envelope. An **envelope** is a portion of the host-cell membrane acquired as the virus leaves the cell by a **budding** process. The envelope is derived from the cell membrane in two steps. First, glycoproteins specified by the viral genome are inserted into the membrane. Then the virion capsid attaches to the cytoplasmic ends of the glycoproteins, causing the membrane to adhere to the capsid. The enveloped virus pinches off from the cell surface without creating a hole in the cell membrane. To infect another cell, an infective virus particle (**virion**) attaches to a specific **receptor** on the host animal cell membrane, either by capsid proteins of a naked virion or by the viral glycoproteins extending from the surface of an enveloped virion. The attached virion is then engulfed by the host cell and the viral genome becomes **uncoated** (removal of the capsid) inside the cell.

The genomes of animal viruses may be DNA or RNA, single-stranded or double-stranded. Double-stranded DNA viral genomes may be either linear or circular. Circular double-stranded DNA may be covalently closed on one or both strands. All known double-stranded RNA viral genomes are segmented (i.e., consisting of multiple RNA molecules, each carrying a different set of genes). Some single-stranded RNA genomes are also known to be segmented. There are no known segmented DNA viruses or circular RNA genomes. Most DNA viruses replicate in the nucleus, using the host's RNA polymerase and other enzymes for capping, splicing, and adding poly-A tails in processing their transcripts. Most RNA viruses (except influenza virus) replicate in the cytoplasm.

The great diversity of animal viruses has been classified into 15–20 viral families based on characteristics such as type and structure of nucleic acid, virion morphology, and common antigenic determinants. Because of the dependent relationship of the viral genome on its mRNAs for replication, animal viruses have been recognized as falling into seven groups as summarized in Fig. 14-4.

Example 14.30. All adenoviruses have a double-stranded DNA genome of about 36 kbp and a naked icosahedral capsid of 252 subunits with prominent spikes at the vertices. Their mRNAs are transcribed directly from their genomes and their genomes replicate directly from their double-stranded DNA templates. Although the nucleotide sequences vary considerably among the members of this family, they all have the above characteristics in common regardless of the host species from which they are isolated.

There are three major types of viral infection. The most common type is a lytic infection that causes death of the host cell when it ruptures to release progeny virions. The second type involves lysogeny similar to that of bacterial viruses (phages) as discussed in Chapter 12. The third type involves virions

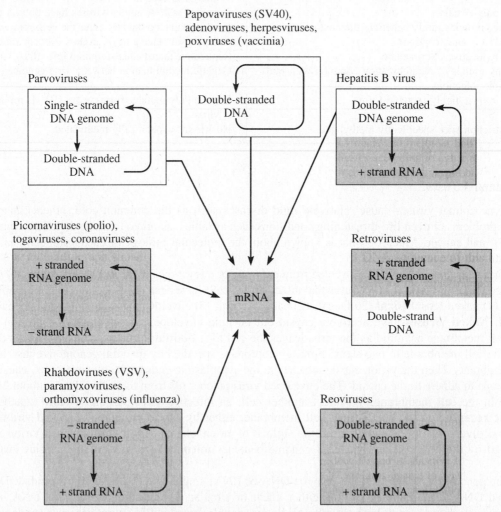

Fig. 14-4. A classification of animal viruses based on replication mechanism and the origin of mRNA. Arrows within each box indicate flow of information during replication. Arrows to mRNA originate at the template for mRNA synthesis. (After J. D. Watson et al., 1987, *Molecular Biology of the Gene,* 4th ed., Benjamin/Cummings Publishing Company, Inc.)

that bud from the cell surface without lysing or killing the host cell. As it buds from the cell, the virion acquires a lipid envelope of host membrane. Prior to becoming encapsulated, certain viral proteins have been synthesized and become incorporated into the host cell membrane. Thus the viral envelope contains viral proteins that enable the virion to attach to another host cell and spread the infection.

(a) **DNA Viruses.**   A typical double-stranded DNA (dsDNA) virus attaches to a cell receptor and then is taken into the cell, where its capsid is removed (uncoated). The viral DNA is replicated using host-cell enzymes. The viral DNA is also transcribed by host enzymes into mRNAs, which in turn are translated (by the host's ribosomes and enzymes) into viral capsid proteins or (in some cases) into enzymes that favor viral DNA replication over that of host DNA. The capsomeres become organized into a capsid around the viral DNA to form progeny virions. The virions are released from the host cell by lysis or by budding. Deviations from this generalized life cycle exist in the dsDNA hepatitis B virus and in the ssDNA parvoviruses.

(b) **RNA Viruses.**   Few host cells contain the enzymes necessary to replicate or repair RNA (rare exceptions are mentioned with viroids later in this chapter). Thus, the genes of RNA viruses have much higher mutation rates (e.g., 10^{-3} to 10^{-4}) than DNA viruses, and they must either code for these enzymes or carry these enzymes with them when they infect a host cell. RNA viruses with single-stranded genomes that function as mRNAs are said to have **positive** or **plus (+) strand** genomes specifying (minimally) the coat proteins and the enzyme(s) needed for replication. RNA viruses with **negative** or **minus (−) strand** genomes have DNA that is complementary to the genomic or mRNA strand, and so cannot be translated into an mRNA transcriptase. Such viruses must, therefore, encode a transcriptase that can synthesize a + RNA strand from a − RNA template, and this enzyme must be packaged in the virion together with the viral RNA genome.

For all RNA viruses except the retroviruses, double-stranded RNA is always an intermediate in viral RNA replication even if the infective virion contains only single-stranded RNA (ssRNA). Double-stranded RNA is replicated in the same manner as DNA; i.e., each RNA strand serves as a template for making a complementary RNA strand. The viral enzyme that replicates viral RNA in this way is an RNA-dependent RNA polymerase called **RNA replicase.** Four model life cycles for the RNA viruses are easily recognized.

Model 1. If the viral RNA is double-stranded (dsRNA), the + strand is transcribed to produce RNA replicase. This enzyme not only replicates viral dsRNA (using both + and − strands as templates) to form dsRNA progeny genomes, but also makes many + copies using the − strands as templates. These extra + strands are required as mRNA templates for translating viral proteins in a relatively short period of time.

Model 2. If the viral RNA is a single + strand, the virion enters the host cell, becomes uncoated, and the + strand RNA is translated to produce an RNA replicase. The replicase then synthesizes a complementary − RNA strand using the + strand as a template, thereby forming a double-stranded RNA replicative intermediate. The − strands are needed as templates for the synthesis of + genomic strands of progeny virions. Some of the + strands are translated by the host cell's machinery into capsid proteins, membrane proteins, etc.

Model 3. If the viral RNA is a single − strand, it cannot serve as a translational template (mRNA) for making RNA replicase. Hence this enzyme must be brought into the host cell along with the viral RNA. The RNA replicase uses the − strand as a template to produce a complementary + strand. More − strands are produced using the plus strand(s) as templates and more + strands are produced using the minus strand(s) as templates. The + strands serve as mRNAs for making viral proteins. The − strands then associate with the capsid proteins and RNA replicase to be packaged into progeny virions.

Model 4. None of the above three model RNA virus life cycles involve DNA as a replicative intermediate. However, the single + strands of RNA viruses known as retroviruses require a DNA replicative intermediate. Retroviruses are discussed later in this chapter under the subject of cancer.

(c) **Prions.**   Two degenerative brain diseases in humans (kuru and Creutzfeldt-Jakob disease) and a similar disease in sheep (scrapie) seem to be caused by a proteinaceous infectious particle (**prion**) devoid of nucleic acid. Little else is presently known about prions.

2. Plant Viruses.

Plant viruses also exist in rod and polyhedral shapes. Most plant viruses have genomes consisting of a single RNA strand of the (+) type. The best-known plant virus is the rod-shaped tobacco mosaic virus (TMV; Fig. 14-5), having a single-stranded (+) RNA genome of 6395 nucleotides. Some viruses with + genomes, however, cannot replicate unless the host cell is infected with two different virions. Such viruses are said to have **segmented genomes.** If the genomic fragments reside in different capsids, the virus is said to be **heterocapsidic;** if the fragments reside in the same capsid, the virus is said to be **isocapsidic.**

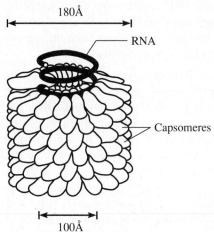

Fig. 14-5. Section of tobacco mosaic virus (3000 Å long) showing its single-stranded RNA genome and its associated capsomers.

Example 14.31. The heterocapsidic genome of the cowpea mosaic virus consists of two RNA chains, each encoding different proteins essential for replication. Each of these RNA chains is encapsulated into separate virions. The virus can only replicate in a host cell that has been infected by both kinds of virions.

Relatively few plant viruses have DNA genomes. There are only two classes of DNA plant viruses. The cauliflower mosaic virus belongs to the first class, which contains a double-stranded DNA genome in a polyhedral capsule. The second class of DNA plant viruses contains the geminiviruses (gemini = twins), characterized by a connected pair of capsids, each containing a circular, single-stranded DNA molecule of about 2500 nucleotides. The paired genomes may be identical in some viruses and markedly different in others.

Plant **viroids** have a very small RNA genome of 240–350 nucleotides in a single-stranded circle that can form extensive internal base pairing. This gives it essentially a stiff, double-helical structure and renders it resistant to digestion by ribonuclease enzymes that usually cut only at unpaired ribonucleotides. The genome is too small to code for any proteins. In the potato spindle tuber viroid there are no AUG initiation codons, and frequent stop codons occur in all reading frames. At least some plant cells (unlike animal cells) are known to contain enzymes capable of replicating RNA. Viroids are not encapsulated in a protein coat. They do not pass through a DNA stage in their life cycle and are not integrated into the host chromosomes. Little else is known of their life cycles.

The variations within each class of plant and animal virus are too numerous to even mention here. Details of the life cycles of specific viruses can be found in more comprehensive volumes.

CANCER

A **tumor** is a swelling or enlargement of a body part due to abnormal cell proliferation. Tumors are not necessarily life-threatening (e.g., warts or galls) and may occur in both plants and animals. **Cancers,** however, are animal diseases characterized by uncontrolled cellular proliferation and spread (**metastasis**) of the abnormal cells into other tissues. Plants do not have cancers because their cell walls prevent metastasis of tumor cells. **Oncogenesis** is the process by which a normal cell becomes cancerous; **oncology** is the study of cancers. It is not that cancer cells grow faster than normal cells; their growth is simply unregulated, and they "forget where they belong" and go wandering off to other body parts. A **neoplasm** is a population of potentially cancerous cells growing out of control. If the neoplasm is confined to its place of origin and has no tendency to recur after removal, it is a **benign** neoplasm. If it metastasizes from its site of origin, it becomes a life-threatening **malignant** neoplasm. A **carcinogen** is any agent (e.g., mutagenic chemicals, ionizing radiations, and certain viruses) that can induce cancer. Aside from the irritant fibers of asbestos, all carcinogens are thought to be mutagenic (causing damage to DNA), but not all mutagens are carcinogenic.

> **Example 14.32.** **Xeroderma pigmentosum** is a genetic syndrome characterized by extreme sensitivity to ultraviolet light and the tendency to develop multiple skin cancers. It is inherited as an autosomal recessive trait that produces a defective enzyme. Individuals with this genotype are unable to repair ultraviolet-induced DNA damage. This disease provides strong evidence that cancer originates in cells that have sustained permanent damage to DNA.

Cancer is generally conceded to involve at least two major steps. The first step, termed **initiation,** results from a single exposure to a carcinogen. The second step, called **promotion,** involves one or more exposures to the same initiator or even to unrelated substances called **promoters** that complete the conversion of a cell to the neoplastic state. In general, the time interval between the exposure to an initiator and a promoter is not critical. However, the order of application is critical; the individual must be exposed to the initiator first, followed by the promoter. The promotion stage is a gradual process, often requiring many weeks in rodents and years in humans. Phorbol esters are among the most well-known promoters. Further heritable changes of an unknown nature are thought to be experienced during the promotion phase. Some substances [e.g., benzo(a)pyrene and polycyclic hydrocarbons, at relatively high doses] can both initiate and promote tumor formation.

Many carcinogens must undergo chemical alteration within the exposed individual before they are capable of becoming an initiator or a promoter. This process is called **metabolic activation.** Enzymes in various tissues, especially those in the liver, are responsible for converting the inactive **precarcinogens** into active carcinogens (see Problem 12.24). Not all species have the enzymes necessary to convert a given precarcinogen into a carcinogen; hence, such a species would not be susceptible to induction of cancer by that substance. Most chemical carcinogens are electrophilic and tend to react with negatively charged substances such as DNA.

1. *In Vitro* Phenomena.

Cancer can be studied either *in vivo* or *in vitro*, the latter being in **cell cultures** or **tissue cultures.** Fibroblast cells (responsible for the formation of extracellular fibers such as collagen in connective tissue) are the easiest cell type to grow in tissue culture; other cell types grow poorly or not at all. After placing some cells into a glass or treated plastic flat-bottomed vial containing a nutrient-rich medium, the cells settle and attach to the bottom of the container and begin to grow. This is called a **primary culture.** The cells may divide a few times, but they eventually reach a **crisis period** in which most of them die. After maintaining the few survivors for many months in fresh medium, some cells may start to grow again, producing an **established cell line.** Cells of an established line have become **immortalized** and can (given fresh nutrients and removal of waste products) continue to divide indefinitely. However, if they are not continually subcultured, most of the cells stop growing when they have formed a confluent monolayer on the bottom of the container. Their growth is arrested by **contact inhibition** or **density-dependent growth.** If forced to grow for many generations at high density, or if treated with carcinogens, some of the cells undergo **neoplastic transformation** and lose contact inhibition. Such transformed cells are thought to resemble or be identical with a tumorigenic condition *in vivo*. Growth of transformed cells causes them to break out of a cultured monolayer and pile up on each other, forming a **focus** (**foci,** plural). Neoplastically transformed cells have several other important properties that distinguish them from normal cells:

(1) They can grow in cell suspension; they no longer require surface contact for growth and may lose their affinity for attachment to substrates. *In vivo* this property fosters metastasis.

(2) They require less supplementation in the nutrient medium.

(3) They have disorganized microfilaments (part of the cytoskeleton), and therefore have a tendency to take on a spherical shape.

(4) They may concentrate certain molecules to high levels.

(5) Tumor antigens may appear on the cell surface.

(6) They often form tumors when injected into an animal of the same species from which they were derived.

(7) Their chromosome number always exceeds the normal diploid number (euploidy or aneuploidy).

(8) If neoplastically transformed by either a DNA or RNA virus, the cell always contains integrated viral DNA.

One of the most important uses of established cell lines has been in the production of **monoclonal antibodies** (MA) by use of the somatic cell hybridization technique discussed in Chapter 6. A **myeloma** is a plasma cell tumor that grows well *in vitro*. Plasma cells are mature lymphocytes that secrete a single kind of antibody (Example 14.23). It is possible to fuse a mouse myeloma cell (defective in its ability to make antibodies) with a mouse plasma cell to produce a **hybridoma** able to multiply indefinitely in cell culture and also able to secrete a single kind of antibody (**monospecific**). Commonly the plasma cells are derived from spleens of mice that have been immunized with a specific antigen. If the myeloma cells are mutant with regard to their ability to make the enzyme HGPRT, they cannot grow in HAT medium, but they can grow if fused with normal plasma cells that can make this enzyme. The plasma cells, however, usually grow so poorly in HAT medium that they either die or are rapidly outgrown by the hybrid cells. The hybridoma clones that survive in HAT medium can then be assayed for antibodies reactive with the immunizing antigen. Once the desired clones are found, they can be frozen for later use or propagated indefinitely in cell culture or by injection into **syngeneic** mice (genetically identical to the plasma cell source) to produce MA-secreting tumors.

Many different plasma cell clones are usually stimulated to respond to the same antigen, each clone producing an antibody that is reactive to a different component or determinant of the antigen (e.g., to different parts of the same antigenic protein molecule). Even antibodies of different clones that recognize the same antigenic determinant may differ in their antigen-binding strengths and in the degree to which they cross-react with related determinants. The monoclonal antibodies produced by a given hybridoma are identical in all respects and can be economically made in virtually unlimited quantities. They are in great demand for a variety of diagnostic, medical, industrial, and research purposes.

2. *In Vivo* Phenomena.

To become malignant, a transformed cell must undergo several further changes in order to metastasize *in vivo*. Some cells of a tumor must burrow their way into a blood vessel or into a vessel of the lymphatic system and then at some other location must reverse the process and burrow out into a tissue again. Basement membranes underlie the epithelial cells from which the common cancers are derived, and consist of a complex of proteins, including collagen IV, laminin, and fibronectin. They also surround the smooth muscles in blood vessel walls. Metastatic cells must produce new protease enzymes to digest the basement membrane (e.g., type IV collagenase, transin). Solid tumors must recruit a rich network of blood vessels to supply them with nutrients for their growth. The process that stimulates formation of these blood vessels is called **angiogenesis.** Tumor cells are known to produce angiogenic factors that enhance the growth of blood vessels toward the tumor. To form a new tumor, the replicated metastasized cells must regain the ability to clump together. This has been attributed in some tumors to the presence of large amounts of a sugar-binding protein on the surface of the tumor cells. During all of this movement and tumor reestablishment, cancer cells have had to undergo additional mutations that allow them to avoid being destroyed by the killer cells and/or antibodies of the immune system (e.g., a mutation might alter the proteins in the cell membrane that normally mark the cell for destruction by the immune system).

Cell division (mitosis) is a very complicated process that is likely to be controlled by many different genes (some stimulatory; others inhibitory). Interference with the timing at which these genes act, the amount of gene product produced, or the activity of the gene product could lead to cancer. Thus, normal cells have genes (called **protooncogenes**) that, if mutated, could change into **oncogenes** that predispose the cells to neoplastic transformation.

Example 14.33.   A particular human protooncogene that was mutated at one base by the carcinogen nitrosomethylurea became an oncogene responsible for a human bladder cancer. A different mutation at that same position in an otherwise identical rat protooncogene created an oncogene responsible for mammary carcinomas in the rat.

Example 14.34.   A type of blood cell cancer known as chronic myelogenous leukemia is associated with a reciprocal translocation involving the tip of the long arm of chromosome 9 and a portion of the long arm of chromosome 22. The chromosome 22 bearing a piece of chromosome 9 is called a Philadelphia chromosome (Example 8.22). A cellular protooncogene called *c-abl* (normally located on chromosome 9) becomes activated to oncogenic status when translocated to chromosome 22. A homologus gene (*v-abl*) exists in the highly oncogenic Abelson murine (mouse) leukemia virus.

Oncogenes can be grouped into five classes based on the nature of their protein products: (1) altered peptide hormones, (2) altered cell receptors, (3) altered G-proteins, (4) altered protein kinases, and (5) altered DNA regulatory proteins. An oncogene that produces cancer by an altered protein or by overproduction of a normal protein would be dominant to its homologous protooncogene; i.e., only one altered gene is required to induce cancer. **Cancer suppressor genes,** on the other hand, must have both gene copies mutated (recessive genotype) in order to lose control over cellular proliferation. A genetic locus on human chromosome 17 is usually associated with colorectal cancer; most of these cancer cells lose one copy of the gene and the other copy has a single base pair mutation. Cancers like this that are associated with the absence of at least one normal gene copy are hypothesized to develop because the normal gene encodes a **tumor suppression factor.**

3. Oncogenic Viruses.

Some viruses are involved in neoplastic transformation; they are called **oncogenic viruses.** Among the vertebrates, about 50 oncogenic viruses have been found to contain DNA and about 150 contain RNA. Several families of DNA viruses contain oncogenic viruses, but among the RNA viruses only some of the **retroviruses** produce tumors. Retroviruses are so named because they contain an enzyme that synthesizes DNA from an RNA template, thus reversing the cellular dogma that all cellular DNA is made from DNA templates. Table 14.3 displays some of the major differences between DNA and RNA oncogenic viruses.

Example 14.35.   The Rous sarcoma virus (RSV) is the best understood retrovirus. Upon entry into a host cell, reverse transcriptase, contained within the RSV virion, produces a double-stranded DNA (dsDNA) from the single-stranded virion RNA. This molecule then circularizes and becomes integrated into the host chromosome as a provirus. Progeny virion RNA is synthesized from the provirus by host-cell RNA polymerase II. The provirus is rarely excised. Its presence does not seem to inhibit cell division, so daughter cells inherit the provirus and continue to produce active virions. In contrast to a lambda phage lysogen, the RSV provirus does not make a repressor, and progeny virions are produced continuously without the necessity of deintegration of the provirus.

Unlike bacterial lysogeny, where all phage genes except the one responsible for repressor of lytic functions are silenced, genes of the proretrovirus (viral DNA integrated into the host chromosome) are transcribed to produce proteins, some of which are involved in the induction of cancer, and others of which are involved in replication of viral RNA genomes. The integration of viral dsDNA into a host chromosome is an essential step in the life cycle of *all* oncogenic viruses. The retroviruses are enveloped

Table 14.3.   A Comparison of the Two Major Classes of Oncogenic Viruses

DNA Tumor Viruses	Oncogenic Retroviruses
Some of these viruses cause a **productive infection** (producing progeny virions) in cells of one species **(permissive cells)** and a tumor in another species **(nonpermissive cells)**	Usually cause tumors in most species in which they can cause a productive infection
Infection of most nonpermissive cells by these viruses is abortive; very few of these cells become cancerous	Most infected permissive cells are tumor cells
Prophage integration involves loss of viral genes; progeny virions cannot then be produced	Integration of viral DNA is obligatory for the production of virions
Some of these viruses contain oncogenes that encode essential early proteins for viral replication	All oncogenes of these viruses are nonessential for production of progeny virions
No virus-induced protein kinases are known in DNA tumor viruses	Some of these viruses produce virus-induced protein kinases

(membrane-bound) virions containing a single + strand RNA genome and an RNA-dependent DNA polymerase called *reverse transcriptase*. This enzyme synthesizes a − DNA strand using the + viral RNA genomic strand as a template. The same enzyme then degrades the viral RNA and synthesizes a complementary + DNA strand using the − DNA strand as a template, thereby forming a dsDNA replicative intermediate. The viral dsDNA is then integrated into a host chromosome in the same manner as DNA oncogenic viruses.

Oncogenic viruses cause cancer by two general mechanisms: (1) insertional inactivation and (2) oncogenes. In insertional mutagenesis, the viral DNA causes a mutation simply by becoming integrated into the host's DNA. Some of these mutations might inactivate cancer-suppressor genes. Alternatively, by inserting near a host gene involved in initiation of the normal cell cycle, the activity of that gene might be stimulated to overproduction of its product (e.g., a growth factor).

Many retroviruses contain oncogenes that are identical or very similar (perhaps differing by only one or a few nucleotides) to normal cellular genes involved in control of the cell cycle (protooncogenes). It is generally believed that retroviruses have, in the course of their evolution, acquired their oncogenes from normal (probably essential) cellular counterparts called protooncogenes. These former cellular protooncogenes may become viral oncogenes by integrating into the viral genome in such a way as to be regulated by a powerful viral promoter, causing overproduction of a normal or near-normal growth factor, and resulting in excessive cell proliferation. Alternatively, some of these retroviral oncogenes code for kinase enzymes that phosphorylate specific amino acids in proteins. Normal host-cell kinases phosphorylate proteins at their serine or threonine residues. Retroviral kinases, however, phosphorylate tyrosine residues. Some host-cell growth factors normally stimulate cell division by causing the phosphorylation of tyrosine in the same proteins activated by retroviral kinases. Other oncogenes code for DNA-binding proteins and growth factor receptors, the overproduction or untimely production of which may lead to uncontrolled cell division.

Example 14.36.   Rous sarcoma virus (RSV) is a retrovirus containing an oncogene *v-src* (for *v*irus, *s*arcoma-producing) that can transform cells. All vertebrates possess DNA sequences similar to *v-src*, and these are called *c-src* (*c*ellular origin). The product of *v-src* is a phosphoprotein (pp) enzyme, namely, phosphokinase called pp60-*v-src* (60 = 60,000 daltons molecular weight). Most cellular protein kinases phosphorylate the amino acid serine or threonine, but pp60-*v-src* is tyrosine-specific. Phosphorylation can activate some proteins and inactivate others. Thus, one kinase may affect several proteins in different ways. The number of such proteins affected by pp-60-*v-src* and their normal functions in control of cell division are not yet known.

Example 14.37.   The oncogene *v-sis*, carried by *s*imian *s*arcoma virus, encodes a protein similar to the platelet-derived growth factor (PDGF) made by the cellular protooncogene *c-sis*. It is believed that the excess PDGF produced by the virus overwhelms the normal controls on cell division.

4. Interferons.

Interferons are host-cell proteins that nonspecifically enhance the resistance of animal cells to many kinds of viruses. Host cells are stimulated by viral infection to synthesize and secrete interferons. Interferons stimulate the production of three enzymes: a kinase, an oligonucleotide synthetase, and an endonuclease. The kinase phosphorylates and inactivates an initiation factor for viral protein translation. The oligonucleotide synthetase forms a compound called 2,5 A from ATP; the 2,5 A activates the endonuclease that degrades viral mRNA. This inhibition of viral protein synthesis by interferons prevents efficient viral replication with little effect on nondividing host cells. Unfortunately, the early hopes that interferons might be used to prevent or treat cancers have not been realized to date.

Solved Problems

14.1. There are approximately 6.4×10^9 nucleotide pairs per diploid human cell. If the average length of a human chromosome at metaphase is about 6 micrometers, what is the average packing ratio (i.e., the ratio of extended DNA to condensed DNA lengths)?

Solution:

Each nucleotide pair occupies 3.4 angstroms of the DNA double helix. Therefore the total extended length of DNA per cell is

$$(3.4 \text{ angstroms/nucleotide pair}) \times (6.4 \times 10^9 \text{ nucleotide pairs}) = 2.2 \times 10^{10} \text{ angstroms}$$

Since 1 angstrom unit $= 10^{-10}$ meter, and 100 centimeters $= 1$ meter,

$$(2.2 \times 10^{10} \text{ angstroms}) \times (10^{-10} \text{ meter/angstrom}) = 2.2 \text{ meters or } 220 \text{ centimeters}$$

Because there are 23 chromosome pairs in a human diploid cell, the average extended length of DNA per chromosome is 220 centimeters/46 chromosomes $= 4.8$ centimeters/chromosome. A micrometer is one-millionth of a meter (10^{-6} meter) or 10^{-4} centimeters. Thus, the packing ratio of an average human chromosome is

$$\text{(Extended DNA length)/(condensed DNA length)} = 4.8 \text{ centimeters}/(6 \times 10^{-4} \text{ centimeter})$$
$$= 8.0 \times 10^3$$

or 8000 times longer when extended than when condensed in metaphase.

14.2. *Chironomus* is a genus of fly, having about 4.3×10^{-13} gram of DNA per diploid cell and 3.4×10^{-9} gram per polytene nucleus. (*a*) Determine the average number of DNA molecules contained in a polytene chromosome of these flies. (*b*) Estimate the number of replications that a single DNA molecule (or chromatid) must undergo to attain the copy number in a polytene chromosome.

Solution:

(*a*) If each chromatid contains a single DNA molecule, the number of DNA replicas per chromosome in a polytene nucleus is

$$(3.4 \times 10^{-9} \text{ gram})/(4.3 \times 10^{-13} \text{ gram}) = 0.79 \times 10^4$$

However, each polytene "chromosome" actually is formed by pairing of homologues, followed by replication of chromatids. Thus, each polytene "chromosome" contains twice the number of chromatids in one homologue.

$$2(0.79 \times 10^4) = 1.6 \times 10^4$$

(*b*) At every replication, the number of chromatids doubles in a chromosome of a polytene nucleus. If we let *n* represent the number of replications (or doublings) required to generate such a chromosome, then

$$2^n = 0.79 \times 10^4$$
$$n = \frac{\log 7900}{\log 2} = \frac{3.897}{0.301} = 12.947$$
$$n = 13 \text{ (to the nearest whole number)}$$

14.3. A single cell, the fertilized egg, is **totipotent,** i.e., it has the capacity to produce a complete, normal adult individual. Repetitive mitotic divisions convert the zygote into the multicelled organism. During this cellular proliferation, many cells differentiate into types with different morphologies and physiological functions. These differences are associated with the different kinds of proteins made by these cells. For example, the protein hormone insulin is made only by the beta cells in the islets of Langerhans in the pancreas, whereas hemoglobin is made only by erythropoietic cells. (*a*) Explain the two major hypotheses that historically have been offered to explain the observation that different proteins are made by different cell types. (*b*) Devise an experiment to test the validity of the above two hypotheses. (*c*) Are differentiated cells totipotent? Devise an experiment that might provide a positive answer to this question. (*d*) In an experiment of the kind described in part (*c*), if the egg nucleus is exposed to ultraviolet light, a positive result might be due to failure of the radiation to destroy the native egg nucleus. Propose an experiment that might prove this was not the cause of the positive result.

Solution:

(*a*) According to one hypothesis, the cells of a developing embryo become genetically differentiated by the loss of all the genes except those producing the proteins characteristic of a given cell type. This is termed **mosaic development.** Thus, the genes for hemoglobin would not be present in a fully differentiated cell of the pancreas and the gene for insulin would be absent in the stem cells that produce erythrocytes. An alternative hypothesis proposes that cells do not lose any genetic material during differentiation. Rather, different groups of genes are silenced or activated in each cell type. This is termed **regulative development.**

(*b*) Extract DNA from pancreatic cells and probe it with labeled hemoglobin mRNA. If the hemoglobin gene is present, the probe should hybridize with it and reveal itself by autoradiography.

(*c*) Remove (by micropipette) or destroy (e.g., by radiation) the nucleus of a fertilized egg. Then transplant a diploid nucleus from a differentiated cell of the same species into the enucleated egg. If a complete, normal adult organism can develop from such an egg, then development in this species must be totipotent. We cannot generalize these results to all species because different species may not give similar results in such transplant experiments.

(*d*) Transplant a conspecific (same species) nucleus containing a genetic marker that differs from that of the recipient individual. If all cells of the resulting adult organism contain only the marker of the transplant, the native egg nucleus must have been destroyed by the ultraviolet light treatment.

14.4. The direction in which the shell coils in the snail *Limnaea peregra* can be *dexteral* like a right-hand screw or *sinistral* like a left-hand screw. The maternal genotype organizes the cytoplasm of the egg in such a way that embryological cleavage divisions of the zygote will follow either of these two patterns regardless of the genotype of the zygote. If the mother has the dominant gene s^+, all her progeny will coil dextrally; if she is of genotype ss, all her progeny will coil sinistrally. This coiling pattern persists for the life of the individual. *Limnaea* is a hermaphoditic snail that can reproduce either by crossing or by self-fertilization. A homozygous dextral snail is fertilized with sperm from a homozygous sinistral snail. The heterozygous F_1 undergoes two generations of self-fertilization. (*a*) What are the phenotypes of the parental individuals? (*b*) Diagram the parents, F_1, and two selfing generations, showing phenotypes and genotypes and their expected ratios.

Solution:

(*a*) Although we know the genotypes of the parents, we have no information concerning the genotype of the immediate maternal ancestor that was responsible for the organization of the egg cytoplasm from which our parental individuals developed. Therefore we are unable to determine what phenotypes these individuals exhibit. Let us assume for the purpose of diagramming part (*b*) that the maternal parent is dextral and the paternal parent is sinistral.

(*b*) Let D = dextrally organized cytoplasm, S = sinistrally organized cytoplasm.

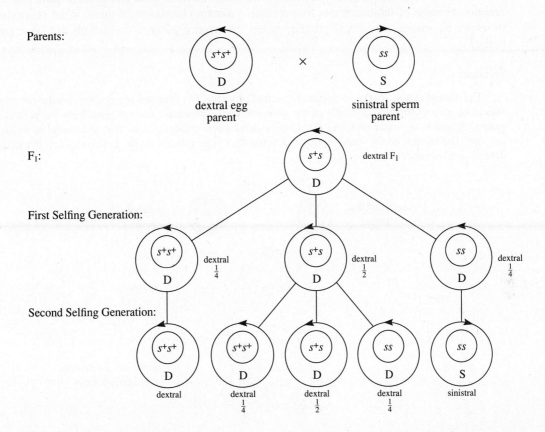

Parents:

s^+s^+ D — dextral egg parent

×

ss S — sinistral sperm parent

F$_1$: s^+s D — dextral F$_1$

First Selfing Generation:

s^+s^+ D dextral $\frac{1}{4}$ s^+s D dextral $\frac{1}{2}$ ss D dextral $\frac{1}{4}$

Second Selfing Generation:

s^+s^+ D dextral s^+s^+ D dextral $\frac{1}{4}$ s^+s D dextral $\frac{1}{2}$ ss D dextral $\frac{1}{4}$ ss S sinistral

Notice that the F$_1$ is coiled dextrally, not because its own genotype is s^+/s, but because the maternal parent possessed the dominant dextral gene s^+. Likewise in the first selfing generation, all are phenotypically dextral regardless of their own genotype because the F$_1$ was s^+/s. In the second selfing generation, we expect the following:

First Selfing Generation		Second Selfing Generation			Summary Genotypes			Phenotypes
$\frac{1}{4}\,s^+s^+$	×	all s^+s^+	=	$\frac{1}{4}\,s^+s^+$	s^+s^+	$=\frac{1}{4}+\frac{1}{8}$	$=\frac{3}{8}$	$\left.\rule{0pt}{12pt}\right\}\frac{5}{8}$ dextral
		$\left\{\begin{array}{l}\frac{1}{4}\,s^+s^+\\ \frac{1}{2}\,s^+s\\ \frac{1}{4}\,ss\end{array}\right.$	$\begin{array}{l}=\\ =\\ \end{array}$	$\begin{array}{l}\frac{1}{8}\,s^+s^+\\ \frac{1}{4}\,s^+s\\ \frac{1}{8}\,ss\end{array}$	s^+s	$=\frac{1}{4}$	$=\frac{2}{8}$	
$\frac{1}{2}\,s^+s$	×				ss	$=\frac{1}{8}+\frac{1}{4}$	=	$\frac{3}{8}$ sinistral
$\frac{1}{4}\,ss$	×	all ss	=	$\frac{1}{4}\,ss$				

14.5. Slow-growing yeast cells called *neutral petites* lack normal activity of the respiratory enzyme cytochrome oxidase associated with the mitochrondria. Petites can be maintained indefinitely in vegetative cultures through budding, but can sporulate only if crossed to wild type. When a haploid neutral petite cell fuses with a haploid wild-type cell of opposite mating type, a fertile wild-type diploid cell is produced. Under appropriate conditions, the diploid cell reproduces sexually (sporulates). The four ascospores of the ascus (Fig. 6-2) germinate into cells with a 1:1 mating type ratio (as expected for nuclear genes), but they are all wild type. The petite trait never appears again, even after repeated backcrossings of both mating types to petite. The mitochondrial factors for petite are able to perpetuate themselves vegetatively, but are "swamped," lost or permanently altered in the presence of wild-type factors. Neutral petite behaves the same in reciprocal crosses regardless of mating type. Assume that a neutral petite yeast has the chromosomal genes for normally functioning mitochondria, but has structurally defective mitochondria. Another kind of yeast is known, called *segregational petite,* which has structurally normal mitochondria that cannot function because of inhibition due to a recessive mutant chromosomal gene. What results would be expected among the sexual progeny when the neutral petite crosses with the segregational petite?

Solution:

The diploid zygote receives structurally normal mitochondria from the segregational petite parent which should be able to function normally in the presence of the dominant nuclear gene from the neutral petite parent. Sporulation would probably distribute at least some structurally normal mitochondria to each ascospore. The nuclear genes would segregate 1 normal : 1 segregational petite. Let shaded cytoplasm contain defective mitochondria.

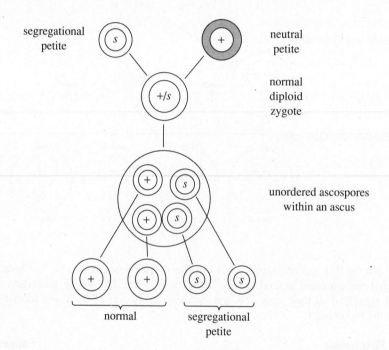

14.6. A condition called "poky" in *Neurospora* is characterized by slow growth due to an abnormal respiratory enzyme system similar to that of petite yeast. The poky trait is transmitted through the maternal (protoperithecial) parent. A chromosomal gene F interacts with poky cytoplasm to produce a faster growing culture called "fast-poky" even though the enzyme system is still abnormal. Poky cytoplasm is not permanently modified by transient contact with an F genotype in the zygote. It returns to the poky state when the genotype bears the alternative allele F'. Gene F has no phenotypic expression in the presence of a normal cytoplasm. If the maternal parent is fast-poky and the paternal (conidial) parent is normal, predict the genotypes and phenotypes of the resulting ascospores.

Solution:

Let shaded cytoplasm contain poky mitochondria. The chromosomal alleles segregate in a 1:1 ratio, but poky cytoplasm follows the maternal (protoperithecial) line. The recovery of poky progeny indicates that poky cytoplasm has not been altered by its exposure to the F gene in the diploid zygotic stage.

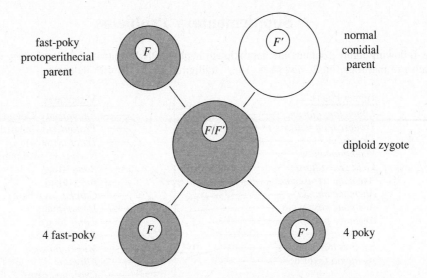

fast-poky
protoperithecial
parent

normal
conidial
parent

diploid zygote

4 fast-poky

4 poky

14.7. Commercial corn results from a "double-cross." Starting with four inbred lines (A, B, C, D), a single cross is made between A and B by growing the two lines together and removing the tassels from line A so that A cannot self-fertilize, and thus receives only B pollen. In another locality the same procedure is followed for lines C and D. The yield of single-cross hybrid seed is usually low because the inbred parent lacks vigor and produces small cobs. Plants that germinate from single-cross seed are usually vigorous hybrids with large cobs and many kernels. It is undesirable for the single-cross hybrid to self-fertilize, as this inbreeding process commonly produces less vigorous progeny. Therefore a double cross is made by using only pollen from the CD hybrid on the AB hybrid. Detasseling is a laborious and expensive process. A cytoplasmic factor that prevents the production of pollen (male-sterile) is known. There also exists a dominant nuclear gene R that can restore fertility in a plant with male-sterile cytoplasm. Propose a method for eliminating hand detasseling in the production of double-cross hybrid commercial seed.

Solution:

Let S = male sterile cytoplasm, F = male fertile cytoplasm. The ABCD double-cross hybrid seed develops on the large ears of the vigorous AB hybrid. When these seeds are planted they will grow into plants, half of which carry the gene for restoring fertility so that ample pollen will be shed to fertilize every plant.

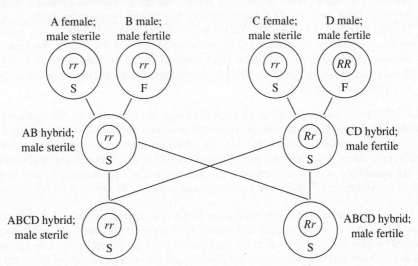

A female;
male sterile

B male;
male fertile

C female;
male sterile

D male;
male fertile

AB hybrid;
male sterile

CD hybrid;
male fertile

ABCD hybrid;
male sterile

ABCD hybrid;
male fertile

Supplementary Problems

14.8. The following figure contains the approximate haploid DNA content in cells of some selected organisms relative to that found in *E. coli* (4×10^{-12} milligram $= 2.4 \times 10^9$ daltons).

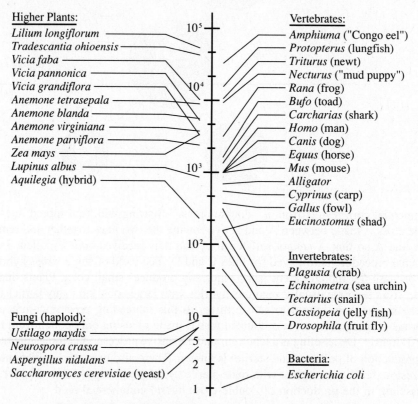

Data from R. Holliday, *Symp. Soc. Microbiol.* 20(1970):362

(*a*) How many times more DNA is found in human cells than in *E. coli*? (*b*) What is the approximate molecular weight (daltons) of DNA in a human cell? (*c*) Approximately how many milligrams of DNA are in a human cell? (*d*) What is the milligram equivalent of 1000 daltons of DNA? (*e*) One might expect that the more complex organisms would have more DNA than more primitive forms of life. For example, some people believe that humans are the pinnacle of evolution. Evaluate this notion in terms of DNA content. (*f*) Approximately how many times more DNA is in the "Congo eel" (*Amphiuma*) than in humans? (*g*) Of the organisms represented in the figure, what generalization can be made regarding vertebrates vs. invertebrates? (*h*) From the data in the figure, which eucaryotic phylum (or division) has the lowest DNA content? (*i*) Do the data in the table support the contention that the amount of selfish DNA tends to accumulate in ancient (less evolved) species? Give examples to support your response.

14.9. About 10^{12} ribosomes are stored in an amphibian egg in preparation for the extraordinarily high rate of protein synthesis needed to sustain the rapid cell divisions during early embryological development. The rate of ribosome production in the oocyte is increased primarily by an approximately 10^3-fold rRNA gene amplification. These genes are also transcribed in oocytes at nearly maximum rate, whereas in somatic cells they are transcribed at only a fraction of the maximum rate. Approximately how many years would be required to synthesize 10^{12} ribosomes at an average somatic cell rate of 3×10^6 ribosomes per day?

14.10. The haploid genome of *Drosophila melanogaster* contains approximately 1.4×10^8 nucleotide pairs. The chromosomes of a polytene nucleus collectively have about 5000 bands. Assuming that 95% of the DNA is located in these bands and 5% is in the interband regions (*a*) determine the average number of nucleotide pairs in each band and interband region and (*b*) estimate the average number of genes per band and interband if an average gene contains 10^3 nucleotide pairs.

14.11. The puffing pattern of *Drosophila* polytene chromosomes seems to change in a predictable pattern during larva development. (*a*) It has been suggested that these puffs are the sites of active genes. How could this hypothesis be tested experimentally? (*b*) The synthesis of a particular protein coincides with the appearance of a specific puff in one of the polytene chromosomes. What inference can be made from this observation?

14.12. A sex-linked mutation results in deficiency of the enzyme glucose-6-phosphate dehydrogenase (G6PD). Some individuals with this enzyme defect are more resistant to malaria than are those without this enzyme defect. Among those parasitized, approximately half of the blood cells of the resistant females contain the causative parasite; the cells of G6PD-deficient males are not parasitized. How can these observations be explained?

14.13. The red blood cells of some women contain two forms of the enzyme G6PD that are easily identified by electrophoresis. The gene locus for G6PD is on the X chromosome. Could this information be used to determine whether chronic myelocytic leukemia (a cancer of erythropoietic stem cells) has a single-cell origin in such women?

14.14. Different mRNA molecules have characteristic half-lives. Propose a method for estimating the half-life of a specific mRNA.

14.15. If a certain protein is found in the Golgi apparatus, how can you explain the fact that its cytoplasmic mRNA transcript contains 24 codons at its 5′ end that are not represented by corresponding amino acids at the amino terminus of the protein?

14.16. The gonads of *Drosophila* develop from material in the posterior end of the oocyte cortex (outer layer) that contains densely staining polar granules. An autosomal recessive mutation (*gs*) when homozygous causes adult females to produce oocytes without polar granules; progeny that develop from such eggs do not develop gonads. If parents are of genotype *gs⁺/gs*, predict the results for the next two generations.

14.17. Identical human twins develop from a single fertilized egg by the separation of embryonic cells at an early stage. Completely normal identical quintuplets have been produced. Through how many cleavage (mitotic) divisions after fertilization is the human genetic information thus known to have been faithfully reproduced?

14.18. A mutant gene in *Drosophila* called *antennapedia* causes legs to develop on the head where antennae normally appear. To what class of developmental control genes does *antennapedia* belong? Offer an explanation as to how this mutation might cause abnormal development.

14.19. Why are translation controls optional for all eucaryotic genes, but essential for many procaryotic genes?

14.20. The N terminus of a polypeptide destined to cross a membrane contains a signal sequence or signal peptide that is removed by a signal peptidase enzyme sometime during the passage of the rest of the polypeptide through the membrane. (*a*) What kinds of amino acids would be expected to predominate in the signal peptide? (*b*) Why is protein translocation through the mitochondrial or chloroplast membranes potentially more complex than that through the endoplasmic reticulum? (*c*) In what major respect does the nuclear membrane differ from the membranes of other organelles?

14.21. If the concentration of cytoplasmic mRNA is higher after than before activation of its gene, does this observation indicate that transcription control of that gene is operative? Explain.

14.22. Pseudogenes are nontranscribed DNA sequences that are highly homologous in nucleotide sequence to functional genes found elsewhere in the same genome. One class of pseudogenes, known as "processed pseudogenes," is characterized by absence of introns and upstream promoter sequences and presence of 3′ terminal poly-A tracts. (*a*) Propose a mechanism that might account for the origin of processed pseudogenes. (*b*) What major problem exists with the mechanism proposed in part (*a*)?

14.23. The diagram below represents a spread of nucleolar chromatin, showing a segment from a tandemly arranged series of nucleolar rRNA genes. They give the appearance of a linear series of Christmas-tree-like structures, first identified by O. L. Miller and B. R. Beatty, and have been subsequently referred to as "Miller trees." Identify the following structures or regions. (*a*) The limits of an rRNA gene for the 38S rRNA precursor molecule. (*b*) A nontranscribed spacer DNA region between the rDNA repeats. (*c*) Promoter or initiator region. (*d*) Terminator of an rDNA gene. (*e*) RNA polymerase molecules. (*f*) 5' end of an rRNA transcript.

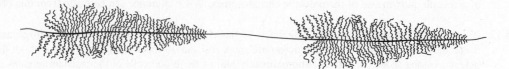

14.24. A recessive chromosomal gene produces green and white stripes in the leaves of maize, a condition called "japonica." This gene behaves normally in monohybrid crosses giving a 3 green : 1 striped ratio. Another striped phenotype was discovered in Iowa, named "iojap" (a contraction of Iowa and japonica), which is produced by a recessive gene *ij* when homozygous. If a plant with iojap striping serves as the seed parent, then the progeny will segregate green, striped, and white in irregular ratios regardless of the genotype of the pollen parent. Backcrossing striped progeny of genotype *Ij/ij* to a green pollinator of genotype *Ij/Ij* produces progeny that continue to segregate green, striped, and white in irregular ratios. White plants die due to lack of functional chloroplasts. Green plants produce only green progeny except when the genotype of the progeny is *ij/ij;* striping then reappears. Interpret this information to explain the inheritance of iojap.

14.25. If a woman contracts German measles during the first trimester of pregnancy, the child may be seriously affected even though the mother herself suffers no permanent physical effects. Such anomalies as heart and liver defects, deafness, cataracts, and blindness often occur in the affected children at birth. Can these phenotypic results be considered hereditary abnormalities?

14.26. A snail produced by a cross between two individuals has a shell with right-hand twist (dextral). This snail produces only left-hand (sinistral) progeny by selfing. Determine the genotype of this snail and its parents. See Problem 14.4.

14.27. Most strains of *Chlamydomonas* (Fig. 5-1) are sensitive to streptomycin. A strain is found that requires streptomycin in the culture medium for its survival. How could it be determined whether streptomycin-dependence is due to a chromosomal gene or to a cytoplasmic element?

14.28. A yeast (Fig. 6-2) culture, when grown on medium containing acriflavine, produces numerous minute cells that grow very slowly. How could it be determined whether the slow growth was due to a cytoplasmic factor or to a nuclear gene?

14.29. The nuclear gene *F* in the presence of "poky" cytoplasm produces a fast-poky phenotype (Problem 14.3). In the presence of normal cytoplasm it has no phenotypic expression. How could a strain of *Neurospora* with normal growth be tested for the presence of *F* or its allele, *F'*?

14.30. Determine the genotypes and phenotypes of sexual progeny in *Neurospora* from the following crosses: (*a*) fast-poky male × normal female of genotype *F'*, (*b*) poky female × fast-poky male, (*c*) fast-poky female × poky male.

14.31. The cells of a *Neurospora* mycelium are usually multinucleate. Fusion of hyphae from different strains results in the exchange of nuclei. A mycelium which has genetically different nuclei in a common cytoplasm is called a *heterokaryon*. Moreover, the union results in a mixture of two different cytoplasmic systems called a *heteroplasmon* or a *heterocytosome*. The mycelia of two slow-growing strains, each with an aberrant cytochrome spectrum, fuse to form a heteroplasmon that exhibits normal growth. Abnormal cytochromes *a* and *b* are still produced by the heteroplasmon. Offer an explanation for this phenomenon.

14.32. Male sterile plants (Problem 14.7) in corn may be produced either by a chromosomal gene or by a cytoplasmic factor. (*a*) At least 20 different male-sterile genes are known in maize, all of which are recessive. Why? Predict the F_1 and F_2 results of pollinating (*b*) a genetic male sterile by a normal, and (*c*) a cytoplasmic male sterile by a normal.

14.33. Given seed from a male sterile line of corn, how would you determine if the sterility was genic or cytoplasmic?

14.34. A bacterial spirochaete that is passed to the progeny only from the maternal parent has been found in *Drosophila willistoni*. This microorganism usually kills males during embryonic development but not females. The trait is called "sex ratio" (SR) for obvious reasons. Occasionally, a son of an SR female will survive. This allows reciprocal crosses to be made. The SR condition can be transferred between *D. equinoxialis* and *D. willistoni*. The spirochaete is sensitive to high temperatures, which inactivates them, forming "cured" strains with a normal sex ratio. (*a*) What would you anticipate to be the consequence of repeated backcrossing of SR females to normal males? (*b*) A "cured" female is crossed to a rare male from an SR culture. Would the sex ratio be normal? Explain.

14.35. Devise a plan for detecting those cells in a *Drosophila* embryo where a specific gene is being expressed.

14.36. The evolution of mitochondrial DNA occurs at a rate much faster than that of nuclear DNA. Hence there is much greater variation from one person to another in mitochondrial DNA sequences than in nuclear DNA sequences. Of all the existing human populations, there appears to be greater variation in those of Africa than any other place on earth. Furthermore, all the human mitochondrial DNA sequences can be arranged into a single phylogenetic tree. Assuming that the mitochondrial DNA of our most ancient ancestors had the same amount of individual variation as that of modern mitochondrial DNA, what are the evolutionary implications of these facts?

14.37. Give at least two mechanisms whereby RNA viruses produce mRNA.

14.38. With regard to retroviruses: (*a*) specify their defining characteristic, (*b*) name the enzyme contained in their virions and list three biochemical activities of that enzyme, (*c*) identify the template for synthesis of retroviral mRNA, (*d*) identify the cellular location of their replication, (*e*) specify those attributes suggesting that their DNA-insertion mechanism is related to transposition.

14.39. The life cycles of eucaryotic viruses and bacteriophages have many similarities, including the establishment of new replication and transcription systems, regulation of gene action (e.g., early vs. late transcription), and synthesis of large quantities of structural proteins. There are certain aspects of viral life cycles, however, that are not (or only rarely) found in the life cycles of phage. Specify some of these unique aspects.

14.40. Some viruses contain an enzyme as part of the infective virion and introduce it into its host cell upon infection. (*a*) Give an example of a virus that carries an enzyme for DNA synthesis. (*b*) Give an example of a virus that carries an enzyme for mRNA synthesis.

14.41. The single-stranded phage ϕX174 of *E. coli* contains 5386 nucleotides coding for 11 proteins with a combined molecular weight of 262,000. (*a*) If an average amino acid has a molecular weight of 110, by how many amino acids is the coding capacity of the phage exceeded? (*b*) How can ϕX174 code for more proteins than it has coding triplets? (*c*) Several animal viruses make more proteins than for which they seem to have coding triplets. Suggest some ways by which they might accomplish this feat if a single reading frame is used.

14.42. All tests of the oncogenic potential of viruses have been made with an established mouse cell line called NIH 3T3 because it had been used for many years to study viral transformation and chemical carcinogens. If cancer is a multistep process, how can the introduction of a single active viral oncogene transform these cells into cancerous cells?

14.43. Some slow-transforming viruses (such as avian leukemia virus) do not contain oncogenes. Offer an explanation as to how they might transform cells.

14.44. Cellular protooncogenes usually contain introns; viral oncogenes do not. (*a*) Propose a scenario for the origin of a viral oncogene. (*b*) Why is it more probable that oncogenes originate in cells rather than in viruses?

14.45. Suppose that a hypothetical cellular protooncogene (*c-pro*) has a viral oncogene counterpart (*v-pro*). It is hypothesized that *c-pro* is amplified in colon cancer cells. (*a*) Devise a plan for testing this hypothesis. (*b*) It is thought that *c-pro* is excessively transcribed in colon cancer cells. Propose an experimental test of this hypothesis.

14.46. A virus is suspected to be involved in the development of breast cancer in certain strains of mice. The virus is transmitted through the milk to the offspring. In crosses where the female carries the "milk factor" and the male is from a strain free of the factor, about 90% of the female progeny develop breast cancer prior to 18 months of age. The virus usually does not initiate cancer development in the infected mouse until she enters the nursing stage, and then only in conjunction with a hormone (estrone) from the ovaries. Males from a virus infected strain are crossed with females from a virus-free strain. (*a*) Predict the proportion of the offspring from this cross that, if individually isolated from weaning to 18 months of age, will probably exhibit breast cancer. (*b*) Predict the proportion of offspring from this cross that will probably exhibit breast cancer if housed in a group from weaning to 18 months of age. (*c*) Answer part (*a*) when the reciprocal

14.47. Another case in which a disease is acquired through the milk (see Problem 14.46) is hemolytic anemia in newborn horses. A mare may produce two or three normal offspring by the same stallion and the next foal may develop severe jaundice within about 96 hours after birth and die. Subsequent matings to the same stallion often produces the same effect. Subsequent matings to another stallion could produce normal offspring. It has been found that if nursed for the first few days on a foster mother the foal will not become ill and develops normally. Evidently something is in the early milk (colostrum) that is responsible for this syndrome. If the foal should become ill, and subsequently recovers, the incompatibility is not transmitted to later generations. (*a*) How might this disease be generated? (*b*) How is the acquisition of this disease different from that of breast cancer in mice?

Review Questions

Vocabulary   For each of the following definitions, give the appropriate term and spell it correctly. Terms are single words unless indicated otherwise.

1.   DNA regions so different from the rest of chromatin that they are easily separated by differential centrifugation.

2.   The product of the first level of DNA packaging, involving histone octomers.

3.   A mobile genetic element, characterized by inverted terminal repeats.

4.   A DNA sequence in cis position with a structural gene that potentiates the transcriptional activity of a gene on that same DNA molecule even though it may be far distant upstream or downstream from the gene it influences.

5.   A genelike DNA sequence bearing close resemblance to a functional gene at a different locus, but rendered nonfunctional by additions or deletions in its structure that prevents its transcription and/or translation.

6.   The conversion of cultured eucaryotic cells to a state of unregulated growth. (One or two words.)

7.   An eucaryotic gene that functions in controlling the normal proliferation of cells, but that can be altered to become a gene that promotes cancer.

8.   A stimulus (usually chemical) that, while not carcinogenic by itself, enhances the production of malignant tumors in cells that have been exposed to a carcinogen.

9.   Descriptive of genes that cause a normal body part to develop in an abnormal location.

10.   The name of a theory that explains the origin of mitochondria and chloroplasts in eucaryotic cells.

True-False Questions   Answer each of the following statements either true (T) or false (F).

1. Histones are highly heterogeneous, acidic chromosomal proteins.

2. Proteins are synthesized on the puffs of polytene chromosomes.

3. A given puff on a polytene chromosome may represent the activity of more than one gene.

4. Middle repetitive DNA sequences are produced by multiple-gene families of homologous DNA sequences.

5. In both procaryotes and eucaryotes, most proteins are coded by unique DNA sequences.

6. The genetic systems of chloroplasts and mitochondria contain all the genes for proteins found within these organelles.

7. Cells that have experienced neoplastic transformation usually undergo a finite number of cell divisions in the best-tended cultures.

8. Most eucaryotic genes are transcribed by their own specific RNA polymerases.

9. All cells that respond to a given hormone have specific receptors for that hormone on the outer surface of their plasma membranes.

10. A large amplification of a hormonal signal can be produced by using cAMP as a second messenger.

Multiple-Choice Questions   Choose the one best answer.

1. Which of the following is not characteristic of heterochromatin?   (*a*) associated with active genes (*b*) usually found in centromeric regions (*c*) identifiable in at least some interphase chromosomes (*d*) located in the dark bands of polytene chromosomes   (*e*) more than one of the above

2. Which of the following statements about mitochondria is incorrect? (*a*) Mitochondrial DNA has a higher mutation rate than nuclear DNA. (*b*) Replication of mitochondrial DNA is synchronized with that of chromosomal DNA. (*c*) The size of mitochondrial DNA varies considerably from one species to another. (*d*) Mitochondria contain a protein-synthesizing system of their own. (*e*) Mitochondria usually follow a maternal inheritance pattern.

3. Differentiation of most somatic cells does not appear to involve the loss of genes or recombination of DNA segments. The most striking exception to this rule is found in   (*a*) histone genes   (*b*) rDNA   (*c*) mitochondrial DNA   (*d*) immunoglobulin genes   (*e*) hemoglobin genes

4. Specific gene amplification is associated with   (*a*) maturation of red blood cells   (*b*) mitochondrial reproduction   (*c*) oogenesis   (*d*) spermatogenesis   (*e*) antibody production

5. Hormones are thought to regulate gene activity primarily at the level of   (*a*) transcription   (*b*) mRNA processing   (*c*) transport of RNA from nucleus to cytoplasm   (*d*) translation   (*e*) post-translation processing of protein

6. Which of the following is not characteristic of most mRNA processing in eucaryotes?   (*a*) addition of a poly-A tail at the 3' end   (*b*) addition of an unusual guanine to the 5' end   (*c*) removal of exons and splicing together of introns   (*d*) removal of leader and trailer sequences   (*e*) more than one of the above

7. There are three kinds of RNA polymerases (I, II, III) in eucaryotic cells, each specific for one class of RNA molecule (mRNA, tRNA, rRNA). Which of the following is a correct match?   (*a*) I = rRNA, II =

tRNA (b) II = mRNA, III = rRNA (c) I = tRNA, III = rRNA (d) I = rRNA, II = mRNA
(e) none of the above

8. Which of the following is not characteristic of eucaryotic viruses? (a) Tailed forms are unknown. (b) Genetic recombination between viral genomes is common. (c) All known double-stranded RNA viral genomes are segmented. (d) All known restriction endonuclease sites are nonmethylated. (e) 3' ends of ssRNA animal viruses have poly-A tails.

9. Cells that have been transformed into tumor cells exhibit the following characteristic(s). (a) If transformed by an oncogenic virus, the virus may or may not be integrated into host DNA. (b) Tumor-specific antigens always appear on the cell surface. (c) They always form tumors when injected into an animal of the same species from which they were derived. (d) Their chromosome number always exceeds the normal diploid number. (e) More than one of the above.

10. Which of the following statements regarding oncogenic retroviruses is incorrect? (a) They usually cause tumors in most species in which they can cause a productive infection. (b) Most infected permissive cells become tumor cells. (c) Integration of viral DNA into host DNA is obligatory for the production of progeny viruses. (d) All oncogenes of these viruses are nonessential for the production of progeny virions. (e) None of the above.

Answers to Supplementary Problems

14.8. (a) 1000 times more

(b) 2.4×10^9 molecular weight in *E. coli* $\times 10^3 = 2.4 \times 10^{12}$ molecular weight

(c) 4×10^{-12} milligram $\times 10^3 = 4 \times 10^{-9}$ milligram

(d) $\dfrac{4 \times 10^{-12} \text{ milligram}}{2.4 \times 10^9 \text{ molecular weight}} = \dfrac{x \text{ milligram}}{10^3 \text{ molecular weight}}$;

$x = 1.67 \times 10^{-18}$ milligram per 1000 molecular weight

(e) There are several "lower" species (especially lily, amphibians, and lungfish) that have much more DNA than humans. DNA content is therefore not a reliable index of organismal "complexity" or position on the phylogenetic (evolutionary) scale.

(f) $(2.5 \times 10^4)/10^3 = 25$ times more.

(g) Most invertebrates have lower DNA contents than vertebrates.

(h) Fungi

(i) The data are inconclusive. For example, alligators have remained relatively unchanged since the Mesozoic era (age of dinosaurs) and yet they have less DNA than the more rapidly evolving mammals. On the other hand, amphibians (as a group) are more ancient than alligators and yet amphibians have more DNA.

14.9. 10^{12} ribosomes/$(3 \times 10^6$ ribosomes/day) $= 3.3 \times 10^5$ days:

$$\frac{3.3 \times 10^5 \text{ days}}{365 \text{ days/year}} = 913 \text{ years}$$

14.10. (a) $(1.4 \times 10^8$ nucleotide pairs $\times 0.95)/(5 \times 10^3$ bands) $= 3 \times 10^4$ nucleotide pairs per band.
$(1.4 \times 10^8$ nucleotide pairs $\times 0.05)/(5 \times 10^3$ bands) $= 1 \times 10^3$ nucleotide pairs per interband.

(b) $(3 \times 10^4$ nucleotide pairs per band)/$(10^3$ nucleotide pairs per gene) $= 30$ genes per band;
$(1 \times 10^3$ nucleotide pairs per interband)/$(10^3$ nucleotide pairs per gene) $= 1$ gene per interband.

14.11. (a) Affix the cells containing the polytene chromosomes to a slide and expose them to radioactive uracils. Active genes will synthesize RNAs containing the labeled uracils. Then wash the slide to remove any unincorporated label and cover it with photographic film sensitive to the radiation (autoradiography). If dots on the developed film are concentrated in the puffed areas, the hypothesis would be confirmed.

(*b*) It might be tempting to speculate that one or more genes in the puffed regions is actively synthesizing the protein. However, it is also possible that the protein itself might be responsible for the change in the puff pattern; or perhaps some other protein synthesized at the same time might be responsible. Thus, cause and effect cannot be established from this observation.

14.12. In most female mammals, including humans, one of the X chromosomes is inactivated. In females that are heterozygous for the mutation, about half of the cells would be expected to have an inactive X chromosome containing the normal G6PD gene and an active X chromosome containing the mutant gene; these cells would have a deficiency of G6PD and would not be parasitized. In the remainder of these female cells, the other X chromosome bearing the normal gene would be active, would not be G6PD deficient, and therefore would be parasitized. Males do not inactivate their single X chromosome. Males hemizygous for G6PD deficiency would therefore not be parasitized.

14.13. One of the X chromosomes in each female mammal is inactivated early in embryological development. Once an X chromosome has been inactivated in a cell, all the descendant cells will also inactivate the same X chromosome. Thus, if the leukemic cells contain both forms of G6PD the cancer must have arisen in at least two cells. If the cancer arose in only one cell, then all leukemic cells of that individual would have only one form of the enzyme. However, it is possible that the same G6PD gene might be inactivated in different stem cells. If cancer developed in 2 or more of such cells, only one form of the enzyme would be present in the leukemic cells. In other words, two enzyme forms would be diagnostic of a multicellular origin of the cancer, whereas a single enzyme form would not be diagnostic of a single-cell origin.

14.14. Expose cells to one or more radioactive ribonucleotides for a defined short period of time (a **pulse**) followed by large amounts of unlabeled ribonucleotides (the **chase**). After various lengths of chase, expose all of the labeled mRNAs to a single-stranded cDNA that is of a nucleotide sequence complementary to that of the mRNA species under consideration. Measure the amount of radioactivity in the mRNA-cDNA hybrids trapped on a nitrocellulose filter. For any given chase time, the relative stability of an mRNA should be directly related to the amount of radioactivity detected in the hybrids.

14.15. Proteins that are destined to cross the endoplasmic reticulum (which contributes to the Golgi apparatus) contain an N-terminal leader sequence called the signal peptide. This peptide is cleaved after it has performed its job of aiding the polypeptide in passing through the ER membrane.

14.16. Offspring bearing the normal gene gs^+ are fertile and can produce a second generation. F_1 females of genotype gs/gs produce offspring (regardless of the genotype of their mates) that will be sterile; hence those F_1 females cannot have "grandchildren." The name of this mutation is "grandchildless."

14.17. Through at least three cleavage divisions. The first cleavage division produces 2 cells, the second produces 4 cells, the third produces 8 cells (3 cells more than necessary for identical quintuplets).

14.18. *Antennapedia* is a homeotic (also spelled homoeotic) gene in which mutation causes transformation of one body part into another. In other words, it makes the right structure in the wrong place. Homeotic genes contain a regulatory sequence that responds to signals from other control genes. In embryonic cells of the imaginal (imago = adult insect) leg disks, the wild-type *antennapedia* gene is normally active; in cells of the imaginal antennae disks, the gene is normally inactive (silenced). A mutant *antennapedia* gene might fail to respond to the signals that normally turn off its normal allele in the antennae discs, and thus it is somehow able to direct development of legs instead of antennae.

14.19. All eucaryotic cytoplasmic mRNAs are monocistronic, whereas many procaryotic mRNAs are polycistronic. Thus, within a bacterial operon, if the product of one structural gene is needed and another is not, then gene expression must be controlled at the translation level (or perhaps posttranslationally).

14.20. (*a*) Hydrophobic amino acids are expected in the signal peptide so that it can easily be inserted into the hydrophobic lipid membrane bilayer to initiate transport of the attached protein.
   (*b*) Because these organelles are surrounded by a double membrane system, whereas the endoplasmic reticulum membrane consists of a single membrane.
   (*c*) There are pores in the nuclear membrane.

14.21. Transcriptional control may be operative. However, posttranscription regulation may be solely responsible or in conjunction with transcription control. Primary eucaryotic mRNA transcripts are subject to 5′ capping, 3′ polyadenylation, intron removal and splicing of exons, RNA degradation, and transport across the nuclear envelope; each operation presents a potential control point.

14.22. (a) If cytoplasmic mRNA could be copied into DNA, it would have the characteristics described for processed pseudogenes. The retroviral enzyme reverse transcriptase can make DNA from viral RNA, and this cDNA can then become integrated into the host's genome, thus providing a model for the origin of processed pseudogenes.

   (b) Recall that DNA synthesis occurs by extension from an RNA primer. It is difficult to understand why a full-length cDNA copy of a polyadenylated mRNA would be primed on the 3′ poly-A tract rather than internally.

14.23.

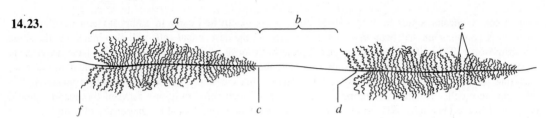

14.24. It appears that the chromosomal gene *ij* when homozygous induces irreversible changes in normal plastids. The plastids exhibit autonomy in subsequent generations, being insensitive to the presence of *Ij* in single or double dose. Random distribution of plastids to daughter cells could give all normal plastids to some, all defective plastids to others, and a mixture of normal and defective plastids to still others. All plastids are not rendered defective in the presence of *ij/ij* as this would produce only white (lethal) seedlings.

14.25. It is important to distinguish between *congenital* defects (recognizable at birth) that are acquired from the environment during embryonic development and genetic defects that are produced in response to the baby's own genotype. The former may be produced by infective agents such as the virus of German measles, which is not really a part of the baby's genotype but is acquired through agents external to the developing individual. An active case of this disease usually produces immunity so that subsequent children of this mother should not be susceptible to the crippling influences of this virus. A hereditary disease is one produced in response to instructions of an abnormal gene belonging to the diseased individual and that can be transmitted in Mendelian fashion from generation to generation.

14.26. Parents: $s^+s\,♀ \times s/?\,♂$; F_1: *ss*

14.27. Cross $ss\ mt^-$ (male) $\times sd\ mt^+$ (female); if chromosomal, 25% of the sexual progeny should be $ss\ mt^-$, 25% $ss\ mt^+$, 25% $sd\ mt^-$, 25% $sd\ mt^+$; if cytoplasmic, almost all of the progeny should follow the maternal line (streptomycin-dependent) as in Example 14.25, while mating type segregates $1\ mt^- : 1\ mt^+$.

14.28. From a cross of minute × normal, a nuclear gene will segregate in the spores in a 1 : 1 ratio (e.g., segregational petite in Problem 14.5). If an extranuclear gene is involved, segregation will not be evident and all spores will be normal (e.g., neutral petite in Example 14.26).

14.29. Use the unknown as conidial parent on a standard poky strain. If the unknown carries *F*, half of the ascospores will be poky and half fast-poky. If the unknown carries *F′*, all of the sexual progeny will be poky.

14.30. (a) All phenotypically normal; $\frac{1}{2}F′$ (normal cytoplasm) : $\frac{1}{2}F$ (normal cytoplasm). (b) and (c) $\frac{1}{2}$ fast-poky; *F* (poky cytoplasm) : $\frac{1}{2}$ poky; *F′* (poky cytoplasm)

14.31. One strain may have an abnormal cytochrome *a* but a normal cytochrome *b*. The other strain might have an abnormal cytochrome *b* but a normal cytochrome *a*. The normal cytochromes in the heteroplasmon complement each other to produce rapid growth.

14.32. (*a*) A plant in which a dominant genic male sterile gene arose by mutation of a normal gene would be unable to fertilize itself and would be lost unless cross-pollinated by a fertile plant. The gene would be rapidly eliminated from heterozygotes within a few generations by continuous back crossing to normal pollen parents. (*b*) F_1: $+/ms$, fertile; F_2: $\frac{1}{4}+/+$, $\frac{1}{2}+/ms$, $\frac{1}{4}ms/ms$; $\frac{3}{4}$ fertile, $\frac{1}{4}$ male sterile. (*c*) Male sterile cytoplasm is transmitted to all F_1 progeny; a selfed F_2 cannot be produced because none of the F_1 plants can make fertile pollen.

14.33. Plant the seeds and pollinate the resulting plants with normal pollen from a strain devoid of male sterility. If the F_1 is sterile, then it is cytoplasmic; if the F_1 is fertile, it is genic.

14.34. (*a*) If interspecific crosses can transmit the spirochaete, it is probably relatively insensitive to the chromosomal gene complement. Backcrossing would cause no change in the SR trait; indeed, this is how the culture is maintained. (*b*) The sex ratio would probably be normal. It is unlikely that the spirochaete would be included in the minute amount of cytoplasm that surrounds the sperm nucleus.

14.35. Expose thin slices of the embryo to a radioactive probe (single-stranded cDNA of complementary nucleotide sequence to the mRNA of interest). Any cells containing the specific mRNA gene product should hybridize with the probe (*in situ* hybridization), and the hybrids can then be detected by autoradiography.

14.36. Africa was probably the place where humans first evolved, and our ancestors emigrated from there to populate the world. Mitochondria are maternally inherited. From this fact and the single family tree for mitochondrial DNA, it has been inferred that there probably was a single ancestral woman (our "mitochondrial Eve") from which all humans derived their mitochondrial DNA.

14.37. (1) Minus-strand RNA viruses transport into the cell a replicase enzyme that synthesizes mRNA from the $(-)$ strand template.
    (2) Plus-strand RNA viruses (other than retroviruses) use their infective strand as a template for synthesizing mRNA using host RNA polymerase.
    (3) Retroviruses use their $(+)$ strand as a template for DNA synthesis, which is then transcribed into mRNA.
    (4) Double-stranded RNA viruses bring a replicase into the host cell that copies double-stranded RNA and synthesizes a $(+)$ strand that functions as mRNA.

14.38. (*a*) They replicate from a DNA intermediate.
    (*b*) RNA-dependent DNA polymerase (reverse transcriptase). Enzyme functions: (1) converting the single-stranded viral RNA to a DNA-RNA hybrid, (2) digesting RNA from a DNA-RNA hybrid, and (3) copying a primed single-stranded DNA to form a double-stranded DNA.
    (*c*) The double-stranded DNA that is formed by reverse transcription from retroviral RNA.
    (*d*) The DNA-RNA hybrid is made in the cytoplasm. The hybrid is converted to double-stranded DNA and becomes inserted into a host chromosome. Messenger RNA is made from the proviral DNA in the nucleus by host RNA polymerase.
    (*e*) Their integrated proviral DNA is terminated at each end by a long terminal repeat and a short inverted repeat (like a composite transposon), which in turn is flanked by a short, direct repeat (like a target sequence).

14.39. (1) Viral proteins usually enter the infected cell along with the viral genome.
    (2) The RNA of some viruses is converted to DNA.
    (3) The mRNA of viruses is processed just like the cellular mRNA of their eucaryotic hosts.
    (4) Polyproteins are produced by some viruses.

14.40. (*a*) Retroviruses (such as human immunodeficiency virus, HIV) that make DNA from an RNA genome; vaccinia virus that replicates its genome in the cytoplasm where no host DNA polymerases reside.
    (*b*) Any virus whose genetic material cannot be translated by cellular enzymes. For example, $(-)$ strand RNA viruses such as influenza virus, and double-stranded RNA viruses like rheovirus.

14.41. (*a*) (262,000 molecular weight/110 molecular weight per amino acid) $-$ (5386 bases/3 bases per codon) $= 586.5$ amino acids.

(b) Some phage genes are overlapping; i.e., the same sequence can be transcribed in different reading frames. The only structural feature responsible for gene overlap is the location of each AUG start codon.

(c) By alternative intron cleavage sites from the same primary transcript, two proteins could be produced having the same N terminus but different C termini. A polyprotein could also be enzymatically cleaved in more than one way to produce different products.

14.42. An established cell line has already experienced one or more early steps (e.g., immortalization) in the induction of neoplastic transformation before exposure to the effects of the oncogene.

14.43. These viruses might become integrated into the host DNA near a cellular protooncogene and activate it, via a viral enhancer sequence, to become an oncogene.

14.44. (a) A retrovirus becomes integrated as a provirus adjacent to a cellular protooncogene. The provirus and the adjacent protooncogene are transcribed into a single transcript. The RNA transcript is processed to remove introns and becomes packaged into a viral capsid. The infective virus is released from the host cell and infects another cell.

(b) Each of the steps in part (a) involves known genetic mechanisms. There is no known mechanism by which introns from viruses can be inserted into cellular protooncogenes.

14.45. (a) Extract the DNA from colon cancer cells and from normal human cells. Cut them into fragments with a restriction endonuclease and then electrophorese the fragments. Transfer the fragments from the gel to nitrocellulose paper by the Southern blotting technique. Probe the blot with radioactive *v-pro* DNA from the virus. After radiography, if the emission intensities of bands from the colon cancer cells are greater than those from normal cells, we infer that the *c-pro* oncogene has been amplified in the cancer cells.

(b) Extract RNAs from the colon cancer cells and from normal cells. Separate these molecules by electrophoresis and then transfer them from gel to paper by the northern blotting technique. Probe the blot with radioactive *v-pro* DNA. Following autoradiography, if the cancer cell RNA bands are more intense than those from normal cells, we infer that the *c-pro* oncogene has been excessively transcribed in cancer cells.

14.46. (a) (b) None of the progeny is expected to develop breast cancer because noninfected females have nursed them. (c) None of the progeny is expected to develop breast cancer because in isolation the infected females could never produce a litter and subsequently enter a lactation period, a prerequisite for expression of the milk factor. (d) 50% females × 90% of females develop breast cancer = approximately 45%.

14.47. (a) This disease is similar to the Rh blood group system incompatibility between a human mother and her baby. In this case, antibodies are transferred to the offspring through the milk rather than across the placenta. (b) The particular stallion that is used has an immediate effect on the character. This is not true in the acquisition of breast cancer in mice. The incompatibility disease in horses cannot be transmitted to later generations, so there is no evidence of a specifically self-duplicating particle like the infective agent that causes cancer in mice.

Answers to Review Questions

Vocabulary

1. satellites or satellite DNA
2. nucleosomes
3. transposon or transposable element
4. enhancer
5. pseudogene
6. neoplastic transformation
7. protooncogene
8. promoter
9. homeotic (homoeotic)
10. endosymbiosis

True-False Questions

1. F (Nonhistone chromosomal proteins have these characteristics.)

2. F (Chromosomal puffs synthesize RNA; proteins are synthesized from mRNA in the cytoplasm.)

3. T   4. T   5. T

6. F (The genomes of these organelles are too small to code for all their proteins; most of their proteins are encoded by nuclear genes and synthesized on cytoplasmic ribosomes.)

7. F (Transformed cells can divide indefinitely; they have become "immortalized.")

8. F (There are only 3 RNA polymerases; they are neither gene- nor tissue-specific.)

9. F (For example, steroid hormone receptors are in the cytoplasm.)

10. T

Multiple-Choice Questions

1. *a*   2. *b*   3. *d*   4. *c*   5. *a*   6. *e* (*c* and *d*)   7. *d*   8. *b*   9. *d*   10. *e*

Index

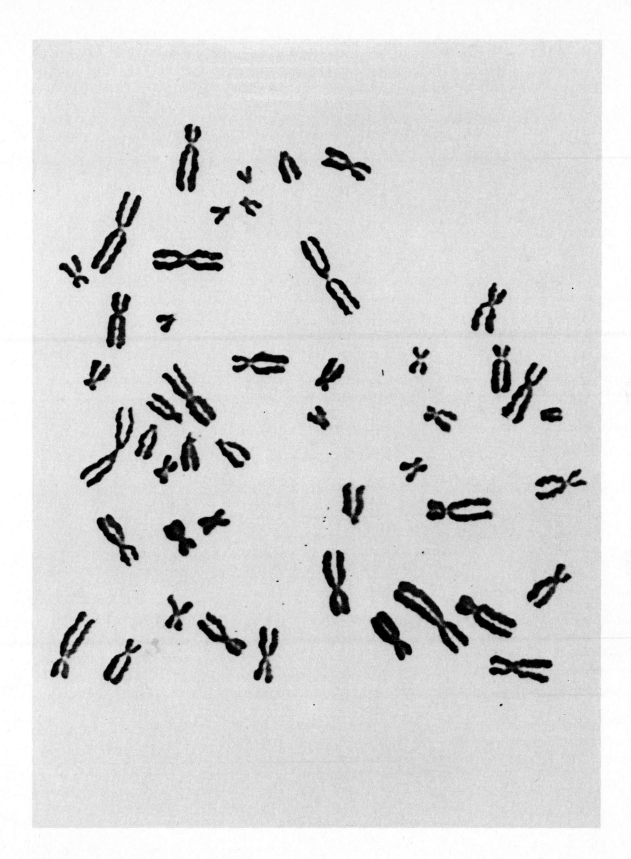

Photograph accompanying Problem 8.45. See p. 203.